新编汉英中医药分类词典

CLASSIFIED DICTIONARY OF TRADITIONAL CHINESE MEDICINE

(New Edition)

谢竹藩　编著

By **Zhu-Fan Xie**

外文出版社

FOREIGN LANGUAGES PRESS　BEIJING

First Edition 2002

ISBN 7-119-03126-0

Published by Foreign Languages Press
24 Baiwanzhuang Road, Beijing 100037, China
Website: http://www.flp.com.cn
Email Address: Info@flp.com.cn
Sales@flp.com.cn

Distributed by China International Book Trading Corporation
35 Chegongzhuang Xilu, Beijing 100044, China
P.O.Box 399, Beijing, China

Printed in the People's Republic of China

原 序

中国医药学是世界医学的一部分，它是一个伟大的宝库。近年来，通过东西方文化的交流，国外已有不少人认识到这门医学的重要性。例如针灸，被人们誉为“医术中的奇迹”，又如中药，由于有确切的疗效而较少毒副作用，也日益受到重视。世界各地有越来越多的人对学习中医抱着极大的热忱，迫切需要这方面的书籍。

为了促使中医学能顺利地传入西方社会，亟需一本系统全面而又精炼的词典以满足中外医学界的需要。本书的编著者以此为己任，在他们过去编写出版的辞书的基础上重新改写，这本《汉英中医药分类词典》就是他们通力合作的结果。

全书共分十八章，内容基本上包括中医学的各个方面。对于每个词条，除有对应的译文外，多数都加简要的注释，使读者能明确了解其含义。在每章之中，词条的排列有序，力求符合中医药学本身的论述规律。因此本书不仅是一本可供查询的工具书，同时也是一本可供阅读的参考书，尤其是对于只谙英语、不能阅读中文的西方人士，本书可作为一本中医药学的简明教材，通读之后将会对中医学的全貌得到一个基本的概念。

本书的编著者都是国内一流的专家，精通中、西医学和英语。在编写本书的过程中他们尽力使各词条的译文符合原意，同时又符合英语的正确用法和习惯，使之易被西方人士所接受，特别是注意避免含混和误解。为了推广应用世界卫生组织推荐的标准针灸名词术语，举凡这类词条均用此标准译名作为正式译文。

由于中医药学具有独特的理论和概念，不少名词的英译具有极大的难度，尽管本书在编写中显然是经过逐字逐句的推敲，仍可能存在着这样或那样的缺点。希望今后能根据实际应用的效果不断改进，逐步形成一套公认的英译中医药名词术语。

张文康

1994年1月

(张文康，现任中华人民共和国卫生部部长；1994年时任中华人民共和国卫生部副部长、中华人民共和国国家中医药管理局局长。)

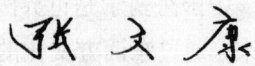

FOREWORD

(Old Edition)

Traditional Chinese medicine, as a part of medicine in the world, is a great treasure-house. In recent years, through the cultural exchanges between the East and the West, many people in the Western countries have recognized the importance of this system of medicine. Some of its component parts, such as acupuncture and moxibustion, have become known abroad as "wonder-making art of healing," and the Chinese herbal medicine has aroused an increasing interest among Westerners because of its confirmed therapeutic effects and less toxic and side effects. A great zeal is shown by a rapidly growing number of people from all parts of the world for knowledge about traditional Chinese medicine as well as an increasing demand for books on the subject.

To facilitate the process of introducing traditional Chinese medicine to the Western world and to meet the ever-increasing demand of medical professionals, Chinese and foreign, for a systematic concise reference book, the compilers take it their duty and something within their capacity to prepare an all-embracing yet kept to the essentials new dictionary of proper size on the basis of their previous publications with substantial innovations and improvements. The present edition of *Classified Dictionary of Traditional Chinese Medicine* is the result of their joint efforts.

The new dictionary has 18 chapters, covering almost all fields of traditional Chinese medicine. The English equivalent of each entry is given in boldface, and for most of the entries, expositions are added for better comprehension. The chapters and entries of each chapter are so arranged that a natural and logical sequence of theoretical exposition of traditional Chinese medicine is maintained and kept perceptible to the readers. For Western readers who have interest in learning traditional Chinese medicine but do not know Chinese, this dictionary can be used as a concise textbook, from which they can get a general idea about this system of medicine without much difficulty.

The compilers of this book are all top-ranking specialists in China, who are experts at both traditional Chinese and modern Western medicine as well as English language. While preparing this dictionary, they pay special attention to the exposition of the terms, and make great efforts to keep the English translation as close as possible to the original sense and at the same time as acceptable as possible to the Western readers. Great care is taken to avoid ambiguity, confusion, misconception, and misleading. In order to promote the unified use of the standard nomenclature of acupuncture proposed by the World Health Organization (1991) all the English names used in this nomenclature are adopted as the equivalents of the relevant terms.

Because of the uniqueness of traditional Chinese medicine, the English translation of the Chinese terms in this dictionary, though well deliberated, can by no means be considered as all perfect. There is still room for improvement. It is hoped that this dictionary can serve as a foundation to develop a complete set of generally accepted English nomenclature of traditional Chinese medicine.

张文康

Professor Zhang Wenkang

January, 1994

Professor Zhang Wenkang, Minister of Health of P.R.C. at present, and Vice-Minister of Health, Director-General of State Administration of Traditional Chinese Medicine of P.R.C. in 1994

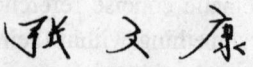

新版序

中国医药学已越来越受到全世界的关注，如何尽快使之走向世界是时代的使命。西方想学习了解中医药学的人很多，但文化背景的差异，特别是文字上的障碍，给他们造成了许多困难。目前国内外用英文出版的中医药书籍正在迅速增多，由于用词不一，几乎每个中医名词术语都有多种译法，这常使读者困惑不解，甚至误解中医原意。因此，对中医药名词术语当前亟需要有公认的正确英译。

我校谢竹藩教授是国内著名的中西医结合专家，在国际上也享有盛名，曾三次被聘为世界卫生组织传统医学顾问，并多次应邀在国外医学院校讲授中医，对如何用英语准确表达中医学的概念和知识有深刻的体会。早在二十世纪八十年代初他就与我校楼之岑、黄孝楷等教授共同编写了汉英常用中医药词汇，出版后深受欢迎；不久又由香港商务印书馆改名为《中医药词典》（*Dictionary of Traditional Chinese Medicine*）出版，进一步引起了国际上的重视。其后，他们在教学科研之余继续从事这方面的研究，1994 年出版的《汉英中医药分类词典》即为其成果之一。由于该书早已脱销，特别是近两年谢竹藩教授承担了有关中医名词术语标准化研究的任务，故在其研究成果的基础上重新编写。

与 1994 年旧版比较，新版有很大变化。首先是词汇量大幅度增加；在编排上也更切合实用，例如将中医名词术语与常用的格言谚语分别处理。对于词条的注释则尽量按照词典的规格，力求使之定义化。更为突出的是中医名词术语的英译对应词，多数译名都是经过对国内外现有多种译法进行研究比较后选定的。这种博采众长的做法，必然会使新版中的英译词汇被多数人所接受。

北京大学常务副校长
北京大学医学部主任　　韩 启 德
中 国 科 学 院 院 士

2002 年 7 月

FOREWORD TO NEW EDITION

Traditional Chinese medicine (TCM) has been arousing more and more interest abroad. It is a mission of the times to facilitate the spread of this system of medicine throughout the world. Many Occidentals want to learn it but have met a lot of difficulties owing to different cultural backgrounds, particularly the language barriers. At present, the number of TCM books written in English is rapidly increasing, but standardized English terminology is lacking. Almost every Chinese medical term has been translated in several different ways. This perplexes the readers and leads to misunderstanding. Therefore, there is an urgent need for developing generally recognized English equivalents.

Professor Xie Zhufan is an outstanding scholar well known both at home and abroad, specializing in the integration of Chinese and Western medicine. He was appointed three times as consultant on traditional medicine by the World Health Organization and was repeatedly invited to give lectures on Chinese medicine at overseas medical schools. He has much experience of expressing Chinese medical concepts and knowledge in English. In early 1980s, collaborating with Professors Lou Zhicen and Huang Xiaokai, he compiled a book entitled *Common Terms of Traditional Chinese Medicine in English* and published by Beijing Medical College Press. Since it was well accepted by the readers, the Commercial Press (Hong Kong) republished it soon afterwards and renamed it *Dictionary of Traditional Chinese Medicine*. The latter exerted more impact abroad. Professor Xie and his collaborators continued their study in this respect, and published *Classified Dictionary of Traditional Chinese Medicine* in 1994 as one of their achievements. Because the *Classified Dictionary* has been out of stock for a long time, and particularly because Professor Xie was assigned a research project on the standardization of TCM nomenclature in 2000, he has rewritten the dictionary on the basis of his research.

In comparison with the edition of 1994, the new edition has the following changes: The vocabulary is greatly increased. The layout is more convenient for practical use, for example, the citations and maxims are separated from the technical terms. The annotations are given in the form of definition as far as possible, concisely stating the exact meaning of the entries. The most distinctive feature is the English equivalent. For most technical terms the equivalents are selected according to the comparative study of various translations that appear in the recent publications both at home and abroad. The extensive reference to different ways of translation will certainly make the selected equivalents widely acceptable.

Professor Han Qide

July, 2002

Professor Han Qide, Executive Vice-President of Peking University, President of Peking University Health Science Center, and Academician, Chinese Academy of Sciences

编者序

本书系在 1994 年出版的《汉英中医药分类词典》的基础上重新编写而成。二书主要区别如下：

一、书中所收集的条目较前增加了 30%，现为 7,010 条。其中 6,630 条为中医药名词术语，380 条为常引用的文句。词条按基础理论、诊断学、治疗学、临床各科和医学史五大类重新排列。

二、词条的增补和编排主要系参照中医学教科书。例如，基础理论部分增添了精气学说一节；诊断学部分增加了若干证名，以与病机术语区分；中药部分按中药学和方剂学教材重新拟定和编排条目。很多格言谚语，具有完整的句型，不宜作为名词术语对待，但又很实用，故按引文另行编排，附于有关章节之后。

三、释义部分系参考 1995 年起陆续出版的“普通高等教育中医药类规划教材”和 1997 年发布的《中华人民共和国国家标准中医临床诊疗术语（证候部分、疾病部分、治法部分）》，按照词典的要求编写或修订的。绝大多数词条的释义均力求定义化，同时更加注重突出中医的特点，避免与西医概念混淆，例如中药和方剂的功能、主治完全按中医论述改写。

四、最艰巨的工作在于名词术语的英译对应词。目前的情况是多数中医名词术语的英译并非阙如，而是译法多种多样，缺乏标准英译。同一名词术语出现多种译法，严重影响中医药学的国际交流。要使之逐步达到统一，切实可行的办法就是对现有的各种译法进行比较，从中选出最贴切的译法。编者自 2000 年 4 月受命于国家中医药管理局科技教育司进行“中医药名词术语英译标准化”的研究以来，对12种汉英中医药词典和50部在国外有影响的英文中医药著作或译作中的词汇做了调查、分析和比较，本书中名词术语的英译对应词即反映了这项研究的结果。至于中药的名称则以《中华人民共和国药典》（英文版，1997）为准。

共同编写1994年版《汉英中医药分类词典》的楼之岑、黄孝楷两教授均于该书出版后不久辞世。编者在对这两位良师益友的缅怀中进行了本书的重新编写工作，并以此书的出版作为对他们的纪念。

北京大学第一临床医学院教授
北京大学中西医结合研究所名誉所长 **谢竹藩**

2002年6月

AUTHOR'S PREFACE

This book is a revised and expanded edition of *Classified Dictionary of Traditional Chinese Medicine,* which was published in 1994. The major differences between the two editions are as follows.

The new edition increases the entries by 30%, reaching a total of 7,010, in which 6,630 are technical terms and 380 are commonly used citations and maxims. The entries are rearranged into five categories: fundamental theories, diagnostics, therapeutics, clinical medicine, and medical history.

The entries are supplemented and rearranged with reference to modern textbooks of traditional Chinese medicine. For example, a new section of essential-*qi* theory is added to the fundamental theories, a large number of syndrome names are inserted to clarify the distinction between pathogenetic and diagnostic terminologies, and the contents of the chapter Chinese Pharmaceuticals are expanded and rearranged accordingly. Since the citations and maxims expressed in sentences, though useful, are beyond the scope of terminology, they are laid out as attachments to the relevant sections.

In the new edition, the explanation of the terminology is compiled or revised in the light of the programmed textbooks for colleges and universities of traditional Chinese medicine (published in 1995 and afterwards), and *State Standard Terminology of Traditional Chinese Medical Diagnosis and Treatment — Syndromes, Diseases, and Therapeutic Methods* (promulgated in 1997). For most entries of the new edition the explanation is written in the form of definition. In addition, the Chinese medical features are stressed and confusion with western concepts is avoided. For instance, the function and indications of Chinese medicines and formulas are all revised in accordance with the Chinese medical concepts.

The most arduous work is the determination of English equivalents. To date, except a limited number of acupuncture terminologies that have been standardized and recommended by the World Health Organization, most traditional Chinese medical terms have no standardized English equivalents. On the other hand, for the majority of Chinese medical terms there are too many different translations instead of none. When the same Chinese medical terms are translated in different ways, the divergence in terminology causes much difficulty in the international exchange of Chinese medicine. In most instances the practical way to standardize the English equivalent of Chinese medical terms is the selection of the most appropriate one from the existing translations. In April 2000, the author was assigned by the Department of Science, Technology and Education, State Administration of Traditional Chinese Medicine a research project on the standardization of English translation of Chinese medical terminology. Comparative studies have been performed on the glossaries collected from 12 Chinese-English dictionaries and 50 influential books of Chinese medicine translated or written in English. The results of the studies are partly reflected in this book. As for the nomenclature of Chinese herbal medicine, the Latin and English names are compiled according to *Pharmacopoeia of the People's Republic of China* (English Edition 1997).

The 1994's edition was accomplished with the collaboration of Professors Zhi-Cen Lou and Xiao-Kai Huang. Both of them passed away in the late nineties of the last century. The new edition is compiled and published also in memory of Professors Lou and Huang.

Zhu-Fan Xie

June, 2002

Zhu-Fan Xie, Professor of the First Clinical Medical College, and Honorary Director of Institute of Integrated Chinese and Western Medicine, Peking University

凡　例

全书的条目按教材的顺序分类排列，共计二十四章，并为五大门类：基础理论、诊断学、治疗学、临床各科和医学史，不仅便于查找，且可作为微缩的中医全书对待。

引文（包括格言谚语）具有完整句型，不属名词术语，故另行分出，附于有关章节之后。

每个条目包括汉字原文、注音（汉语拼音加方括号）、对应英译（用黑体字）和释义，但少数名词术语和多数引文因意义不言自明，故无释义。

少数条目有两种以上公认的译法难作取舍者，则予并列，并以分号隔开。

凡一个条目有两种以上含义者，则予并列，用数码分开，并分别释义。

凡一个条目有两种以上含义属不同医学范畴者，则有关章节均可见该条目。

原文和译文中凡用圆括号括起的字属于可加可不加，用方括号括起的字表示可与括号前的字置换。

部分名词术语迄今尚无适当英译，只能暂用汉语拼音。但拼音汉语仍为汉语，故与其它非英语的文字（如拉丁文）同等对待，用斜体印刷。已被承认为英语者则不在此例。

Guide to the Use of the Dictionary

The entries are arranged in 24 sections, which are grouped into five categories: fundamental theories, diagnostics, therapeutics, clinical medicine, and medical history. The arrangement is basically in accordance with modern series of textbooks of Chinese medicine, so that this book is not only easy to consult, but can also be taken as an encyclopedia of Chinese medicine in miniature.

The entries contain technical terms and commonly used citations (including maxims). Since the citations are beyond the scope of terminology, they are separately arranged as attachments to relevant sections.

Each entry consists of the term or citation in Chinese characters, Chinese phonetic transcriptions (*pinyin* in square brackets), English translation (in boldface) and explanations, but for a few terms and most citations there is no explanation as the translation is self-explanatory.

Some terms may have two or more select translations. In this case the translations are placed abreast and separated by semicolon.

If a term has two or more meanings, the different meanings are given separately and marked with numerals to distinguish one from the other.

If a term has two or more different meanings belonging to different branches of medicine, the same term will appear in different chapters.

In the original texts and translations, the word put in round brackets can be deleted if necessary, and the word put in square brackets can be used to replace the word preceding the brackets.

To date, no equivalents have been found for some terms of Chinese medicine, and only *pinyin* can be used for the time being. Han characters in *pinyin* are still Chinese language, and so they are printed in italics as other foreign languages such as Latin. However, this does not include the words of foreign origin that have already been generally accepted as English.

目 录

CONTENTS

基础理论　FUNDAMENTAL THEORIES

哲学基础　Philosophical Basis

精气学说　Theory of Essential *Qi*

精气学说 [jīng qì xué shuō]

theory of essential *qi*: an ancient Chinese philosophical system which explains the formation of the universe by an invisible substance called *qi*. The ceaseless movement of *qi* causes all kinds of changes, and the essential part of *qi* gives rise to life.

精气 [jīng qì]

essential *qi*: the *qi* of the essence, from which life originated and by which it is maintained

精 [jīng]

essence: (1) the essential part of *qi*; (2) all the substances useful for the human body, e.g.，food essence from diet; (3) the essential substance stored in the kidney, also called kidney essence

气 [qì]

***qi*:** the invisible basic substance that forms the universe and produces everything in the world through its movement and changes.

神 [shén]

vitality; spirit: liveliness derived from essential *qi*, referring to (1) manifestations of vital functioning; (2) domination of all life activities; (3) spiritual and mental activities

三宝 [sān bǎo]

three treasures: a collective name for essence, *qi* and vitality

精气互化 [jīng qì hù huà]

mutual transformation of essence and *qi*: Essence can be transformed into invisible *qi*, and *qi* can be transformed into visible essence.

气机 [qì jī]

***qi* movement:** constant movement of *qi* in the human body that maintains the vital activities

气化 [qì huà]

***qi* transformation:** changes produced by the movement of *qi*, viz, metabolism of essence, *qi*, blood, and body fluids as well as their mutual transformation

生化 [shēng huà]

generation and transformation: a term used in Chinese medicine to indicate the production and changes of things

升、降、出、入 [shēng, jiàng, chū, rù]

ascending, descending, exiting, and entering: the various directions of *qi* movement, the coordination of which maintains normal life

形 [xíng]

physique: the form or structure of a person's body, opposite to but inseparable from spirit

常用引文 **Commonly Used Citations**

万物之生，皆禀元气。[wàn wù zhī shēng, jiē bǐng yuán qì]

Everything is produced with the endowments of genuine *qi*.

气始而生化，气散而有形，气布而蕃育，气终而象变，其致一也。[qì shǐ ér shēng huà, qì sàn ér yǒu xíng, qì bù ér fān yù, qì zhōng ér xiàng biàn, qí zhì yī yě]

When *qi* starts, there is generation and transformation; when *qi* moves, the shape of a thing is formed; when *qi* spreads; there is multiplication, when *qi* ends, the shape of a thing is changing: all things are alike.

生之来谓之精，两精相搏谓之神。[shēng zhī lái wèi zhī jīng, liǎng jīng xiāng bó wèi zhī shén]

The original substance of life is called essence, and when yin essence and yang essence combine, vitality is produced.

积精全神 [jī jīng quán shén]

Preserve the essence and perfect the spirit.

得神者昌，失神者亡。[dé shén zhě chāng, shī shén zhě wáng]

A patient with vitality is apt to recover from the illness, while there is a poor prognosis for a patient without vitality.

升降出入，无器不有。[shēng jiàng chū rù, wú qì bù yoù]

In all visible things, *qi* ascends, descends, goes out and comes in.

根于中者，命曰神机，神去则机息。根于外者，命曰气立，气止则化绝。

[gēn yú zhōng zhě, mìng yuē shén jī, shén qù zé jī xī。gēn yú wài zhě, mìng yuē qì lì, qì zhǐ zé huà jué]

When the source of vitality stays inside, it is called the mechanism of the spirit; if the spirit moves away, the mechanism ceases. When the source of vitality stays outside, it is called establishment of *qi*; if *qi* stops, transformation is ended.

阴阳学说 Theory of Yin-Yang

阴阳学说 [yīn yáng xué shuō]

theory of yin-yang: an ancient Chinese philosophical concept of naive dialectics, expressing the law of the unity of opposites

阴阳 [yīn yáng]

yin and yang: the two fundamental principles or properties in the universe, ever opposing and complementing each other, the ceaseless motion of which gives rise to all the changes in the world — an ancient philosophical concept used in traditional Chinese medicine for indicating various antitheses in anatomy, physiology, pathology, diagnosis and treatment, and for explaining the health and disease processes

阴 [yīn]

yin: the female or negative principle, the structural or material aspect of an effective position

阳 [yáng]

yang: the male or positive principle, the active or functional aspect of an effective position

阴中之阳，阴中之阴 [yīn zhōng zhī yáng, yīn zhōng zhī yīn]

yang within yin and yin within yin: Yin may be further divided into yang and yin. The resultant yang and yin are called yang within yin and yin within yin respectively, e.g., night is regarded as yin in relation to day, the period from nightfall to midnight is said to be yang within yin, and the period of the small hours is said to be yin within yin.

阳中之阳，阳中之阴 [yáng zhōng zhī yáng, yáng zhōng zhī yīn]

yang within yang and yin within yang: Yang may be further divided into yang and yin. The resultant yang and yin are called yang within yang and yin within yang respectively, e.g., day is regarded as yang in relation to night, the period from dawn to noon is said to be yang within yang, and the afternoon is said to be yin within yang.

阴阳交感 [yīn yáng jiāo gǎn]

intercourse of yin and yang: interaction and combination of yin *qi* and yang *qi*, by which things, living and non-living, are thus produced

阴阳互根 [yīn yáng hù gēn]

interdependence of yin and yang: the existence of one being the prerequisite for the existence of the other. Without "brightness" (yang), there would be no "darkness" (yin); without "interior" (yin), there would be no "exterior" (yang).

阴阳对立 [yīn yáng duì lì]

opposition of yin and yang: Yin and yang are always in a state of opposing each other, e.g., feminine, interior, cold, and inhibition being yin while masculine, exterior, heat, and excitement are yang.

阴阳转化 [yīn yáng zhuǎn huà]

transformation of yin and yang: The property of the same thing can be transformed from yin to yang, or from yang to yin, e.g., the heat syndrome of a disease can be transformed into a cold one, and vice versa.

阴阳消长 [yīn yáng xiāo zhǎng]

waxing and waning of yin and yang: Of the two opposites of a single entity, increase of the one is usually associated with decrease of the other, e.g., functional activities (yang) consume nutrient substances (yin) — waning of yin with waxing of yang. Formation and storage of nutrient substances consume functional energy — waxing of yin with waning of yang.

阴阳平衡 [yīn yáng píng héng]

balance between yin and yang; yin-yang balance: a harmonious state of yin and yang by which health is guaranteed

阴阳调和 [yīn yáng tiáo hé]

harmony between yin and yang; yin-yang harmony: a state of yin and yang by which health is guaranteed, same as yin-yang balance

阴阳失调 [yīn yáng shī tiáo]

disharmony between yin and yang; yin-yang disharmony: a state of yin and yang which is regarded as the general pathogenesis of disease

阴阳不和 [yīn yáng bù hé]

imbalance between yin and yang; yin-yang imbalance: a state of yin and yang which is regarded as the general pathogenesis of disease, same as yin-yang disharmony

阴阳乖戾 [yīn yáng guāi lì]

perversion of yin and yang; yin-yang perversion: a state of yin and yang which is regarded as the general pathogenesis of disease, same as yin-yang disharmony

阴阳离决 [yīn yáng lí jué]

divorce of yin and yang; yin-yang divorce: a state of yin and yang that indicates the end of life

阴阳自和 [yīn yáng zì hé]

restoration of yin-yang balance; restoration of yin-yang harmony: a state of yin and yang indicating recovery of a person from illness

阴阳偏胜 [yīn yáng piān shèng]

relative preponderance of yin or yang: any morbid condition marked by yin or yang higher than the normal level — presence of heat when yang is preponderant, and presence of cold when yin is preponderant

阴阳偏衰 [yīn yáng piān shuāi]

relative decline of yin or yang: any morbid condition marked by yin or yang lower than the normal level: — presence of cold when yang is deficient, and presence of heat when yin is deficient

阴阳胜复 [yīn yáng shèng fù]

alternative preponderance of yin and yang: a hypothesis put forward in ancient times to explain natural changes and disease processes such as the periodic changes of the seasons and the periodic prevalence of certain diseases

阳损及阴 [yáng sǔn jí yīn]

yang impairment involving yin: a morbid condition in which impairment of yang impedes generation of yin, e.g., deficiency of vital function often complicated by deficiency of vital essence in advanced cases

阴损及阳 [yīn sǔn jí yáng]

yin impairment involving yang: a morbid condition in which impairment of yin impedes generation of yang, e.g., deficiency of vital essence often complicated by deficiency of vital function in advanced cases

常用引文 Commonly Used Citations

阴阳者，天地之道也，万物之纲纪，变化之父母，生杀之本始。[yīn yáng zhě, tiān dì zhī dào yě, wàn wù zhī gāng jì, biàn huà zhī fù mǔ, shēng shā zhī běn shǐ]

Yin-yang is the law of nature, the principle of all things, the mother of all changes, and the root of life and death.

天为阳，地为阴；日为阳，月为阴。[tiān wéi yáng, dì wéi yīn; rì wéi yáng, yuè wéi yīn]

Heaven pertains to yang, while Earth pertains to yin; the sun pertains to yang, while the moon pertains to yin.

水为阴，火为阳。[shǐ wéi yīn, huǒ wéi yáng]

Water pertains to yin, while fire pertains to yang.

生之本，本于阴阳。[shēng zhī běn, běn yú yīn yáng]

Life is based on yin and yang.

阴阳者，万物之能始也。 [yīn yáng zhě, wàn wù zhī nēng shì yě]

All things are initiated by yin and yang.

阳化气，阴成形。[yáng huà qì, yīn chéng xíng]

Yang gives rise to activity, and yin makes the configuration.

外者为阳，内者为阴。[wài zhě wéi yáng, nèi zhě wéi yīn]

What exists outside pertains to yang, and what exists inside pertains to yin.

阴中有阳，阳中有阴。[yīn zhōng yǒu yáng, yáng zhōng yǒu yīn]

There is yang in yin, and there is yin in yang.

背为阳，阳中之阳，心也。[bèi wéi yáng, yáng zhōng zhī yáng, xīn yě]

As the back of the body is yang, the heart is yang within yang.

背为阳，阳中之阴，肺也。[bèi wéi yáng, yáng zhōng zhī yīn, fèi yě]

As the back of the body is yang, the lung is yin within yang.

腹为阴，阴中之阴，肾也。[fù wéi yīn, yīn zhōng zhī yīn, shèn yě]

As the abdomen is yin, the kidney is yin within yin.

腹为阴，阴中之阳，肝也。[fù wéi yīn, yīn zhōng zhī yáng, gān yě]

As the abdomen is yin, the liver is yang within yin.

腹为阴，阴中之至阴，脾也。[fù wéi yīn, yīn zhōng zhī zhì yīn, pí yě]

As the abdomen is yin, the spleen is extreme yin within yin.

阴在内，阳之守也。阳在外，阴之使也。[yīn zài nèi, yáng zhī shǒu yě。yáng zài wài, yīn zhī shǐ yě]

Yin, existing in the interior, is the basis of yang; yang, existing in the exterior, is the activity of yin.

阳根于阴，阴根于阳。[yáng gēn yú yīn, yīn gēn yú yáng]

Yang is rooted in yin, and yin is rooted in yang.

阴平阳秘，精神乃治。[yīn píng yáng mì, jīng shén nǎi zhì]

If one keeps yin even and yang firm, one's spirit will be sound.

阴阳离决，精气乃绝。[yīn yáng lí jué, jīng qì nǎi jué]

If one's yin and yang fail to communicate, his essential *qi* will be exhausted.

重阴必阳，重阳必阴。[chóng yīn bì yàng, chóng yáng bì yīn]

Yin in its extreme gives rise to yang, while yang in its extreme gives rise to yin. — a mechanism of yin-yang transformation, e.g., severe loss of fluids (yin) may show symptoms of yang nature, such as feeling hot and restlessness, and intense heat may bring on cold symptoms such as chills and cold limbs

阴胜则阳病，阳胜则阴病。[yīn shèng zé yáng bìng, yáng shèng zé yīn bìng]

Yin in excess makes yang suffer, and yang in excess makes yin suffer. — a mechanism of disease explained by yin-yang theory, e.g., excessive cold (yin) impairs yang *qi*, and exuberant heat consumes body fluids (yin)

阳胜则热，阴胜则寒。[yáng shèng zé rè, yīn shèng zé hán]

Excess yang causes heat, and excess yin causes cold.

阴阳者，数之可十，推之可百，数之可千，推之可万，万之大不可胜数，然其要一也。[yīn yáng zhě, shǔ zhī kě shí, tuī zhī kě bǎi, shǔ zhī kě qiān, tuī zhī kě wàn, wàn zhī dà bù kě shèng shǔ, rán qí yào yī yě]

Yin and yang can be counted from one to ten, and inferred from ten to one hundred, counted from one hundred to one thousand, and inferred from one thousand to ten thousand and even to infinity, but the principle of yin-yang is just one (i.e., the unity of opposites).

谨察阴阳所在而调之，以平为期。[jǐn chá yīn yáng suǒ zài ér tiáo zhī, yǐ píng wéi qī]

One must carefully observe the positions of yin and yang, and apply treatment properly until they are balanced.

阳常有余，阴常不足。[yáng cháng yǒu yú, yīn cháng bù zú]

Yang is usually redundant, while yin is ever deficient. — a theory advocated by Zhu Danxi (1281-1358), according to which the method of replenishing yin is recommended as a basic principle for treating diseases

阴静阳躁 [yīn jìng yáng zào]

Yin is quiescent, and yang vigorous.

五行学说 Theory of the Five Elements

五行学说 [wǔ xíng xué shuō]

theory of five elements: one of the basic theories in traditional Chinese medicine, introduced from ancient natural philosophy concerning the composition and evolution of the physical universe

五行 [wǔ xíng]

five elements: wood, fire, earth, metal and water, with their characteristic properties and their generating and restricting relationships — an ancient natural philosophy purporting to explain the composition and phenomena of the physical universe, and used in traditional Chinese medicine to expound the correspondence between man and the universe, and the physiological and pathological relationships between the internal organs

五行归类 [wǔ xíng guī lèi]

classification according to the five elements: classification of things according to the properties of the five elements either by analogy or by deduction, e.g., the liver, heart, spleen, lung, and kidney are classified into the categories of wood, fire, earth, metal, and water, respectively

五行相生 [wǔ xíng xiāng shēng]

generation in the five elements: the generating relationships of the five elements in the following sequence — wood, fire, earth, metal and water — in which each element is conceived as producing or promoting the subsequent one, i.e., wood generates fire, fire generates earth, earth generates metal, and so forth

五行相克 [wǔ xíng xiāng kè]

restriction in the five elements: the restricting relationships of the five elements in the following sequence — water, fire, metal, wood and earth — in which each element is conceived as restricting or checking the subsequent one, i.e., water restricts fire, fire restricts metal, and so forth

五行制化 [wǔ xíng zhì huà]

inhibition and generation in the five elements: the producing and checking relationships of the five elements which form a self-limiting balanced process, e.g., wood checks earth which produces metal that will check wood in turn, and so forth

五行相乘 [wǔ xíng xiāng chèng]

subjugation in the five elements: abnormally severe restriction of the five elements in the same sequence as ordinary restriction

五行相侮 [wǔ xíng xiāng wù]

reverse restriction in the five elements: restriction opposite to that of the ordinary restricting sequence of the five elements

五行母子相及 [wǔ xíng mǔ zǐ xiāng jí]

"mother-child" relationship in the five elements: Disease of the "mother" may involve the "child", and vice versa.

母 [mǔ]

"mother": the element that generates in the generation sequence of the five elements, e.g., wood being the "mother" of fire

母气 [mǔ qì]

***qi* of the "mother" (organ):** *qi* of the organ that generates in the generation sequence of the five elements, e.g., for the heart (fire), liver (wood) *qi* being the *qi* of the "mother" organ, and for the liver (wood), kidney (water) *qi* being the *qi* of the "mother" organ

子 [zǐ]

"child": the element that is generated in the generation sequence of the five elements, e.g., fire being the "child" of wood

子气 [zǐ qì]

***qi* of the "child" (organ):** *qi* of the organ that is generated in the generation sequence of the five elements, e.g., for the heart (fire), spleen (earth) *qi* being the *qi* of "child" organ, and for the spleen (earth), lung (metal) *qi* being the *qi* of the "child" organ

木克土 [mù kè tǔ]

wood restricting earth: (1) the physiological relationship between the liver (wood) and the spleen and stomach (earth); (2) a pathological condition in which a hyperactive liver impairs the functions of the spleen and stomach, also known as wood subjugating earth (木乘土 [mù chèng tǔ])

木乘土 [mù chèng tǔ]

wood subjugating earth, same as wood restricting earth (木克土 [mù kè tǔ])

木旺乘土 [mù wàng chèng tǔ]

exuberant wood subjugating earth: a pathological change involving disharmony between the liver and the spleen and stomach, in which hyperactivity of the former is primary, while insufficiency of the latter is secondary (cf. 土虚木乘 [tǔ xū mù chèng])

土虚木乘 [tǔ xū mù chèng]

wood subjugating asthenic earth: a pathological change involving disharmony between the liver and the spleen and stomach, in which hyperactivity of the former is secondary, while insufficiency of the latter is primary (cf. 木旺乘土 [mù wàng chèng tǔ])

木火刑金 [mù huǒ xíng jīn]

wood fire torturing metal: a pathological change expressed in the light of the five-elements theory that excessive liver fire consumes lung yin, causing dry cough and chest pain or even hemoptysis accompanied by irritability, bitterness in the mouth and blood-shot eyes

火不生土 [huǒ bù shēng tǔ]

fire failing to generate earth: a pathological change expressed in the light of the five-elements theory that fire of the life gate (i.e., kidney yang) is insufficient to warm the spleen and stomach, bringing on such symptoms as diarrhea, indigestion, intolerance of cold and edema

土不制水 [tǔ bù zhì shuǐ]

earth failing to control water: a pathological change expressed in the light of the five-elements theory that a weak spleen unable to control the water flow may leads to flood, manifested by edema or retained fluid

土虚水侮 [tǔ xū shuǐ wù]

reversed restriction of water on asthenic earth: an expression for insufficiency of the spleen with anasarca according to the five-elements theory

金寒水冷 [jīn hán shuǐ lěng]

coldness of metal and water: a figurative expression for deficiency-cold of both the lung and kidney

水不涵木 [shuǐ bù hán mù]

water failing to moisten wood: a pathological change expressed in the light of the five-elements theory that kidney yin deficiency deprives the liver of its nourishment, resulting in insufficiency of liver yin with stirring of liver wind

五运 [wǔ yùn]

five circuit phases: a collective term referring to wood, fire, earth, metal and water in motion

五常 [wǔ cháng]

five normal phases, same as five circuit phases (五运 [wǔ yùn])

六气 [liù qì]

six *qi*; six climatic factors: a collective term for wind, cold, summer-heat, dampness, dryness and fire

运气 [yùn qì]

circuit *qi*: an abbreviation for the five circuit phases and six climatic factors

天干 [tiān gān]

Heavenly stems: a sequence of symbols, ten in number, used as serial numbers and also in combination with the twelve Earthly branches to designate years, months, days and hours

地支 [dì zhī]

Earthly branches: a sequence of symbols, twelve in number, used in combination with the ten Heavenly branches to designate years, months, days and hours

常用引文 Commonly Used Citations

木曰曲直。[mù yuē qū zhí]

Wood is that which can be bent and straightened.

火曰炎上。[huǒ yuē yán shàng]

Fire is that which flames upward.

土爰稼啬。[tǔ yuán jià sè]

Earth is the sowing and reaping.

金曰从革。[jīn yuē cóng gé]

Metal is a product of smelting.

水曰润下。[shuǐ yuē rùn xià]

Water is moistening and descending. — a metaphor to explain the downward tendency of pathological changes due to dampness such as diarrhea, and edema of the lower extremities，also known as 水性流下 [shuǐ xìng liú xià]

水性流下 [shuǐ xìng liú xià]

Water tends to flow downwards.

木喜条达 [mù xǐ tiáo dá]

Wood (or tree) tends to spread out freely. — a figure of speech to explain the physiological function of the liver in smoothing the flow of *qi*

and blood

土喜温燥 [tǔ xǐ wēn zào]

Earth prefers warmth and dryness. — a figure of speech to explain the physiological property of the spleen, which functions well in warm and dry conditions and is liable to be impaired by cold and dampness

土生万物 [tǔ shēng wàn wù]

Earth engenders the myriad things. — a metaphor to explain that the spleen and stomach provide the material foundation for the whole body by digesting food and supplying nutrients

金气肃降 [jīn qì sù jiàng]

Metal *qi* is depurative and descending. — a figure of speech to explain the functional property of the lung, whose disorder often leads to cough, dyspnea and expectoration

金破不鸣 [jīn pò bù míng]

"A broken gong does not sound." — an expression figuratively referring to hoarseness due to impairment function of the lung

金实不鸣 [jīn shí bù míng]

"A muffled gong does not sound." — an expression figuratively referring to sudden onset of hoarseness due to attack on the lung by exogenous pathogens such as wind-cold or wind-heat

亢则害，承乃制。[kàng zé hài, chéng nǎi zhì]

Hyperactivity will do harm, so restriction is necessary.

所不胜，克我者也。[suǒ bù shèng, kè wǒ zhě yě]

The restraining is what checks me.

所胜，我所克也。[suǒ shèng, wǒ suǒ kè yě]

The restrained is what I check.

母病及子 [mǔ bìng jí zǐ]

Disease of the "mother " (organ) affects her "son" (organ). — an explanation of a group of pathological conditions using the five-elements theory, e.g., hyperactivity of liver yang developing into exuberant heart fire, weakness of spleen *qi* leading to deficiency of lung *qi*

子病及母 [zǐ bìng jí mǔ]

Disease of the "child" (organ) affects its "mother" (organ). — an explanation of a group of pathological conditions using the five-elements theory, e.g., lung *qi* deficiency developing into spleen *qi* deficiency with failure of the transporting function

子盗母气 [zǐ dào mǔ qì]

A "child" (organ) robs its "mother" (organ) *qi*. — another expression for 子病及母 [zǐ bìng jí mǔ]

天人相应 Correspondence between Human and the Universe

天人相应 [tiān rén xiāng yìng]

correspondence between human and the universe: one of the basic theories in traditional Chinese medicine, according to which the physical structure and physiological phenomena of the human body as well as the pathological changes are in adaptive conformity with the variations of the natural environment, and hence in diagnosis and treatment the influences of environmental factors such as climatic conditions, geographical localities, should be considered

顺应四时 [shùn yìng sì shí]

adaptation to seasonal changes: one of the major points in the theory of correspondence between human and the universe that the human body should keep in adaptation to the climatic variations of the different seasons

因时制宜 [yīn shí zhì yí]

being suited to the time: a principle of treatment based on the correspondence between human and the universe that the patient should be treated in accordance with the climatic variations of the different seasons

因地制宜 [yīn dì zhì yí]

being suited to the place: a principle of treatment based on the correspondence between human and the universe that the patient should be treated in accordance with the geographical features of different areas

常用引文 Commonly Used Citations

人与天地相参。[rén yǔ tiān dì xiāng cān]

Human, Heaven and Earth are a trinity.

人以天地之气生，四时之法成。[rén yǐ tiān dì zhī qì shēng, sì shí zhī fǎ chéng]

Human depends on the *qi* of Heaven and Earth to exist, and develops along with the law of the four seasons.

五脏应四时。[wǔ zàng yìng sì shí]

The five *zang*-organs correspond to the four seasons.

春夏养阳，秋冬养阴。[chūn xià yǎng yáng, qiū dōng yǎng yīn]

One should cultivate yang in spring and summer, and nourish yin in autumn and winter.

四变之动，脉与之上下，以春应中规，夏应中矩，秋应中衡，冬应中权。[sì biàn zhī dòng, mài yǔ zhī shàng xià, yǐ chūn yīng zhòng guī, xià yīng zhòng jù, qiū yīng zhòng héng, dōng yīng zhòng quán]

A normal pulse varies with the seasonal changes: It should be round and smooth in spring, square and full in summer, float to the surface in autumn, and sink to the interior in winter.

必先岁气，无伐天和。[bì xiān suì qì, wú fá tiān hé]

One must know in advance the condition of the year's *qi* to avoid attack on the harmony of man and nature.

夫百病者，多以旦慧昼安，夕加夜甚。[fū bǎi bìng zhě, duō yǐ dàn huì zhòu ān, xī jiā yè shèn]

Most diseases are light in the morning, calm in the day, aggravated in the evening, and worse at night.

脏腑 *Zang-Fu* Organs

脏腑 [zàng fǔ]

***zang-fu* organs; viscera:** a collective term for all internal organs, including *zang* organs, *fu* organs, and extra *fu* organs

脏 [zàng]

***zang* organs:** the internal organs that produce, transform and store essential *qi*

腑 [fǔ]

***fu* organs:** the internal organs that receive, contain and transmit food and drink

五脏 [wǔ zàng]

five *zang* organs: a collective term for the heart, liver, spleen, lung and kidney

六腑 [liù fǔ]

six *fu* organs: a collective term for the gallbladder, stomach, large intestine, small intestine, urinary bladder, and triple energizer, all related to food digestion and fluid transmission.

阳脏 [yáng zàng]

yang *zang* organs: the *zang* organs of yang nature, referring to the heart and the liver, distinguished for their preponderant yang quality, also known as 牡脏 [mǔ zàng]

牡脏 [mǔ zàng]

male viscera: another name for yang *zang* organs (阳脏 [yáng zàng])

阴脏 [yīn zàng]

yin *zang* organs: the *zang* organs of yin nature, referring to the spleen, the lung and the kidney, distinguished for their preponderant yin quality, also known as 牝脏 [pìn zàng]

牝脏 [pìn zàng]

female viscera: another name for yin *zang* organs (阴脏 [yīn zàng])

心 [xīn]

heart: a *zang* organ that controls blood circulation and mental activities

心气 [xīn qì]

heart *qi*: *qi* of the heart, which propels the blood through the vessels and also serves as the motive force of mental activities

心血 [xīn xuè]

heart blood: the part of the blood that nourishes the heart and serves as the material basis of mental activities

心阴 [xīn yīn]

heart yin: the yin-fluid of the heart, closely related to heart blood physiologically and pathologically

心阳 [xīn yáng]

heart yang: the yang-*qi* of the heart, closely related to heart *qi* physiologically and pathologically

肝 [gān]

liver: a *zang* organ that stores blood, smoothes the flow of *qi*, and is closely related to the functions of the tendons and eyes

肝气 [gān qì]

liver *qi*: (1) the visceral *qi* that serves as the motive force of the liver's activities; (2) an abbreviation for liver *qi* stagnation (肝气郁滞 [gān qì yù zhì])

肝血 [gān xuè]

liver blood: the blood that is stored in the liver and nourishes the liver system, including the liver itself, liver meridian, eyes, tendons and nails

肝阴 [gān yīn]

liver yin: the blood and fluid of the liver that coordinates with liver yang

肝阳 [gān yáng]

liver yang: yang-*qi* of the liver, referring chiefly to the flourishing and *qi*-smoothing function of the liver

脾 [pí]

spleen: one of the *zang* organs, which shares with the stomach the function of digesting food, transports and distributes nutrients and water, reinforces *qi*, keeps the blood flowing within the vessels, and is closely related to the limbs and muscles

脾气 [pí qì]

spleen *qi*: *qi* of the spleen that serves as the motive force of the transportation, distribution and ascension of nutrients and water, and keeps the blood flowing within the blood vessels

脾阳 [pí yáng]

spleen yang: the yang aspect of the spleen, which refers to the promotion of the spleen functions including transportation, distribution, ascension and warming

脾阴 [pí yīn]

spleen yin: (1) yin-fluid (including blood and fluid) of the spleen; (2) the yin aspect of the spleen, in contrast to spleen yang; (3) a term referring to the spleen itself as the stomach pertaining to yang

肺 [fèi]

lung: a *zang* organ that controls respiration, dominates *qi*, regulates fluid circulation, and is closely related to the functions of the nose and skin surface

肺气 [fèi qì]

lung *qi*: motive force of the various functions of the lung

肺阴 [fèi yīn]

lung yin: yin-fluid that moistens the lung, coordinating with lung *qi*

肺津 [fèi jīn]

lung fluid: the fluid that moistens the lung, synonymous with lung yin (肺阴 [fèi yīn])

肺阳 [fèi yáng]

lung yang: the yang aspect of the lung, referring to the warming, moving, ascending and diffusing functions of the lung

肾 [shèn]

kidney: a *zang* organ that installs vital essence, takes charge of the growth, development, reproduction, and urinary functions, and also has a direct effect on the conditions of the bone and marrow, activities of the brain, hearing, and inspiratory function of the respiratory system

肾阴 [shèn yīn]

kidney yin: the yin aspect of the kidney, which has a moistening and nourishing effect on all the organs; also called kidney water (肾水 [shèn shuǐ]), genuine water (真水 [zhēn shuǐ]), original yin (元阴 [yuán yīn]), or genuine yin (真阴 [zhēn yīn])

肾水 [shèn shuǐ]

kidney water: another name for kidney yin (肾阴 [shèn yīn])

真水 [zhēn shuǐ]

genuine water: another name for kidney yin (肾阴 [shèn yīn])

元阴 [yuán yīn]

original yin: another name for kidney yin (肾阴 [shèn yīn]), stressing the latter's importance

真阴 [zhēn yīn]

genuine yin: another name for kidney yin (肾阴 [shèn yīn]), stressing the latter's importance

肾阳 [shèn yáng]

kidney yang: the yang aspect of the kidney, which warms and activates all the organs; also called original yang (元阳 [yuán yáng]), genuine yang (真阳 [zhēn yáng]) and genuine fire (真火 [zhēn huǒ])

元阳 [yuán yáng]

original yang: another name for kidney yang (肾阳 [shèn yáng]), stressing its importance

真阳 [zhēn yáng]

genuine yang: another name for kidney yang (肾阳 [shèn yáng])

真火 [zhēn huǒ]

genuine fire: another name of kidney yang (肾阳 [shèn yáng])

心包络 [xīn bāo luò]

pericardium: the sac that surrounds the heart and protects the latter against the attack of exogenous pathogenic factors, usually abbreviated as

心包 [xīn bāo]

心包 [xīn bāo]

pericardium, same as 心包络 [xīn bāo luò]

命门 [mìng mén]

(1) life gate; vital gate: the house of water and fire as the root of life, closely related to the kidney both physiologically and pathologically. The genuine fire in the life gate, i.e. life gate fire, refers to kidney fire, and the genuine water in the life gate refers to kidney yin. **(2) *mingmen* (GV4):** an acupoint on the lower back and on the posterior midline, in the depression below the spinous process of the 2nd lumbar vertebra

胆 [dǎn]

gallbladder: a *fu* organ that connected with the liver, stores and discharges bile

胃 [wèi]

stomach: a *fu* organ that receives and preliminarily digests food, and expels the chyme into the small intestine

胃脘 [wèi wǎn]

stomach cavity: the space or potential space within the stomach extending from the cardia to the pylorus

上脘 [shàng wǎn]

(1) upper stomach cavity: the upper part of the stomach cavity, including the cardia; **(2) *shangwan* (CV13):** an acupoint on the upper abdomen and on the anterior midline, 5 *cun* above the center of the umbilicus

中脘 [zhōng wǎn]

(1) middle stomach cavity: the middle part of the stomach cavity; **(2) *zhongwan* (CV12):** an acupoint on the upper abdomen and on the anterior midline, 4 *cun* above the center of the umbilicus

下脘 [xià wǎn]

(1) lower stomach cavity: the lower part of the stomach cavity, including the pylorus; **(2) *xiawan* (CV10):** an acupoint on the upper abdomen and on the anterior midline, 2 *cun* above the center of the umbilicus

胃气 [wèi qì]

stomach *qi*: (1) referring to the function of food intake and preliminary digestion; (2) referring to the material basis of the normal pulse

胃阳 [wèi yáng]

stomach yang: the yang aspect of the stomach, referring to its warming and digestive functions

胃阴 [wèi yīn]

stomach yin: the yin aspect of the stomach, referring to (1) the stomach fluid; (2) the body fluid as a whole

胃津 [wèi jīn]

stomach fluid: fluid produced by the stomach, a part of stomach yin

大肠 [dà cháng]

large intestine: a *fu* organ that has the function of passing the waste in the alimentary tract

小肠 [xiǎo cháng]

small intestine: a *fu* organ that receiving food content from the stomach, further digests it, absorbs the useful and excretes the waste

膀胱 [páng guāng]

bladder: a *fu* organ that stores and discharges urine

三焦 [sān jiāo]

triple energizer: a collective term for the three portions of the body cavity, through which *qi* and fluids are transmitted

上焦 [shàng jiāo]

upper energizer: the upper portion of the body cavity, i.e., the portion above the diaphragm housing the heart and lung

中焦 [zhōng jiāo]

middle energizer: the middle portion of the body cavity, i.e., the portion between the diaphragm and the umbilicus housing the spleen and stomach

下焦 [xià jiāo]

lower energizer: the lower portion of the body cavity, i.e., the portion below the umbilicus cavity housing the kidney, bladder, small and large intestines, and including the liver owing to its patho-physiologic relation to the kidney

形脏 [xíng zàng]

organs containing visible substances: a group of organs including the stomach, small and large intestines, and bladder

奇恒之腑 [qí héng zhī fǔ]

extraordinary organs: a collective term for the brain, marrow, bones, blood vessels, gallbladder and uterus. They are so called because their physiological properties are different from both ordinary *zang* and *fu* organs.

脑 [nǎo]

brain: one of the extraordinary organs contained within the cranium where the marrow converges, also known as sea of marrow (髓海 [suǐ hǎi])

髓海 [suǐ hǎi]

sea of marrow: another name for the brain (脑 [nǎo])

髓 [suǐ]

marrow: an extraordinary organ including bone marrow and spinal marrow, both of which are nourished by kidney essence

骨 [gǔ]

bone: one of the extraordinary organs forming the framework of the body, closely related to the kidney function and nourished by the marrow

髓之府 [suí zhī fǔ]

house of marrow: a euphemistic name for bone

脉 [mài]

(1) blood vessel: the conduit through which *qi* and blood pass; **(2) pulse:** beating of the artery as felt at the wrist

血之府 [xuè zhī fǔ]

house of blood: a euphemistic name for blood vessels

女子胞 [nǚ zǐ bāo]

uterus; womb: an organ in the female for carrying and nourishing offspring during development before birth, also called 胞宫 [bāo gōng], 子脏 [zǐ zàng] and 胞脏 [bāo zàng]

胞宫 [bāo gōng]

another name for the uterus (女子胞 [nǚ zǐ bāo])

子脏 [zǐ zàng]

"offspring's viscus": another name for the uterus (女子胞 [nǚ zǐ bāo])

胞脏 [bāo zàng]

"viscus for fetus": another name for the uterus (女子胞 [nǚ zǐ bāo])

四海 [sì hǎi]

four seas; four reservoirs: the sea (reservoir) of marrow (the brain), the sea (reservoir) of blood (the conception vessel), the sea (reservoir) of *qi* (the pectoral region) and the sea (reservoir) of water and grain (the stomach)

气海 [qì hǎi]

(1) sea of *qi*; reservoir of *qi*: the central part of the chest or the pectoral region as the upper one and the region just below the umbilicus as the lower one; **(2) *qihai* (CV6):** an acupoint on the conception vessel, 1.5 *cun* below the umbilicus

血海 [xuè hǎi]

(1) sea of blood; reservoir of blood: (a) the conception vessel; (b) the liver; **(2) *xuehai* (SP10):** an acupoint on the medial side of the thigh, 2 *cun* above the superior medial corner of the patella, on the prominence of the medial head of the quadriceps muscle of the thigh

水谷之海 [shuǐ gǔ zhī hǎi]

reservoir of water and grain: a euphemistic term for the stomach

血室 [xuè shì]

blood chamber: a term referring to (1) the uterus; (2) the liver; (3) the conception vessel

脏象 [zàng xiàng]

visceral manifestation: the outward manifestation of internal organs through which physiological functions as well as pathological changes can be detected and the state of health judged

传化之腑 [chán huà zhī fǔ]

transmissive-transformative *fu* organs: *fu* organs that have the function of transmitting and transforming food and water, i.e., the stomach, small intestine, large intestine, triple energizer, and bladder

五脏所恶 [wǔ zàng suǒ wù]

intolerance of the five *zang* organs: The heart, lung, liver, spleen and kidney are intolerant of heat, cold, wind, dampness and dryness, respectively.

五脏所主 [wǔ zàng suǒ zhǔ]

charges of the five *zang* organs: The heart, lung, liver, spleen and kidney are in charge of the vessels, skin, tendons, muscles and bones, respectively.

五脏所藏 [wǔ zàng suǒ cáng]

storage of the five *zang* organs: The heart, lung, liver, spleen and kidney store the mind, spirit, mood, idea and memory, respectively

五味所入 [wǔ wèi suǒ rù]

accessibility of the five sapors (flavors): The sour, bitter, sweet, pungent and salty flavors are accessible to the liver, heart, spleen, lung and kidney, respectively.

五志 [wǔ zhì]

five emotions: (1) joy, anger, anxiety, grief, and fear assigned to the heart, liver, spleen, lung and kidney respectively; (2) various emotional changes

脏腑相合 [zàng fǔ xiāng hé]

connection between the *zang* and *fu* organs: the interrelation and mutual influence between the *zang* and *fu* organs, which are connected by the corresponding meridians

脏气 [zàng qì]

***qi* of *zang* organs:** the functional activities of the *zang* organs

心肾相交 [xīn shèn xiāng jiāo]

coordination of the heart and kidney: mutual helping and checking relationship between the heart and the kidney, also known as 水火相济 [shuǐ huǒ xiāng jì]

水火相济 [shuǐ huǒ xiāng jì]

coordination of water and fire: an expression synonymous with coordination of the heart and the kidney (心肾相交 [xīn shèn xiāng jiāo]) for the heart corresponds to fire and the kidney to water

中精之腑 [zhōng jīng zhī fǔ]

***fu* organ with refined juice:** the gallbladder that contains bile

传导之官 [chuán dǎo zhī guān]

organ in charge of transmission: the large intestine that conveys the waste

命门之火 [mìng mén zhī huǒ]

fire of the life gate: a synonym for kidney yang (肾阳 [shèn yáng])

先天之火 [xiān tiān zhī huǒ]

inborn fire: another name for genuine fire (真火 [zhēn huǒ]) or kidney yang (肾阳 [shèn yáng])

肾之府 [shèn zhī fǔ]

residence of the kidney: the loin or lumbar region where the kidneys are situated

相火 [xiàng huǒ]

ministerial fire: (1) a kind of physiological fire originating in the kidney and attached to the liver, gallbladder and triple energizer, which, in cooperation with the king fire (or monarch fire) from the heart warms the viscera and promotes their activities; (2) the part of fire controlled by the kidney that promotes sexual potency

三焦气化 [sān jiāo qì huà]

activity of the triple energizer: distribution, dissemination and excretion of fluid and movement of *qi* that depend on the normal functioning of the triple energizer

中渎之腑 [zhōng dú zhī fǔ]

***fu* organ for water communication:** a euphemism for the triple energizer

常用引文 **Commonly Used Citations**

五脏为实，藏而不泄。 [wǔ zàng wéi shí, cáng ér bù xiè]

The five *zang* organs are solid, installing but not discharging.

六腑为空，泄而不藏。 [liù fǔ wéi kōng, xiè ér bù cáng]

The six *fu* organs are hollow, discharging but not installing.

脏行气于腑。 [zàng xíng qì yú fǔ]

The *zang* organs provide the *fu* organs with *qi*.

腑输精于脏。 [fǔ shū jīng yú zàng]

The *fu* organs supply the *zang* organs with nutrients.

五脏藏精气而不泄。 [wǔ zàng cáng jīng qì ér bù xiè]

The five *zang* organs install but do not discharge the essential *qi*.

六腑传化物而不藏。 [liù fǔ chuán huà wù ér bù cáng]

The six *fu* organs transmit but do not store food contents.

心包络与三焦相表里。 [xīn bāo luò yǔ sān jiāo xiāng biǎo lǐ]

The pericardium and triple energizer are interior-exteriorly related.

三焦者，决渎之官。 [sān jiāo zhě, jué dú zhī guān]

The triple energizer is an organ that controls water communication.

心属火。 [xīn shǔ huǒ]

The heart pertains to fire.

心主血脉。 [xīn zhǔ xuè mài]

The heart controls blood circulation.

心主神明。 [xīn zhǔ shén míng]

The heart is in charge of mental activities.

心，其华在面。 [xīn, qí huá zài miàn]

The heart is manifested in the complexion.

心开窍于舌。 [xīn kāi qiào yú shé]

The heart opens into the tongue. The condition of the heart is often reflected in the tongue.

舌为心之苗。 [shé wéi xīn zhī miáo]

The tongue signifies the heart.

心藏神。 [xīn cáng shén]

The heart houses the mind.

心在志为喜。 [xīn zài zhì wéi xǐ]

Joy is related to the heart.

心恶热。 [xīn wù rè]

The heart is intolerant of heat.

心合小肠。 [xīn hé xiǎo cháng]

The heart is functionally connected with the small intestine.

心与小肠相表里。 [xīn yǔ xiǎo cháng xiāng biǎo lǐ]

The heart and small intestine are interior-exteriorly related.

小肠主受盛。 [xiǎo cháng zhǔ shòu chéng]

The small intestine receives food contents (from the stomach).

小肠化食，泌别清浊。 [xiǎo cháng huà shí, mì bié qīng zhuó]

The small intestine digests food, and separates the clear [useful] from the turbid [waste].

肝属木。 [gān shǔ mù]

The liver pertains to wood.

肝藏血。 [gān cáng xuè]

The liver stores blood.

肝主疏泄。 [gān zhǔ shū xiè]

The liver ensures the free movement of *qi*.

肝主升发。 [gān zhǔ shēng fà]

The liver is predisposed to flourishing growth.

肝主筋。 [gān zhǔ jīn]

The liver governs the tendons.

肝，其华在爪。 [gān, qí huá zài zhǎo]

The liver is manifested in the nails. Lustrous nails signify a sound liver.

爪为筋之余。 [zhǎo wéi jīn zhī yú]

The nails are the odds and ends of the tendons. The nail reflects the condition of the liver which supplies the tendon with blood and nutrients.

肝开窍于目。 [gān kāi qiào yú mù]

The liver opens into the eyes. Normal eyesight depends upon proper functioning of the liver.

肝主目。 [gān zhǔ mù]

The liver governs the eyes.

肝藏魂。 [gān cáng hún]

The liver houses the ethereal soul. Patients with liver disease often complain of dreadful dreams and restlessness.

肝主怒。 [gān zhǔ nù]

Irritability is a chief symptom of liver disease.

肝在志为怒。 [gān zài zhì wéi nù]

Anger is related to the liver.

肝恶风。 [gān wù fēng]

The liver is intolerant of wind.

肝为风木之脏。 [gān wéi fēng mù zhī zàng]

The liver is a viscus of wind and wood. It is so said because the liver smoothes the flow of *qi* and blood, like tree branching out freely and, if diseased, it gives rise to symptoms of wind such as vertigo, tremor or even convulsions.

肝为血海。 [gān wéi xuè hǎi]

The liver is a sea of blood.

发为血之余。 [fà wéi xuè zhī yú]

Hair is the odds and ends of blood.

肝为刚脏。 [gān wéi gāng zàng]

The liver is a viscus of the temperament. It is so said because a patient with a liver disease is apt to become excited, fiery, and hard to be put under control or restraint.

肝为牡脏。 [gān wéi mǔ zàng]

The liver is a male organ. It is so said because the liver is preponderantly of an active and effective position, in contrast to the spleen and the lung (e.g., it checks the function of the spleen, and its fire can make the lung suffer).

肝体阴而用阳。 [gān tǐ yīn ér yòng yáng]

The liver is substantially yin but functionally yang. It is so said because the liver stores the blood (yin factor) and, on the other hand, its physiological functions and pathological manifestations (e.g., normal and abnormal motility) are of yang nature.

肝肾同源。 [gān shèn tóng yuán]

The liver and the kidney have a common source. It is so said because: (1) the liver and the kidney store, respectively, the blood and the vital essence that have a common source; (2) the essence of the liver and the kidney can reinforce each other, and deficiency of one will result in deficiency of the other.

肝合胆。 [gān hé dǎn]

The liver communicates with the gallbladder.

肝与胆相表里。 [gān yǔ dǎn xiāng biǎo lǐ]

The liver and gallbladder are interior-exteriorly related.

胆主决断。 [dǎn zhǔ jué duàn]

The gallbladder has the power of making decisions.

胆者,中正之官。 [dǎn zhě, zhōng zhèng zhī guān]

The gallbladder is analogous to a mediator.

脾属土。 [pí shǔ tǔ]

The spleen pertains to earth.

脾主运化。 [pí zhǔ yùn huà]

The spleen is in charge of transportation and transformation.

脾藏营。 [pí cáng yíng]

The spleen stores nutrients.

脾气主升。 [pí qì zhǔ shēng]

Spleen *qi* keeps ascending.

脾主升清。 [pí zhǔ shēng qīng]

The spleen sends clarity upward.

脾统血。 [pí tǒng xuè]

The spleen keeps the blood within the vessels.

脾主肌肉。 [pí zhǔ jī ròu]

The spleen nourishes the flesh. One with a healthy spleen usually has a full figure, while a diseased spleen makes one lose flesh.

脾主四肢。 [pí zhǔ sì zhī]

The spleen nourishes the limbs. The strength of the limbs depends upon the nourishment guaranteed by the normal functioning of the spleen. A diseased spleen usually causes weakness of the limbs.

脾,其华在唇。 [pí, qí huá zài chún]

The spleen is manifested in the lips. Red and lustrous lips signify normal functioning of the spleen.

脾开窍于口。 [pí kāi qiào yú kǒu]

The spleen opens into the mouth.

脾藏意。 [pí cáng yì]

The spleen stores idea. Excessive scrupulosities may impair the spleen, bringing on such symptoms as anorexia.

脾在志为思。 [pí zài zhì wéi sī]

Pensiveness (or worry) is related to the spleen.

脾恶湿。 [pí wù shī]

The spleen is intolerant of dampness. Dampness is apt to impair the transporting and transforming function of the spleen, leading to diarrhea, lassitude, edema, etc.

脾为生化之源。 [pí wéi shēng huà zhī yuán]

The spleen is the source of production and transformation. This is because the spleen has the functions of digestion, assimilation, transportation and distribution of nutrients.

脾主后天。 [pí zhǔ hòu tiān]

The spleen determines the acquired constitution.

脾胃为后天之本。 [pí wèi wéi hòu tiān zhī běn]

The spleen and stomach provide the material basis of the acquired constitution.

脾胃为仓廪之官。 [pí wèi wéi cāng lǐn zhī guān]

The spleen and stomach are "barn" organs. They store and supply nutrients for the body.

脾合胃。 [pí hé wèi]

The spleen is connected to the stomach.

脾与胃相表里。 [pí yǔ wèi xiāng biǎo lǐ]

The spleen and stomach are interior-exteriorly related.

胃主受纳。 [wèi zhǔ shòu nà]

The stomach governs the food intake.

胃为水谷之海。 [wèi wéi shuǐ gǔ zhī hǎi]

The stomach serves as the reservoir of water and grains (food).

胃主腐熟。 [wèi zhǔ fǔ shú]

The stomach digests food into chyme.

胃主降浊。 [wèi zhǔ jiàng zhuó]

The stomach sends chyme downward.

胃气主降。 [wèi qì zhǔ jiàng]

Stomach *qi* goes downward.

肺属金。 [fèi shǔ jīn]

The lung pertains to metal.

肺主气，司呼吸。 [fèi zhǔ qì, sī hū xī]

The lung governs *qi* and performs respiration.

肺为气之主。 [fèi wéi qì zhī zhǔ]

The lung is the governor of *qi*.

肺主宣发。 [fèi zhǔ xuān fā]

The lung has a diffusing and disseminating function.

肺主肃降。 [fèi zhǔ sù jiàng]

The lung has a cleansing and down-bringing function.

肺朝百脉。 [fèi cháo bǎi mài]

The lung faces all blood vessels. All the blood must pass through the lung.

肺主行水。 [fèi zhǔ xíng shuǐ]

The lung controls the movement of water.

肺主通调水道。 [fèi zhǔ tōng tiáo shuǐ dào]

The lung regulates the water course.

肺为水之上源。 [fèi wéi shuǐ zhī shàng yuán]

The lung is the upper source of water.

肺合皮毛。 [fèi hé pí máo]

The lung is interrelated with the skin and body hair.

肺主皮毛。 [fèi zhǔ pí máo]

The lung controls the skin and body hair.

肺主一身之表。 [fèi zhǔ yī shēn zhī biǎo]

The lung is in charge of the body surface.

肺主声。 [fèi zhǔ shēng]

The lung controls the voice.

肺开窍于鼻。 [fèi kāi qiào yú bí]

The lung opens into the nose.

肺为华盖。 [fèi wéi huá gài]

The lung is the canopy of the viscera.

肺为娇脏。 [fèi wéi jiāo zàng]

The lung is a delicate organ.

肺藏魄。 [fèi cáng pò]

The lung houses the corporeal soul.

肺在志为悲。 [fèi zài zhì wéi bēi]

Sadness is related to the lung.

肺在志为忧。 [fèi zài zhì wéi yōu]

Grief is related to the lung.

肺恶寒。 [fèi wù hán]

The lung is intolerant of cold.

肺与大肠相表里。 [fèi yǔ dà cháng xiāng biǎo lǐ]

The lung and the large intestine are interior-exteriorly related.

肺合大肠。 [fèi hé dà cháng]

The lung is functionally connected to the large intestine.

大肠主传导。 [dà cháng zhǔ chuán dǎo]

The large intestine governs conveyance of waste.

肾属水。 [shèn shǔ shuǐ]

The kidney pertains to water.

肾为气之根。 [shèn wéi qì zhī gēn]

The kidney is the root of *qi*.

肾主纳气。 [shèn zhǔ nà qì]

The kidney controls the reception of *qi*. The kidney promotes inspiration.

肾主生殖。 [shèn zhǔ shēng zhí]

The kidney is in charge of reproduction.

肾为先天之本。 [shèn wéi xiān tiān zhī běn]

The kidney is the foundation of the inborn constitution. It is so said because the function of the kidney is related to growth, development and reproduction.

腰为肾之府。 [yāo wéi shèn zhī fǔ]

The lumbus is the seat of the kidney.

肾藏志。 [shèn cáng zhì]

The kidney houses the will (or memory).

肾在志为恐。 [shèn zài zhì wéi kǒng]

Fear is related to the kidney.

肾藏精。 [shèn cáng jīng]

The kidney stores essence.

肾主水。 [shèn zhǔ shuǐ]

The kidney governs water.

肾司开阖。 [shèn sī kāi hé]

The kidney regulates excretion and retention (of water).

肾为水脏。 [shèn wéi shuǐ zàng]

The kidney is an organ of water. It is so said because the kidney corresponds to water according to the five elements theory, and regulates water metabolism in the body.

肾其充在骨，骨充则髓实。 [shèn qí chōng zài gǔ, gǔ chōng zé suǐ shí]

The kidney supplies the bones with marrow, and the bone marrow is full if the kidney is in good condition.

肾主骨。 [shèn zhǔ gǔ]

The kidney governs the bones.

齿为骨之余。 [chǐ wéi gǔ zhī yú]

The teeth are the odds and ends of bone.

肾主命门之火。 [shèn zhǔ mìng mén zhī huǒ]

The kidney controls the fire of the life gate.

肾司二阴。 [shèn sī èr yīn]

The kidney controls the two private parts [the urethra and anus].

肾恶燥。 [shèn wù zào]

The kidney is intolerant of dryness.

肾开窍于二阴。 [shèn kāi qiào yú èr yīn]

The kidney opens into the uro-genital orifice and the anus.

肾与膀胱相表里。 [shèn yǔ páng guāng xiāng biǎo lǐ]

The kidney and the bladder are interior-exteriorly related.

肾合膀胱。 [shèn hé páng guāng]

The kidney is connected to the bladder.

肾，其华在发。 [shèn, qí huá zài fà]

The kidney is manifested in the hair of the head. The function of the kidney is reflected in the thickness and glossiness of the hair of the head.

肾开窍于耳。 [shè kāi qiào yú ěr]

The kidney opens into the ears.

肾气通于耳。 [shèn qì tōng yú ěr]

Kidney *qi* reaches the ears.

六腑以通为用。 [liù fǔ yǐ tōng wéi yòng]

The six *fu* organs function well when they are unobstructed.

膀胱者，州都之官。 [páng guāng zhě, zhōu dū zhī guān]

The bladder serves as a reservoir.

膀胱主藏津液。 [páng guāng zhǔ cáng jīn yè]

The bladder is in charge of storing fluid [urine].

三焦有名无形。 [sān jiāo yǒu míng wú xíng]

The triple energizer is an unsubstantial name without particular shape.

上焦如雾。 [shàng jiāo rú wù]

The upper energizer works like a sprayer (to spread nutrients and *qi* throughout the body).

中焦如沤。 [zhōng jiāo rú òu]

The middle energizer works like a fermentation tub (to digest food).

下焦如渎。 [xià jiāo rú dú]

The lower energizer works like a gutter (to drain off waste and surplus water.)

三焦为营卫之源。 [sān jiāo wéi yíng wèi zhī yuán]

The triple energizer is the source of both nutritive and defensive *qi*.

上焦主纳。 [shàng jiāo zhǔ nà]

The upper energizer is in charge of reception.

中焦主化。 [zhōng jiāo zhǔ huà]

The middle energizer is in charge of transformation.

下焦主出。 [xià jiāo zhǔ chū]

The lower energizer is in charge of excretion.

脑为元神之府。 [nǎo wéi yuán shén zhī fǔ]

The brain is the seat of mentality.

髓海有余，则轻劲多力，自过其度。 [suǐ hǎi yǒu yú, zé qīng jìn duō lì, zì guò qí dù]

If one's sea of marrow is in surplus, one will be nimble and vigorous, and able to endure unusually hard work.

髓海不足，则脑转耳鸣。 [suǐ hǎi bù zú, zé nǎo zhùan ěr míng]

If one's sea of marrow is insufficienct, vertigo and tinnitus will occur.

官窍与形体

Sense Organs and Other Body Structures

五官 [wǔ guān]

five (sense) organs: a collective term for the nose, eyes, ears, mouth and throat

孔窍 [kǒng qiào]

orifice: outer opening in the body, e.g. nasal orifices

七窍 [qī qiào]

seven orifices: a collective term for the eyes, ears, nostrils and mouth

九窍 [jiǔ qiào]

nine orifices: (1) a collective term for the eyes, ears, nostrils and mouth, plus the urethral orifice and anus; (2) eyes, ears, nostrils and mouth plus tongue and throat

上窍 [shàng qiào]

upper orifices: the orifices on the head

下窍 [xià qiào]

lower orifices: the urethral opening and anus

苗窍 [miáo qiào]

signal orifices: the body openings serving as windows, through which pathological changes of the internal organs can be detected. The nose, eyes, mouth (lips), tongue and ears are the specific body openings (or windows) of the lung, liver, spleen, heart and kidney, respectively.

鼻 [bí]

nose: that part of the face above the mouth, used for breathing, smelling, and assisting in vocalization, and taken as the "specific opening" of the lung

鼻窍 [bí qiào]

nasal orifice: the outer opening of the nasal cavity, taken as a specific opening related to the lung

鼻孔 [bí kǒng]

nostrils: the external openings in the nose through which the breath passes, also known as the opening of the nasal cavity (鼻洞 [bí dòng])

鼻洞 [bí dòng]

opening of the nasal cavity, see nostrils (鼻孔 [bí kǒng])

鼻翼 [bí yì]

ala nasi: expanded outer wall on each side of the nose

鼻准 [bí zhǔn]

apex nasi: the tip of the nose

鼻尖 [bí jiān]

tip of the nose, same as apex nasi (鼻准 [bí zhǔn])

鼻根 [bí gēn]

radix nasi: the root of the nose

鼻隧 [bí suì]

passage of the nose: that part of the nose including vestibulum nasi and posterior naris

鼻梁 [bí liáng]

dorsum nasi: that part of the nose formed by the junction of the lateral surfaces, also known as 鼻茎 [bí jīng]

鼻茎 [bí jīng]

bridge of the nose, same as dorsum nasi (鼻梁 [bí liáng])

鼻柱 [bí zhù]

(1) dorsum of the nose: same as dorsum nasi (鼻梁 [bí liáng]); **(2) nasal septum:** the dividing wall between the nasal cavities

鼻柱骨 [bí zhù gǔ]

bony nasal septum: the body part of the nasal septum

鼻毛 [bí máo]

vibrissa: hair growing in the nasal cavity

口 [kǒu]

mouth: the opening through which one takes in food, and regarded as the specific orifice for the spleen

唇 [chún]

lip: the fleshy margin of the mouth, also called "flying door" (飞门 [fēi mén]), the color of which reflects the condition of the spleen

飞门 [fēi mén]

flying door: the lip (唇 [chún])

齿 [chǐ]

tooth: hard bony structure rooted in the gum, used for biting, chewing, and assisting in vocalization

真牙 [zhēn yá]

wisdom tooth: third molar tooth

龈 [yín]

gum: flesh at the base of the teeth, pertaining to the stomach meridian

舌 [shé]

tongue: movable organ in the mouth, used in tasting and assisting in swallowing, mastication and vocalization

舌旁 [shé páng]

side of the tongue, also known as edge of the tongue (舌边 [she biān])

舌边 [shé biān]

edge of the tongue; border of the tongue: the outside boundary of the tongue, which may reflect the condition of the liver and gallbladder

舌端 [shé duān]

apex of the tongue, also known as the tip of the tongue (舌尖 [shé jiān])

舌尖 [shé jiān]

tip of the tongue: the point or thin end of the tongue, which may reflect the condition of the heart and lung

咽 [yān]

pharynx: the passage between the mouth and the larynx and esophagus, also called 嗌 [yì]

嗌 [yì]

same as 咽 [yān]

咽门 [yān mén]

opening of the pharynx: that part of the throat through which food passes from the mouth into the esophagus

咽底 [yān dǐ]

retropharynx: the posterior pharyngeal wall

咽喉 [yān hóu]

laryngopharynx; throat: the potential cavity at the back of the root of the tongue, connected with the mouth, nose, and the respiratory and alimentary tracts, and through which many meridians run

悬雍垂 [xuán yōng chuí]

uvula palatina; palatine uvula: the small fleshy mass hanging from the soft palate above the root of the tongue, also called "small tongue" (小舌 [xiǎo shé]), or uvula (蒂丁 [dì dīng]; 蒂中 [dì zhōng])

小舌 [xiǎo shé]

"small tongue": another name for uvula palatina (悬雍垂 [xuán yōng chuí])

蒂丁 [dì dīng]; 蒂中 [dì zhōng]

uvula: pendent flashy mass, usually referring to uvula palatina (悬雍垂 [xuán yōng chuí])

颃颡 [háng sǎng]

nasopharynx: upper part of the pharynx continuous with the nasal passages

喉核 [hóu hé]

tonsils: a pair of prominent masses that lie one on each side of the throat

喉关 [hóu guān]

throat pass: that part of the throat formed by the tonsils, uvula and back of the tongue

肺系 [fèi xì]

lung system: (1) a collective term for the lungs and their appendages, including the nose, larynx, trachea and bronchi; (2) the tract connecting the lung with the larynx; (3) the larynx and trachea

会厌 [huì yàn]

epiglottis: a thin lamella of cartilage that serves to cover the glottis during the act of swallowing

七冲门 [qī chōng mén]

seven portals: the seven important doorways or openings along the alimentary tract — lips (飞门 [fēi mén]), teeth (户门 [hù mén]), epiglottis (吸门 [xī mén]), cardia (贲门 [bēn mén]), pylorus (幽门 [yōu mén]), ileocecal conjunction (阑门 [lán mén]), and anus (魄门 [pò mén])

户门 [hù mén]

"house door": the teeth, one of the seven portals (七冲门 [qī chōng mén])

吸门 [xī mén]

"inhalation door": the epiglottis, one of the seven portals (七冲门 [qī chōng mén])

贲门 [bēn mén]

cardia: the orifice between the esophagus and the stomach, one of the seven portals (七冲门 [qī chōng mén])

幽门 [yōu mén]

pylorus: the distal (duodenal) aperture of the stomach, one of the seven portals (七冲门 [qī chōng mén])

阑门 [lán mén]

ileocecal conjunction: the part of the intestines where the small and large intestines join, one of the seven portals (七冲门 [qī chōng mén])

魄门 [pò mén]

corporeal-soul opening: the anus，one of the seven portals (七冲门 [qī chōng mén]). It is so called because the anus is the lower opening of the large intestine which is exterior-interiorly related to the lung — the *zang* organ that stores the corporeal soul.

皮毛 [pí máo]

skin with hair: the body surface which is closely related to the lung in function

毫毛 [háo máo]

down: fine hair of the skin

腠[凑]理 [còu lǐ]

striated layer: a collective term for the skin, sweat pores, subcutaneous tissues and muscles

肌腠[凑] [jī còu]

muscular striae: a general term for the superficial layer of the human body under the skin

肌 [jī]

muscle: tissue that produces movement and strength

肉 [ròu]

flesh: soft tissue between the skin and bones, consisting of muscle and fat

分肉 [fēn ròu]

muscle boundary: the boundary between muscles and subcutaneous fat

玄府 [xuán fǔ]; **元府** [yuán fǔ]

sweat pore: the opening of the duct of the sweat gland on the surface of the skin, literally meaning "mysterious residence", so named because the opening is too minute to be visible, also known as 气门 [qì mén] or 鬼门 [guǐ mén]

气门 [qì mén]

"*qi* portal": another name for sweat pore (玄府 [xuán fǔ])

鬼门 [guǐ mén]

"devil's portal": another name for sweat pore (玄府 [xuán fǔ])

膈[鬲] [gé]

diaphragm: musculo-membranous partition separating the chest and abdomen

筋 [jīn]

tendon; sinew: tough band or cord of tissue that joins muscle to bone

膜原 [mó yuán];

(1) pleurodiaphragmatic interspace; (2) interior-exterior interspace: space between the interior and exterior of the body, a concept used in the diagnosis of febrile diseases

募原 [mù yuán]

same as 膜原 ([mó yuán])

膏肓 [gāo huāng]

(1) *gaohuang*; infracardio-supradiaphragmatic space: space below the heart and above the diaphragm, the innermost part of the body. A disease involving this part is said to be beyond cure. **(2)** ***gaohuang*** **(BL43):** a point on the bladder meridian

丹田 [dān tián]

elixir fields; ***dantian*****:** three regions of the body to which one's mind is focused while practicing *qigong*: the lower elixir field — the region located on the upper 2/3 of the line joining the umbilicus and symphysis pubis; the middle elixir field — the xiphoid area; and the upper elixir field — the region between the eyebrows

精明之府 [jīng míng zhī fǔ]

house of intelligence: a euphemistic term for the head

诸阳之会 [zhū yáng zhī huì]

confluence of all the yang meridians: the site where all the yang meridians meet, i.e. the head

头颅骨 [tóu lú gǔ]

cranium: skull

巅顶 [diān dǐng]

vertex cranii: the top of the head, often abbreviated as 巅 [diān]

巅 [diān]

vertex: an abbreviation of vertex cranii (top of the head) (巅顶 [diān dǐng])

囟门 [xìn mén]; **囟** [xìn]

fontanel: the membrane-covered space remaining in the incompletely ossified skull of an infant

发际 [fà jì]

hairline: the edge of the scalp round the face and over the neck

前发际 [qián fà jì]

anterior hairline: the edge of the scalp above the forehead

后发际 [hòu fà jì]

posterior hairline: the edge of the scalp above the neck

天庭 [tiān tíng]

mid-frons: the middle of the forehead

阙中 [què zhōng]; **阙** [què]

ophryon: the mid-point between the eyebrows, inspection of which serves as a guide to diagnosing lung diseases

印堂 [yìn táng]

(1) ophryon: same as 阙中 [què zhōng]; **(2)** ***yintang*** **(EX-HN3):** an extra point located between the eyebrows

阙上 [què shàng]

supra-ophryon area: the area above the mid-point between the eyebrows, inspection of which serves as a guide to diagnosing diseases of the throat

额 [é]

forehead: the part of the face above the eyebrows and below the hairline, also known as 额颅 [é lú]

额颅 [é lú]

frons, same as the forehead (额 [é])

额角 [é jiǎo]

forehead corner: the area where the corner of the forehead meets the hairline

颞颥 [niè rú]

anterior temple: the region lateral and posterior to the orbit, corresponding to the temporal side of the sphenoid bone

太阳 [tài yáng]

(1) temporal region; (2) *taiyang* (EX-HN5): an acupoint on the temporal part of the head

锐发 [ruì fà]

sideburns: patches of hair growing on the face in front of the ears

眉棱骨 [méi léng gǔ]

supra-orbital ridge: the prominence of the frontal bone over the supra-orbital arch

眉心 [méi xīn]

center of the eyebrows: the midpoint between the eyebrows

目 [mù]

eye: the organ of sight, which is closely related functionally to all *zang-fu* organs and meridians, particularly the liver

目眶 [mù kuàng]

orbit: the bony cavity beneath the frontal bone on each side, which encloses and protects the eye

泪窍 [lèi qiào]

lacrimal punctum: the opening of the lacrimal duct at the inner canthus of the eye

五轮 [wǔ lún]

five orbiculi: a collective term for the eyelid, canthus, the white of the eye, the black of the eye and the pupil. A theory of ophthalmology holds that each of the *zang* organs is physio-pathologically related to one of the orbiculi respectively. (cf. 肉轮 [ròu lún], 血轮 [xuè lún], 气轮 [qì lún], 风轮 [fēng lún], 水轮 [shuǐ lún])

肉轮 [ròu lún]

"flesh orbiculus": the eyelid, one of the five orbiculi, which is believed to be closely related to the spleen

血轮 [xuè lún]

"blood orbiculus": the canthus, one of the five orbiculi, which is believed to be closely related to the heart

气轮 [qì lún]

"*qi* orbiculus": the white of the eye, one of the five orbiculi, which is believed to be closely related to the lung

风轮 [fēng lún]

"wind orbiculus": the black of the eye, one of the five orbiculi, which is believed to be closely related to the liver

水轮 [shuǐ lún]

"water orbiculus": the pupil, one of the five orbiculi, which is believed to be closely related to the kidney

八廓 [bā kuò]

eight regions of the eye: an ancient hypothesis of dividing the eye into eight regions, each of which is thought to be related to a particular internal organ pathologically. This hypothesis is obsolete because of controversies on the location of the regions and their relationship to the internal organs.

胞睑 [bāo jiǎn]

palpebra: the eyelid

目眦 [mù zì]

canthus (of the eye): the corner of the eye formed by the meeting of the upper and lower eyelids

目内眦 [mù nèi zì]

inner canthus (of the eye): the medial corner of the eye, also called the medial canthus

目锐眦 [mù ruì zì]

outer canthus (of the eye): the lateral corner of the eye, also called the lateral canthus

内眦 [nèi zì]

medial canthus, same as the inner canthus

外眦 [wài zì]

outer canthus, same as the lateral canthus

目纲 [mù gāng]

tarsal plate: thc plate that forms the framework of the eyelid

睑弦 [jiǎn xián]

palpebral margin: the edge of the free margin of the eyelid, from which the eyelashes rise

目弦 [mù xián]

margin of the eyelid, same as the palpebral margin (睑弦 [jiǎn xián])

目上胞 [mù shàng bāo]

upper eyelid: the superior of the paired movable folds that protect the anterior surface of the eyeball

目上弦 [mù shàng xián]

margin of the upper eyelid: the edge of the free margin of the upper eyelid

目下胞 [mù xià bāo]

lower eyelid: the inferior of the paired movable folds that protect the anterior surface of the eyeball

目下弦 [mù xià xián]

margin of the lower eyelid: the edge of the free margin of the lower eyelid

睑内 [jiǎn nèi]

palpebral conjunctiva: the membrane that lines the inner side of the eyelid

白睛 [bái jīng]

white of the eye: the white part of the eyeball, also called 白仁 [bái rén]

白仁 [bái rén]

"white kernel": another name for the white of the eye (白睛 [bái jīng])

目系 [mù xì]

ocular system: the cord connecting the eye with the brain, including the ocular nerve and blood vessels associated with the eye

耳 [ěr]

ear: the organ of hearing, to which the kidney *qi* flows to, and is known as the orifice of the kidney

耳廓 [ěr kuò]

auricle: the portion of the external ear not contained within the head, including the helix, anthelix and earlobe, also known as the auricula (耳壳 [ěr qiào])

耳壳 [ěr qiào]

auricula, same as auricle (耳廓 [ěr kuò])

耳轮 [ěr lún]

helix: the incurved rim of the external ear

耳垂 [ěr chuí]

earlobe: the pendent part of the external ear

耳孔 [ěr kǒng]

ear-hole: opening of the external ear

耳道 [ěr dào]

external acoustic meatus: the auditory canal leading from the opening of the external ear to the eardrum, also called 耳窍 [ěr qiào]

耳窍 [ěr qiào]

external auditory meatus, same as the external acoustic meatus (耳道 [ěr dào])

耳膜 [ěr mó]

eardrum: the tympanic membrane

耳门 [ěr mén]

(1) tragus: the cartilaginous projection before the external meatus of the ear; **(2)** ***ermen*** **(TE21):** acupoint on the face, anterior to the supratragic notch, in the depression behind the posterior border of the condyloid process of the mandible

颧 [quán]

malar eminence: the prominence of the cheekbone

颊 [jiá]

bucca: the area of the cheek inferior and lateral to the malar eminence and anterior to the ear lobe

颊车 [jiá chē]

(1) angle of the mandible: the angle formed at the junction of the posterior edge of the ramus and the lower edge of the mandible; **(2)** ***jiache*** **(ST6):** acupoint on the face, in the depression where the masseter muscle is prominent

曲颊 [qū jiá]

mandibular arch: the curved structure of the lower jaw

颐 [yí]

lower cheek: the portion of the face between the corner of the mouth and the mandibular angle

人中 [rén zhōng]]

(1) philtrum: the middle vertical groove below the nose and above the upper lip; **(2) *renzhong* (GV26):** acupoint on the face, at the junction of the upper third and middle third of the philtrum, also called *shuigou* (GV26) (水沟 [shuǐ gōu])

承浆 [chéng jiāng]

(1) middle of the mental labial groove; (2) *chengjiang* (CV24): acupoint located at the middle of the mental labial groove

吻 [wěn]

corner of the mouth: the part of the mouth where the upper and lower lips meet

颌 [hé]

mandible: the lower jaw with its surrounding soft parts

颔 [hàn]

chin: the lower portion of the face below the lower lip, including the front part of the lower jaw

颈 [jǐng]

neck: the part of the body that connects the head to the shoulders

颈骨 [jǐng gǔ]

cervical vertebra: the vertebra of the neck

结喉 [jié hóu]

laryngeal prominence: the Adam's apple

枕骨 [zhěn gǔ]

occipital bone: the bone that forms the posterior part of the cranium

项 [xiàng]

nape: the back part of the neck

肩 [jiān]

shoulder: the part of the body by which the arm is connected to the trunk

肩胛 [jiān jiǎ]

scapula: the shoulder-blade

胂 [shèn]

prominent muscle: (1) the paravertebral muscle; (2) the muscle below the iliac crest

臂 [bì]

(1) arm: the upper limb from the shoulder to the hand; **(2) forearm:** the part of the arm from the elbow to the wrist

臂内廉 [bì nèi lián]

inner arm: (1) the medial aspect of the forearm; (2) the medial aspect of the entire upper limb

臂外廉 [bì wài lián]

outer arm: (1) the lateral aspect of the forearm; (2) the lateral aspect of the entire upper limb

臑 [nào]

(1) humeral region: the region of the arm below the shoulder and above the elbow; **(2) anterior brachial muscle**

臑骨 [nào gǔ]

humerus: the bone extending from the shoulder to the elbow

肱 [gōng]

upper arm: the part of the arm from the shoulder to the elbow

缺盆 [quē pén]

(1) supraclavicular fossa: the depression on either side of the neck behind the clavicle; **(2)** ***quepen*** **(ST12):** acupoint at the center of the supraclavicular fossa

上横骨 [shàng héng gǔ]

suprasternal notch: the jugular notch of the sternum

虚里 [xū lǐ]

(1) area of the apex beat; (2) great collateral of the spleen

膻中 [dàn zhōng]

(1) thoracic center: the central part of the chest, between the two nipples; (2) ***danzhong*** **(GV17):** point on the chest and on the anterior midline, at the midpoint of the line connecting the nipples

鸠尾 [jiū wěi]

(1) xiphoid process: the pointed process of cartilage, connected with the lower part of the body of the sternum; **(2)** ***jiuwei*** **(CV15):** acupoint on the anterior midline, 1 *cun* below the xiphisternal synchondrosis

膺 [yīng]

pectoral muscle: the muscle on the ventral wall of the chest, also known as 臆 [yì]

臆 [yì]

another name for the pectoral muscles (膺 [yīng])

胁 [xié]

costal region: the upper part of the side of the human body from the armpit to the twelfth rib

季肋 [jì lèi]

hypochondrium; hypochondriac region: either of the superolateral regions of the abdomen, lateral to the epigastric region, overlying the costal cartilages of the 11th and 12th ribs, also called 季胁 [jì xié]

季胁 [jì xié]

same as 季肋 [jì lèi]

腹 [fù]

abdomen: the part of the body below the chest and diaphragm

大腹 [dà fù]

upper abdomen: the part of the abdomen above the umbilicus

小腹 [xiǎo fù]

lower abdomen: the part of the abdomen below the umbilicus

少腹 [shào fù]

(1) lower abdomen, same as 小腹 [xiǎo fù]; **(2) inguinal region:** either of the lateral regions of the lower abdomen

神阙 [shén què]

(1) umbilicus: the navel; **(2)** ***shenque*** **(CV8):** point at the center of the umbilicus

横骨 [héng gǔ]

(1) pubic bone: the anterior inferior part of the hip bone on either side, articulating with its fellow in the anterior midline at the pubic symphysis; **(2)** ***henggu*** **(KI 11):** acupoint on the lower abdomen, 5 *cun* below the center of the umbilicus and 0.5 *cun* lateral to the anterior midline

曲骨 [qū gǔ]

(1) pubic symphysis: the joint formed by the union of the bodies of the pubic bones; **(2)** ***qugu*** **(CV2):** acupoint on the anterior midline at the midpoint of the upper border of the pubic symphysis

会阴 [huì yīn]

(1) perineum: the area between the anus and the posterior part of the external genitalia; **(2)** ***huiyin*** **(CV1):** a point in the center of the perineum

毛际 [máo jì]

pubes margin: the border of the region where the pubic hair grows

气街 [qì jiē]

path of *qi*: (1) the femoral artery at the groin; (2) the path through which *qi* circulates

前阴 [qián yīn]

front private parts: the external genitalia including the external orifice of the urethra

后阴 [hòu yīn]

back private part: the anus

二阴 [èr yīn]

two private parts: the front and back private parts, i.e., the external genitalia including the external urethral orifice and anus

产门 [chǎn mén]

vaginal orifice (of a parturient): the external opening of the vagina during childbirth

阴户 [yīn hù]

vaginal orifice: the external opening of the vagina

子门 [zǐ mén]

orifice of the uterine cervix: the opening through which the fetus passes out of the uterus during delivery

廷孔 [tíng kǒng]

external urethral orifice (of the female)

阴器 [yīn qì]

external genitals

阴囊 [yīn náng]

scrotum: the external pouch that contains the testes, also called 肾囊 [shèn náng]

肾囊 [shèn náng]

another name for the scrotum (阴囊 [yīn náng])

睾 [gāo]

testis; testicle: male sex organ in which sperm-bearing fluid is produced

阴茎 [yīn jīng]; **茎** [jīng]

penis: the cylindrical organ with which a male copulates and urinates

茎垂 [jīng chuí]

penis and testes

宗筋 [zōng jīn]

(1) confluent tendon; (2) penis

宗筋之会 [zōng jīn zhī huì]

(1) confluence of tendons; (2) male genitals

精窍 [jīng qiào]

male urinary meatus: the external orifice of the male urethra

肛门 [gāng mén]

anus: the opening through which waste matter from the alimentary tract passes out of the body, also called the corporeal-soul opening (魄门 [pò mén])

腰 [yāo]

lumbus; loin: the part of the back between the thorax and the pelvis

精室 [jīng shì]

essence chamber: the part of the body where the essence is stored in the male and to which the uterus is linked in female, also known as life gate (命门 [mìng mén])

交骨 [jiāo gǔ]

"union bone": (1) sacrococcygeal joint; (2) pubis of the female

股 [gǔ]

thigh: the part of the leg between the knee and the hip

膝 [xī]

knee: the joint between the thigh and the lower part of the leg

筋之府 [jīn zhī fǔ]

house of tendons: the knee where *yanglingquan* (GB34), the influential point of tendons, is located

膝髌 [xī bìn]

kneecap; patella: a thick flat movable bone that forms the anterior point of the knee

膝腘 [xī guó]

post-patellar fossa: the popliteal fossa

腘 [guó]

popliteal fossa: the depression in the posterior region of the knee

胫 [jìng]

shin: (1) the part of the lower limb between the knee and the ankle; (2) the anterior aspect of the leg

腓腨 [féi chuǎi]

calf: the fleshy back part of the leg below the knee, also known as 腨 [chuǎi]

腨 [chuǎi]
abbreviation for 腓腨 [féi chuǎi]

内踝 [nèi huái]
internal malleolus; medial malleolus: the process of the tibia that projects on the medial side of its lower extremity at the ankle, also known as 合骨 [hé gǔ]

合骨 [hé gǔ]
another name for the internal malleolus (内踝 [nèi huái])

外踝 [wài huái]
external malleolus; lateral malleolus: the expanded projection of the fibula on the lateral side of the leg at the ankle, also known as 核骨 [hé gǔ]

核骨 [hé gǔ]
another name for the external malleolus (外踝 [wài huái])

踵 [zhǒng]
heel: the back part of the human foot below the ankle and behind the arch

百骸 [bǎi hái]
skeleton: the bones of the body collectively, forming the framework supporting the human body

脊 [jǐ]
spine: the spinal column

颈骨 [jǐng gǔ]
neck bone: the cervical vertebra

柱骨 [zhù gǔ]
columnar bone: (1) the clavicle; (2) the cervical vertebra

腰骨 [yāo gǔ]
lumbar bone: the lumbar vertebra

髁骨 [kē gǔ]
hip bone: the pelvic bone, also called 髋骨 [kuān gǔ]

髋骨 [kuān gǔ]
hip bone, same as 髁骨 [kē gǔ]

高骨 [gāo gǔ]
eminent bone: the styloid process of the radius

辅骨 [fǔ gǔ]
subsidiary bone: (1) the radius; (2) the fibula

骺骨 [héng gǔ]

leg-bone: a collective term for the fibula and tibia

骭骨 [gàn gǔ]

shinbone; tibia: the inner of the two bones of the leg between the knee and ankle

髀 [bì]

thigh: the part of the leg from the hip to the knee

髀骨 [bì gǔ]

thigh-bone; femur: the proximal bone of a lower limb extending from the hip to the knee, also called 楗 [jiàn]

楗 [jiàn]

another name for the thigh bone (髀骨 [bì gǔ])

髀枢 [bì shū]

trochanteric region: the part over the major trochanter of the femur

尾骶 [wěi dǐ]

sacrococcygeal region: the region of the back overlying the sacrum and coccyx

尾骶骨 [wěi dǐ gǔ]

sacrococcyx: the caudal extremity of the vertebral column formed by the union of the five fused vertebrae and the coccygeal bone

尾闾 [wěi lǘ]

tail bone; coccyx: the small bone caudad to the sacrum

尻 [kāo]

sacral region: the region of the back overlying the sacrum

尻骨 [kāo gǔ]

sacrum: the part of the spinal column that forms the dorsal wall of the pelvis and consists of five fused vertebrae

外辅骨 [wài fǔ gǔ]

fibula: the outer of the two bones between the knee and the foot

胫骨 [jìng gǔ]

tibia: shin bone

足跗 [zú fū]

instep: the back of the foot, abbreviated as 跗 [fū]

跗 [fū]

abbreviation of 足跗 [zú fū]

跗骨 [fū gǔ]

metatarsal bones: the five bones extending from the tarsus to the phalanges of the toes

百节 [bǎi jié]

all joints: the joints of the body on the whole

十二节 [shí èr jié]

twelve joints: the joints of the shoulder girdle, elbow and wrist on the upper limbs and the joints of the thigh, knee and ankle on the lower limbs, altogether twelve in number

大节 [dà jié]

"large joints": (1) the large joints of the human skeleton; (2) the proximal joints of the fingers and toes

八溪 [bā xī]

eight joints: the joints at the elbow, wrist, knee and ankle

本节 [běn jié]

basic (digital) joints: the eminences of the metacarpophalangeal and metatarsophalangeal joints

虎口 [hǔ kǒu]

"tiger's mouth": the area between the thumb and the index finger, so called because it looks like an opening mouth of a tiger

赤白肉际 [chì bái ròu jì]

dorso-ventral boundary (of the hand or foot): the boundary between the palm or sole (red in color) and the back of the hand or foot (white in color)

丛毛 [cóng máo]

clustered hair: hairs growing on the back of the proximal phalange of the big toe

气、血、精、津液 *Qi*, Blood, Essence and Body Fluids

气 [qì]

***qi* (*ch'i*):** the basic element that constitutes the cosmos and, through its movements, changes and transformations, produces everything in the world, including the human body and life activities. In the field of medicine, *qi* in its physiological sense is referred to as the basic element or energy which makes up the human body and supports its vital activities, such as 水谷之气 [shuǐ gǔ zhī qì], *qi* of foodstuff, i.e., food energy, 呼吸

之气 [hū xī zhī qì], *qi* of respiration, i.e., the breathed air. Since *qi* is invisible and its existence in the human body can only be perceived through its resultant activities as expressed through organs and tissues, it is more frequently used in the sense of functional activities, such as 脏腑之气 [zàng fŭ zhī qì], i.e., the functional activities of the *zang-fu* organs. The term *qi* can also be used in a pathological sense, e.g., 邪气 [xié qì], which means pathogenic factor.

水谷之气 [shuĭ gŭ zhī qì]

food *qi*: essential substance and energy derived from foodstuffs

谷气 [gŭ qì]

same as 水谷之气 [shuĭ gŭ zhī qì]

水谷 [shuĭ gŭ]

water and grains: food or diet

大气 [dà qì]

air: the earth's atmosphere, especially that which is breathed

呼吸之气 [hū xī zhī qì]

breathed air: air inhaled and exhaled through respiration

先天之气 [xiān tiān zhī qì]

inborn *qi*; innate *qi*: the *qi* that exists in a person from birth

后天之气 [hòu tiān zhī qì]

acquired *qi*: the *qi* that is acquired after birth and is formed from food *qi* obtained by the spleen and stomach in combination with the fresh air (oxygen) inhaled by the lung

原[元]气 [yuán qì]

original *qi*: the *qi* derived from the innate essence and supplemented by acquired *qi*, acting as the primary motive force for life activities

真气 [zhēn qì]

genuine *qi*: the combination of inborn *qi* and acquired *qi*, serving as the dynamic force of all vital functions

正气 [zhèng qì]

(1) normal *qi*; healthy *qi*: a synonym for 真气 [zhēn qì], particularly referring to the body resistance opposing pathogenic factors; **(2) normal weather**

宗气 [zōng qì]

pectoral *qi*: a combination of essential *qi* derived from food with the inhaled air, stored in the chest, serving as the dynamic force of blood circulation, respiration, voice, and bodily movements

营气 [yíng qì]

nutritive *qi*: the *qi* that moves within the vessels and nourishes all the organs and tissues

营阴 [yíng yīn]

nutritive yin: another name for nutritive *qi* as the *qi* that moves inside the vessels pertains to yin while that which moves outside the vessels pertains to yang

卫气 [wèi qì]

defensive *qi*; protective *qi*: the *qi* that moves outside the vessels, permeating the body surface and warding off exogenous pathogens

卫阳 [wèi yáng]

nutritive yang: another name for defensive *qi* as the *qi* that moves outside the vessels pertains to yang while that which moves inside the vessels pertains to yin

津气 [jīn qì]

fluid *qi*: (1) a synonym for 津 [jīn]; (2) a collective term for body fluid and yang *qi*

精气 [jīng qì]

essential *qi*: the *qi* of the essence, from which life originates and is maintained, including the *qi* derived from reproductive essence, food essence, and essence of *zang-fu* organs, generally equivalent to normal *qi* or healthy *qi* (正气 [zhèng qì])

肾间动气 [shèn jiān dòng qì]

motive *qi* between the kidneys: that part of genuine *qi* as the motive force necessary for the activities of the *zang-fu* organs and meridian system

脏气 [zàng qì]

***zang*-organ *qi*:** the functional activities of a *zang* organ

腑气 [fǔ qì]

***fu*-organ *qi*:** the functional activities of a *fu* organ

心气 [xīn qì]

heart *qi*: the functional activities of the heart

肝气 [gān qì]

liver *qi*: (1) the functional activities of the liver; (2) an abbreviation for stagnation of liver *qi*

脾气 [pí qì]

spleen *qi*: the functional activities of the spleen

肺气 [fèi qì]

lung *qi*: (1) the functional activities of the lung; (2) air breathed, including pectoral *qi*

肾气 [shèn qì]

kidney *qi*: the functional activities of the kidney

胆气 [dǎn qì]

gallbladder *qi*: the functional activities of the gallbladder

胃气 [wèi qì]

stomach *qi*: (1) the functional activities of the stomach; (2) the reflection of the functional activities of the stomach in the pulse

清气 [qīng qì]

clear *qi*: (1) fresh air, usually referring to the air inspired in the lung, especially oxygen; (2) the clarified thin part of food essence, i.e., the nutrient; (3) to clear up the *qi* system, a method of treating febrile diseases with heat in the *qi* system

浊气 [zhuó qì]

turbid *qi*: (1) the dense part of food essence; (2) waste gas, e.g., air expired or flatus discharged

阳气 [yáng qì]

yang *qi*: the yang aspect of *qi*, often referring to functional activity in opposition to yin-*qi* as substance

阴气 [yīn qì]

yin *qi*: the yin aspect of *qi*, often referring to substance in opposition to yang-*qi* as functional activity

清阳 [qīng yáng]

lucid yang: light and clear yang-*qi* that usually exists in the upper or exterior part of the body, including the fresh air inhaled and the superficial resistance

经络之气 [jīng luò zhī qì]

meridian *qi*: the *qi* that constitutes the structure and particularly that which maintains the functional activities of the meridian system

经气 [jīng qì]

an abbreviation for meridian *qi* (经络之气 [jīng luò zhī qì])

卫气营血 [wèi qì yíng xuè]

defense, *qi*, nutrient, and blood: four systems denoting the four portions or strata of the body from the superficial to the deep, to show the location, seriousness, stage or phase of an acute febrile disease as a guide to diagnosis

卫分 [wèi fèn]

defense system; superficial defensive system: the most superficial stratum of the body apt to be invaded at the initial stage of an acute febrile disease, often abbreviated as 卫 [wèi]

卫 [wèi]

(1) an abbreviation of defense system (卫分 [wèi fèn]); (2) an abbreviation of defense *qi* (卫气 [wèi qì])

气分 [qì fèn]

***qi* system:** the second stratum of the body deeper than the superficial defensive system, often referring to the lung, gallbladder, spleen, stomach or large intestine

营分 [yíng fèn]

nutrient system: that stratum of the body further deeper than the *qi* system, often abbreviated as 营 [yíng]

营 [yíng]

(1) an abbreviation of nutrient system (营分 [yíng fèn]); (2) an abbreviation of nutrient *qi* (营气 [yíng qì]) or nutritive yin (营阴 [yíng yīn])

血分 [xuè fèn]

blood system: the deep stratum of the body involved in the severest stage of an acute febrile disease, often abbreviated as 血 [xuè]

气机 [qì jī]

***qi* movement:** the constant movement of *qi* (ascending, descending, exiting and entering) that promotes and facilitates various physiological activities, maintaining life

气化 [qì huà]

***qi* transformation:** a general term referring to various transforming changes through the activity of *qi*, namely the metabolism and mutual transformation between essence, *qi*, blood and fluids. In other words, *qi* transformation corresponds to metabolism, substance transformation and energy transformation.

中气 [zhōng qì]

middle *qi*: an abbreviation for *qi* of the middle energizer, i.e., *qi* of the spleen and stomach

血 [xuè]

blood: the red fluid circulating through the blood vessels and nourishing the body tissues

精血 [jīng xuè]

essence-blood: a combined term indicating both the essence and the blood owing to their close relationship, and often representing all the nourishing substances necessary for maintaining human life

营血 [yíng xuè]

(1) nutrient-blood: a synonym of blood as the nutrient, being the *qi* of blood; **(2) nutrient and blood:** the later two stages of an acute febrile disease in which both the nutrient system and blood system are involved

血脉 [xuè mài]

blood vessel: any channel for carrying blood

血气 [xuè qì]

blood *qi*: the *qi* of blood, referring to the functions of blood

精 [jīng]

(1) essence: the fundamental substance that builds up the physical structure and maintains the body function; **(2) semen,** known also as reproductive essence 生殖之精 [shēng zhí zhī jīng]

水谷之精 [shuǐ gǔ zhī jīng]

food essence: the essential substance derived from food, which is required for the maintenance of life activities and the metabolism of the human body, also known as 水谷精微 [shuǐ gǔ jīng wēi]

水谷精微 [shuǐ gǔ jīng wēi]

same as 水谷之精 [shuǐ gǔ zhī jīng]

精微 [jīng wèi]

refined essence: usually referring to the refined nutritious substances derived from foodstuffs through digestion

先天之精 [xiān tiān zhī jīng]

innate essence: the original substance which is essential for construction of the body, often referring to the reproductive essence (生殖之精 [shēng zhí zhī jīng])

后天之精 [hòu tiān zhī jīng]

acquired essence: the fundamental substance derived from food to maintain the body functions and replenish physical construction

生殖之精 [shēng zhí zhī jīng]

reproductive essence: the fundamental substance for reproduction, referring to semen and ovum

肾精 [shèn jīng]

kidney essence: the original essence stored in the kidney, including the reproductive essence

浊阴 [zhuó yīn]

turbid yin: heavy and turbid matter in the body, chiefly referring to the urine and feces, but also to the concentrated and turbid part of food essence

精汁 [jīng zhī]

refined juice: the juice contained in the gallbladder, referring to bile

神 [shén]

(1) mind: condition of one's mental faculties, including consciousness, attention, and thinking; **(2) vitality**: liveliness or vigor

形体 [xíng tǐ]

configuration and constitution; physique: general appearance and condition of a person's body

形 [xíng]

an abbreviation for 形体 [xíng tǐ]

精神 [jīng shén]

spirit: state of mind or mood

魂 [hún]

ethereal soul: the moral and spiritual part of man, as distinguished from his intellect

魄 [pò]

corporeal soul: the animating part of the mind

意 [yì]

thought: act or power of thinking

志 [zhì]

(1) will: mental power by which a person can direct his thoughts and actions; **(2) memory:** power to remember

津 [jīn]

(1) (thin) fluid: the fluid that circulates with *qi* and blood. It is mainly distributed over the exterior part of the body, and can be secreted as tears, saliva, sweat, etc. **(2) saliva**

液 [yè]

(thick or **mucous) fluid:** the fluid that does not circulate together with *qi* and blood, but is stored in body cavities such as the articular and cranial cavities

津液 [jīn yè]

(1) (body) fluids: a general term for all fluids in the body, including secretions such as saliva, tears, sweat, etc. **(2) liquid nutrients**

阴液 [yīn yè]

yin fluids: all kinds of nutrient fluid in the body, especially that of the internal organs

清浊 [qīng zhuó]

clarity and turbidity: often referring to the essence and the waste of digested food

五液 [wǔ yè]

five kinds of fluid: sweat, tears, snivel, slobber and spittle

五脏化液 [wǔ zàng huà yè]

secretion from the five *zang* organs: sweat derived from the heart, tears from the liver, saliva from the spleen, snivel from the lung, and spittle from the kidney

汗 [hàn]

sweat: a product of fluid metabolism discharged from the pores

泪 [lèi]

tear: one of the five kinds of fluid, which cleanses and moistens the eyeballs, and excessive discharge of which, if not during weeping, is often related to the liver meridian

涎 [xián]

slobber; (thin) saliva: liquid produced in the mouth that helps one chew and digest, one of the five kinds of fluid that is closely related to the functions of the spleen

涕 [tì]

snivel: nasal mucus

唾 [tuò]

spittle; (thick) saliva: a part of liquid produced in the mouth, one of the five kinds of fluid that is closely related to the functions of the kidney

常用引文 Commonly Used Citations

泪为肝液。 [lèi wéi gān yè]

Tears are the fluid of the liver. It is so said because tears come from the eyes, which reflect the condition of the liver as its specific opening. Lack of tears with dry eyes is a common symptom indicating deficiency of essence and blood in the liver.

汗为心液。 [hàn wéi xīn yè]

Sweat is the fluid of the heart. It is so said because sweat comes from blood, which is controlled by the heart. Clinically, spontaneous sweating is commonly seen when heart yang is insufficient, while night sweating usually suggests heart yin deficiency.

涎为脾液。 [xián wéi pí yè]

Slobber is the fluid of the spleen. It is so said because the spleen has its specific body opening in the mouth. Clinically, dry mouth is frequently seen in cases of inadequacy of fluid in the spleen and stomach, and dysfunction of the spleen in sending up fluid.

涕为肺液。 [tì wéi fèi yè]

Snivel is the fluid of the lung. It is so said because the nose is the specific body opening of the lung. Clinically, a dry nose is usually due to heat or dryness in the lung, while patients with impeded functions of the lung often have a running nose.

唾为肾液。 [tuò wéi shèn yè]

Spittle is the fluid of the kidney. It is so said because the kidney meridian runs through the sublingual area. Clinically, excessive spittle can be cured by using kidney tonics.

血汗同源。 [xuè hàn tóng yuán]

Blood and sweat have one and the same source. It is so said because sweat comes from blood.

精血同源。 [jīng xuè tóng yuán]

Essence and blood have a common source. Both essence and blood constitute the material basis of the human body; blood comes from congenital essence and is nourished by acquired food essence.

津血同源。 [jīn xuè tóng yuán]

Body fluids and blood are derived from a common source. Both body fluids and blood are derived from water and food, so they are closely related physiologically and pathologically.

气为血帅。 [qì wéi xuè shuài]

***Qi* is the commander of blood.** It is so said because *qi* serves as the dynamic force of blood flow, keeps the blood circulating within the vessels, and promotes blood regeneration; and hence, stagnancy of *qi* is apt to cause blood stasis, and deficiency of *qi* may lead to chronic bleeding or deficiency of blood.

血为气母。 [xuè wéi qì mǔ]

Blood is the mother of *qi*. It is so said because blood is the material basis of *qi*, deficiency of blood usually leads to insufficient *qi* (vital energy), and massive loss of blood may cause prostration of *qi* manifested as collapse.

气行血行。 [qì xíng xuè xíng]

***Qi* in motion keeps the blood circulating.**

卫气者，所以温分肉，充皮肤，肥腠理，司开合者也。[wèi qì zhě, suǒ yǐ wēn fēn ròu, chōng pí fū, féi còu lǐ, sī kāi hé zhě yě]

Defense *qi* warms the flesh, flushes the skin, replenishes the interstices and controls the opening and closing of the pores.

宗气积于胸中，出于喉咙，以贯心脉，而行呼吸。[zōng qì jī yú xiōng zhōng, chū yú hóu lóng, yǐ guàn xīn mài, ér xíng hū xī]

Pectoral *qi* accumulates in the chest, issues through the throat, goes through the heart and vessels, and conducts respiration.

营气者，泌其津液，注之于脉，化以为血，以荣四末，内注五脏六腑。[yíng qì zhě, mì qí jīn yè, zhù zhī yú mài, huà yǐ wéi xuè, yǐ róng sì mò, nèi zhù wǔ zàng liù fǔ]

Nutrient *qi* secretes fluids, discharges them into the vessels and turns them into blood, to nourish the limbs and supply the *zang-fu* organs.

夫精者，身之本也。[fū jīng zhě, shēn zhī běn yě]

Essence is the basis of the body.

生之来谓之精，两精相搏谓之神。[shēng zhī lái wèi zhī jīng, liǎng jīng xiāng bó wèi zhī shén]

What enables human generation is called essence; when yin essence and yang essence combine, life activity exists, which is called spirit.

恬淡虚无，真气从之，精神内守，病从安来。[tiǎn dàn xū wú, zhēn qì cóng zhī, jīng shén nèi shǒu, bìng cōng ān lái]

When one has a tranquil mind content in nothingness, genuine *qi* will come in the wake of it; and when one concentrates one's spirit

internally, how can any illness occur?

病因 Cause of Disease

病因 [bìng yīn]

cause of disease: that which produces disease

三因 [sān yīn]

three categories of etiological factors: exogenous, endogenous, and non-exo-endogenous – an ancient classification of causes of disease

外因 [wài yīn]

exogenous factors: etiological factors that originate outside the body, referring chiefly to the six excessive and untimely climatic influences and pestilential pathogens

内因 [nèi yīn]

endogenous factors: etiological factors that arise within the body, referring chiefly to excessive emotional changes

不内外因 [bù nèi wài yīn]

non-exo-endogenous factors: etiological factors other than the exogenous and endogenous ones, referring chiefly to such factors as improper diet, overwork, trauma, sexual overindulgence, animal bite, etc.

邪气 [xié qì]

pathogenic *qi*; evil *qi*: factors that are harmful to the body and capable of causing disease

邪 [xié]

pathogen; evil: abbreviation of pathogenic or evil *qi* (邪气 [xié qì])

外邪 [wài xié]

exogenous pathogens: pathogenic factors from without, including the six excesses and various infectious factors

客邪 [kè xié]

intruding pathogen: pathogenic factor from without, same as 外邪[wài xié]

时邪 [shí xié]

seasonal pathogen: a general designation for the pathogenic factors causing seasonal diseases

外感 [wài gǎn]

external affection; external contraction: catching or developing a disease caused by any of the exogenous pathogens

六气 [liù qì]

six *qi*: (1) the six vital substances for human life: essence, *qi* , nutrient, fluid, blood and vessels; (2) the six climatic influences: wind, cold, summer heat, dampness, dryness, and fire

六淫 [liù yín]

six excesses: (1) the six excessive or untimely climatic influences as exopathogenic factors: wind, cold, summer heat, dampness, dryness, and fire; (2) the six pathogenic factors: wind, cold, heat, dampness, dryness, and fire either exogenous or endogenous

淫气 [yín qì]

excessive *qi*: excessive climatic influence or overabundance of yin or yang of the body which causes disease

四时不正之气 [sì shí bù zhèng zhī qì]

abnormal weather changes of the four seasons: those which are unfavorable to the normal growth and development of living beings and often cause disease

疠气; 戾气 [lì qì]

pestilential *qi*; pestilential pathogen: pathogen that causes a virulent contagious or infectious disease, called also 疫疠之气 [yì lì zhī qì], 疫毒 [yì dú], 异气 [yì qì] , 杂气 [zá qì]

疫疠之气 [yì lì zhī qì]

the full name of 疠气 [lì qì]

疫毒 [yì dú]

epidemic toxin: another name for pestilential pathogen 疠气 [lì qì] or 疫疠之气 [yì lì zhī qì]

异气 [yì qì]

abnormal *qi*: another name for pestilential pathogen 疠气 [lì qì]

杂气 [zá qì]

impure *qi*: another name for pestilential pathogen 疠气 [lì qì]

时行戾气 [shí xíng lì qì]

prevalent pestilential pathogen: pathogen that causes an epidemic of pestilence

恶气 [è qì]

malign *qi*: (1) a general term for pathogenic *qi*, including the six excesses and pestilential factors; (2) a pathological product derived from stagnation of *qi* and blood

贼风 [zéi fēng]

evil wind: wind as a pathogenic factor that invades an unprotected body

阴邪 [yīn xié]

yin pathogens: (1) pathogenic factors of yin nature, i.e., cold and dampness, which tend to impede and injure yang; (2) pathogenic factors that attack the yin meridians

阳邪 [yáng xié]

yang pathogens: (1) pathogenic factors of yang nature, i.e., wind, summer heat, dryness and fire, which tend to take the form of heat and injure yin (body fluid and essence); (2) pathogenic factors that attack the yang meridians

合邪 [hé xié]

combined pathogen: a combination of two or more pathogenic factors invading the human body simultaneously

伏气 [fú qì]

latent *qi*: (1) latent pathogen, another name for 伏邪 [fú xié]; (2) an abbreviation of 伏气温病 [fú qì wēn bìng], i.e., a warm disease caused by a latent pathogen

伏邪 [fú xié]

latent pathogen: pathogen concealed in the body, which causes disease after an incubation period, also called 伏气 [fú qì]

风 [fēng]

wind: (1) one of the six excesses as a pathogenic factor, also called pathogenic wind (风邪 [fēng xié]); (2) abbreviation of wind syndrome (风证 [fēng zhèng])

风邪 [fēng xié]

pathogenic wind: full name of wind (风 [fēng]) as a pathogenic factor

风气 [fēng qì]

wind *qi*: (1) wind as one of the natural climatic influences: (2) wind as a pathogenic factor

风痰 [fēng tán]

wind-phlegm: (1) a syndrome marked by vertigo, numbness, and hemiplegia; (2) pathogenic factor that causes such a syndrome

内风 [nèi fēng]

internal wind; endogenous wind: (1) a morbid condition caused by excessive heat or deficiency of blood or essence and marked by dizziness, fainting, convulsion, tremor, numbness, hemiplegia, etc., also known as liver wind; (2) pathogenetic factor that produces such a condition

外风 [wài fēng]

external wind; exogenous wind: one of the six excesses as a pathogenic factor

伤风 [shāng fēng]

wind affection: (1) syndrome of *taiyang* meridian affected by wind; (2) common cold

寒 [hán]

cold: (1) one of the six excesses as a pathogenic factor, also called 寒邪 [hán xié]; (2) abbreviation of cold syndrome (寒证 [hán zhèng]), usually marked by aversion to cold, cold limbs, preference for warmth, loose stool, pale tongue with whitish coating, etc.

寒邪 [hán xié]

pathogenic cold: full name of cold (寒 [hán]) as a pathogenic factor

外寒 [wài hán]

external cold; exogenous cold: (1) cold pathogen from outside in an external contraction; (2) outer manifestation of yang-*qi* insufficiency such as cold limbs and aversion to cold

内寒 [nèi hán]

internal cold; endogenous cold: (1) a morbid condition caused by yang-*qi* insufficiency of the internal organs, especially of the kidney and spleen, marked by watery diarrhea, abdominal pain, cold limbs, intolerance of cold, and slow and sunken pulse; (2) pathogenetic factor that produces such a condition

中寒 [zhòng hán]

direct attack of cold: attack of cold directly to the stomach and intestines, marked by abdominal pain, borborygmi and diarrhea, accompanied by chills or cold limbs

中寒 [zhōng hán]

cold in the middle (energizer): morbid condition caused by deficiency of the spleen and stomach yang, marked by abdominal pain which can be relieved by warmth, intolerance of cold, cold limbs, loss of appetite, and loose bowels

暑 [shǔ]

summer-heat: one of the six excesses as a pathogenic factor, which exists only in summer and brings on symptoms such as fever, headache, thirst, fidgetiness, sweating, and rapid gigantic pulse, also called summer *qi* (暑气 [shǔ qì]) or pathogenic summer-heat (暑邪 [shǔ xié])

暑气 [shǔ qì]

summer *qi*: summer heat as a pathogenic factor

暑邪 [shǔ xié]

pathogenic summer-heat: summer heat as a pathogenic factor, often abbreviated as summer heat (暑 [shǔ])

暑热 [shǔ rè]

summer heat: (1) same as 暑邪 [shǔ xié]; (2) heat syndrome due to invasion of pathogenic summer-heat

暑湿 [shǔ shī]

summer-damp: (1) a combined pathogenic factor in summer causing fever with stuffy sensation in the chest and epigastrium, and yellow greasy tongue coating; (2) disease caused by summer heat and dampness

湿 [shī]

dampness; damp: (1) one of the six excesses as a pathogenic factor, which is apt to disturb the flow of *qi* and normal functioning of the spleen and stomach, also called damp *qi* (湿气 [shī qì]); (2) pathological product due to disordered water metabolism, which may in turn become a pathogenic factor, also called endogenous dampness (内湿 [nèi shī])

湿气 [shī qì]

damp *qi*: damp as a pathogenic factor

湿浊 [shī zhuó]

damp turbidity; turbid damp: a synonym of damp *qi* (湿气 [shī qì]), so named because of the turbid and sticky property of pathogenic damp

湿邪 [shī xié]

pathogenic damp: damp as a pathogenic factor, often abbreviated as damp (湿 [shī])

外湿 [wài shī]

external damp(ness); exogenous damp(ness): a pathogenic factor attacking a person living and working in damp places, bringing on symptoms such as headache as if the head were tightly bound, lassitude, heaviness in the limbs, fullness in the chest, joint pains and swelling with sensation of heaviness

内湿 [nèi shī]

internal damp(ness); endogenous damp(ness): (1) retention of water within the body caused by deficiency of spleen and kidney yang with disturbance in the water metabolism and distribution, manifested by loss of appetite, diarrhea, abdominal distension, oliguria and edema; (2) the pathological product due to disordered water metabolism, which turns into a pathogenic factor affecting the function of the internal organs, particularly the spleen and stomach

水气 [shuǐ qì]

water *qi*: (1) pathogenetic factor derived from water retention in a case of kidney insufficiency and causes edema; (2) edema

燥 [zào]

dryness: (1) one of the six pathogenic factors, which prevails in autumn and impairs body fluid, bringing on dryness of the nasal cavity, parched lips, dry cough, constipation, etc., called also dryness *qi* (燥气 [zào qì]); (2) abbreviation of dryness syndrome (燥证 [zào zhèng])

燥气 [zào qì]

dryness *qi*: dryness as a pathogenic factor

燥邪 [zào xié]

pathogenic dryness: dryness as a pathogenic factor

凉燥 [liáng zào]

cool-dryness: (1) disease marked by a syndrome of wind-cold together with dryness; (2) pathogenic factor that causes such a disease

温燥 [wēn zào]

warm-dryness: (1) disease marked by a syndrome of wind-heat together with dryness; (2) pathogenic factor that causes such a disease

燥热 [zào rè]

dryness-heat: pathogenic heat transformed from dryness

燥火 [zào huǒ]

dryness-fire: pathogenic fire transformed from dryness

外燥 [wài zào]

external dryness; exogenous dryness: climatic influence as a pathogenic factor marked by dryness

内燥 [nèi zào]

internal dryness; endogenous dryness: (1) syndrome of dryness due to consumption of body fluid; (2) pathological condition resulting from fluid consumption as a pathogenetic factor for the development of complications

火 [huǒ]

fire: (1) one of the five elements; (2) physiological energy of life; (3) one of the six excesses as a pathogenic factor, called also pathogenic fire (火邪 [huǒ xié]); (4) pathological manifestation of intense heat such as flushed face, bloodshot eyes or acute local inflammation, resulting from excessive functional activities, immoderate emotional influences or affection by various pathogenic factors

火邪 [huǒ xié]

pathogenic fire: fire as a pathogenic factor

热 [rè]

heat: (1) one of the six excesses as a pathogenic factor of the same property as fire, called also pathogenic heat (热邪 [rè xié]); (2) an abbreviation of heat syndrome (热证 [rè zhèng]), usually marked by fever, aversion to heat, thirst with desire for cold drinks, scanty concentrated urine, constipation, reddened tongue with yellow coating, and rapid pulse

热邪 [rè xié]

pathogenic heat: heat as a pathogenic factor

温热 [wēn rè]

(1) warmth-heat: pathogenic factor causing febrile diseases, same as pathogenic warmth (温邪 [wēn xié]) and pathogenic heat (热邪 [rè xié]). In the strict sense, pathogenic warmth attacks insidiously, causes milder diseases and prevails in winter and spring, while pathogenic heat causes severe disease with sudden onset and prevails in summer. **(2) warm-heat disease:** any epidemic febrile disease, same as 温病 [wēn bìng]

温邪 [wēn xié]

warm pathogen: a collective term for various pathogens causing acute febrile diseases

风温 [fēng wēn]

wind-warm: (1) wind and warm combined as a pathogenic factor, also called 风温邪气 [fēng wēn xié qì]; (2) disease caused by wind-warm pathogen

风温邪气 [fēng wēn xié qì]

wind-warm pathogen: full name of wind-warm (风温 [fēng wēn]) as a pathogenic factor

风寒 [fēng hán]

wind-cold: (1) wind and cold combined as a pathogenic factor, also called pathogenic wind-cold (风寒邪气 [fēng hán xié qì]), which causes marked chilliness with mild fever, headache, general aching, nasal congestion and discharge, and floating, tense pulse when invading the exterior of the body; (2) abbreviation of wind-cold syndrome (风寒证 [fēng hán zhèng]), i.e. syndrome caused by attack of wind and cold in combination

风寒邪气 [fēng hán xié qì]

wind-cold pathogen: full name of wind-cold (风寒 [fēng hán]) as a pathogenic factor

风热 [fēng rè]

wind-heat: (1) wind and heat combined as a pathogenic factor, also called pathogenic wind-heat (风热邪气 [fēng rè xié qì]), which causes high fever with slight aversion to wind, mild thirst, and floating, rapid pulse when invading the exterior of the body; (2) abbreviation of wind-heat syndrome (风热证 [fēng rè zhèng]), i.e. syndrome caused by attack of wind and heat in combination

风热邪气 [fēng rè xié qì]

wind-heat pathogen: full name of wind-heat (风热 [fēng rè]) as a pathogenic factor

风火 [fēng huǒ]

wind-fire: wind and fire combined as a pathogenic factor

风湿 [fēng shī]

wind-damp: (1) wind and damp combined as a pathogenic factor, also called pathogenic wind-damp (风湿邪气 [fēng shī xié qì]), which often blocks the collateral meridians, causing general aching, arthralgia and impaired movements; (2) abbreviation of wind-damp syndrome (风湿证 [fēng shī zhèng]), i.e. syndrome caused by attack of wind and damp in combination

风湿邪气 [fēng shī xié qì]

pathogenic wind-damp, see wind-damp (风湿 [fēng shī])

风寒湿 [fēng hán shī]

wind-cold-damp: combined pathogenic factor of wind, cold and dampness, which often causes rheumatic and rheumatoid arthritis, also called pathogenic wind-cold-damp (风寒湿邪 [fēng hán shī xié])

风寒湿邪 [fēng hán shī xié]

pathogenic wind-cold-damp: full name of wind-cold-damp (风寒湿 [fēng hán zhī]) as a pathogenic factor

寒湿 [hán shī]

cold-damp: (1) combined pathogenic factor of cold and damp that often causes muscle and joint pains; (2) abbreviation of cold-damp syndrome (寒湿证 [hán shī zhèng])

湿热 [shī rè]

damp-heat: (1) combined pathogenic factor of damp and heat; (2) abbreviation of damp-heat disease 湿热病 [shī rè bìng] or damp-heat syndrome 湿热证 [shī rè zhèng]

湿火 [shī huǒ]

damp-fire: fire that comes from stagnant damp and impairs spleen and stomach yin

风燥 [fēng zào]

wind-dryness: (1) combined pathogenic factor of wind and dryness, generally prevailing in autumn; (2) abbreviation of wind-dryness syndrome 风燥证 [fēng zào zhèng]

燥热 [zào rè]

dryness-heat: (1) combined pathogenic factor of dryness and heat, also called dryness-fire 燥火 [zào huǒ]; (2) abbreviation of dryness-heat syndrome 燥热证 [zào huǒ zhèng]

燥火 [zào huǒ]

dryness-fire: (1) combined pathogenic factor of dryness and fire; (2) abbreviation of dryness-fire syndrome 燥火证 [zào huǒ zhèng]

毒 [dú]

(1) toxin: a common pathogenic factor in pyogenic inflammations; **(2) poison:** substance that kills or harms an organism

热毒 [rè dú]

heat toxin: toxin derived from retained pathogenic heat

火毒 [huǒ dú]

fire toxin: (1) toxin that originates from stagnation of pathogenic fire or heat, mostly occurring in inflammations of external diseases; (2) toxin that causes infection of burns

湿毒 [shī dú]

damp toxin: toxin that comes from retained damp and causes an intractable lesion with abundant exudation

寒毒 [hán dú]

cold toxin: pathogen of cold-induced diseases

麻毒 [má dú]

measles toxin: the pathogen that causes measles

内毒 [nèi dú]

endogenous toxin: toxin arising inside the body, which may cause a bscess, eruption, bleeding, and even impairment of consciousness

胎毒 [tāi dú]

fetal toxicosis: toxic fire affecting the fetus, which causes a variety of inflammatory or eruptive diseases of the infant after birth

蛊毒 [gǔ dú]

parasitic toxin: the pathogenic factor that causes diseases marked by tympanites and ascites

内伤 [nèi shāng]

internal injury: (1) a general term for the pathogenic factors that impair the internal organs (2) a term designating injury to the deep tissue or internal organs

七情 [qī qíng]

seven emotions: joy, anger, worry, anxiety, sadness, fear and fright, taken as endogenous factors causing diseases if in excess

五志 [wǔ zhì]

five emotions: a collective term for joy, anger, anxiety, grief and fear, which may turn into fire if in excess

喜 [xǐ]

joy: one of the seven emotions that in excess may make the heart *qi* sluggish, resulting in absent-mindedness, and even mental disturbance

怒 [nù]

anger: one of the seven emotions that in excess may cause the liver *qi* to ascend, resulting in headache, flushed face, blood-shot eyes, or hematemesis, and even sudden fainting

忧 [yōu]

(1) worry: one of the seven emotions, which often arises together with anxiety, and in excess may cause injury to the spleen; **(2) grief:** deep sorrow that may injure the lung

思 [sī]

anxiety: one of the seven emotions that in excess may cause stagnation of spleen *qi*, resulting in anorexia, abdominal distension, and loose stool

悲 [bēi]

sadness: one of the seven emotions that in excess may consume lung *qi*, resulting in shortness of breath, listlessness and fatigue

恐 [kǒng]

fear: one of the seven emotions that in excess may cause kidney *qi* to sink, resulting in incontinence of urine and stool, or even syncope

惊 [jīng]

fright: one of the seven emotions that in excess may disturb heart *qi*, resulting in palpitations or spirit confusion

五志过极 [wǔ zhì guò jí]

five emotions in excess: excessive joy, anger, anxiety, grief and fear may disturb the normal flow of *qi* and blood of the internal organs, causing morbid conditions

五志化火 [wǔ zhì huà huǒ]

transformation of the five emotions into fire: Uncontrolled overflow of the five emotions (joy, anger, anxiety, grief and fear) may disturb the natural flow of *qi* and injure genuine yin, giving rise to fire symptoms, such as irritability, insomnia, bitterness in the mouth, chest pain, and hemoptysis.

邪火 [xié huǒ]

evil fire: pathogenic or pathological fire as opposed to physiological fire

郁火 [yù huǒ]

stagnancy-fire: fire derived by stagnancy of yang *qi*

六郁 [liù yù]

six kinds of stagnancy: stagnancy of *qi*, blood, dampness, fire, phlegm (mucus) and food

饮食劳倦 [yǐn shí láo juàn]

improper diet and overstrain: a group of pathogenic factors that cause internal injuries, including dietary irregularities, abnormal degree of fatigue, etc.

饮食不节 [yǐn shí bù jié]

improper diet: diet harmful to health, including ingestion of raw, cold or unclean food, voracious eating or excessive hunger, predilection for a special food, alcohol addiction, etc.

饮食不洁 [yǐn shí bù jié]

unclean food: food contaminated by disease-carrying substances

贪食生冷 [tān shí shēng lěng]

overindulgence in raw and cold food: eating too much cold and uncooked food, which is apt to impair the functions of the spleen and stomach

膏粱厚味 [gān liáng hòu wèi]

rich food: food containing a large amount of fat and spices, which may produce phlegm and heat

五味偏嗜 [wǔ wèi piān shì]

flavor partiality; flavor predilection: habitual preference for a particular flavor or taste that may give rise to disease, e.g., partiality for pungent food that induces oral ulceration, constipation and hemorrhoids

癖嗜 [pǐ shì]

addiction: habitual preference

酒癖 [jiǔ pǐ]

alcohol addiction: alcoholism, in which dependence is present

劳倦 [láo juàn]

overstrain: abnormal degree of fatigue brought about by excessive activity

房事过度 [fáng shì guò dù]

excess of sexual activity: excessive sexual intercourse that consumes kidney essence

房事不节 [fáng shì bù jié]

intemperance in sexual activity, synonymous with excess of sexual activity (房事过度 [fáng shì guò dù])

房劳 [fáng láo]

sexual consumption: exhaustion due to sexual overindulgence

劳复 [láo fù]

relapse due to fatigue: relapse of disease due to over-fatigue

女劳复 [nǚ láo fù]

relapse due to sex: relapse of disease due to intemperance in sexual life

食复 [shí fù]

relapse due to diet: relapse of disease due to improper diet

跌打损伤 [diē dǎ sǔn shāng]

(injury from) knocks and falls

烫火伤 [tàng huǒ shāng]

burns and scalds

虫兽伤 [chóng shòu shāng]

insect or animal bite

癫狗咬伤 [diān gǒu yǎo shāng]

rabid dog bite

瘀血 [yū xuè]

stagnant blood: a pathological product of blood stagnation, including extravasated blood and blood moving sluggishly in circulation or congested in a viscus, all of which may turn into pathogenic factors

痰 [tán]

phlegm: (1) pathologic secretions of diseased respiratory organs, also called "phlegm visible" (有形之痰 [yǒu xíng zhī tán]) since it is visible when expectorated; (2) a pathological product of diseased internal organs, especially the spleen, which, in turn, may cause various troubles, e.g., nausea and vomiting when the stomach is affected, palpitation, impairment of consciousness or even mania when the heart is invaded, and scrofula when accumulating subcutaneously, also known as "phlegm invisible" (无形之痰 [wú xíng zhī tán]) in these cases

有形之痰 [yǒu xíng zhī tán]

visible phlegm: phlegm in the respiratory tract, especially the sputum expectorated

无形之痰 [wú xíng zhī tán]

invisible phlegm: phlegm that exists in the body except the respiratory tract

湿痰 [shī tán]

damp-phlegm: phlegm as a pathogenic factor produced by long-standing retention of dampness due to deficiency of spleen *qi*, which brings on such symptoms as profuse frothy sputum, nausea, fullness in the chest, cough and dyspnea, and plump tongue with slippery or greasy coating, also called phlegm-damp (痰湿 [tán shī])

痰湿 [tán shī]

phlegm-damp, same as 湿痰 [shī tán]

痰浊 [tán zhuó]

phlegm turbidity: a term referring chiefly to stagnated phlegm, particularly phlegm that causes apoplexy, epilepsy or mania

顽痰 [wán tán]

pertinacious phlegm: phlegm existing persistently, serving as the cause of a stubborn illness

饮 [yǐn]

retained fluid: (1) a general term for various types of retained-fluid syndromes; (2) pathogenic factor that causes such syndromes

浊邪 [zhuó xié]

turbid pathogen: pathogenic damp-turbidity

秽浊 [huì zhuó]

filthy turbidity: a common term for various turbid pathogens and filthy *qi*, including miasma

中毒 [zhòng dú]

poisoning: illness caused by a poison

中恶 [zhòng è]

attack of noxious factor: a condition occurring in children, characterized by sudden onset of syncope or mental disorder

水土不服 [shuǐ tǔ bù fú]

non-acclimatization: illness due to temporary unadaptability of a person to the climate of a new dwelling place, with symptoms such as loss of appetite, abdominal distension, diarrhea, menstrual complaints in women, etc.

诸虫 [zhū chóng]

parasitic worms: worms living in the human body, especially in the intestines

瘴气 [zhàng qì]

miasma: noxious mountainous vapor alleged to be the cause of malaria, also known as toxic miasma 瘴毒 [zhàng dú] or mountainous miasma 山岚瘴气 [shān lán zhàng qì]

瘴毒 [zhàng dú]

toxic miasma, same as miasma (瘴气 [zhàng qì])

山岚瘴气 [shān lán zhàng qì]

mountainous miasma, same as miasma (瘴气 [zhàng qì])

先天不足 [xiān tiān bù zú]

congenital defect: imperfection existing before birth

后天失调 [hòu tiān shī tiáo]

lack of proper care after birth

病机 Mechanism of Disease

病机 [bìng jī]

mechanism of disease; pathogenesis: the mechanism of the origination, development and outcome of a disease

病机十九条 [bìng jī shí jiǔ tiáo]

nineteen guiding rules of pathogenesis: the general rules of the origination and development of diseases as summarized in the *Canon of Medicine*

病能 [bìng néng]

state of disease: an ancient term referring comprehensively to clinical manifestations, cause of disease and pathogenesis

正邪相争 [zhèng xié xiāng zhēng]

struggle between normal and pathogenic *qi*: basic pathogenesis in which any disease process is considered as the process of struggle between normal and pathogenic *qi* and the rise and decline of either of them

邪正盛衰 [xié zhèng shèng shuāi]

exuberance and decline of pathogenic or normal *qi*: the key factor that determines the process and prognosis of a patient, namely, rise of normal *qi* with decline of pathogenic *qi* leading to improvement and cure, while exuberance of pathogenic *qi* with decline of normal *qi* results in deterioration and even death

正虚邪实 [zhèng xū xié shí]

insufficiency of the normal and excessiveness of the pathogenic: a pathological condition in which healthy *qi* is undermined while pathogenic factors are prevailing, denoting that the patient is in an unfavorable state with lowered resistance

阳虚阴盛 [yáng xū yīn shèng]

yang insufficiency with yin preponderance: excessive yin resulting from insufficient yang of the spleen and kidney which fails to warm up all other internal organs, usually manifested as intolerance of cold, cold limbs, diarrhea and edema

阴盛阳衰 [yīn shèng yáng shuāi]

yin preponderance with yang insufficiency: decline of yang resulting from endogenous excessive cold, usually manifested as intolerance of cold, cold limbs, and diarrhea

阳盛 [yáng shèng]

yang exuberance: any pathological state characterized by preponderance of yang with excessive functional activity, increased metabolism, enhanced bodily reactivity, and surplus of heat, occurring typically in excess-heat syndromes

阴盛 [yīn shèng]

yin preponderance: any pathological state characterized by preponderance of yin with decreased function, insufficient heat production, and accumulation of disease products, occurring typically in excess-cold syndromes

阴虚阳亢 [yīn xū yáng kàng]

yin deficiency with exuberant yang: Deficiency of vital essence, blood or body fluid may lead to a breakdown of the equilibrium between yin and yang, resulting in exuberance of the latter, with such symptoms as headache, dizziness, malar flush, heat sensation in the chest, palms and soles, afternoon fever, night sweats, hemoptysis, irritability, insomnia, increased libido, or nocturnal emission.

阴虚火旺 [yīn xū huǒ wàng]

yin deficiency with up-flaming fire: exuberance of fire due to deficiency of yin, often causing such symptoms as flushed cheeks, irritability, sore throat or increased libido

阴阳格拒 [yīn yáng gé jù]

repelling of yin or yang: a special form of pathological change in which extremely excessive yin in the interior forces asthenic yang to spread outward or extremely exuberant yang in the interior keeps insufficient yin on the outside, forming pseudo-heat or pseudo-cold phenomena

阳盛格阴 [yáng shèng gé yīn]

exuberant yang repelling yin: a pathological condition in which extremely exuberant yang trapped in the interior keeps insufficient yin in the exterior, usually referring to high fever with pseudo-cold symptoms

格阴 [gé yīn]

repelled yin: an abbreviation of exuberant yang repelling yin (阳盛格阴 [yáng shèng gé yīn])

阴盛格阳 [yīn shèng gé yáng]

excessive yin repelling yang: a pathological condition in which extremely excessive yin entrenched in the exterior forces the asthenic yang to float on the body surface, usually referring to intense endogenous cold with pseudo-heat symptoms

格阳 [gé yáng]

repelled yang: an abbreviation of exuberant yin repelling yang (阴盛格阳 [yīn shèng gé yáng])

阴阳两虚 [yīn yáng liǎng xū]

yin-yang dual deficiency: deficiency of both yin and yang, usually denoting a serious stage of a disease

亡阴 [wáng yīn]

yin collapse: a pathological change caused by a sudden massive loss of fluid leading to collapse

亡阳 [wáng yáng]

yang collapse: a pathological change where yang *qi* is suddenly exhausted, resulting in abrupt failure of bodily functions, usually manifested by dripping sweat, cold clammy skin, and hardly perceptible pulse

脱阴 [tuō yīn]

yin prostration: a prostration state of essence and fluid of the internal organs, especially of the liver and kidney, leading to sudden deterioration of eyesight, usually occurring at the late stage of a febrile disease, malnutrition, or postpartum weakness

脱阳 [tuō yáng]

yang prostration: (1) a prostration state due to excessive consumption of yang with such symptoms as profuse sweating, hallucination, illusion or other psychic disorders; (2) prostration of the male during or after sexual intercourse

虚阳上浮 [xū yáng shàng fú]

upward floating of asthenic yang: one of the pathogenetic mechanisms to explain endogenous cold with superficial pseudo-heat manifestations

孤阳上越 [gū yáng shàng yuè]

upward floating of desolate yang, same as 虚阳上浮 [xū yáng shàng fú]

表气不固 [biǎo qì bù gù]

insecurity of superficial *qi*: lowered superficial resistance, which makes one susceptible to exogenous pathogenic factors, especially cold, and liable to perspire spontaneously

卫气不固 [wèi qì bù gù]

insecurity of defensive *qi*, same as 表气不固 [biǎo qì bù gù]

温邪上受 [wēn xié shàng shòu]

upper attack of warm pathogen: the mechanism of the onset of most acute febrile diseases starting from the upper respiratory tract

温邪犯肺 [wēn xié fàn fèi]

attack of warm pathogen to the lung: the mechanism of the initial stage of an acute febrile disease that the warm pathogen invades the lung and the superficial defensive system, causing fever, cough, sore throat, thirst, and rapid floating pulse

逆传心包 [nì chuán xīn bāo]

adverse transmission to the pericardium: the mechanism of impairment of consciousness or coma occurring soon after the onset of an acute febrile disease, when a warm pathogen is transmitted directly to the pericardium instead of to the *qi* system

阳虚水泛 [yáng xū shuǐ fàn]

water flooding due to yang deficiency: a mechanism of generalized edema, when yang deficiency of the spleen and kidney leads to retention of water in the body

营卫不和 [yíng wèi bù hé]

disharmony between nutrient and defense: the mechanism that explains certain forms of abnormal sweating, particularly spontaneous sweating in an exterior syndrome, as the defense system regulates the excretion of sweat while the nutrient system provides fluid for the formation of sweat

卫弱营强 [wèi ruò yíng qiáng]

weak defense with strong nutrient: the mechanism of spontaneous sweating without fever

卫强营弱 [wèi qiáng yíng ruò]

strong defense with weak nutrient: the mechanism of sweating that occurs only during fever

卫气同病 [wèi qì tóng bìng]

dual disease of defense and *qi*: pathological change that causes high fever, thirst and irritability together with intolerance of cold and wind, and general pains in the case of an acute febrile disease

卫营同病 [wèi yíng tóng bìng]

dual disease of defense and nutrient: pathological change that causes high fever and delirium together with chills, headache and general aching in the case of an acute febrile disease

气营两燔 [qì yíng liǎng fān]

blazing of both *qi* and nutrient: intense heat in both *qi* and nutrient systems that causes high fever, thirst, mental irritability, delirium and barely visible skin eruption in the case of an acute febrile disease

气血两燔 [qì xuè liǎng fān]

blazing of both *qi* and blood: intense heat in both the *qi* and blood systems that causes high fever, delirium, hemoptysis, epistaxis, skin eruptions, and even convulsions in the case of an acute febrile disease

热邪阻肺 [rè xié zǔ fèi]

heat pathogen obstructing the lung: a pathological change that causes fever, cough, thick, yellowish or blood-stained sputum, dyspnea, chest pain, reddened tip of the tongue with dry yellow coating, and full and rapid pulse

热迫大肠 [rè pò dà cháng]

heat compelling the large intestine: a pathological change that causes acute diarrhea with abdominal pain, burning sensation in the anus, scanty dark urine, and dry yellow tongue coating

热入心包 [rè rù xīn bāo]

heat into the pericardium: a pathological change that causes high fever with delirium or even coma in the case of an acute febrile disease

热入血分 [rè rù xuè fèn]

heat into the blood system: a pathological change that causes fever, restlessness, delirium, skin eruption and bleeding (hematemesis, epistaxis or hematochezia) in the late and severest stage of an acute febrile disease

血分热毒 [xuè fèn rè dú]

heat toxin in the blood system: (1) penetration of heat into the blood system in the case of an epidemic febrile disease, causing high fever, delirium, skin eruption, or hematuria; (2) common mechanism of acute pyogenic infections marked by recurrent local inflammation or boil formation

热入血室 [rè rù xuè shì]

heat into the blood chamber: a pathological change with penetration of heat into the uterus, usually causing abdominal pain, menstrual disturbances, alternate fever and chills, and delirium at night

热邪内结 [rè xié nèi jié]

heat pathogen accumulating in the interior: a general term referring to accumulation of heat pathogen in internal organs

热结下焦 [rè jié xià jiāo]

heat accumulating in the lower energizer: accumulation of heat in the intestines and bladder that causes lower abdominal distention and pain, constipation, dark urine or even hematuria, and sometimes tenderness in the lower abdomen accompanied by restlessness

热盛伤津 [rè shèng shāng jīn]

exuberant heat consuming fluid: consumption of body fluid by excess of heat, causing fluid consumption syndrome

热灼肾阴 [rè zhuó shèn yīn]

heat scorching kidney yin: a pathological change with consumption of kidney yin by heat, that causes low fever, heat sensation in palms and soles, dry mouth, impairment of hearing, dry and deep red tongue without coating, and thready and rapid pulse, occurring at the later stage of an acute febrile disease

热伤筋脉 [rè shāng jīn mài]

heat damaging muscles and tendons: a pathological change that leads to cramps, flaccidity or paralysis of limbs in cases of high fever or prolonged fever

瘀热 [yū rè]

stagnant heat: (1) heat and phlegm dampness accumulating in the interior of the body which causes fever; (2) heat produced by stagnated blood

伏热 [fú rè]

insidious heat: pathological change occurring in the case of a febrile disease with the heat pathogen hidden deeply in the interior

伏热在里 [fú rè zài lǐ]

insidious heat in the interior: a pathological change that usually causes dry throat, foul breath, reddened tongue, constipation and scanty dark urine

血分瘀热 [xuè fèn yū rè]

stagnant heat in blood system: (1) heat accumulated in the blood system with deep penetration into internal organs including the heart, liver and kidney; (2) heat produced by stagnated blood

热极生风 [rè jí shēng fēng]

extreme heat producing wind: pathological mechanism referring to the occurrence of convulsions and opisthotonus in a case of high fever

热盛风动 [rè shèng fēng dòng]

exuberant heat stirring up wind, same as 热极生风 [rè jí shēng fēng]

血虚生风 [xuè xū shēng fēng]

blood deficiency producing wind: pathological mechanism referring to dizziness, twitching or tremor resulting from persistent anemia or profuse bleeding

风湿相搏 [fēng shī xiāng bó]

conjoint invasion of wind and damp: a pathological change resulting in muscle aches and joint pain, usually occurring in wind-damp affection

风火相煽 [fēng huǒ xiāng shān]

mutual stirring-up of wind and fire: a pathological change that causes hyperexia and convulsions in the most advanced stage of an acute febrile disease

湿郁肌表 [shī yù jī biǎo]

damp stagnating in superficies: stagnation of damp in the superficial portion of the body, usually impeding the circulation of *qi* and blood and causing a sensation of heaviness and aching of the limbs

湿蔽清阳 [shī bì qīng yáng]

damp shading the head: a pathological change that causes dizziness and heaviness sensation as if the head were bound tight

湿邪困脾 [shī xié kùn pí]

damp pathogen disturbing the spleen: a pathological change that results in anorexia, epigastric distension, lassitude and heaviness of the limbs

湿郁化热 [shī yù huà rè]

stagnant damp transforming into heat: a pathological change that causes heat symptoms together with damp syndrome

湿热内蕴 [shī rè nèi yùn]

damp-heat accumulating in the interior: a general term for the accumulation of damp-heat in the internal organs, especially in the stomach, spleen, liver and gallbladder, causing persistent fever, heaviness of the body, lassitude, loss of appetite, abdominal distension or jaundice

湿热下注 [shī rè xià zhù]

damp-heat pouring downward: a pathological change that causes mucous and bloody discharge with dysentery stool, turbid urine in urinary infections, morbid leukorrhea in pelvic infections, etc.

湿毒流注 [shī dú liú zhù]

spilling of damp-toxin: a pathological change characterized by flow of damp-toxin into muscles and skin, causing ulcers or festering sores on the shanks

燥伤肺气 [zào shāng fèi qì]

dryness damaging lung *qi*: a pathological change that may lead to dry cough, hemoptysis, diabetes mellitus, and even flaccidity of limbs due to inadequate distribution of body fluid to the muscles and tendons

燥伤津液 [zào shāng jīn yè]

dryness damaging body fluid: a pathological change that may result in upward adverse flow of stomach *qi* when the stomach is involved, constipation when the intestinal fluid is impaired, and diabetes when kidney fluid is consumed

津枯肠燥 [jīn kū cháng zào]

fluid consumption with intestinal dryness: one of the mechanisms for constipation

燥气寒化 [zào qì hán huà]

dryness *qi* transforming into cold: a pathological process often occurring in patients with a yang-insufficient or yin-exuberant constitution

燥气化热 [zào qì huà rè]

dryness *qi* transforming into heat: a pathological process often occurring in patients with a yin-insufficient or yang-exuberant constitution

虚火上炎 [xū huǒ shàng yán]

flaring up of asthenic fire: a pathological change occurring in kidney yin deficiency, causing dry and sore throat, dizziness, restlessness, red eyes or oral ulcers

火伤血络 [huǒ shāng xuè luò]

fire damaging blood vessels: a pathological change that causes hemoptysis, hematemesis, and epistaxis

寒热错杂 [hán rè cuò zá]

interlocking of cold and heat: a pathological change that causes complicated heat and cold conditions such as heat in the upper part with cold in the lower part of the body or cold in the exterior and heat in the interior of the body

寒邪外束 [hán xié wài shù]

cold pathogen fettering the exterior: a pathological process that causes chills, general aching, headache, absence of sweating, and floating tense pulse

寒从中生 [hán cóng zhōng shēng]

generation of cold from the interior: a pathological process where an interior-cold syndrome results from yang deficiency of an internal organ

化热 [huà rè]

transformation into heat: transformation of pathogenic factors such as wind, cold or dryness into heat, resulting in intolerance of heat, thirst, irritability, reddened tongue with yellow fur, and rapid pulse

化火 [huà huǒ]

transformation into fire: transformation of intense heat into fire, producing such symptoms as persistent thirst, blood-shot eyes, flushed face, parched lips, dry and sore throat, hemoptysis, epistaxis, hematuria, and even impairment of consciousness or raving madness

胃热化火 [wèi rè huà huǒ]

transformation of stomach-heat into fire: a pathological change that usually causes ulceration of the mouth in addition to the symptoms of stomach heat

化风 [huà fēng]

transformation into wind: occurrence of wind symptoms such as dizziness, convulsions or tremors in the course of a febrile disease

化燥 [huà zào]

transformation into dryness: a pathological process in which pathogenic heat or loss of blood gives rise to impairment of body fluid, manifested by thirst, dry throat and lips, constipation and dry cough

气机失调 [qì jī shī tiáo]

disorder of *qi* movement: a general term for disordered activity of *qi* in ascending, descending, exiting and entering that may cause various pathological changes such as stagnation of *qi*, reversed flow of *qi*, sinking of *qi*, blockage of *qi*, and collapse of *qi*

气机不利 [qì jī bù lì]

disturbance of *qi* movement: a general term for disorder of *qi*, referring to dysfunction of the internal organs at large, especially functional derangement in sending things up or down, as manifested by hiccups, stuffy feeling in the chest, abdominal distension, or diarrhea

气机郁滞 [qì jī yù zhì]

depression and stagnation of *qi* movement: depressed and stagnant flow of *qi* occurring in a certain part of the body or in an internal organ, which usually causes local distention and pain and may lead to further pathological changes such as blood stasis or formation of phlegm and retained fluid

气郁 [qì yù]

***qi* depression:** an abbreviation of depression and stagnation of *qi* movement (气机郁滞 [qì jī yù zhì])

气郁化火 [qì yù huà huǒ]

transformation of depressed *qi* into fire: a pathological change of long-standing depression of *qi* that transforms into fire and leads to such symptoms as emotional depression, irritability, irascibility, distention and burning pain in the chest, and reddened tongue with yellow coating

气化不利 [qì huà bù lì]

disturbance of *qi* transformation: a general term for dysfunction of internal organs, particularly referring to that of the triple energizer in water metabolism

气逆 [qì nì]

reversed flow of *qi*: dysfunction of *qi* in descending that leads to upward disturbance of *qi* with such manifestations as cough, asthma, hiccups, belching, nausea, vomiting and regurgitation

气陷 [qì xiàn]

sinking of *qi*: a pathological change of *qi* marked by failure in its lifting or holding function, often leading to visceroptosis

升降失常 [shēng jiàng shī tiáo]

disturbance in ascending and descending: a general term referring to disturbance of ascending and descending movement of visceral *qi*, e.g., dysfunction of the spleen in sending up food essence and water, which causes diarrhea and abdominal distention, and dysfunction of the stomach in sending down food contents, giving rise to nausea, vomiting, and regurgitation

下陷 [xià xiàn]

sinking: another expression for sinking of *qi*, usually due to deficiency of spleen *qi*, resulting in prolapse of visceral organs (cf. 中气下陷 [zhōng qì xià xiàn])

内陷 [nèi xiàn]

penetration: a term referring to penetration of pathogenic factors into the interior of the body

肝气不和 [gān qì bù hé]

disharmony of liver *qi*: a pathological change of the liver in its smoothing and discharging function, causing irritability, hypochondriac, mammary or lower abdominal distention and pain, and irregular menstruation

肝气不舒 [gān qì bù shū]

constraining of liver *qi*: a pathological change that causes functional disturbance of the liver, manifested by irritability, irascibility, stuffy feeling in the chest, hypochondriac and lower abdominal distension and pain, and in women distending pain of the breast and menstrual complaints

肝气横逆 [gān qì héng nì]

transverse drive of liver *qi*: a pathological change in which hyperactive liver *qi* runs transversely, impairing the spleen and stomach

肝气犯胃 [gān qì fàn wèi]

liver *qi* invading the stomach: a pathological change in which the hyperactive *qi* running transversely impairs the stomach function and results in epigastric distention and pain, frequent sighing, belching, acid regurgitation, or nausea and vomiting

肝气犯脾 [gān qì fàn pí]

liver *qi* invading the spleen: a pathological change in which hyperactive *qi* running transversely impairs the spleen function and results in hypochondriac, epigastric and abdominal distention and pain, anorexia and diarrhea

肝气上逆 [gān qì shàng nì]

upward drive of liver *qi*: a pathological change in which the hyperactive liver *qi* running upward, attacks the upper portion of the body, and causes dizziness, headache, tinnitus, deafness, pain and distension of the chest and hypochondrium, and even hematemesis

肝阳化火 [gān yáng huà huǒ]

transformation of liver yang into fire: a pathological change in which hyperactive liver yang is transformed into fire, and causes such symptoms as dizziness, flushing of the face, bitterness in the mouth, irritability and irascibility

心气不足 [xīn qì bù zú]

insufficiency of heart *qi*, same as heart *qi* deficiency (心气虚 [xīn qì xū])

心气不宁 [xīn qì bù níng]

unsteadiness of heart *qi*: a pathological change of heart *qi* marked by uneasiness, palpitation, susceptibility to fright, vexation, and insomnia

心气不固 [xīn qì bù gù]

insecurity of heart *qi*: a pathological change of heart *qi* marked by floating of the mind, susceptibility to fright, forgetfulness, spontaneous sweating, or sweating upon mild exertion

心气不收 [xīn qì bù shōu]

dispersion of heart *qi*, same as 心气不固 ([xīn qì bù gù])

心血不足 [xīn qì bù zú]

insufficiency of heart blood: a pathological change of the heart that causes abstraction, insomnia, dream-disturbed sleep, palpitation, and thready weak pulse, also called heart blood deficiency (心血虚 [xīn xuè xū])

心血瘀阻 [xīn xuè yū zhǔ]

stasis of heart blood: a pathological change of the heart in which the blood flow in the heart vessels is impeded, causing a feeling of suffocation and precordial pain

心阴不足 [xīn yīn bù zú]

insufficiency of heart yin: a pathological change of the heart in which deficiency of yin fails to check yang and results in relative preponderance of heart yang with such manifestations as mental unsteadiness, insomnia, night sweats, and feverish sensation in the palms of the hands and soles of the feet, also called heart yin deficiency (心阴虚 [xīn yīn xū])

心阳不足 [xīn yáng bù zú]

insufficiency of heart yang: a pathological change referring to diminution of the heart function in controlling blood and vessels and in governing the mental activities associated with deficiency of yang *qi* that causes cold manifestations, also called heart yang deficiency (心阳虚 [xīn yáng xū])

心营过耗 [xīn yíng guò hào]

over-consumption of heart nutrient: a pathological change in which the nutrient in the heart blood is excessively consumed by heat, causing emaciation, night fever, and vexation

热伤神明 [rè shāng shén míng]

heat damaging the mind: a pathological change marked by damage to the mental activity by heat, same as heat into the pericardium (热入心包 [rè rù xīn bāo])

痰蒙心包 [tán méng xīn bāo]

phlegm clouding the pericardium: a pathological change marked by mental confusion caused by phlegm

痰迷心窍 [tán mí xīn qiào]

phlegm misting the heart: a pathological change of the heart that causes mental derangement or even coma accompanied by phlegmatic sounds in the throat

心神失养 [xīn shén shī yǎng]

impaired nourishment of the heart: a pathological change that may lead to palpitation, dysphoria, insomnia and amnesia

神不守舍 [shén bù shǒu shě]

mind failing to keep to its abode: a pathological change that may result in insomnia and mental derangement

心火亢盛 [xīn huǒ kàng shèng]

exuberance of heart fire: a pathological change that may cause insomnia, dysphoria, or even impairment of consciousness and delirium

心火上炎 [xīn huǒ shàng yán]

flaring-up of heart fire: a pathological change in which fire flares upward along the heart meridian, causing oral or lingual erosion

心火内炽 [xīn huǒ nèi chì]

internal flaming of heart fire: a pathological change in which intense heat disturbs the mental activity, causing vexation, insomnia, throbbing palpitation, restlessness, or even mania

心火内焚 [xīn huǒ nèi fén]

internal deflagration of heart fire, same as 心火内炽 [xīn huǒ nèi chì]

痰火扰心 [tán huǒ rǎo xīn]

phlegm-fire agitating the heart: agitation of the heart by phlegm-fire that causes mental derangement or mania

心移热于小肠 [xīn yí rè yú xiǎo cháng]

shifting of heart fire to the small intestine: a pathological change characterized by transmission of pathological fire of the heart to the small intestine, resulting in ardor urinae, urodynia, hematuria, etc.

脾不运化 [pí bù yùn huà]

spleen failing to transport and transform: dysfunction of the spleen in transporting and transforming nutrients and water, resulting in dyspepsia, diarrhea, emaciation, lassitude and even edema of the limbs, also known as 脾不健运 [pí bù jiàn yùn]

脾不健运 [pí bù jiàn yùn]

dysfunction of the spleen in transportation, same as 脾不运化 [pí bù yùn huà]

脾失健运 [pí shī jiàn yùn]

failure of the spleen in transportation, same as 脾不健运 [pí bù jiàn yùn]

脾不统血 [pí bù tǒng xuè]

spleen failing to control blood: a pathological change of the spleen that usually results in chronic hemorrhage

脾气不升 [pí qì bù shēng]

spleen *qi* failing to ascend: dysfunction of the spleen in sending up nutrients, usually due to spleen *qi* deficiency, retention of dampness or stagnation of food

胃气不和 [wèi qì bù hé]

stomach *qi* disharmony: general term referring to various functional disorders of the stomach, called also stomach disharmony (胃不和 [wèi bù hé])

胃不和 [wèi bù hé]

stomach disharmony: same as stomach *qi* disharmony (胃气不和 [wèi qì bù hé])

胃气不降 [wèi qì bù jiàng]

stomach *qi* failing to descend: dysfunction of the stomach in sending down its contents, causing such symptoms as anorexia, nausea, vomiting, belching, and stuffiness over the epigastric region

胃失和降 [wèi shī hé jiàng]

stomach failing to send downward harmoniously, same as 胃气不降 [wèi qì bù jiàng]

胃气上逆 [wèi qì shàng nì]

upward reversal of stomach *qi*: a pathological change of the stomach function that causes belching, hiccups, regurgitation, and vomiting

中气不足 [zhōng qì bù zú]

insufficiency of middle *qi*: deficiency of *qi* in the middle energizer, leading to general weakness and diminished transporting and transforming function of the spleen and stomach

中阳不振 [zhōng yáng bù zhèn]

devitalized yang in the middle: weakened yang in the middle energizer (the spleen and stomach), resulting in dyspepsia, vomiting, diarrhea, cold limbs, and sallow face, often seen in cases of chronic dyspepsia and chronic dysentery

肺气不利 [fèi qì bù lì]

dysfunction of lung *qi*: disturbance of the functional activities of the lung, especially referring to its function in maintaining water metabolism, giving rise to oliguria and edema together with respiratory symptoms

肺气不宣 [fèi qì bù xuān]

obstruction of lung *qi*: impediment of the functional activities of the lung, usually leading to nasal obstruction, sneezing and cough

肺津不布 [fèi jīn bù bù]

lung failing to distribute fluid: failure of the lung to distribute essence and fluid, leading to production of sputum and causing cough and asthma

肺失清肃 [fèi shī qīng sù]

failure of lung in purifying: one of the common mechanisms of lung diseases that gives rise to cough, dyspnea, expectoration of sputum, fullness in the chest, etc.

肺气上逆 [fèi qì shàng nì]

upward reversal of lung *qi*: one of the common mechanisms of lung diseases that causes cough, dyspnea and asthma

痰浊阻肺 [tán zhuó zǔ fèi]

phlegm-turbidity obstructing the lung: a pathological change that impairs the lung's functional activities, causing cough with profuse expectoration or dyspnea with full sensation in the chest associated with white greasy tongue coating and slippery pulse

风寒束肺 [fēng hán shù fèi]

wind-cold fettering the lung: a pathological change often occurring in colds and at the initial stage of acute febrile diseases in which wind-cold attacks the superficies of the body as well as the lung, causing such symptoms as congested nose with sneezing and watery discharge, headache, aversion to cold, mild fever, and floating pulse

热伤肺络 [rè shāng fèi luò]

injury to the lung vessels by heat: a pathological change characterized by pathogenic heat that injures the lung vessels and causes bloody sputum or hemoptysis

大肠传导失职 [dà cháng chuán dǎo shī zhí]

dysfunction of the large intestine in transmission: a pathological change that may cause diarrhea or constipation

大肠实热 [dà cháng shí rè]

excess-heat of the large intestine: a pathological change of the large intestine meridian in which excessive heat in the meridian causes fever, flushed face, cough, dyspnea, and fullness in the abdomen

肾精不足 [shèn jīng bù zú]

insufficiency of kidney essence: a pathological change of the kidney due to congenital weakness, old age, and malnutrition or after protracted illness, causing retarded growth and development in children, delayed sexual development in adolescents, and hypogonadism and impotence in adults, as well as impaired mentality, weak legs and slow reflexes

封藏失职 [fēng cáng shī zhí]

dysfunction in essence-storing: failure of the kidney to install essence and control urination and defecation, causing spermatorrhea, premature ejaculation, incontinence of urine, frequent urination at night, and diarrhea before dawn

相火妄动 [xiāng huǒ wàng dòng]

frenetic stirring of ministerial fire: hyperactivity of ministerial fire of the liver and kidney, usually due to deficiency of yin and resulting in dizziness, headache, tinnitus and irritability if the liver is chiefly involved, and feverish feeling in the chest, palms of the hands and soles of the feet, aching in the loins, and hyperaphrodisia if the kidney is chiefly involved

命门火衰 [mìng mén huǒ shuāi]

decline of the fire of life gate, synonymous with decline of kidney yang (肾阳虚衰 [shèn yáng xū shuāi])

肾阳虚衰 [shèn yáng xū shuāi])

decline of kidney yang: a pathological change of the kidney that causes chronic diarrhea, especially diarrhea daily before dawn, chills in the back, edema of the legs, lowered sexual ability, and frequent micturition at night

膀胱不利 [páng guāng bù lì]

dysfunction of the bladder: disordered function of the bladder in storing and discharging urine that may cause frequency and urgency of urination, dribbling of urine, anuria or enuresis and incontinence of urine

膀胱气闭 [páng guāng qì bì]

blockage of bladder *qi*: a pathological change of the urinary bladder that often caused dysuria

气化不利 [qì huà bù lì]

disturbance in *qi* activity: (1) in a broad sense, denoting metabolic disorders of all sorts of vital essence and energy; (2) in a narrow sense, denoting disturbance in urine excretion due to dysfunction of the kidney and the urinary bladder – one of the causes of edema and difficulty in urination

气化无权 [qì huà wú quán]

inability of *qi* activity, same as 气化不利 [qì huà bù lì]

寒凝气滞 [hán níng qì zhì]

congealing cold and stagnating *qi*: *qi* stagnation caused by cold with a congealing effect which impedes the flow of *qi*, often manifested clinically by spasms and pains

气滞血瘀 [qì zhì xuè yū]

(1) *qi* stagnation and blood stasis: coexistence of the two pathological states which exert an influence on each other, as stagnant *qi* makes the blood flow sluggish while stagnant blood impedes the flow of *qi*;

(2) **blood stasis due to *qi* stagnation:** a pathological change in which a long-standing or severe stagnation of *qi* leads to blood stasis, often manifested, e.g., by aggravation of local pain originally caused by *qi* stagnation, and change of the distending and scurrying character of the pain into a stabbing and fixed one with tenderness, or even accompanied by mass formation

气虚不摄 [qì xū bù shè]

insufficient *qi* failing to control blood: a pathological change of *qi* deficiency in which *qi* is unable to keep the blood flowing within the vessels, thus resulting in bleeding

气虚血瘀 [qì xū xuè yū]

(1) *qi* deficiency and blood stasis: coexistence of *qi* deficiency and blood stasis; **(2) blood stasis due to *qi* deficiency:** a pathological change of *qi* deficiency in which *qi* is insufficient to drive the blood flow, thus forming blood stasis

气虚中满 [qì xū zhōng mǎn]

***qi* deficiency with abdominal distention:** a pathological change of *qi* deficiency in which *qi* is insufficient for normal transportation in the middle energizer, thus causing abdominal distension

气血失调 [qì xuè shī tiáo]

disharmony of *qi* and blood: mechanism of disease marked by a lack of normal coordination between *qi* and blood, e.g., *qi* in insufficiency leading to blood stasis instead of promoting blood flow

血脱气脱 [xuè tuō qì tuō]

prostration of blood with (*qi*) collapse: a pathological change in which massive loss of blood leads to collapse, marked by pale complexion, cold extremities, profuse sweating, thready and barely perceptible pulse, called also 气随血脱 [qì suí xuè tuō]

气随血脱 [qì suí xuè tuō]

***qi* collapse following blood prostration,** same as 血脱气脱[xuè tuō qì tuō]

血随气陷 [xuè suí qì xiàn]

bleeding following sinking of *qi*: a pathological change that incessant bleeding such as uterine bleeding or bleeding per rectum occurs following sinking of *qi*

血不归经 [xuè bù guī jīng]

escape of blood from vessels: basic mechanism of various hemorrhages

血不循经 [xuè bù xún jīng]

blood failing to circulate in vessels, same as 血不归经 [xuè bù guī jīng]

血热妄行 [xuè rè wàng xíng]

frenetic movement of blood due to heat: one of the mechanisms of bleeding

冲任损伤 [chōng rèn sǔn shāng]

damage to the thoroughfare and conception vessels: a pathological change in cases of gynecological diseases, usually caused by infection, intemperance in sexual life or frequent pregnancy, resulting in dysmenorrhea, pain in the lower abdomen and loins, uterine bleeding, or abortion

冲任不固 [chōng rèn bù gù]

insecurity of the thoroughfare and conception vessels: a pathological change in cases of gynecological diseases, usually causing uterine bleeding or abortion

经隧失职 [jīng suí shī zhí]

dysfunction of meridians: a pathological change of meridians that causes impeded circulation of *qi* and blood

经气逆乱 [jīng qì nì luàn]

disturbance of meridian *qi*: a pathological change of meridians in which the adverse flow of meridian *qi* leads to disordered circulation of *qi* and blood

常用引文 Commonly Used Citations

风善行而数变。 [fēng shàn xíng ér shuò biàn]

Wind moves swiftly and is changeable.

风胜则动。 [fēng shèng zé dòng]

When wind prevails, involuntary movements occur.

风为百病之长。 [fēng wéi bǎi bìng zhī zhǎng]

Wind is the chief of many diseases.

寒为阴邪，易伤阳气。 [hán wéi yīn xié, yì shāng yáng qì]

Cold, as a yin pathogen, is likely to damage yang *qi*.

寒性凝滞。 [hán xìng níng zhì]

Cold is congealing and tends to cause stagnation.

寒性收引。 [hán xìng shōu yǐn]

Cold is characterized by contraction.

湿性重着。 [shī xìng zhòng zhuó]

Dampness is characterized by heaviness and stickiness.

湿性粘滞。 [shī xìng nián zhì]

Dampness is viscous and tends to stagnate.

湿胜则阳微。 [shī shèng zé yáng wēi]

When dampness prevails, yang is debilitated.

湿胜则濡泻。 [shī shèng zé rú xiè]

When dampness prevails, diarrhea occurs.

燥胜则干。 [zào shèng zé gān]

When dryness prevails, desiccation occurs.

火性炎上。 [huǒ xìng yán shàng]

Fire is characterized by flaring up.

气有余便是火。 [qì yǒu yú biàn shì huǒ]

***Qi* in excess will turn into fire.**

喜伤心。 [xǐ shāng xīn]

(Excessive) joy injures the heart.

喜则气缓。 [xǐ zé qì huǎn]

Joy makes (heart) *qi* relax.

怒伤肝。 [nù shāng gān]

Anger injures the liver.

怒则气上。 [nù zé qì shàng]

Anger makes (liver) *qi* rise.

忧伤肺。 [yōu shāng fèi]

Worry injures the lung.

忧则气郁。 [yōu zé qì yù]

Worry makes *qi* stagnate.

悲则气消。 [bēi zé qì xiāo]

Sadness makes (lung) *qi* disperse.

思伤脾。 [sī shāng pí]

Anxiety injures the spleen.

思则气结。 [sī zé qì jié]

Anxiety makes (spleen) *qi* stagnate.

恐伤肾。 [kǒng shāng shèn]

Fear injures the kidney.

恐则气下。 [kǒng zé qì xià]

Fear makes (kidney) *qi* descend.

惊则气乱。 [jīng zé qì luàn]

Fright makes *qi* disturbed.

寒则气收。 [hán zé qì shōu]

Cold makes *qi* compact.

炅则气泄。 [jiǒng zé qì xiè]

Heat makes *qi* dispersed.

劳则气耗。 [láo zé qì hào]

Strain makes *qi* consumed.

诸风掉眩，皆属于肝。 [zhū fēng diào xuán, jiē shǔ yú gān]

All wind with vertigo and shaking is ascribed to the liver.

诸寒收引，皆属于肾。 [zhū hán shōu yǐn, jiē shǔ yú shèn]

All cold with contraction is ascribed to the kidney.

诸气膹郁，皆属于肺。 [zhū qì fèn yù, jiē shǔ yú fèi]

All *qi* rushing and oppression is ascribed to the lung.

诸湿肿满，皆属于脾。 [zhū shī zhǒng mǎn, jiē shǔ yú pí]

All dampness with swelling and fullness is ascribed to the spleen.

诸热瞀瘛，皆属于火。 [zhū rè mào chì, jiē shǔ yú huǒ]

All fever with impaired consciousness and convulsion is ascribed to fire.

诸痛痒疮，皆属于心。 [zhū tòng yǎng chuāng, jiē shǔ yú xīn]

All painful and itching sores are ascribed to the heart.

诸厥固泄，皆属于下。 [zhū jué gù xiè, jiē shǔ yú xià]

All cold extremities, constipation and diarrhea are ascribed to the lower part.

诸痿喘呕，皆属于上。 [zhū wěi chuǎn ǒu, jiē shǔ yú shàng]

All atrophy, dyspnea and vomiting are ascribed to the upper part.

诸禁鼓栗，如丧神守，皆属于火。 [zhū jìn gǔ lì, rú sàng shén shǒu, jiē shǔ yú huǒ]

All trismus with shivering chills and delirium is ascribed to fire.

诸痉项强，皆属于湿。 [zhū jìng xiàng jiàng, jiē shǔ yú shī]

All spasms and neck rigidity are ascribed to dampness.

诸逆冲上，皆属于火。 [zhū nì chōng shàng, jiē shǔ yú huǒ]

All disorders with upward perversion are ascribed to fire.

诸胀腹大，皆属于热。 [zhū zhàng fù dà, jiē shǔ yú rè]

All abdominal distension and fullness is ascribed to heat.

诸躁狂越，皆属于火。 [zhū zào kuáng yuè, jiē shǔ yú huǒ]

All states of agitation and mania are ascribed to fire.

诸暴强直，皆属于风。 [zhū bào jiāng zhí, jiē shǔ yú fēng]

All sudden muscular spasm and rigidity is ascribed to wind.

诸病有声，鼓之如鼓，皆属于热。 [zhū bìng yǒu shēng, gǔ zhī rú gǔ, jiē shǔ yú rè]

All abdominal distension like a drum with borborygmi is ascribed to heat.

诸病胕肿，疼酸惊骇，皆属于火。 [zhū bìng fù zhǒng, téng suān jīng hài, jiē shǔ yú huǒ]

All illnesses with swelling and aching of the instep and mental strain are ascribed to fire.

诸转反戾，水液混浊，皆属于热。 [zhū zhuǎn fǎn lì, shuǐ yè hún zhuó, jiē shǔ yú rè]

All cramps, rigidity, and turbid urine are ascribed to heat.

诸病水液，澄澈清冷，皆属于寒。 [zhū bìng shuǐ yè, chéng chè qīng lěng, jiē shǔ yú hàn]

All thin, clear and watery discharge is ascribed to cold.

诸呕吐酸，暴注下迫，皆属于热。 [zhū ǒu tù suān, bào zhù xià pò, jiē shǔ yú rè]

All acid eructation and spouting diarrhea with urgency for evacuation are ascribed to heat.

邪气盛则实。 [xié qì shèng zé shí]

Excess syndromes occur when the pathogenic factors are in abundance.

精气夺则虚。 [jīng qì duó zé xū]

Deficiency syndromes occur when the patient's essential *qi* is severely damaged.

阴盛则寒。 [yīn shèng zé hán]

Preponderance of yin gives rise to cold syndrome.

阳盛则热。 [yáng shèng zé rè]

Exuberance of yang gives rise to heat syndrome.

阳虚则外寒。 [yáng xū zé wài hán]

Deficiency of yang brings on external cold.

阴虚则内热。 [yīn xū zé nèi rè]

Deficiency of yin brings on internal heat.

气虚则寒。 [qì xū zé hán]

Deficiency of *qi* brings on cold.

热盛则肿。 [rè shèng zé zhǒng]

Exuberant heat brings on swelling.

久热伤阴。 [jiǔ rè shāng yīn]

Longstanding heat injures yin.

风盛则动。 [fēng shèng zé dòng]

Fierce wind produces involuntary movement.

寒极生热。 [hán jí shēng rè]

Extreme cold leads to heat.

热极生寒。 [rè jí shēng hán]

Extreme heat leads to cold.

壮火食气。 [zhuàng huǒ shí qì]

Vigorous fire consumes *qi*.

诊断学 DIAGNOSTICS

诊断学 [zhěn duàn xué]

diagnostics: the science and practice of diagnosis

诊断 [zhěn duàn]

diagnosis: determination of the nature of a disease and the state of health of the patient based on information collected through inspection, inquiry and examination

诊病 [zhěn bìng]

disease identification: determination of the category of a disease, also called disease differentiation (辨病 [biàn bìng])

辨病 [biàn bìng]

disease differentiation: act of distinguishing one category of disease from others, synonymous with disease identification (诊病 [zhěn bìng])

辨证 [biàn zhèng]

syndrome differentiation; pattern identification: determination of the location, cause and nature of a disease as well as the trend of its development at a certain period of a case in the light of traditional Chinese medical theories

证型 [zhèng xíng]

syndrome pattern: one of the commonly encountered and typical syndromes with a well-established name

证候 [zhèng hòu]

syndrome manifestation: manifestation of a syndrome, including symptoms and signs

诊法 Diagnostic Methods

诊法 [zhěn fǎ]

diagnostic method: method of examining a patient and collecting information for diagnosis

四诊 [sì zhěn]

four examinations: inspection, auscultation-olfaction, interrogation (history taking), and palpation (including pulse taking)

望诊 [wàng zhěn]

inspection: examination by using the eyes, including inspection of vitality, complexion, expression, behavior, body surface, tongue, excreta, secretions, etc.

望神 [wàng shén]

inspection of vitality: inspection of the state and power of living, especially the general condition of mental and physical activities such as consciousness, thinking, facial expression, speech, and response to external stimuli

得神 [dé shén]

presence of vitality, one's general state marked by fullness of vigor, with lustrous eyes, resonant voice, radiant face, easy breathing, and quick movements

少神 [shào shén]

lack of vitality: one's general state marked by listlessness, with dull eyes, reluctance to talk, and slow movements, also called insufficiency of vital *qi* (神气不足 [shén qì bù zú])

神气不足 [shén qì bù zú]

insufficiency of vital *qi*: a synonym for lack of vitality (少神 [shào shén])

失神 [shī shén]

loss of vitality: one's general state marked by apathy and inertness, with dim eyes, incoherent speech, difficulty in movement, and even impaired consciousness

假神 [jiǎ shén]

false vitality: transient spiritedness in a critical case, often indicating impending death with manifestation of divorced yang

回光反照 [huí guāng fǎn zhào]

flash of lucidity of the dying: momentary recovery of consciousness just before death

神昏 [shén hūn]

clouding of consciousness: a form of mental state with impairment of the cognitive function and reduced awareness of the environment

神志不清 [shén zhì bù qīng]

disordered consciousness: a synonym for clouding of consciousness (神

昏 [shén hūn])

不省人事 [bù xǐng rén shì]

loss of consciousness: a state of unconsciousness from which the patient cannot be aroused

循衣摸床 [xún yī mō chuáng]

floccillation: aimless semiconscious fumbling and picking at the bedclothes by a critically ill patient

神乱 [shén luàn]

mental disturbance: derangement of the mind and abnormal mentality

谵妄 [zhān wàng]

delirium: disturbance of consciousness characterized by confusion, disordered speech, and hallucination

躁狂 [zào kuáng]

mania: type of mental disorder characterized by expansiveness, elation, agitation, hyperactivity and hyperexcitability

烦躁 [fán zào]

vexation-restlessness: vexation followed by restlessness, either due to yang deficiency or yin excess

躁烦 [zào fán]

restlessness-vexation: restlessness followed by vexation, seen in a critical case of yin deficiency

心中懊憹 [xīn zhōng ào nóng]

distress in the heart: distressing heat sensation in the heart and chest

心烦 [xīn fán]

vexation: state of being vexed, often indicating depressed heat in the heart

望色 [wàng sè]

inspection of color: observation of the patient's skin color, particularly the color of the face

气色 [qì sè]

complexion: natural color and appearance of the face

常色 [cháng sè]

normal color: normal color of the skin of the face

主色 [zhǔ sè]

individual's normal color: one's normal natural color of the skin of the face

客色 [kè sè]

varied normal color: climatically varied normal natural color of the skin of the face

病色 [bìng sè]

morbid color: abnormal color of the face caused by disease

善色 [shàn sè]

favorable color: complexion indicating a favorable prognosis

恶色 [è sè]

unfavorable color: complexion indicating an unfavorable prognosis

面黄肌瘦 [miàn huáng jī shòu]

sallow complexion with emaciation: a complexion often seen in a chronically debilitated patient with consumption of *qi* and blood

面色淡白 [miàn sè dàn bái]

pallid complexion: a complexion often indicating blood deficiency or loss of blood

面色苍白 [miàn sè cāng bái]

pale complexion: a complexion often caused by yang collapse or exuberance of cold

面色㿠白 [miàn sè huāng bái]

bright pale complexion: a complexion often seen in cases of yang deficiency

面色黎黑 [miàn sè lí hēi]

darkish complexion: a complexion indicating kidney insufficiency, cold syndrome, or blood stasis

面红 [miàn hóng]

flushed face: a sign indicating the presence of heat

面尘 [miàn chén]

dusty complexion: dark-gray complexion as if covered with dust, which indicates latent pathogens in excess syndromes, and consumption of liver and kidney yin in deficiency syndromes

五色 [wǔ sè]

five colors: blue (or green), red, yellow, white and black, which, according to the theory of the five elements, corresponding to the liver (wood), heart (fire), spleen (earth), lung (metal) and kidney (water), respectively

青色 [qīng sè]

bluish discoloration: cyanosis of the skin or complexion, usually due to stagnant blood circulation, seen in cold syndrome, and cases of severe pain, *qi* stagnation, blood stasis, and convulsions

黄色 [huáng sè]

yellow discoloration: A yellow complexion suggests spleen insufficiency or presence of dampness; yellow discoloration of the whole body surface including the sclera, i.e., jaundice, signifies the presence of damp-heat if the color is bright yellow, and the presence of cold-damp if the color is dark yellow.

萎黄 [wěi huáng]

sallowness: sallow color of the skin, especially the face, which usually occurs in cases of spleen *qi* deficiency

赤色 [chì sè]

red discoloration: Reddening of the complexion usually indicates the presence of heat.

白色 [bái sè]

white discoloration: White complexion usually indicates cold or deficiency.

黑色 [hēi sè]

black discoloration: Black or dark gray complexion is often seen in severe and chronic cases of blood stasis, pain, and kidney yang deficiency.

五色主病 [wǔ sè zhǔ bìng]

diagnostic significance of the five colors: (1) The five colors — blue (or green), red, yellow, white, and black — indicate disorders of the liver, heart, spleen, lung and kidney respectively. (2) Blue indicates wind, cold, pain, convulsion, or blood stasis; red indicates the presence of heat; yellow reveals dampness; white implies deficiency of *qi* and blood or presence of cold; black indicates pain, exhaustion or blood stasis.

真脏色 [zhēn zàng sè]

visceral-exhaustion color: color reflected in the face indicating exhaustion of essence and *qi* of *zang* organs with unfavorable prognosis

望形体 [wàng xíng tǐ]

observation of physical build: a method of detecting the nature of a disease by observation of the patient's stature, constitution, and body pattern

望姿态 [wàng zī tài]

observation of posture: a method of finding out the patient's condition by observing his (her) posture, gesture, and movement

仰卧伸足 [yǎng wò shēn zú]

lying supine with legs stretched: a posture often taken by a patient with excessive heat

蜷卧缩足 [juǎn wò suō zú]

lying on the side with the knees drawn up: a posture often taken by a patient with deficiency-cold

手足蠕动 [shǒu zú rú dòng]

wriggling of the extremities: a type of involuntary movement of the extremities, usually indicating stirring of internal wind due to yin deficiency

手足颤动 [shǒu zú chàn dòng]

trembling of the extremities: a type of involuntary movement of the extremities, often due to blood deficiency involving the tendons or chronic alcoholism, but sometimes being a premonitory sign of convulsion

项强 [xiàng jiàng]

nape rigidity: stiffness or inflexibility of the back of the neck

角弓反张 [jiǎo gōng fǎn zhāng]

opisthotonus: a form of spasm consisting of extreme hyperextension of the body, with the head and the heels bent backward and the body bowed forward

转筋 [zhuàn jīn]

systremma: a cramp in the muscles of the calf of the leg

拘挛 [jū luán]

contracture: a condition of high resistance to the passive stretch of a muscle

拘急 [jū jí]

contraction: shortening of a muscle or muscles with increased tonicity

抽筋 [chōu jīn]

spasm: a sudden, violent, involuntary contraction of a muscle or group of muscles

筋惕肉瞤 [jīn tì ròu rún]

twitching of the muscles: a condition of short spastic muscular contractions

身瞤动 [shēn rún dòng]

twitching of the body: sudden rapid involuntary movement of the body

刚痉 [gāng jìng]

tonic convulsion: convulstion accompanied by rigidity of the neck and even opisthotonos, occurring in cases of febrile diseases

口㖞 [kǒu wāi]

wry mouth: deviation of the angle of the mouth to one side

口眼㖞斜 [kǒu yǎn wāi xié]

deviation of eye and mouth: a sign indicating attack of wind-phlegm to the meridian

审苗窍 [shěn miáo qiào]

inspection of the signaling orifices: inspection of the eyes, ears, nose, mouth and tongue which can indicate changes in the *zang-fu* organs

望目 [wàng mù]

inspection of the eyes: inspection including observation of the luster, color, appearance, and motility of the eyes, not only for diagnosing eye diseases, but also for determining the condition of the *zang-fu* organs

察目 [chá mù]

examination of the eyes: a synonym for observation of the eyes (望目 [wàng mù])

目窠上微肿 [mù kē shàng wēi zhǒng]

mild edema of the eyelids: an early sign of edematous disease

目下有卧蚕 [mù xià yǒu wò cán]

puffiness under the eyes: sign of edema due to spleen insufficiency

目胞浮肿 [mù bāo fú zhǒng]

edema of eyelids: sign of edema due to spleen insufficiency, as the eyelids pertain to the spleen

目下肿 [mù xià zhǒng]

edema under the eyes: a synonym for puffiness under the eyes (目下有卧蚕 [mù xià yǒu wò cán])

目窠肿 [mù kē zhǒng]

edema of the eye sockets: a synonym for edema of the eyelids (目胞浮肿 [mù bāo fú zhǒng])

两眼无光 [liǎng yǎn wú guāng]

lusterless eyes: eyes without luster and sluggish in motion, often seen in a seriously ill person

神光耗散 [shén guāng hào sàn]

spiritless eyes: eyes without spirit, dull, clouded and inflexible in motion, often seen in a critically ill person

眼珠干涩 [yǎn zhū gān sè]

dryness of the eyes: a condition of the eyes that lack secretion and tears, indicating consumption of body fluids in cases of febrile diseases

眼珠牵斜 [yǎn zhū qiān xié]

strabismus; squint: deviation of the eye which the patient cannot overcome

眼珠塌陷 [yǎn zhū tā xiàn]

sunken eyes: a sign indicating consumption of body fluids or deficiency of *qi* and blood

眼窝凹陷 [yǎn wō āo xiàn]

sunken sockets, same as sunken eyes (眼珠塌陷 [yǎn zhū tā xiàn])

眼球突出 [yǎn qiú tū chū]

protrusion of the eyeballs: a sign indicating obstruction of the lung by phlegm-turbidity if there is accompanying dyspnea, and indicating accumulation of phlegm and *qi* if there is accompanying goiter

瞪目直视 [dēng mù zhí shì]

staring straight ahead: a sign that indicates that the patient is critically ill, particularly when there is loss of consciousness as well

横目斜视 [héng mù xié shì]

staring sideways: a sign often occurring in the stirring-up of liver wind

两眼翻上 [liǎng yǎn fān shàng]

supraduction: upward rotation of the eyes around the horizontal axis

胞睑下垂 [bāo jiǎn xià chuí]

blepharoptosis: drooping of one or both upper eyelids

废睑 [fèi jiǎn]

another name for blepharoptosis (胞睑下垂 [bāo jiǎn xià chuí])

昏睡露睛 [hūn shuì lù jīng]

lethargic sleeping with the eyes open: a sign indicating failure of the spleen and stomach in children with consumption of body fluids due to severe vomiting and diarrhea

白睛色诊 [bái jīng sè zhěn]

inspection of the white of the eyes: observing the change in color of the white of the eye, e.g., redness in lung fire or external contraction of wind-heat, yellowness in jaundice

白睛发黄 [bái jīng fā huáng]

yellow discoloration of the white of the eye: a major sign of jaundice

望耳 [wàng ěr]

inspection of the ear: a diagnostic method to detect not only local pathological changes but also the general condition, particularly the condition of the kidney and gallbladder

耳轮淡白 [ěr lún dàn bái]

pale helix, frequently seen in cases of deficiency of *qi* and blood

耳轮红肿 [ěr lún hóng zhǒng]

red swollen helix, seen in cases of damp-heat of the liver and gallbladder or attack of heat toxin

耳轮青黑 [ěr lún qīng hēi]

bluish dark helix, seen in cases of excessive interior cold or severe pain

耳轮干枯 [ěr lún gān gū]

withering of the helix: a sign of extreme consumption of kidney yin

耳轮萎缩 [ěr lún wěi suō]

atrophy of the helix: a sign indicating exhaustion of kidney *qi* in a critical case

耳轮甲错 [ěr lún jiǎ cuò]

scaly dry helix: a sign of blood stasis

望鼻 [wàng bí]

inspection of the nose: a diagnostic method to detect pathological changes in the lung, spleen, stomach, and other visceral organs by inspecting the color, form, structure and discharge of the nose

鼻翼煽动 [bí yì shān dòng]

flaring nares: a sign indicating dyspnea

鼻流清涕 [bí liú qīng tì]

thin nasal discharge: a symptom that usually occurs in cases of wind-cold

鼻流浊涕 [bí liú zhuó tì]

turbid nasal discharge: a symptom that usually occurs in cases of wind-heat

久流浊涕 [jiǔ liú zhuó tì]

chronic turbid nasal discharge: a symptom that frequently appears in cases of nasal sinusitis

鼻色主病 [bí sè zhǔ bìng]

indications of the color of the nose: Blue, yellow, white, red and grey indicate abdominal pain, damp-heat in the interior, loss of blood, heat in the spleen and lung, and retention of fluid, respectively.

鼻出血 [bí chū xuè]

nosebleed: bleeding from the nose

鼻衄 [bí nǜ]

epistaxis: bleeding from the nose, same as nosebleed (鼻出血 [bí chū xuè])

舌诊 [shé zhěn]

tongue diagnosis: diagnosis made according to information obtained by inspection of the tongue

望舌 [wàng shé]

inspection of the tongue: one of the most important contents of examinations for diagnosis, in which the tongue proper and its coating are carefully observed

舌的分部 [shé de fēn bù]

partition of the tongue: The tongue is usually divided into the following parts, i.e., the tip, middle, root and borders, revealing pathologic changes of the heart and lung, the spleen and stomach, the kidney, and the liver and gallbladder, respectively.

舌尖 [shé jiān]

tip of the tongue, often reflecting the condition of the heart and lung

舌边 [shé biān]

borders of the tongue, often reflecting the condition of the liver and gall-bladder

舌中 [shé zhōng]

middle part of the tongue, often reflecting the condition of the spleen and stomach

舌心 [shé xīn]

central part of the tongue, same as 舌中 [shé zhōng]

舌根 [shé gēn]

root of the tongue, often reflecting the condition of the kidney

舌本 [shé běn]

base of the tongue, same as 舌根 [shé gēn]

舌体 [shé tǐ]

tongue body: a synonym for the tongue proper (舌质 [shé zhì])

舌质 [shé zhì]

tongue proper; tongue substance: the muscular and vascular structure of the tongue, also called the tongue body (舌体 [shé tǐ])

舌下脉络 [shé xià mài luò]

sublingual vein: the vein under the tongue on either side of the frenulum

舌色 [shé sè]

tongue color: color of the tongue body, which reflects the condition of *qi* and blood and functional state of the *zang-fu* organs

淡红舌 [dàn hóng shé]

pale-red tongue: tongue of normal color

舌淡白 [shé dàn bái]

pale tongue, seen in cases of *qi* and blood deficiency or yang deficiency, also called 舌淡 [shé dàn]

舌淡 [shé dàn]

an abbreviation of 舌淡白 [shé dàn bái]

红舌 [hóng shé]

red tongue: tongue redder than normal, indicating presence of heat

舌红 [shé hóng]

redness of the tongue, same as 红舌 [hóng shé]

绛舌 [jiàng shé]

deep-red tongue: a sign of intense heat, also called 舌绛 [shé jiàng]

舌绛 [shé jiàng]

deep-redness of the tongue, same as 绛舌 [jiàng shé]

紫舌 [zǐ shé]

purple tongue: a sign indicating impaired circulation of *qi* and blood

青舌 [qīng shé]

blue tongue: a sign indicating congealing cold with blood stasis

舌青紫 [shé qīng zǐ]

cyanosis of the tongue: bluish purple discoloration of the tongue due to blood stasis, penetration of toxic heat into nutrient-blood, or *qi* stagnation with sluggish blood flow

舌有瘀点 [shé yǒu yū diǎn]

tongue with purple spots: a sign of blood stasis

舌有瘀斑 [shé yǒu yu ban]

tongue with ecchymosis: a sign of blood stasis

瘦薄舌 [shòu báo shé]

thin tongue: a tongue which is thinner than normal, usually due to deficiency of *qi* and blood if the tongue is thin and pale, and due to yin deficiency if it is thin and red

胖大舌 [pàng dà shé]

enlarged tongue: a tongue larger than normal due to accumulation of fluid, often seen in deficiency of *qi* or yang

舌胖 [shé pàng]

plump tongue: a synonym for enlarged tongue (胖大舌 [pàng dà shé])

舌体胖大 [shé tǐ pàng dà]

plump tongue body: a synonym for enlarged tongue (胖大舌 [pàng dà shé])

肿胀舌 [zhǒng zhàng shé]

swollen tongue: a reddened tongue distended and larger than normal, often caused by exuberant fire of the heart and spleen or externally contracted damp-heat, but sometimes by congenital vascular anomaly

齿痕舌 [chǐ hén shé]

tooth-marked tongue: a tongue with dental indentations on its edges, seen in cases of retention of water-damp when the tongue is enlarged as well, also called 舌有齿痕 [shé yǒu chǐ hén]

舌有齿痕 [shé yǒu chǐ hén]

tongue with tooth-marks, same as 齿痕舌 [chǐ hén shé]

点刺舌 [diǎn cì shé]

speckled tongue: a tongue with red spots formed by swollen fungiform papillae, indicating the presence of exuberant heat

舌起芒刺 [shé qǐ máng cì]

prickles on the tongue: thorn-like protruding swollen fungiform papillae formed on the surface of the tongue

芒刺舌 [máng cì shé]

prickled tongue: a tongue with thorn-like protrusions on its surface, indicating the presence of exuberant heat

裂纹舌 [liè wén shé]

cracked tongue: a tongue with cracks on its surface, often indicating consumption of fluids or yin

舌裂 [shé liè]

fissured tongue: appearance of fissures on the surface of the tongue, cf. cracked tongue (裂纹舌 [liè wén shé])

舌肿 [shé zhǒng]

swelling of the tongue: abnormal enlargement of the tongue, usually reddened in color, cf. swollen tongue (肿胀舌 [zhǒng zhàng shé])

重舌 [chóng shé]

double tongue: hypertrophy of the bilateral sublingual glands resembling a smaller tongue lying under the original one

强硬舌 [jiàng yìng shé]

stiff tongue: a tongue difficult to move freely, seen in cases of high fever with impairment of consciousness or loss of fluid, and also in cases of apoplexy, known also as 舌强 [shé jiàng]

舌强 [shé jiàng]

stiffness of the tongue, same as 强硬舌 [jiàng yìng shé]

舌謇 [shé jiǎn]

sluggish tongue: a curling tongue, sluggish in motion with difficulty in speaking, also called 舌蹇 [shé jiǎn]

舌蹇 [shé jiǎn]

same as 舌謇 [shé jiǎn]

颤动舌 [chàn dòng shé]

trembling tongue: a sign of wind caused by deficiency of *qi* and blood, stirred up by extreme heat, or transformed from liver yang, also known as 舌战 [shé zhàn]

舌战 [shé zhàn]

tremor of the tongue: a synonym for trembling tongue (颤动舌 [chàn dòng shé])

痿软舌 [wěi ruǎn shé]

flaccid tongue: a tongue that is flabby and cannot move easily, seen in impairment of yin or deficiency of *qi* and blood

舌痿 [shé wěi]

flaccidity of the tongue: a synonym for flaccid tongue (痿软舌 [wěi ruǎn shé])

歪斜舌 [wāi xié shé]

deviated tongue: a tongue that deviates to one side when extended, indicating the presence of liver wind with phlegm or obstruction of the meridian by phlegm and stagnant blood

舌歪 [shé wāi]

deviation of the tongue: a synonym for deviated tongue (歪斜舌 [wāi xié shé])

短缩舌 [duǎn suō shé]

shortened tongue: a tongue that cannot be fully extended from the mouth and appears to be contracted, usually seen in critically ill patients

舌短 [shé duǎn]

shortness of the tongue: a synonym for shortened tongue (短缩舌 [duǎn suō shé])

舌卷囊缩 [shé juǎn náng suō]

curled tongue and retracted testicles: a sign that may occur in a critical case of febrile disease or apoplexy

木舌 [mù shé]

wooden tongue: a swollen, hard tongue resembling a piece of wood, seen in infantile glossitis

吐舌 [tǔ shé]

protruding tongue: tongue that extends out of the mouth, with licking of the lips

弄舌 [nòng shé]

moving tongue: one which moves from one side to the other when extended, or moves without stopping

吐弄舌 [tǔ nòng shé]

protruding and moving tongue: a sign seen in children with defective development of the brain, also in febrile diseases with stirring-up of wind

舌苔 [shé tāi]

tongue coating: a layer of moss-like material covering the tongue, inspection of which can provide information about the nature, depth and location of the pathogenic factor, the strength and integrity of normal *qi*, and the degree of fluid consumption

苔色 [tāi sè]

tongue coating color: the color of the tongue coating, which reflects not only the heat or cold nature of the condition, but also the interior or exterior characteristics and the degree of penetration of the disease

白苔 [bái tāi]

white coating: a sign indicating presence of cold, but thin white coating often seen in normal persons

黄苔 [huáng tāi]

yellow coating: a sign indicating presence of heat

薄白苔 [bó bái tāi]

thin white coating: a form of tongue coating often seen in normal persons or in the early stage of an exterior syndrome

薄黄苔 [bó huáng tāi]

thin yellow coating: a form of tongue coating often seen in cases of exterior heat syndrome or early stage of interior heat

白腻苔 [bái nì tāi]

white greasy coating: a form of tongue coating indicating damp-phlegm or retained food

黄腻苔 [huáng nì tāi]

yellow greasy coating: a form of tongue coating indicating accumulation of damp-heat, phlegm-heat or retained food with heat

黑苔 [hēi tāi]

black coating: a tongue coating indicating either excessive cold (if the coating is moistened and the tongue body pale), or extreme heat (if the coating is dry and the tongue body reddened)

灰苔 [huī tāi]

gray coating: a tongue coating with similar clinical significance to 黑苔 (black coating)

染苔 [rǎn tāi]

stained coating, often caused by food or medicine

苔的厚薄 [tāi de hòu bó]

thickness of the tongue coating: A thin coating usually indicates absence of severe illness or only the exterior portion of the body being attacked by pathogenic factors, while a thick coating suggests inward penetration of pathogenic factors or presence of retained food or phlegm.

苔的润燥 [tāi de rùn zào]

moisture of the tongue coating: A moist coating indicates that the body fluid is not impaired, while a dry coating is a sign of impairment of body fluid.

腐苔 [fǔ tāi]

curdy coating: a coating consisting of coarse granules like bean dregs, capable of being wiped off, reflecting retention of food in the stomach

腻苔 [nì tāi]

greasy coating: a dense, sticky, slimy tongue coating, thick in the center, thin on the sides, and hard to wipe off, indicating presence of phlegm-damp or stagnancy of food

滑苔 [huá tāi]

slippery coating: a moist tongue coating with excessive fluid and an oily appearance, indicating presence of dampness

燥苔 [zào tāi]

dry coating: a sign generally indicative of damage to the body fluids

糙苔 [cāo tāi]

rough coating: a tongue coating that is so dry that it looks rough, indicating severe damage to the body fluids

白砂苔 [bái shā tāi]

white sandy coating: white, thick and dry tongue coating as rough as sand, indicating rapid transformation of heat into dryness with severe impairment of body fluids before the coating turns yellow

剥苔 [bō tāi]

peeled coating: a tongue with its coating peeled off

舌苔脱落 [shé tāi tuó luò]

peeling of tongue coating: complete or partial peeling of the tongue coating, usually due to impairment of stomach *qi*, consumption of stomach yin, deficiency of *qi* and blood, or general debility

光剥舌 [guāng bō shé]

sudden peeling of coating: a tongue with its coating suddenly peeled, usually indicative of exhaustion of stomach yin and severe damage to stomach *qi*

镜面舌 [jìng miàn shé]

mirror-like tongue: a completely peeled tongue resembling a mirror, indicating collapse of stomach *qi* or exhaustion of stomach yin

有根苔 [yǒu gēn tāi]

rooted coating: tongue coating with root, closely attached to the tongue surface

无根苔 [wú gēn tāi]

rootless coating: tongue coating without root, which can be easily wiped or scraped off

口唇干裂 [kǒu chún gān liè]

cracked lips: a sign of impairmenf of body fluids by dryness-heat or yin deficiency, also called 唇裂 [chún liè]

唇裂 [chún liè]

cracked lips, same as 口唇干裂 [kǒu chún gān liè]

口角流涎 [kǒu jiǎo liú xián]

dripping from the corner of the mouth: excessive flow of saliva from the corner of the mouth, often due to spleen dampness or stomach heat in children, or appearing in stroke patients with a wry mouth

口唇糜烂 [kǒu chún mí làn]

erosion of lips: a sign of upward steaming of accumulated heat in the spleen and stomach

口张 [kǒu zhāng]

opened mouth: one that is puckered open, like the mouth of a fish, indicating failure of the spleen

口噤 [kǒu jìn]

lockjaw: inability to open the mouth, mainly caused by liver wind, seen in cases of convulsive diseases and tetanus

口撮 [kǒu cuō]

tightening of the lips: a sign of infantile convulsion

口僻 [kǒu pì]

wry mouth, same as 口㖞 [kǒu wāi]

口振 [kǒu zhèn]

trembling of the lips: a sign of violent struggle between normal and pathogenic *qi*

口动 [kǒu dòng]

moving mouth: one that opens and closes frequently and involuntarily, signifying weakness of stomach *qi*

唇紫 [chún zǐ]

purple lips: a sign of blood stasis in patients with decline of heart yang and severe dyspnea

望齿 [wàng chǐ]

inspection of the teeth, including the gums, not only for diagnosing local illnesses, but also for detecting diseases of the internal organs, particularly disorders of the kidney and stomach, and impairment of body fluids

齿燥 [chǐ zào]

dryness of the teeth: a sign of excessive fire in the lung and stomach with severe consumption of fluid in acute cases, or serious impairment of kidney yin in chronic cases

齿槁 [chǐ gǎo]

withering of the teeth: a sign of exhaustion of kidney yin, seen in febrile diseases at the late stage

齿焦 [chǐ jiāo]

scorching of the teeth: a sign of severe loss of fluid in critical cases

齿衄 [chǐ nǜ]

bleeding from the gums

齿摇 [chǐ yáo]

looseness of teeth, often suggesting kidney insufficiency

齿龈肿痛 [chǐ yín zhǒng tòng]

painful swelling of the gums, often indicating excessive heat in the stomach

望痰 [wàng tán]

inspection of sputum: examination of the color, quality and quantity of the sputum to detect conditions of the visceral organs and features of pathogenic factors

痰稀 [tán xī]

thin sputum: phlegm of cold nature

痰如泡沫 [tán rú pào mò]

frothy sputum, indicating presence of cold

痰多 [tán duō]

profuse sputum, usually indicating dampness, also known as 痰盛 [tán shèng]

痰盛 [tán shèng]

abundant expectoration, same as 痰多 [tán duō]

黄痰 [tán huáng]

yellow sputum: phlegm of heat nature

咯血 [kǎ xuè]

hemoptysis: expectoration of blood or blood-stained sputum

咳血 [ké xuè]

coughing of blood: bringing-up of blood or bloody sputum when coughing

血痰 [xuè tán]

bloody sputum: sputum containing blood, also known as 痰中带血 [tán zhōng dài xuè]

痰中带血 [tán zhōng dài xuè]

blood-stained sputum, same as 血痰 [xuè tán]

血丝痰 [xuè sī tán]

blood-streaked sputum: sputum containing streaks of blood

望指纹 [wàng zhǐ wén]

inspection of finger venules: a diagnostic method for children under 3, in which the extension and color of the superficial venules on the palmar side of the index finger are examined and taken as reference for diagnosis, e.g., red venules with yellowish tint, faintly visible, not extending beyond the proximal segment of the finger indicating health, deep red venules suggesting presence of heat, dark venules signifying blood stasis, purple and blue venules often occurring in cases of convulsion and pain

三关 [sān guān]

three passes: a collective term for the three segments of the index finger used for measuring the extension of the visible venules, i.e., "wind pass" (the proximal segment), "*qi* pass" (the middle segment) and "life pass" (the distal segment). Venules only visible at the wind pass usually indicate a mild disease. The farther the venules extend, the more serious is the case.

风关 [fēng guān]

wind pass: the proximal segment of the index finger

气关 [qì guān]

***qi* pass:** the middle segment of the index finger

命关 [mìng guān]

life pass: the distal segment of the index finger

透关射甲 [tòu guān shè jiǎ]

extension (of visible venules) through the passes toward the nail, often indicating that a child is critically ill, also known as 通关射甲 [tōng guān shè jiǎ]

通关射甲 [tōng guān shè jiǎ]

shooting through the passes to the nail, same as 透关射甲 [tòu guān shè jiǎ]

望皮肤 [wàng pí fū]

inspection of the skin: an examination not only for skin diseases, but also for the condition of *qi*, blood and visceral organs

肿胀 [zhǒng zhàng]

swelling: an abnormal protuberance or distension of a body part or area

水肿 [shuǐ zhǒng]

edema: an abnormal excess accumulation of fluid under the skin, often showing prolonged existence of the pits produced by pressure

脚肿 [jiǎo zhǒng]

edema of the lower extremities: a sign indicating yin edema

跗肿 [fū zhǒng]

instep edema: edema of the upper surface of the foot in front of the ankle joint

发黄 [fā huáng]

yellow discoloration: a condition in which the skin and the whites of the eyes become abnormally yellow, usually referring to jaundice

黄胖 [huáng pàng]

yellow puffiness: yellow tinge of the skin with puffy face and ankle edema

斑 [bān]

macula: a deep red or dark purple spot on the skin that is not elevated above the surface and does not fade under pressure

阳斑 [yáng bān]

yang macula: macula red-purple in color, accompanied by fever and other manifestations of excess heat, often occurring in cases of epidemic febrile diseases

阴斑 [yīn bān]

yin macula: macula dark purple in color, accompanied by pallor, cold limbs and other manifestations of deficiency cold, often due to spleen insufficiency or decline of yang

疹 [zhěn]

papula: a small circumscribed, superficial, solid elevation of the skin, which fades upon pressure

斑疹 [bān zhěn]

maculo-papula: a collective term for skin eruptions in a generalized disease

水疱 [shuǐ pào]

vesicle: a small circumscribed epidermal elevation containing fluid

白痦 [bái pēi]

miliaria alba: skin eruption of fine white crystalline vesicles appearing on the neck and chest, and sometimes on the limbs, in the course of acute febrile diseases

晶痦 [jīng pēi]

sudamina crystallina: fine white crystalline vesicles appearing on the skin surface due to retention of sweat

肌肤甲错 [jī fū jiǎ cuò]

squamous skin: dried, roughened, and scaling skin, indicating blood stasis

闻诊 [wén zhěn]

auscultation and olfaction: The Chinese character 闻 has dual meanings — hearing and smelling.

闻声音 [wén shēng yīn]

auscultation: listening to the patient's voice, sounds of breathing, coughing, etc.

语声 [yǔ shēng]

voice: sounds formed by a person speaking

语声重浊 [yǔ shēng zhòng zhuó]

deep turbid voice: a change of voice due to nasal congestion in cases of colds

声重 [shēng zhòng]

an abbreviation for deep turbid voice (语声重浊 [yǔ shēng zhòng zhuó])

语声低微 [yǔ shēng dī wēi]

faint low voice: a change of voice in a condition of deficiency

嘶嗄 [sī shà]

hoarseness: rough and harsh voice

失音 [shī yīn]

loss of voice: failure to speak above a whisper

喑（瘖）[yīn]

aphonia, same as loss of voice (失音 [shī yīn])

谵语 [zhān yǔ]

delirious speech: disordered speech in delirium

郑声 [zhèng shēng]

unconscious murmuring: a sign indicating consumption of heart *qi* with mental confusion

独语 [dú yǔ]

soliloquy: talking to oneself during the absence of others, a sign of insufficient heart *qi* with mental derangement

错语 [cuò yǔ]

paraphrasia; paraphasia: a type of dysphasia in which the patient frequently employs wrong words or uses words in wrong and senseless combinations, and is aware of the mistakes after uttering them

呓语 [yì yǔ]

somniloquy: talking while asleep, often caused by heart fire, gallbladder heat or disharmonious stomach *qi*

狂言 [kuáng yán]

raving: furious, incoherent and irrational utterance, seen in mania

语言謇涩 [yǔ yán jiǎn sè]

dysphasia: impeded speech with lack of coordination and difficulty in arranging words in the proper order

呼吸 [hū xī]

breathing: the process of drawing air into and expelling it from the lung

呼吸气粗 [hū xī qì cū]

coarse breathing: breathing that often indicates an excess condition

呼吸气微 [hū xī qì wēi]

feeble breathing: that often indicates insufficiency of lung and kidney *qi*

喘 [chuǎn]

dyspnea: difficult or labored breathing

喘逆 [chuǎn nì]

dyspnea with reversed flow of *qi*: a complex expression of dyspnea (喘 [chuǎn])

上气 [shàng qì]

ascent of *qi*: dyspnea with quick breaths due to obstruction of the airway which causes upward flow of air to the throat

短气 [duǎn qì]

shortness of breath: panting with quick breaths, occurring both in deficiency and excess conditions

少气 [shǎo qì]

asthenic breathing, synonymous with feeble breathing (呼吸气微 [hū xī qì wēi]), occurring only in deficiency condition

咳逆上气 [ké nì shàng qì]

cough with reversed ascent of *qi*: cough and dyspnea with quick breaths due to obstruction of the airway by phlegm

不得偃卧 [bù dé yǎn wò]

inability to lie flat: dyspnea while lying down, relieved by assuming an upright position

喘促 [chuǎn cù]

panting: labored breathing with short quick breaths, also called 喘急 [chuǎn jí]

喘急 [chuǎn jí]

same as 喘促 [chuǎn cù]

喘鸣 [chuǎn míng]

wheezing dyspnea: difficult and labored breathing with a continuous sound in the airway, also called 哮 [xiào]

哮 [xiào]

wheezing, synonymous with wheezing dyspnea (喘鸣 [chuǎn míng])

痰鸣 [tán míng]

phlegm wheezing: wheezing due to obstruction of the airway by phlegm

太息 [tài xī]

sighing: taking a long deep breath that can be heard. Frequent sighing indicates stagnation of live *qi*.

善太息 [shàn tài xī]

frequent sighing: cf. sighing (太息 [tài xī])

咳嗽 [ké sòu]

cough: sudden noisy expulsion of air from the lung, resulting from failure of lung *qi* in descending, abnormal ascending or rushing up of lung *qi* or phlegm in the air passage

咳声重浊 [ké shēng zhòng zhuó]

deep turbid cough: cough that sounds heavy and harsh, indicating excess lung syndrome

咳声清脆 [ké shēng qīng cuì]

clear crisp cough: cough that indicates dryness-heat

咳声不扬 [ké shēng bù yáng]

muffled cough: cough that sounds indistinctly, usually due to the presence of thick phlegm in the air passage, indicating heat syndrome of the lung

咳如犬吠 [ké rú quǎn fèi]

barking cough: cough that sounds sharp and harsh, specifically in cases of inflammation of the throat, particularly diphtheria

干咳 [gān ké]

dry cough: cough with little or no sputum, indicating lung dryness or yin deficiency

久咳 [jiǔ ké]

chronic cough: long-lasting or continually recurring cough, also called 久嗽 [jiǔ sòu]

久嗽 [jiǔ sòu]

chronic cough: a synonym of 久咳 [jiǔ ké]

嗅气味 [xiù qì wèi]

smelling odors: one of the diagnostic methods with special attention to unusual smells

腥臭气 [xīng chòu qì]

stink: horrid and offensive smell as given off by stools in cases of steotorrhea or from cancerous discharge

口气 [kǒu qì]

mouth breath, often referring to malodorous breath

口气臭秽 [kǒu qì chòu huì]

offensive breath: bad smell of breath that often indicates presence of stomach heat

口臭 [kǒu chòu]

halitosis: fetid breath, often indicating dyspepsia, tooth decay or unclean oral cavity

口气酸臭 [kǒu qì suān chòu]

sour foul smel of breath: an abnormal smell of breath that indicates dyspepsia

十问 [shí wèn]

ten questions: the ten questions recommended by Zhang Jie-bin (1563-1640) for a physician to ask of his patient while making diagnosis: (1) about chills and fever; (2) perspiration; (3) head and body; (4) stool and urine; (5) food and drink; (6) chest and abdomen; (7) hearing; (8) thirst; (9) past illnesses; (10) cause of present illness. In addition, inquiry should be made into the efficacy of medicine taken, about menstruation in the case of women, and history of smallpox and measles in the case of children.

问诊 [wèn zhěn]

interrogation: an important way of gaining information for diagnosis by asking the patient about the complaint and the history of the illness

问起病 [wèn qǐ bìng]

inquiry about onset of illness: inquiry about the course of the illness, including the time of onset, predisposing factors, chief complaints, treatment and effects

问现证 [wèn xiàn zhèng]

inquiry about present symptoms: cf. "ten questions" (十问 [shí wèn])

问寒热 [wèn hán rè]

inquiry about chills and fever: asking the patient whether he or she has any chilly or feverish sensation

恶热 [wù rè]

aversion to heat: strong dislike of heat, one of the manifestations of externally contracted febrile diseases, but sometimes also occurring in the case of internal injuries such as yin deficiency with endogenous heat or stomach fire

畏寒 [wèi hán]

intolerance of cold: sensation of cold which can be relieved by wearing more clothes or warming oneself near a source of heat

恶寒 [wù hán]

aversion to cold: sensation of cold which cannot be relieved by warmth

憎寒 [zèng hán]

abhorrence of cold: strong aversion to cold

寒战 [hán zhàn]

rigors: violent chills with trembling

战栗 [zhàn lì]

shivers: fit of trembling, often followed by high fever

恶风 [wù fēng]

aversion to wind: strong dislike of wind, a symptom often resulting from external contraction of pathogenic wind

恶寒发热 [wù hán fā rè]

aversion to cold with fever: simultaneous appearance of aversion to cold together with fever

发热恶寒 [fā rè wù hán]

fever and aversion to cold: a common symptom of various externally contracted febrile diseases, in which aversion to cold usually precedes fever, and disappears when the fever starts, but sometimes may persist together with the fever

但热不寒 [dàn rè bù hán]

fever without chills: a symptom usually caused by interior heat

但寒不热 [dàn hán bù rè]

chills without fever: a symptom usually caused by interior cold, either of excess type or of deficiency type

寒热往来 [hán rè wǎng lái]

alternating fever and chills: a condition in which fever and chills attack alternately

身热 [shēn rè]

generalized fever: elevation of the body temperature or feverish feeling all over the body

发热 [fā rè]

fever: elevation of the body temperature above the normal or subjective feeling of feverishness

壮热 [zhuàng rè]

high fever, usually persistent and without chills

灼热 [zhuó rè]

burning fever: high fever with a burning sensation or with the patient's skin hot to the touch

烦热 [fán rè]

vexing fever: fever with vexation

微热 [wēi rè]

mild fever: low-grade fever, often occurring in certain cases of internal injury or at the late stage of warm diseases

潮热 [cháo rè]

tidal fever: fever with periodic rise and fall of body temperature at fixed hours of the day

日晡潮热 [rì bū cháo rè]

late afternoon (tidal) fever: fever more marked at 3-5 p.m. daily

午后潮热 [wǔ hòu cháo rè]

afternoon (tidal) fever: fever occurring in the afternoon daily

五心烦热 [wǔ xīn fán rè]

vexing heat in the chest, palms and soles: a common symptom of the following conditions: (1) consumptive diseases with deficiency of yin or blood with exuberant endogenous fire, (2) persistent asthenic fire as a sequela of febrile diseases, and (3) internal stagnation of fire-heat

手足心热 [shǒu zú xīn rè]

feverish sensation in the palms and soles: cf. vexing heat in the chest, palms and soles (五心烦热 [wǔ xīn fán rè])

身热不扬 [shēn rè bù yáng]

unsurfaced fever: a sign of damp-heat, when the physician feels the patient's skin to be hot only on extended palpation

问汗 [wèn hàn]

inquiry about sweating

多汗 [duō hàn]

excessive sweating; hyperhidrosis

自汗 [zì hàn]

spontaneous sweating: excessive sweating during the daytime with no apparent cause (such as hot weather, thick clothing) or at the slightest physical exertion

盗汗 [dào hàn]

night sweats: sweating during sleep, a symptom frequently occurring in cases of yin deficiency with endogenous heat

大汗 [dà hàn]

profuse sweating: sweating which may cause excessive loss of body fluids

热汗 [rè hàn]

hot sweats: sweating in the case of a yang syndrome, also called yang sweats (阳汗 [yáng hàn])

阳汗 [yáng hàn]

yang sweats, synonymous with hot sweats (热汗 [rè hàn])

冷汗 [lěng hàn]

cold sweats: profuse sweating accompanied by cold body and limbs and hardly perceivable pulse, a sign of exhaustion of yang

战汗 [zhàn hàn]

shiver sweating: sweating following shivering in the course of a febrile disease, indicating a violent struggle between normal and pathogenic *qi*, which may lead either to subsidence of fever and then recovery, or to collapse

绝汗 [jué hàn]

exhaustion sweating: incessant profuse sweating of a patient in a moribund state

头汗 [tóu hàn]

sweating head: sweating only on the head

额汗 [é hàn]

sweating forehead: sweating most marked on the forehead

半身汗多 [bàn shēn hàn duō]

hemihidrosis: sweating on one side of the body only, usually due to disharmony of *qi* and blood

手足心汗 [shǒu zú xīn hàn]

sweating palms and soles: excessive sweating from the palms and soles, often indicating heat in the yin meridians

阴汗 [yīn hàn]

(1) genital sweating: localized sweating in the genital region, particularly the scrotum; **(2) yin sweating:** another name for cold sweats (冷汗 [lěng hàn])

问头身 [wèn tóu shēn]

inquiry about the head and body: obtaining information about headaches and generalized pain through interrogation

头痛 [tóu tòng]

headache: pain in the head

头重 [tóu zhòng]

heavy-headedness: a subjective feeling of heaviness in the head

头风 [tóu fēng]

head wind: chronic or recurrent headache

偏头痛 [piān tóu tòng]

hemilateral headache: pain on one side of the head

偏头风 [piān tóu fēng]

migraine: recurrent unilateral severe headache

眩晕 [xuàn yūn]

(1) dizziness: a sensation of unsteadiness with a feeling of movement within the head; **(2) vertigo:** illusory sense that either the environment or one's own body is revolving

瞑眩 [míng xuàn]

dimness of vision: temporary dimness of vision with vexation — a side effect of drug therapy

眩冒 [xuàn mào]

dizziness with dim vision: a sensation of unsteadiness with dimness of vision

掉眩 [diào xuàn]

dizziness with shaking: dizziness with shaking of the extremities — a symptom indicating the presence of liver wind

徇蒙招尤 [xuán méng zhāo yóu]

dimmed vision with shaking of the head: a symptom indicating disorder of the liver

健忘 [jiàn wàng]

forgetfulness: diminished ability to recall facts and events

胸痛 [xiōng tòng]

chest pain: pain in the chest

胁痛 [xié tòng]

hypochondriac pain: pain in the hypochondriac region

脘痛 [wǎn tòng]

epigastric pain: pain in the epigastric region

腹痛 [fù tòng]

abdominal pain: pain in the abdomen

身痛 [shēn tòng]

body pain: pain involving the whole body

腰痛 [yāo tòng]

lumbar pain: pain in the lumbar region

腰酸（痠）[yāo suān]

lumbar ache: aching in the lumbar region

背痛 [bèi tòng]

back pain: pain in the posterior part of the trunk

肩痛 [jiān tòng]

shoulder pain: pain in the shoulder

肩臂酸痛 [jiān bì suān tòng]

aching shoulder and arm: aching in the shoulder and arm, often due to contraction of pathogenic wind, cold and damp

肩不举 [jiān bù jǔ]

inability to lift shoulder and arm: a symptom often caused by attack of wind damp, injury or strain

痹痛 [bì tòng]

arthralgia: joint pain due to invasion of pathogenic wind, cold or/and damp

胀痛 [zhàng tòng]

distending pain: pain accompanied by a distending sensation, a symptom caused by *qi* stagnation

刺痛 [cì tòng]

stabbing pain: a sharp pain as if caused by a stab, usually due to blood stasis

走窜痛 [zǒu cuàn tòng]

scurrying pain: a pain which repeatedly changes its location, often occurring in the chest and abdomen

窜痛 [cuàn tòng]

scurrying pain, same as 走窜痛 [zǒu cuàn tòng]

游走痛 [yóu zǒu tòng]

wandering pain: pain in the joints of the extremities with repeated changes of location

固定痛 [gù dìng tòng]

fixed pain: a pain fixed in location, often due to blood stasis when it occurs in the chest and abdomen, and due to obstruction by cold-damp when it occurs in the limbs and joints

冷痛 [lěng tòng]

cold pain: pain accompanied by a cold sensation, often due to obstruction of collaterals by cold pathogen or insufficiency of yang *qi*

灼痛 [zhuó tòng]

burning pain: pain accompanied by a burning sensation, often due to the attack of pathogenic fire

绞痛 [jiǎo tòng]

colicky pain: an acute pain in the chest or abdomen, usually due to obstruction of *qi* movement by pathogenic cold or by a solid such as calculus

隐痛 [yǐn tòng]

dull pain: a pain often continuous but not felt sharply

重痛 [zhòng tòng]

pain with heavy sensation: a pain frequently occurring when *qi* movement is obstructed by dampness

掣痛 [chè tòng]

pulling pain: pain in one part involving other parts along a meridian

空痛 [kōng tòng]

pain with sensation of emptiness: a pain mostly occurring in the head or lower abdomen, often due to deficiency of *qi*, blood and essence

麻木 [mά mù]

numbness: reduced sensitivity to touch

不仁 [bù rén]

loss of sensation: insensitivity to touch

问渴饮 [wèn kě yǐn]

inquiry about thirst and drinking: asking the patient about his (her) desire for drinks and condition of fluid intake

口渴 [kǒu kě]

thirst: symptom often occurring in dryness and heat syndromes

口渴引饮 [kǒu kě yǐn yǐn]

thirst with frequent drinking: a sign of consumption of body fluids

口渴喜冷 [kǒu kě xǐ lěng]

thirst with preference for cold drinks: a sign indicating consumption of body fluids by excessive heat

口干不欲饮 [kǒu gān bù yù yǐn]

dryness in the mouth with no desire to drink: a symptom occurring in spleen insufficiency with retention of dampness

烦渴 [fάn kě]

vexing thirst: dire thirst with desire for voluminous drinking

问二便 [wèn èr biàn]

inquiry about stool and urine: obtaining information about the change of stool and urine through interrogation

问大便 [wèn dà biàn]

inquiry about stool: inquiry about constipation, diarrhea, contents of stool, condition of defecation, etc.

便秘 [biàn bì]

constipation: infrequent or difficult evacuation of the feces, also called 不更衣 [bù gēng yī] in an elegant style of wording

不更衣 [bù gēng yī]

an ancient euphemistic expression for constipation

泄泻 [xiè xiè]

diarrhea: frequent discharges of loose or even watery stools

便溏 [biàn táng]

loose bowels: discharge of soft, unformed stools

溏便 [táng biàn]

loose stool; sloppy stool: soft or semiliquid unformed stool

完谷不化 [wán gǔ bù huà]

undigested food (in stool): a condition in which the stool contains undigested food

溏结不调 [táng jié bù tiáo]

stool sometimes loose and sometimes hard: a symptom often caused by disharmony between the liver and spleen

脓血便 [nóng xuè biàn]

purulent and bloody stool: a symptom indicating dysentery

下痢脓血 [xià lì nóng xuè]

dysentery with purulent and bloody stool: type of dysentery marked by content of pus, mucus and blood in the stool

注泄 [zhù xiè]

watery diarrhea: serious diarrhea with liquid discharge

泄注赤白 [xiè zhù chì bái]

watery diarrhea with blood and mucus: a symptom. indicating dysentery

里急后重 [lǐ jí hòu zhòng]

tenesmus: ineffectual and painful straining at stool

上吐下泻 [shàng tù xià xiè]

simultaneous vomiting and diarrhea: a symptom. often indicating damage to the spleen and stomach by pathogenic damp or improper diet

问小便 [wèn xiǎo biàn]

inquiry about urine: inquiry about the volume of urine, frequency of urination, sensation during urinary discharge, etc.

多尿 [duō niào]

polyuria: discharge of excessive amount of urine

少尿 [shǎo niào]

oliguria: excretion of diminished amount of urine

小便频数 [xiǎo biàn pín shuò]

frequent urination: increased frequency of urination, also called 尿频 [niào pín]

尿频 [niào pín]

frequent urination, same as 小便频数 [xiǎo biàn pín shuò]

尿清长 [niào qīng cháng]

profuse clear urine: a sign of the presence of cold in the body

小便清长 [xiǎo biàn qīng cháng]

long voiding of clear urine, synonymous with profuse clear urine (尿清长 [niào qīng cháng])

尿短赤 [niào duǎn chì]

scanty dark urine: a sign of the presence of heat in the body

小便短赤 [xiǎo biàn duǎn chì]

short voiding of dark urine, synonymous with scanty dark urine (尿短赤 [niào duǎn chì])

小便黄赤 [xiǎo biàn huáng chì]

dark urine: dark yellow or even reddish urine, usually indicating the presence of heat

尿赤 [niào chì]

reddish urine, synonymous with dark urine (小便黄赤 [xiǎo biàn huáng chì])

小便不利 [xiǎo biàn bù lì]

inhibited urination: (1) difficulty in urination; (2) deficient secretion of urine

小便涩痛 [xiǎo biàn sè tòng]

difficult and painful urination: a major symptom of stranguria

小便灼热 [xiǎo biàn zhuó rè]

burning sensation during urination: a sign of the presence of heat in stranguria

尿血 [niào xuè]

hematuria: blood in the urine

溲血 [sōu xuè]

hematuria, same as 尿血 [niào xuè]

小便失禁 [xiǎo biàn shī jìn]

urinary incontinence: failure of voluntary control of urination

小便淋漓 [xiǎo biàn lín lì]

dribbling urination: dribbling charge of urine with inability to achieve a full stream

余沥不尽 [yú lì bù jìn]

dribbling after voiding: continued dribbling discharge of urine after voiding

遗尿 [yí niào]

enuresis: involuntary discharge of urine

失溲 [shī sōu]

enuresis, synonymous with 遗尿 [yí niào]

问胸腹 [wèn xiōng fù]

inquiry about chest and abdomen: inquiry about problems in the chest and abdomen

心悸 [xīn jì]

palpitation: a subjective sensation of rapid beating of the heart

心动悸 [xīn dòng jì]

throbbing palpitation: palpitation with visible throbbing of the heart

怔忡 [zhēng zhōng]

fearful throbbing: throbbing palpitation with fear

心痛彻背 [xīn tòng chè bèi]

precordial pain radiating to back: severe pain in the precordial region with radiation to the back

胃脘痛 [wèi wǎn tòng]

epigastric pain: pain in the epigastric region, also called 胃痛 [wèi tòng], 脘痛 [wǎn tòng], and 心下痛 [xīn xià tòng]

胃痛 [wèi tòng]

stomachache, synonymous with epigastric pain (胃脘痛 [wèi wǎn tòng])

脘痛 [wǎn tòng]

pain in the stomach, synonymous with epigastric pain (胃脘痛[wèi wǎn tòng])

心下痛 [xīn xià tòng]

pain below heart, synonymous with epigastric pain (胃脘痛 [wèi wǎn tòng])

恶心 [ě xīn]

nausea: an unpleasant sensation with disgust for food and an urge to vomit

泛恶 [fàn ě]

same as 恶心 [ě xīn]

干呕 [gān ǒu]

retching: a strong involuntary effort to vomit, but without bringing anything up from the stomach

反胃 [fǎn wèi]

(1) regurgitation: bringing the stomach contents up into the mouth; **(2) dysphagia:** difficulty in swallowing, with the food returning to the mouth

吐血 [tù xuè]

spitting of blood: sending out blood from the mouth (with no regard to the source of bleeding)

呕血 [ǒu xuè]

hematemesis: vomiting of blood

呕吐清涎 [ǒu tù qīng xián]

vomiting of clear mucus: a symptom. indicating retention of phlegm that obstructs the descending of stomach *qi*

呕吐酸腐 [oǒu tù suān fǔ]

vomiting of sour fetid matter: a symptom. indicating retention of undigested food in the stomach

呕吐宿食 [ǒu tù sù shí]

vomiting of retained food: a sign of retention of food contents in the stomach

朝食暮吐 [zhāo shí mù tù]

evening vomiting of food eaten in the morning: a symptom. due to retention of undigested food with damage to the spleen

暮食朝吐 [mù shí zhāo tù]

morning vomiting of food eaten the previous evening: a symptom. due to retention of undigested food with damage to the spleen

食已即吐 [shí yǐ jí tù]

vomiting immediately after eating: a symptom. occurring in the course of obstruction of the stomach by heat, phlegm-*qi*, undigested food, or stagnant blood

呃逆 [è nì]

hiccup: sudden involuntary stopping of the breath with a peculiar sound, often recurring at short intervals

嘈杂 [cáo zá]

gastric upset: an epigastric discomfort resembling a vague ache but not real pain, seems to be in want of food but not actually hungry, and often makes one suffering and annoyed

烧心 [shāo xīn]

heartburn: a burning discomfort in the lower part of the chest, usually caused by indigestion

吞酸 [tūn suān]

acid swallowing: swallowing of acid contents regurgitated from the stomach

反酸 [fǎn suān]

acid regurgitation: casting up of acid contents from the stomach

嗳气 [ài qì]

belching; eructation: the casting up of gas from the stomach

噫气 [ài qì]

same as 嗳气 [ài qì]

嗳腐 [ài fǔ]

belching with fetid odor: a symptom. often caused by retention of undigested food in the stomach and intestines

纳呆 [nà dāi]

anorexia: loss of appetite

多食善饥 [duō shí shàn jī]

polyphagia with frequent hunger: a symptom. indicating exuberant stomach fire with increased digestion

饥不欲食 [jī bù yù shí]

anorexia despite hunger: a symptom. usually indicating deficiency of stomach yin with endogenous fire

饮食偏嗜 [yǐn shí piān shì]

dietary partiality: partiality for certain kinds of food

腹痛下坠 [fù tòng xià zhuì]

abdominal pain with straining: abdominal pain accompanied by an urge to evacuate the bowels

肠鸣 [cháng míng]

borborygmus: a rumbling sound caused by the movement of gas through the intestines

腹鸣 [fù míng]

borborygmus, same as 肠鸣 [cháng míng]

腹中雷鸣 [fù zhōng léi míng]

thunderous borborygmus: loud rumbling sound caused by propulsion of gas through the intestines

中满 [zhōng mǎn]

fullness in the abdomen: (1) fullness sensation in the epigastric region; (2) abdominal distention

腹胀 [fù zhàng]

abdominal distention: a subjective sensation of distention and fullness in the abdomen

腹满䐜胀 [fù mǎn chēn zhàng]

abdominal fullness and distention: sensation of fullness and distension due to stagnation of *qi* in the abdomen

小腹满 [xiǎo fù mǎn]

fullness in the lower abdomen: abdominal distention and fullness below the umbilicus

少腹拘急 [shào fù jū jí]

lower abdominal cramp: involuntary painful muscular contraction in the lower abdomen

少腹硬满 [shào fù yìng mǎn]

rigidity and fullness in the lower abdomen: a symptom indicating accumulation of heat or retention of blood in the bladder

控睾 [kòng gāo]

radiating pain to the testis: lower abdominal pain radiating to the testis

腹中硬块 [fù zhōng yìng kuài]

solid mass in the abdomen: hard solid mass in the abdomen, usually caused by blood stasis

问口味 [wèn kǒu wèi]

inquiry about tastes in the mouth: inquiry about changes in tastes in the mouth

口中和 [kǒu zhōng hé]

harmony in the mouth: normal taste in the mouth unaffected by illness

口淡 [kǒu dàn]

tastelessness in the mouth: diminished sensitivity of taste, also called 口中无味 [kǒu zhōng wú wèi]

口中无味 [kǒu zhōng wú wèi]

tastelessness in the mouth, same as 口淡 [kǒu dàn]

口甜 [kǒu tián]

sweetness in the mouth: subjective sweet taste, frequently caused by damp-heat, either exogenous or endogenous, also called 口甘 [kǒu gān]

口甘 [kǒu gān]

sweetness in the mouth, same as 口甜 [kǒu tián]

口苦 [kǒu kǔ]

bitterness in the mouth: subjective bitter taste, seen in gallbladder disorders, particularly in cases of exuberant fire of the liver and gallbladder

口酸 [kǒu suān]

sourness in the mouth: subjective sour taste, usually occurs in cases of indigestion

口咸 [kǒu xián]

salty taste in the mouth: subjective salty taste, often due to kidney insufficiency with flooding of water

口粘腻 [kǒu nián nì]

sticky, slimy sensation in the mouth: a subjective sensation in the mouth, frequently caused by retained phlegm or stagnated food

口不仁 [kǒu bù rén]

numbness of the mouth: premonitory symptom of transformation of liver yang into wind or a symptom indicating over-dosage of certain drugs

问睡眠 [wèn shuì mián]

inquiry about sleep: inquiry about disorders of sleep and wakefulness

多梦 [duō mèng]

excessive dreaming: a condition in which sleep is frequently disturbed by dreams

失眠 [shī mián]

insomnia: inability to sleep, also called 不寐 [bù mèi] or 不得眠 [bù dé mián]

不得眠 [bù dé mián]

inability to sleep, same as 失眠 [shī mián]

不寐 [bù mèi]

sleeplessness, same as 失眠 [shī mián]

嗜睡 [shì shuì]

somnolence: excessive sleepiness

嗜卧 [shì wò]

somnolence, same as 嗜睡 [shì shuì]

但欲寐 [dàn yù mèi]

desire only to sleep: an ancient expression for somnolence (嗜睡

[shì shuì])

梦遗 [mèng yí]

nocturnal emission: involuntary discharge of semen during sleep accompanied by erotic dreams

滑精 [huá jīng]

spermatorrhea: involuntary and excessive discharge of semen without copulation

阳萎 [yáng wěi]

impotence: lack of copulative power in the male

早泄 [zǎo xiè]

premature ejaculation: ejaculation of semen consistently occurring prior to or immediately after the penis enters the vagina

胸闷 [xiōng mèn]

thoracic oppression: feeling of oppression in the chest

痞满 [pǐ mǎn]

stuffiness and fullness: a sensation of stuffiness and fullness in the chest or epigastrium but without pain

胸痞 [xiōng pǐ]

thoracic stuffiness: a sensation of stuffiness in the chest

心下痞 [xīn xià pǐ]

epigastric stuffiness: a sensation of stuffiness and fullness over the epigastrium without local rigidity

心下痞硬 [xīn xià pǐ yìng]

epigastric stuffiness and rigidity: a sensation of stuffiness and fullness over the epigastrium with local rigidity

心下逆满 [xīn xià nì mǎn]

epigastric fullness with nausea: a sensation of fullness in the epigastrium with reversed flow of *qi* such as nausea and regurgitation

下坠 [xià zhuì]

straining at stool: incessant but ineffectual desire for defecation

问妇女经带 [wèn fù nǚ jīng dài]

inquiry about menstruation and leukorrhea: inquiry about the condition of the periods, vaginal discharge, pregnancy and labor in women

月经 [yuè jīng]

menstruation: cyclic discharge from the genital tract of women, usually at approximately one-month intervals

月信 [yuè xìn]

menstruation, same as 月经 [yuè jīng]

月经过多 [yuè jīng guò duō]

excessive menorrhea: excessive uterine bleeding occurring at regular intervals

月经过少 [yuè jīng guò shǎo]

scanty menorrhea: menstrual discharge of less than the normal amount occurring at regular intervals, the period of flow being shorter than the usual duration

月经提前 [yuè jīng tí qián]

advanced periods: periods that come one week or more ahead of due time, also called 月经先期 [yuè jīg xiān qī]

月经先期 [yuè jīng xiān qī]

early periods, synonymous with advanced periods (月经提前 [yuè jīng tí qián])

月经错后 [yuè jīng cuò hòu]

delayed periods: periods that come one week or more after due time

月经后期 [yuè jīng hòu qī]

late periods, synonymous with delayed periods (月经错后 [yuè jīng cuò hòu])

经行先后无定期 [jīng xíng xiān hòu wú dìng qī]

irregular periods; irregular menstrual cycle: periods that come in an irregular cycle, more than one week early and late

经闭 [jīng bì]

absence of menstruation: (1) no experience of menstruation in a women over the age of 18; (2) absence of menstruation for more than three months not related to pregnancy, lactation or menopause

经水断绝 [jīng shuǐ duàn jué]

cessation of menstruation: (1) natural cessation of menstruation occurring around the age of 50 in the female; (2) absence of menstruation for more than three months not due to pregnancy, lactation or menopause

经断 [jīng duàn]

cessation of menstruation: an abbreviated expression for 经水断绝 [jīng shuǐ duàn jué]

经绝 [jīng jué]

cessation of menstruation: an abbreviated expression for 经水断绝 [jīng shuǐ duàn jué]

经行腹痛 [jīng xíng fù tòng]

painful menstruation: abdominal pain during menstruation

白带 [bái dài]

leukorrhea: whitish discharge from the vagina

黄带 [huáng dài]

yellowish leukorrhea: yellowish viscid discharge from the vagina

赤白带下 [chì bái dài xià]

reddish leukorrhea: profuse leukorrhea mixed with reddish discharge

带下臭秽 [dài xià chòu huì]

fetid leukorrhea: leukorrhea with foul smell, often indicating damp-heat

切诊 [qiè zhěn]

palpation: examination of the surface of the body by feeling with the hand or fingers, including taking the pulse

脉象 [mài xiàng]

pulse image: the condition of the pulse felt on examination

脉学 [mài xué]

pulse lore: study of the pulse

脉诊 [mài zhěn]

pulse examination: examination of the pulse for making diagnosis

切脉 [qiè mài]

pulse-taking: feeling the pulse

寸、关、尺 [cùn、guān、chǐ]

***cun, guan, chi*; inch, bar, and cubit:** the three sections over the radial artery considered when feeling the pulse. The bar (*guan*) is just over the eminent head of the radius at the wrist, where the tip of the physician's middle finger is placed, the inch (*cun*) is next to it on the distal side where the tip of the physician's index finger rests, and the cubit (*chi*) is on the proximal side where the tip of the physician's ring finger is placed.

举、按、寻 [jǔ、àn、xún]

lifting, pressing, and searching: the three manipulations in pulse taking. By touching is meant resting the fingers on the patient's wrist very lightly; by pressing is meant feeling the pulse with proper force, and by searching is meant varying the force or moving the fingers to get a more distinct pulse reading.

举法 [jǔ fǎ]

lifting: cf. 举、按、寻 [jǔ、àn、xún]

按法 [àn fǎ]

pressing: cf. 举、按、寻 [jǔ、àn、xún]

寻法 [xún fǎ]

searching: cf. 举、按、寻 [jǔ、àn、xún]

推法 [tuī fǎ]

pushing: pushing and moving the finger to examine the pulse

循法 [xún fǎ]

tracing: moving the examining finger along the radial artery to find out the pulse conditions in detail

总按 [zǒng àn]

total palpation: taking the pulse of the three sections with three fingers simultaneously

单按 [dān àn]

individual palpation: taking the pulse at each of the three sections individually

平息 [píng xī]

normal breathing: normal respiratory cycle of the physician, used as a unit for measuring the patient's pulse rate

三部九候 [sān bù jiǔ hóu]

nine readings of three sections: (1) taking the pulse on three portions of the body, the head, and the upper and lower limbs. At each portion the pulses of the following arteries are examined: the temporal artery at point *taiyang* (EX-HN5) for the state of the head, the auricular artery at point *ermen* (TE21) for the ears, the buccal artery at points *dicang* (ST4) and *daying* (ST5) for the mouth and teeth, the radial artery at inch (*cun*) for the lung, the ulnar artery at point *shenmen* (HT7) for the heart. Also, the pulse at point *hegu* (LI4) is examined for the chest, the pulse at points *wuli* (LR10) and *taichong* (LR3) for the liver, the pulse at points *qimen* (LR14) and *chongyang* (ST42) for the spleen and stomach, and the pulse at point *taixi* (KI3) for the kidney – a method of general examination adopted in ancient times; (2) three sections of the radial artery at the wrist for pulse feeling are designated as inch, bar and cubit, each section felt with light, moderate and heavy force to study the superficial, medium and deep pulses, respectively.

寸口 [cùn kǒu]

***cunkou*; wrist pulse:** the pulsation of the radial artery felt at the wrist, also called 气口 [qì kǒu] or 脉口 [mài kǒu]

气口 [qì kǒu]

***qi* opening:** another name for wrist pulse (寸口 [cùn kǒu])

脉口 [mài kǒu]

wrist pulse: another name for *cunkou* (寸口 [cùn kǒu])

寸口脉 [cùn kǒu mài]

radial artery at the wrist: the portion of the radial artery the pulsation of which can be easily felt at the wrist

趺阳脉 [fū yáng mài]

anterior tibial artery: the artery the pulsation of which can be easily felt at the instep close to the ankle joint

人迎脉 [rén yíng mài]

common carotid artery: the artery the pulsation of which can be easily felt beside the Adam's apple

病脉 [bìng mài]

abnormal pulse: a pulse indicating pathological changes

二十八脉 [èr shí bā mài]

twenty-eight pulses: twenty-eight kinds of pulses, i.e., floating, sunken (deep), slow, rapid, slippery, choppy, empty, full, long, short, surging, faint, tense (tight), relaxed, wiry, hollow, tympanic, firm, soggy, weak, scattered, thready (fine), hidden, throbbing, hurried, knotted, intermittent, and large pulses

浮脉 [fú mài]

floating pulse; superficial pulse: a pulse which can be felt by a light touch and grows faint on hard pressure, usually indicating an exterior syndrome

沉脉 [chén mài]

sunken pulse; deep pulse: a pulse which can only be felt when pressing hard, showing that a disease is located in the interior of the body

伏脉 [fú mài]

hidden pulse: a pulse which can only be felt upon pressing to the bone, located even deeper than sunken pulse, seen in cases of syncope, shock, or severe pain

数脉 [shuò mài]

rapid pulse: a pulse with five or six beats to one cycle of the physician's respiration (more than 90 beats per minute), indicating the presence of heat

迟脉 [chí mài]

slow pulse: a pulse with less than four beats to one cycle of the physician's respiration (less than 60 beats per minute), usually indicating a cold syndrome, but occasionally seen in cases of interior accumulation of heat

缓脉 [huǎn mài]

(1) moderate pulse: a pulse with a moderate rate, even rhythm and moderate tension, indicating a normal condition; **(2) relaxed pulse:** a pulse with diminished tension and moderate frequency, seen in cases of dampness or spleen insufficiency

虚脉 [xū mài]

(1) empty pulse: a feeble and void pulse, indicating deficiency of *qi* and blood or consumption of body fluids; **(2) pulse of deficiency type:** a collective term for various pulse conditions showing deficiency

实脉 [shí mài]

(1) full pulse: a pulse feeling vigorous and forceful upon both light and heavy pressure, indicating an excessive syndrome; **(2) pulse of excess type:** collective term for various pulse conditions showing excessiveness

洪脉 [hóng mài]

surging pulse: a pulse beating like dashing waves with forceful rising and gradual decline, usually indicating presence of excessive heat

细脉 [xì mài]

thready pulse; thin pulse; fine pulse: a pulse as thin as a silk thread, straight and soft, feeble yet always perceptible upon hard pressure, indicating deficiency of *qi* and blood, and seen in other kinds of deficiency conditions, but also in cases of a sudden attack of cold or severe pain

微脉 [wēi mài]

faint pulse: a thready and soft pulse, scarcely perceptible, indicating extreme exhaustion

弱脉 [ruò mài]

weak pulse: a deep, soft and thin pulse, seen in debilitated patients with deficiency of *qi* and blood

濡脉 [rú mài]

soggy pulse: a pulse which can felt on light pressure like a thread floating on water, but growing faint upon hard pressure, seen in deficiency conditions or retention of dampness, also called 软脉 [ruǎn mài]

软脉 [ruǎn mài]

soft pulse, same as soggy pulse (濡脉 [rú mài])

滑脉 [huá mài]

slippery pulse: a pulse coming and going smoothly like beads rolling on a plate, seen in patients with phlegm and dampness or stagnation of food, and also in pregnant women and normal persons

涩脉 [sè mài]

choppy pulse: a pulse coming and going unsmoothly with small, fine, slow joggling tempo like scraping bamboo with a knife, indicating sluggishness of blood circulation caused by deficiency of blood and essence or stagnancy of *qi* and blood

革脉 [gé mài]

tympanic pulse: a pulse felt hard and hollow as if touching the surface of a drum, seen after loss of blood or spermatorrhea

牢脉 [láo mài]

firm pulse: a forceful and taut pulse, felt only by hard pressure, seen in cases of accumulation of yin cold and mass formation

长脉 [cháng mài]

long pulse: a pulse with large extent exceeding *cun, guan* and *chi* sections, seen in cases of excessive heat syndrome, but also in normal persons

短脉 [duǎn mài]

short pulse: a pulse with shorter extent, only felt at *cun* or *guan* section, but not perceptible at *chi* section, indicating *qi* disorders

疾脉 [jí mài]

swift pulse: a hasty and swift pulse, 7-8 beats to one cycle of respiration (120-140 beats per minute), seen in severe cases of acute febrile diseases or consumptive conditions

促脉 [cù mài]

hurried pulse: a rapid pulse with irregular intermittence, seen in cases of excessive heat, stagnation of *qi* and blood, retention of phlegm, or indigestion

代脉 [dài mài]

intermittent pulse: a pulse pausing at regular intervals, indicating a decline of the visceral functions

结脉 [jié mài]

knotted pulse: a pulse of moderate rate, pausing at irregular intervals, seen usually in cases of *qi* stagnation

紧脉 [jǐn mài]

tense pulse; tight pulse: a pulse feeling like a tightly stretched cord, usually indicating the presence of pathogenic cold or pain

散脉 [sǎn mài]

scattered pulse: a pulse that feels diffusing and feeble upon a light touch and faint upon hard pressure, indicating exhaustion of *qi* in critical illnesses

弦脉 [xián mài]

wiry pulse: a straight and long pulse, like a musical string, seen usually in liver and gallbladder disorders or cases of severe pain

芤脉 [kōu mài]

hollow pulse: a floating, large, soft, and hollow pulse, like a scallion stalk, formed by sudden decrease of circulating blood volume, as seen in cases of massive loss of blood or severe vomiting and diarrhea

大脉 [dà mài]

large pulse: a pulse with a high wave which lifts the examiner's finger to a greater height than normal, either forceful (seen in cases of excessive heat with undamaged body resistance) or weak (seen in cases of general debility)

动脉 [dòng mài]

throbbing pulse: a quick, jerky pulse, like a bouncing pea, seen in cases of fright or pregnancy

七绝脉 [qī jué mài]

seven moribund pulses: seven kinds of pulses indicating impending death, also known as 七怪脉 [qī guài mài]

七怪脉 [qī guài mài]

seven paradoxical pulses, same as 七绝脉 [qī jué mài]

雀啄脉 [què zhuó mài]

bird-pecking pulse: an abrupt, quick, arrhythmic pulse resembling the pecking of a bird, one of the seven pulses indicating impending death

鱼翔脉 [yú xiáng mài]

fish-swimming pulse: an extremely short pulse resembling a swimming fish with only its tail wagging, one of the seven pulses indicating impending death

虾游脉 [xiā yóu mài]

shrimp-darting pulse: a nearly imperceptible pulse with occasional darting beats, one of the seven pulses indicating impending death

釜沸脉 [fǔ fèi mài]

bubble-rising pulse: an extremely floating and rapid pulse like bubbles rising to the surface in boiling water, one of the seven pulses indicating impending death

屋漏脉 [wū lòu mài]

dripping pulse: an extremely retarded pulse resembling water dripping from a roof crack, one of the seven pulses indicating impending death

弹石脉 [tán shí mài]

flicking pulse: a deep and solid pulse resembling flicking a stone with the finger tips, one of the seven pulses indicating impending death

解索脉 [jiě suǒ mài]

snapping pulse: a rhythmless pulse resembling the snapping of a cord, one of the seven pulses indicating impending death

喜脉 [xǐ mài]

pregnancy pulse: pulse indicating pregnancy

单一脉象 [dān yī mài xiàng]

single-featured pulse: pulse with only one distinct feature, such as slow pulse or slippery pulse

相兼脉象 [xiàng jiān mài xiàng]

multi-featured pulse: pulse with two or more distinct features, such as floating and tense pulse, deep, fine and rapid pulse

反关脉 [fǎn guān mài]

dorsally located pulse: an anatomic anomaly of the radial artery which makes the pulse beat felt on the dorsal aspect of the wrist

斜飞脉 [xié fēi mài]

slantingly located pulse: an anatomic anomaly of the radial artery which makes the pulse beat felt running from the *chi* (cubit) section outward and slantwise to the back of the hand

脉合四时 [mài hé sì shí]

pulse corresponding to the season: change of the pulse in response to the change of season, e.g., normal pulse being slightly taut in spring and somewhat full in summer

脉逆四时 [mài nì sì shí]

pulse contrary to the season: failure of pulse in varying with the change of the season, e.g., floating instead of taut in spring, and deep instead of full in summer, indicating inability of the body to adapt itself to the change of season

胃、神、根 [wèi、shén、gēn]

stomach *qi*, vitality, and root: three qualities for a normal pulse

脉有胃气 [mài yǒu wèi qì]

pulse with stomach *qi*: a pulse beating smoothly with regular rhythm, normal frequency, moderate force, appropriate volume, and situated in median depth (neither floating nor sunken), indicating adequacy of stomach *qi*

脉无胃气 [mài wú wèi qì]

pulse without stomach *qi*: a pulse that has lost its usual rhythm, frequency and evenness, indicating a critical lack of stomach *qi*

脉有神 [mài yǒu shén]

pulse with vitality: pulse beating with moderate but sufficient strength

脉有根 [mài yǒu gēn]

pulse with root: pulse that can be felt upon deep palpation

脉静 [mài jìng]

calm pulse: pulse that becomes gentle and even in the course of an illness, usually indicating improvement of the condition

脉躁 [mài zào]

agitated pulse: pulse that becomes rapid and rushing, usually indicating deterioration of the condition

脉象主病 [mài xiàng zhǔ bìng]

disease indicated by pulse condition: type of pulse indicative of a particular syndrome, e.g., floating pulse of exterior syndrome, deep pulse of interior syndrome, wiry pulse of liver disorder, etc.

脉阴阳俱浮 [mài yīn yáng jù fú]

floating pulse at both yin and yang: floating pulse felt at both the inch (*cun*) and cubit (*chi*) sections, indicating an exterior syndrome

脉阴阳俱紧 [mài yīn yáng jù jǐn]

tense pulse at both yin and yang: tense pulse felt at both the inch (*cun*) and cubit (*chi*) sections, indicating an exterior syndrome caused by cold

真脏脉 [zhēn zàng mài]

visceral exhaustion pulse: a pulse condition indicating exhaustion of *zang* organs, often found in a critically ill patient

脉悬绝 [mài xuán jué]

extremely abnormal pulse: pulse very different from the normal, usually seen in severe cases

色脉合参 [sè mài hé cān]

consideration of both pulse and complexion: making a diagnosis by reviewing the patient's pulse condition together with the complexion

四诊合参 [sì zhěn hé cān]

comprehensive consideration of the four examinations: making a diagnosis by analyzing the results of all the four examinations

脉证合参 [mài zhèng hé cān]

consideration of both pulse and symptoms: making a diagnosis by reviewing the patient's pulse condition together with the symptoms

舍脉从证 [shě mài cóng zhèng]

preference for symptoms over pulse: making a diagnosis on the basis of symptoms rather than the pulse condition

舍证从脉 [shě zhèng cóng mài]

preference for pulse over symptoms: making a diagnosis on the basis of pulse condition rather than symptoms

按诊 [àn zhěn]

touching: examination of the body surface by touch with the hand or fingers

按尺肤 [àn chǐ fū]

palpation of the forearm: examination of the forearm with the hand for determining the texture of the skin, development of the muscles and temperature of the extremities

按肌肤 [àn jī fū]

palpation of the skin: examination of certain area of skin with the hand for determining local temperature, moisture, pain, swelling and other local changes

按胸腹 [àn xiōng fù]

palpation of the chest and abdomen: examination of the chest and abdomen with the hand to determine the location and extent of the affected region and the pathological change of the viscera

按脘腹 [àn wǎn fù]

palpation of the epigastrium and abdomen: examination of the abdomen, including the epigastric region with the hand for local temperature, consistency, distention, mass formation and tenderness

按手足 [àn shǒu zú]

palpation of the hands and feet: examination of the hands and feet chiefly for determining the cold or heat nature of a syndrome

按俞穴 [àn shù xué]

pressing on acupoints: examination of acupoints with the finger to search for tender points which can reflect diseases in corresponding internal organs

拒按 [jù àn]

refusal of pressure: a condition in which pressing can aggravate discomfort or pain

喜按 [xǐ àn]

preference for pressing: a condition in which pressing can relieve discomfort or pain

常用引文 Commonly Used Citations

望而知之谓之神，闻而知之谓之圣，问而知之谓之工，切脉知之谓之巧。

[wàng ér zhī zhī wèi zhī shén，wén ér zhī zhī wèi zhī shèng，wèn ér zhī zhī wèi zhī gōng，qiè mài zhī zhī wèi zhī qiǎo]

It is wonderful to know by observation; it is wise to know by auscultation and olfaction; it is skillful to know by interrogation; and it is ingenious to know by pulse-taking.

欲知病色，必先知常色；欲知常色，必先知常色之变；欲知常色之变，必先知常色变中之变。 [yù zhī bìng sè，bì xiān zhī cháng sè；yù zhī cháng sè，bì xiān zhī cháng sè zhī biàn；yù zhī cháng sè zhī biàn，bì xiān zhī cháng sè biàn zhōng zhī biàn。]

If you want to know what color is abnormal, you must first know the normal color; if you want to know what color is normal, you must first know the range of normal color; if you want to know the range of normal color, you must first know all the modifications of the normal range.

得神者昌。[dé shén zhě chāng]

A patient with vitality is apt to recover from illness.

失神者亡。[shī shén zhě wáng]

A patient losing vitality has a poor prognosis.

司外揣内。[sī wài chuǎi nèi]

One can predict the interior by inspecting the exterior.

见微知著。[jiàn wēi zhī zhù]

From small beginnings, one can see how things will develop.

揆度奇恒。[kúi duó qí héng]

One should assess the generality and the particularity.

肝脉弦。[gān mài xián]

A wiry pulse indicates liver disorder.

心脉洪。[xīn mài hóng]

A surging pulse often occurs in caes of heart disorder.

脾脉缓。[pí mài huǎn]

A relaxed pulse suggests spleen insufficiency.

肺脉浮。[fèi mài fú]

A floating pulse is frequently found in cases of lung disease.

肾脉沉。[shèn mài chén]

A sunken pulse usually signifies kidney insufficiency.

辨证

Syndrome Differentiation (Pattern Identification)

辨证 [biàn zhèng]

syndrome differentiation; pattern identification: the process of overall analysis of clinical data to determine the location, cause and nature of a patient's disease and achieve diagnosis of a syndrome or pattern

证 [zhèng]

syndrome; pattern: diagnostic conclusion of the pathological changes at a certain stage of a disease, including the location, cause, and nature of the disease as well as the trend of development, sometimes also known as 证候 [zhèng hòu]

证候 [zhèng hòu]

(1) syndrome manifestation: symptoms and signs of a syndrome; **(2) syndrome; pattern:** another term for 证 [zhèng] when a disyllabic word is needed

证型 [zhèng xíng]

syndrome pattern; pattern: a common and typical syndrome with a standard name

八纲辨证

Eight-principle Syndrome Differentiation (Eight-principle Pattern Identification)

八纲 [bā gāng]

eight principles: guiding principles of syndrome differentiation (or pattern identification), viz., yin and yang, exterior and interior, cold and heat, deficiency (or insufficiency) and excess

八纲辨证 [bā gāng biàn zhèng]

eight-principle syndrome differentiation; eight-principle pattern identification: the process of diagnosing a syndrome (or pattern) by analyzing the patient's condition according to the eight principles, i.e., differentiating the location of a disease between exterior and interior, distinguishing the nature of a disease between cold and heat, identifying the patient's condition as deficiency or excess, and generalizing the syndrome or pattern as yin or yang

阴阳 [yīn yáng]

yin and yang: two basic principles for the categorization of syndromes or patterns, including categorization of the remaining principles, e.g., interior, cold, and deficiency pertaining to yin, and exterior, heat, and excess pertaining to yang

阴证 [yīn zhèng]

yin syndrome: a collective term for interior, cold and deficiency syndromes with inhibitory, hypofunctional, quiescent or dimmed manifestations, or inward and downward symptoms, as well as diseases caused by pathogenic factors of yin nature

阳证 [yáng zhèng]

yang syndrome: a collective term for exterior, heat and excess syndromes with excitatory, hyperfunctional, restless or bright manifestations, or outward and upward symptoms, as well as diseases caused by pathogenic factors of yang nature

表里 [biǎo lǐ]

exterior and interior: parts of the body, the exterior referring to the skin and body hair, subcutaneous tissues, muscles and superficial meridians, and the interior referring to internal organs and bone marrow. An exogenous affliction only involving the exterior is usually milder than that penetrating into the interior.

表证 [biǎo zhèng]

exterior syndrome: a general term for syndromes that occur chiefly at the early stage of exogenous afflictions or acute infectious diseases invading the human body through the skin surface or respiratory tract and affecting the exterior part of the body

里证 [lǐ zhèng]

interior syndrome: a general term for syndromes that indicate the existence of disease in the *zang-fu* organs, *qi* and blood, or bone marrow

寒热 [hán rè]

(1) cold and heat: a pair of principles for differentiating the nature of disease; **(2) chills and fever**

寒证 [hán zhèng]

cold syndrome: a general term for syndromes caused either by exogenous cold factors or by insufficient yang within the body

热证 [rè zhèng]

heat syndrome: a general term for syndromes resulted either from yang prevalence or from yin deficiency

虚实 [xū shí]

deficiency (or insufficiency) and excess (or excessiveness): a pair of principles for determining the condition of the body resistance to pathogenic factors. Deficiency denotes insufficiency of normal *qi*, while excess indicates the presence of excessive pathogenic factors with intense body reaction or the accumulation of pathological products due to dysfunction of the internal organs

虚证 [xū zhèng]

deficiency syndrome: a general term for syndromes caused by insufficiency of normal *qi* (including yang *qi*, yin fluid, essence, blood, nutrients and defensive *qi*)

实证 [shí zhèng]

excess syndrome: a general term for syndromes caused by exogenous pathogenic factors or by accumulated pathological products due to dysfunction of internal organs, such as phlegm, retained fluid, stagnant blood, and undigested food

表寒 [biǎo hán]

exterior cold: (1) attack on the exterior part of the body by wind-cold; (2) abbreviation for exterior cold syndrome (表寒证 [biǎo hán zhèng])

表寒证 [biǎo hán zhèng]

exterior cold syndrome: a type of exterior syndrome in which the external part of the body is attacked by exogenous cold or wind, manifested by chills or aversion to cold or wind, headache, general aching or joint pains, thin and white tongue coating, and floating and tense pulse

表热 [biǎo rè]

exterior heat: (1) attack on the exterior part of the body by wind-heat; (2) abbreviation for exterior heat syndrome (表热证 [biǎo rè zhèng])

表热证 [biǎo rè zhèng]

exterior heat syndrome: a type of exterior syndrome in which the external part of the body is attacked by exogenous wind-heat, manifested by mild aversion to wind, moderate fever, headache, slight thirst, thin white or thin yellowish tongue coating or red tip of the tongue, and floating rapid pulse

表虚 [biǎo xū]

exterior deficiency: (1) deficiency of defense *qi* in the superficial part of the body, marked by spontaneous sweating or sweating accompanied by aversion to wind, and floating feeble pulse; (2) abbreviation for exterior deficiency syndrome (表虚证 [biǎo xū zhèng])

表虚证 [biǎo xū zhèng]

exterior deficiency syndrome: a type of exterior syndrome resulted from lowered superficial defense *qi*, and manifested by spontaneous sweating, intolerance of wind, and floating feeble pulse.

表实 [biǎo shí]

exterior excess: (1) invasion of exogenous pathogens that causes gathering of defense *qi* in the skin and muscles and blockage of the interstices and pores; (2) abbreviation for exterior excess syndrome (表实证 [biǎo shí zhèng])

表实证 [biǎo shí zhèng]

exterior excess syndrome: an exterior syndrome with forceful or tight floating pulse and no sweating, showing the external part of the body being attacked by exogenous pathogens, yet the patient's defense *qi* is not damaged

里寒 [lǐ hán]

interior cold: abbreviation for interior cold syndrome (里寒证 [lǐ hán zhèng])

里寒证 [lǐ hán zhèng]

interior cold syndrome: a type of interior syndrome caused either by endogenous cold, i.e., deficiency of yang or by exogenous cold transmitted to the interior of the body, mainly manifested by intolerance of cold, pallor, cold limbs, pale tongue with white moistened coating, and deep, slow or fine pulse

里虚寒证 [lǐ xū hán zhèng]

interior deficiency-cold syndrome: an interior cold syndrome resulting from yang deficiency

里热 [lǐ rè]

(1) heat in the interior: accumulation of heat in the internal organs, particularly in the stomach and intestines, in the lung and stomach, and in the liver and gallbladder; **(2) interior heat:** abbreviation for interior heat syndrome (里热证 [lǐ rè zhèng])

里热证 [lǐ rè zhèng]

interior heat syndrome: a type of interior syndrome caused by pathogenic heat in the internal organs, especially in the stomach, intestines, lung, liver and gallbladder, mainly manifested by fever, intolerance of heat, thirst, irritability, scanty and condensed urine, full, rapid and forceful or taut pulse, and reddened tongue with yellow coating

里虚热证 [lǐ xū rè zhèng]

interior deficiency-heat syndrome: interior heat syndrome resulting from yin deficiency

里虚 [lǐ xū]

interior deficiency: a general term for deficiency of *qi*, blood, yin, and yang of the internal organs

里实 [lǐ shí]

(1) excessiveness in the interior: a general term denoting accumulation of pathological products in the body, such as phlegm, retained fluid, stagnant *qi* and blood, intestinal parasites, and undigested food; **(2) interior excess:** abbreviation for interior excess syndrome 里实证 [lǐ shí zhèng]

里实证 [lǐ shí zhèng]

interior excess syndrome: (1) syndrome caused by accumulated heat in the stomach and intestines after an attack of exogenous pathogenic factors; (2) syndrome caused by retention of phlegm, blood stasis, accumulation of undigested food or parasitic worms

表里同病 [biǎo lǐ tóng bìng]

dual exterior-interior syndrome: (1) coexistence of exterior and interior syndromes; (2) syndrome involving both the exterior and the interior

表寒里热 [biǎo hán lǐ rè]

exterior cold and interior heat: (1) cold in the exterior and heat in the interior; (2) abbreviation for exterior cold and interior-heat syndrome (表寒里热证 [biǎo hán lǐ rè zhèng])

表寒里热证 [biǎo hán lǐ rè zhèng]

exterior-cold and interior-heat syndrome: a complicated condition seen either in cases with pre-existing internal heat and affected by exogenous cold and wind in addition, or in cases with the transformation of exogenous cold into heat after having penetrated into the interior of the body while the pathogenic cold in the exterior of the body is still present. Its main symptoms are coexistence of both exterior cold (chills and headache with no sweating) and interior heat (fever with irritability, thirst, scanty condensed urine, and constipation).

表热里寒 [biǎo rè lǐ hán]

exterior heat and interior cold: (1) heat in the exterior and cold in the interior; (2) abbreviation for exterior-heat and interior-cold syndrome (表热里寒证 [biǎo rè lǐ hán zhèng])

表热里寒证 [biǎo rè lǐ hán zhèng]

exterior-heat and interior-cold syndrome: jumbled case with pre-existing deficiency-cold of the spleen and stomach, affected by wind-heat, with symptoms showing the coexistence of exterior heat (fever, headache, and intolerance of wind) and internal cold (cold limbs, loose bowels, etc.)

表虚里实 [biǎo xū lǐ shí]

exterior deficiency and interior excess: (1) deficiency in the exterior and excessiveness in the interior; (2) abbreviation for exterior- deficiency and interior-excess syndrome (表虚里实证 [biǎo xū lǐ shí zhèng])

表虚里实证 [biǎo xū lǐ shí zhèng]

exterior-deficiency and interior-excess syndrome: jumbled case in which symptoms of exterior deficiency such as intolerance of wind and spontaneous sweating exist together with symptoms of interior excess such as abdominal pain with tenderness and constipation

表实里虚 [biǎo shí lǐ xū]

exterior excess and interior deficiency: (1) excess in the exterior and deficiency in the interior; (2) abbreviation for exterior-excess and interior-deficiency syndrome (表实里虚证 [biǎo shí lǐ xū zhèng])

表实里虚证 [biǎo shí lǐ xū zhèng]

exterior-excess and interior-deficiency syndrome: jumbled case in which symptoms of exterior excess such as chills, headache and general aching exist together with symptoms of interior deficiency such as anorexia, lassitude, palpitation, and shortness of breath, usually seen in chronic disease complicated with new exogenous affliction

表里出入 [biǎo lǐ chū rù]

transmission between exterior and interior: transmission of the pathogen in the course of a disease from the exterior to the interior part of the body and vice versa

由表入里 [yóu biǎo rù lǐ]

penetration from the exterior into the interior: development of a disease with the pathogen penetrating from the exterior to the interior of the body

由里出表 [yóu lǐ chū biǎo]

recession from the interior to exterior: process of a disease where the pathogen goes from the interior out to the body surface, e.g., appearance of skin eruption followed by abatement of fever in the course of measles, indicating improvement of the case

表热传里 [biǎo rè chuán lǐ]

transmission of exterior heat into the interior: process of a disease where interior heat syndrome develops along with disappearance of exterior heat symptoms, also known as transmission of pathogenic heat into the interior (热邪传里 [rè xié chuán lǐ])

热邪传里 [rè xié chuán lǐ]

transmission of pathogenic heat into the interior: another way of saying transmission of exterior heat into the interior (表热传里 [biǎo rè chuán lǐ])

寒热转化 [hán rè zhuǎn huà]

conversion of cold and heat: conversion of a cold syndrome into a heat syndrome, and vice versa

入里化热 [rù lǐ huà rè]

conversion into heat after penetration into the interior: transformation of exogenous pathogenic factors into heat after having penetrated into the interior of the body

半表半里 [bàn biǎo bàn lǐ]

half-exterior and half-interior: (1) location between the exterior and the interior; (2) abbreviation for half-exterior and half-interior syndrome (半表半里证 [bàn biǎo bàn lǐ zhèng])

半表半里证 [bàn biǎo bàn lǐ zhèng]

half-exterior and half-interior syndrome: syndrome due to affliction located between the exterior and interior of the body, marked by alternate fever and chills, fullness and choking feeling in the chest and costal region, bitter taste in the mouth, dry throat, nausea and loss of appetite, and taut pulse. The *shaoyang* meridian syndrome belongs to this category.

上寒下热 [shàng hán xià rè]

upper cold and lower heat: (1) cold in the upper and heat in the lower part of the body; (2) abbreviation for upper-cold and lower-heat syndrome (上寒下热证 [shàng hán xià rè zhèng])

上寒下热证 [shàng hán xià rè zhèng]

upper-cold and lower-heat syndrome: jumbled case in which cold symptoms in the upper (e.g. aversion to cold, nausea and vomiting) exist together with heat symptoms in the lower (e.g. constipation, scanty and condensed urine)

上热下寒 [shàng rè xià hán]

upper heat and lower cold: (1) heat in the upper and cold in the lower part of the body; (2) abbreviation for upper-heat and lower-cold syndrome (上热下寒证 [shàng rè xià hán zhèng])

上热下寒证 [shàng rè xià hán zhèng]

upper-heat and lower-cold syndrome: jumbled case in which heat symptoms in the upper (e.g., acid regurgitation with annoying sensation of heat in the chest) appear simultaneously with cold symptoms in the lower (e.g., loose stool and abdominal pain which can be eased by warmth)

上虚下实 [shàng xū xià shí]

upper deficiency and lower excess: abbreviation for upper-deficiency and lower-excess syndrome 上虚下实证 [shàng xū xià shí zhèng]

上虚下实证 [shàng xū xià shí zhèng]

upper-deficiency and lower-excess syndrome: jumbled case with deficiency of normal *qi* in the upper and preponderance of pathogenic factors in the lower part of the body, e.g., a case of cardiac palpitation due to heart insufficiency complicated by damp-heat dysentery

上实下虚 [shàng shí xià xū]

upper excess and lower deficiency: abbreviation for upper-excess and lower-deficiency syndrome (上实下虚证 [shàng shí xià xū zhèng])

上实下虚证 [shàng shí xià xū zhèng]

upper-excess and lower-deficiency syndrome: jumbled case with deficiency of normal *qi* in the lower and preponderance of pathogenic factors in the upper part of the body, e.g., a case of lumbago, weakened legs and nocturnal emission due to kidney insufficiency associated with dizziness, headache and irritability resulting from exuberant liver *qi*

虚中夹实 [xū zhōng jiá shí]

deficiency complicated by excess: deficiency syndrome complicated by excess symptoms while the former is dominant, e.g., a case of consumptive disease with emaciation and other deficiency symptoms complicated by blood stasis with amenorrhea

实中夹虚 [shí zhōng jiá xū]

excess complicated by deficiency: excess syndrome complicated by deficiency symptoms while the former is dominant, e.g., a case of ascites with abdominal distension complicated by emaciation, lassitude, loss of appetite and other deficiency symptoms

虚寒 [xū hán]

deficiency-cold: (1) cold of deficiency type, usually resulting from yang deficiency; (2) abbreviation of deficiency-cold syndrome (虚寒证 [xū hán zhèng]

虚寒证 [xū hán zhèng]

deficiency-cold syndrome: a cold syndrome caused by deficiency of yang, marked by intolerance of cold, epigastric or abdominal pain which can be relieved by heat and pressure, loose bowels, fine thready pulse, and profuse whitish and thin leukorrhea in women

虚热 [xū rè]

(1) deficiency-heat: an abbreviation of deficiency-heat syndrome (虚热证 [xū rè zhèng])； **(2) fever of deficiency type:** fever caused by deficiency of yin, blood or *qi*

虚热证 [xū rè zhèng]

deficiency-heat syndrome: a heat syndrome resulting from deficiency of normal *qi* or impairment of normal *qi* by excessive pathogenic factors

虚火 [xū huǒ]

deficiency-fire: (1) fire syndrome caused by consumption of yin, marked by afternoon fever, heat sensation in the palms and soles, thirst, night sweat, reddened tongue, and fine, rapid pulse; (2) pseudo-heat symptoms resulting from rejection of yang by excess of yin

虚火证 [xū huǒ zhèng]

deficiency-fire syndrome: an abbreviation of 阴虚火旺证 [yīn xū huǒ wàng zhèng]

实寒 [shí hán]

excess cold: (1) cold of excess type; (2) abbreviation of excess-cold syndrome (实寒证 [shí hán zhèng])

实寒证 [shí hán zhèng]

excess-cold syndrome: a syndrome caused by pathogenic cold accumulated in the interior of the body, marked by aversion to cold, cold limbs, abdominal pain, constipation, absence of thirst, whitish thick or greasy coating of the tongue, and deep, taut and forceful pulse

实热 [shí rè]

excess heat: (1) heat of excess type; (2) abbreviation of excess-heat syndrome (实热证 [shí rè zhèng])

实热证 [shí rè zhèng]

excess-heat syndrome: a heat syndrome caused by excessive pathogenic factors while the body resistance is still sufficient, with intense reaction, marked by high fever with restlessness, constipation, and gigantic or slippery and rapid pulse

实火 [shí huǒ]

excess fire: (1) fire of excess type; (2) abbreviation of excess-fire syndrome (实火证 [shí huǒ zhèng])

实火证 [shí huǒ zhèng]

excess-fire syndrome: fire syndrome caused by excessive pathogenic factors, usually marked by blood-shot eyes, bitterness in the mouth, thirst, irritability, constipation, reddened tongue with yellow coating, and gigantic rapid pulse

火热炽盛证 [huǒ rè chì shèng zhèng]

exuberant fire-heat syndrome: a synonym for excess-fire syndrome (实火证 [shí huǒ zhèng]) and excess-heat syndrome (实热证 [shí rè zhèng])

阴虚 [yīn xū]

yin deficiency: (1) consumption of yin fluid, usually associated with internal heat and dryness; (2) an abbreviation of yin deficiency syndrome (阴虚证 [yīn xū zhèng])

阴虚证 [yīn xū zhèng]

yin deficiency syndrome: a syndrome resulting from insufficiency of yin fluid, incapable of restraining yang and usually manifested by afternoon fever, night sweats, malar flush, vexing heat sensation in the palms and soles, dryness of the mouth and throat, reddened tongue with scanty coating, and fine, rapid pulse

阴液亏虚证 [yīn yè kuī xū zhèng]

yin-fluid insufficiency syndrome: a synonym for yin deficiency syndrome (阴虚证 [yīn xū zhèng])

阳虚 [yáng xū]

yang deficiency: (1) insufficiency of yang *qi*, usually associated with decline of warming, driving and moving actions; (2) abbreviation for yang deficiency syndrome (阳虚证 [yáng xū zhèng])

阳虚证 [yáng xū zhèng]

yang deficiency syndrome: a syndrome resulting from deficiency of yang *qi*, usually accompanied by cold symptoms, marked by pallor, intolerance of cold, cold extremities, loose bowels, pale tongue, and feeble pulse

伤阴 [shāng yīn]

damage to yin: impairment of yin, especially that of the liver and kidney in advanced cases of febrile disease, usually manifested as low fever, heat sensation in the palms and soles, emaciation, thirst, malar flush, dry and scarlet red tongue, and fine, feeble and rapid pulse

伤津 [shāng jīn]

damage to fluid: impairment of body fluid, especially that of the lung and the stomach, usually manifested as thirst, dry cough, irritability, scanty urine, and constipation

伤阳 [shāng yáng]

damage to yang: impairment of yang, resulting from various causes such as excessive use of cold-nature drugs, attack of cold on meridians, usually manifested as aversion to cold, cold extremities and other symptoms of yang deficiency

亡阴 [wáng yīn]

yin exhaustion; yin collapse: excessive loss of essence and fluid due to high fever, profuse sweating, vomiting, diarrhea, bleeding, or other consumptive conditions

亡阴证 [wáng yīn zhèng]

yin-exhaustion syndrome: serious syndrome resulting from exhaustion of yin fluid, manifested by thirst and craving for cold drink, flushed face, restlessness, dry tongue and thready, swift pulse

阴脱证 [yīn tuō zhèng]

yin-collapse syndrome: a synonym for yin-exhaustion syndrome (亡阴证 [wáng yīn zhèng])

亡阳 [wáng yáng]

yang exhaustion; yang collapse: a critical condition seen in cases of high fever, profuse perspiration, drastic vomiting and diarrhea, massive bleeding, etc., manifested as dripping of cold sweat, intolerance of cold, cold limbs, exceedingly feeble pulse or rapid, floating and void pulse

亡阳证 [wáng yáng zhèng]

yang-exhaustion syndrome: a serious syndrome resulting from exhaustion of yang *qi*, manifested as pallor, dripping of cold sweat, cold limbs, pale and moistened tongue, and hardly perceptible pulse

阳脱证 [yáng tuō zhèng]

yang-collapse syndrome: a synonym for yang-exhaustion syndrome (亡阳证 [wáng yáng zhèng])

阴证似阳 [yīn zhèng sì yáng]

yin syndrome resembling yang: yin syndrome that appears as a yang syndrome, e.g., an advanced case of yin deficiency showing pseudo-heat symptoms such as feeling hot and thirsty

阳证似阴 [yáng zhèng sì yīn]

yang syndrome resembling yin: yang syndrome that appears as a yin syndrome, e.g., a severe case of febrile disease showing pseudo-cold symptoms such as intolerance of cold and cold limbs

假寒 [jiǎ hán]

pseudo-cold: apparent cold symptom in cases of diseases caused by heat. The patient is intolerant of cold but dislikes to be thickly covered; has cold limbs though the chest and abdomen feel hot.

假热 [jiǎ rè]

pseudo-heat: apparent heat symptom in cases of diseases caused by cold. The patient feels hot yet wishes to be thickly covered, feels thirsty yet drinks little, moves restlessly yet is mentally quiescent.

真寒假热 [zhēn hán jiǎ rè]

true cold with false heat: cold syndrome with pseudo-heat symptoms

真热假寒 [zhēn rè jiǎ hán]

true heat with false cold: heat syndrome with pseudo-cold symptoms

真实假虚 [zhēn shí jiǎ xū]

true excess with false deficiency: excess syndrome with pseudo-deficiency symptoms, e.g., accumulation of damp-heat presenting such signs as lack of strength and weak limbs, also known as "great excessiveness looking like debilitation" (大实如羸状 [dà shí rú léi zhuàng])

真虚假实 [zhēn xū jiǎ shí]

true deficiency with false excess: deficiency syndrome with pseudo-excess symptoms, e.g., severe decline of *zang-fu* functions with such manifestations as abdominal distension, panting and constipation, also known as "extreme insufficiency present signs of exuberance" 至虚有盛候 [zhì xū yǒu shèng hòu]

常用引文 Commonly Used Citations

寒极似热。[hán jí sì rè]

Extreme cold resembles heat.

热极似寒。[rè jí sì hán]

Extreme heat resembles cold.

邪气盛则实。[xié qì shèng zé shí]

Where pathogenic *qi* is exuberant, there is excess.

精气夺则虚。[jīng qì duó zé xū]

Where essential *qi* is despoiled, there is deficiency.

大实如羸状。[dà shí rú léi zhuàng]

Great excessiveness looks like debilitation. cf. 真实假虚 [zhēn shí jiǎ xū]

至虚有盛候。[zhì xū yǒu shèng hòu]

Extreme insufficiency presents signs of exuberance. cf. 真虚假实 [zhēn xū jiǎ shí]

揆度奇恒。[kuí duó qí héng]

observe and judge by the general and particular

六经辨证

Six-meridian Syndrome Differentiation (Six-meridian Pattern Identification)

六经辨证 [liù jīng biàn zhèng]

six-meridian syndrome differentiation; six-meridian pattern identification: differentiation of syndromes (or identification of patterns) in accordance with the theory of the six meridians, applied to the diagnosis of acute febrile diseases at different stages, but also useful for the syndrome differentiation (or pattern identification) of other diseases

六经病证 [liù jīng bìng zhèng]

diseases (or syndromes) of the six meridians: a collective term for diseases (or syndromes) of *taiyang*, *yangming*, *shaoyang*, *taiyin*, *shaoyin* and *jueyin* meridians

太阳病证 [tài yáng bìng zhèng]

taiyang **(greater yang) disease;** ***taiyang*** **syndrome:** disease (or syndrome) characterized by attack of pathogenic wind-cold to the body surface and struggle between the normal and pathogenic factors at the exterior portion of the body

太阳经证 [tài yáng jīng zhèng]

taiyang **(greater yang) meridian syndrome:** one of the syndromes of the six meridians due to attack of pathogenic wind-cold to the *taiyang* meridian of the body surface, usually seen in the initial stage of the contraction, marked by chills and fever, pain in the head and neck, and floating pulse, also known as 太阳经病 [tài yáng jīng bìng]

太阳经病 [tài yáng jīng bìng]

taiyang **(greater yang) meridian disease,** same as 太阳经证 [tài yáng jīng zhèng]

太阳腑证 [tài yáng fǔ zhèng]

taiyang fu**-organ syndrome:** a syndrome in which the urinary bladder (*taiyang fu*-organ) is attacked by the pathogen in an unrelieved *taiyang* meridian syndrome, also known as 太阳腑病 [tài yáng fǔ bìng]

太阳腑病 [tài yáng fǔ bìng]

taiyang fu**-organ disease,** same as 太阳腑证 [tài yáng fǔ zhèng]

太阳蓄水证 [tài yáng xù shuǐ zhèng]

taiyang **water-retention syndrome:** a type of *taiyang fu*-organ syndrome in which the pathogen penetrates and causes retention of water in the bladder, manifested as fever and chills, oliguria, lower abdominal fullness, vomiting immediately after drinking, floating or floating and rapid pulse

太阳蓄血证 [tài yáng xù xuè zhèng]

taiyang **blood-retention syndrome:** a type of *taiyang fu*-organ syndrome in which the pathogen combines with blood and remains in the lower abdomen, manifested as lower abdominal cramps or fullness with rigidity, polyuria, delirium, amnesia, dark stool, and sunken and choppy or sunken and knotted pulse

阳明病证 [yáng míng bìng zhèng]

yangming **(splendid yang) disease;** ***yangming*** **syndrome:** syndrome marked by exuberant yang and dryness-heat in the stomach and intestines occurring in the course of a cold-induced febrile disease

阳明经证 [yáng míng jīng zhèng]

yangming **meridian syndrome:** syndrome caused by exuberant pathogenic heat flooding the *yangming* meridian and spreading over the body but not yet inducing constipation, characteristically manifested as high fever without chills, profuse sweating, dire thirst, and full and gigantic pulse, also known as 阳明经病 [yáng míng jīng bìng]

阳明经病 [yáng míng jīng bìng]

***yangming* meridian disease,** same as 阳明经证 [yáng míng jīng zhèng]

阳明腑证 [yáng míng fǔ zhèng]

***yangming fu*-organ syndrome:** syndrome caused by accumulation of pathogenic heat in the stomach and large intestine, manifested by tidal fever in the afternoon, abdominal pain and tenderness, constipation, deep and forceful pulse, or even delirium, also known as 阳明腑病 [yáng míng fǔ bìng]

阳明腑病 [yáng míng fǔ bìng]

***yangming* fu-organ disease,** same as 阳明腑证 [yáng míng fǔ zhèng]

少阳病证 [shào yáng bìng zhèng]

***shaoyang* (lesser yang) disease; *shaoyang* (lesser yang) syndrome:** disease or syndrome in which the pathogenic heat exists between the exterior and interior of the body, marked by alternate fever and chills, fullness and choking feeling in the chest and hypochondriac region, dry throat, and taut pulse

太阴病证 [tài yīn bìng zhèng]

***taiyin* (greater yin) disease; *taiyin* (greater yin) syndrome:** disease or syndrome characterized by decline of spleen yang with production of cold-damp in the interior, and manifested by abdominal fullness and sometimes abdominal pain, vomiting and diarrhea, anorexia, sunken and relaxed or weak pulse

少阴病证 [shào yīn bìng zhèng]

***shaoyin* disease; *shaoyin* syndrome:** syndrome occurring at the late stage of a cold-induced disease marked by general decline of yin and yang

少阴寒化 [shào yīn hán huà]

***shaoyin* cold transformation:** decline of yang in *shaoyin* syndrome with transformation of the pathogen into yin cold in the interior

少阴寒化证 [shào yīn hán huà zhèng]

***shaoyin* cold-transformation syndrome:** *shaoyin* syndrome with cold transformation of the pathogen which invades the heart and kidney, usually manifested as aversion to cold, cold limbs, sleepiness, lienteric diarrhea, pale tongue and deep faint pulse

少阴热化 [shào yīn rè huà]

***shaoyin* heat transformation:** decline of yin with exuberance of yang in *shaoyin* syndrome with transformation of the pathogen into heat in the interior

少阴热化证 [shào yīn rè huà zhèng]

***shaoyin* heat-transformation syndrome:** *shaoyin* syndrome with heat transformation of the pathogen, manifested by vexation, insomnia, dry mouth and throat, reddened tongue tip, and thready rapid pulse

厥阴病证 [jué yīn bìng zhèng]

***jueyin* (reverting yin) disease; *jueyin* (reverting yin) syndrome:** one of the syndromes of the six meridians occurring at the late stage of a cold-induced disease characterized by interweaving of cold and heat or yin and yang, manifested by fever or a burning sensation in the epigastrium with cold limbs, hunger but no desire to eat

经证 [jīng zhèng]

meridian syndrome: morbid condition of any of the three yang meridians due to attack of pathogenic factors while the related *fu*-organ is not affected

腑证 [fǔ zhèng]

***fu*-organ syndrome:** morbid condition indicating that pathological changes of one or more yang meridians have already affected the respective internal organs: the urinary bladder (*taiyang*), the stomach and large intestine (*yangming*), and the gallbladder (*shaoyang*)

并病 [bìng bìng]

overlapping of syndromes: overlapping of two meridian syndromes, in which they appear in succession and then coexist

二阳并病 [èr yáng bìng bìng]

two-yang overlapping: overlapping of two yang meridian syndromes, e.g., *shaoyang* syndrome (vomiting and fullness in the chest) appearing before the subsidence of *taiyang* syndrome (headache, chills, fever and joint pains)

合病 [hé bìng]

combined syndrome: combination of two or more meridian syndromes appearing at the same time

太阳与少阳合病 [tài yáng yǔ shào yáng hé bìng]

***taiyang-shaoyang* combined syndrome:** simultaneous occurrence of *taiyang* syndrome (headache and fever) and *shaoyang* syndrome (bitterness in the mouth, dry throat, and dizziness)

太阳与阳明合病 [tài yáng yǔ yáng míng hé bìng]

***taiyang-yangming* combined syndrome:** simultaneous occurrence of *taiyang* syndrome (headache and neck rigidity) and *yangming* syndrome (fever and thirst)

阳明与少阳合病 [yáng míng yǔ shào yáng hé bìng]

***yangming-shaoyang* combined syndrome:** simultaneous occurrence of *yangming* syndrome (fever and thirst) and *shaoyang* syndrome (bitterness in the mouth, dry throat, and fullness in the chest)

三阳合病 [sān yáng hé bìng]

three-yang combined syndrome: syndrome caused by transmission of pathogenic heat into the *yangming* meridian from both *taiyang* and *shaoyang* meridians, resulting in a distinctive heat syndrome manifested by fever, thirst, perspiration, abdominal distension, utter loss of appetite, delirium, and incontinence of urine

循经传 [xún jīng chuán]

sequential meridian transmission: transmission of a disease from one meridian to another, by the order of *taiyang*, *yangming*, *shaoyang*, *taiyin*, *shaoyin* and *jueyin*

越经传 [yuè jīng chuán]

skip-over meridian transmission: transmission of a disease from one meridian to another with skipping of one or more meridians, e.g., transmission from *taiyang* to *shaoyang* with *yangming* skipped over

表里传 [biǎo lǐ chuán]

exterior-interior transmission: transmission of a disease between two exterior-interiorly related meridians, e.g., *taiyang* and *shaoyin*, *yangming* and *taiyin*, *shaoyang* and *jueyin*

传经 [chuán jīng]

meridian transmission: transmission of a disease from one meridian to another, with respective change of syndrome

传变 [chuán biàn]

transmission and change: development of a disease, particularly referring to a cold-induced disease

不传 [bù chuán]

non-transmission: no further development of a cold-induced disease

变证 [biàn zhèng]

deteriorated syndrome: deterioration of a case due to improper medication or weakened body resistance

直中 [zhí zhōng]

direct attack: attack of exogenous pathogen directly to the three yin meridians instead of transmission from the yang meridians

卫气营血辨证

Defense-*Qi*-Nutrient-Blood Syndrome Differentiation (Four-aspect Pattern Identification)

卫气营血辨证 [wèi qì yíng xuè biàn zhèng]

defense-*qi*-nutrient-blood syndrome differentiation; four-aspect pattern identification: syndrome differentiation or pattern identification of epidemic febrile diseases in accordance with the theory of defense, *qi*, nutrient and blood which indicate the stages of the clinical course with corresponding pathological changes

卫分证 [wèi fèn zhèng]

defense (*wei*) system syndrome; defense-aspect pattern: the initial stage of an epidemic febrile disease when only the superficial part of the defensive energy is involved, marked by fever, slightly aversion to wind and cold, headache, reddened tongue tip, and floating and rapid pulse

气分证 [qì fèn zhèng]

***qi* system syndrome; *qi*-aspect pattern:** the second stage of an epidemic febrile disease showing invasion of pathogenic heat to the *yangming* meridian or the lung, gallbladder, spleen, stomach or large intestine, marked by high fever without chills, dire thirst, flushed face, dark urine, reddened tongue with yellow coating, and rapid forceful pulse

营分证 [yíng fèn zhèng]

nutrient (*ying*) system syndrome; construction-aspect pattern: serious development of an epidemic febrile disease showing invasion of pathogenic heat to the nutrient yin (or construction aspect) including that of the heart (mind), marked by fever (higher at night), restlessness or delirium, faint skin rashes, and crimson tongue

血分证 [xuè fèn zhèng]

blood system syndrome; blood-aspect pattern: epidemic febrile disease at its severest stage, characterized by severe damage to yin blood, with various forms of bleeding such as hemoptysis, epistaxis, hematuria, hematochezia, in addition to high fever, coma, or convulsion

血热动血 [xuè rè dòng xuè]

blood-heat stirring wind: (1) a pathological change characterized by blood heat causing frenetic movement of blood; (2) abbreviation for syndrome of blood heat stirring blood (血热动血证 [xuè rè dòng xuè zhèng])

血热动血证 [xuè rè dòng xuè zhèng]

syndrome of blood heat stirring blood: a syndrome marked by fever, thirst, vexing insomnia, crimson tongue, and various hemorrhagic disorders

血热风盛 [xuè rè fēng shèng]

blood heat with raging wind: (1) a pathological change characterized by extremely exuberant pathogenic heat which enters the blood system and stirs up violent wind; (2) abbreviation for syndrome of blood heat with raging wind (血热风盛证 [xuè rè fēng shèng zhèng])

血热风盛证 [xuè rè fēng shèng zhèng]

syndrome of blood heat with raging wind: a syndrome marked by high fever, convulsions, opisthotonos, crimson tongue with dry yellow coating, and rapid wiry pulse

血热化燥 [xuè rè huà zào]

blood heat transforming into dryness: (1) a pathological change in which the pathogenic heat entering the blood, impairs yin and induces dryness transformation; (2) abbreviated expression for syndrome of blood heat with dryness transformation (血热化燥证 [xuè rè huà zào zhèng])

血热化燥证 [xuè rè huà zào zhèng]

syndrome of blood heat with dryness transformation: a syndrome marked by dry mouth and throat, constipation, lassitude, fever (higher at night), thirst with not much desire to drink, crimson tongue with scanty coating, and rapid thready pulse

热入营血 [rè rù yíng xuè]

heat entering nutrient-blood: (1) a pathological change characterized by pathogenic heat entering the nutrient-blood and disturbing the heart (mind); (2) abbreviation for syndrome of heat entering nutrient-blood (热入营血证 [rè rù yíng xuè zhèng])

热入营血证 [rè rù yíng xuè zhèng]

syndrome of heat entering nutrient-blood: a syndrome marked by fever (higher at night), vexing insomnia or impaired consciousness, barely visible skin rashes or bleeding, constipation, crimson tongue, and rapid thready pulse

卫气同病证 [wèi qì tóng bìng zhèng]

both defense and *qi* affection syndrome: a condition characterized by the coexistence of syndromes of the defense (*wei*) and *qi* systems, manifested as high fever, slight aversion to wind and cold, thirst, irritability, reddened tongue with whitish or yellowish coating, and rapid floating pulse

气营两燔证 [qì yíng liǎng fān zhèng]

both *qi* and nutrient blazing syndrome: a condition characterized by simultaneous existence of syndromes of *qi* and nutrient systems, manifested as high fever, thirst, mental irritability, delirium and barely visible skin eruption

气血两燔证 [qì xuè liǎng fān zhèng]

both *qi* and blood blazing syndrome: a condition characterized by the coexistence of syndromes of the *qi* and blood systems, manifested as high fever, thirst, delirium, skin eruptions, and various bleeding symptoms

顺传 [shùn chuán]

normal transmission: transmission of a disease in the normal sequence, e.g., from the defense (*wei*) system to the *qi* system

逆传 [nì chuán]

abnormal transmission: transmission of a disease not in the normal sequence, e.g., from the defense (*wei*) system directly to the nutrient (*ying*) system and blood system, instead of by way of the *qi* system

三焦辨证

Triple-Energizer Syndrome Differentiation (Triple-Energizer Pattern Identification)

三焦辨证 [sān jiāo biàn zhèng]

triple-energizer syndrome differentiation; triple-energizer pattern

identification: syndrome differentiation or pattern identification in accordance with the theory of the triple energizer

上焦病证 [shàng jiāo bìng zhèng]

upper-energizer syndrome: syndrome due to invasion of pathogen to the lung meridian at the early stage of an epidemic febrile disease, marked by chills and fever, sweating, headache, and cough, or on the pericardium meridian marked by delirium, and deep red tongue

中焦病证 [zhōng jiāo bìng zhèng]

middle-energizer syndrome: syndrome due to invasion of pathogen to the stomach meridian at the middle stage of epidemic febrile disease, marked by fever without chills, sweating, thirst, and full pulse, or on the spleen meridian marked by continuous moderate fever, aching and heavy feeling in the body, stuffiness in the chest with nausea and vomiting, and greasy tongue coating

下焦病证 [xià jiāo bìng zhèng]

lower-energizer syndrome: syndrome due to impairment of the kidney meridian at the later stage of an epidemic febrile disease, manifested as fever (more remarkable in the palms than on the back of hands), thirst, parched lips and restlessness, or due to impairment of the liver meridian manifested as mental disorders, twitching or convulsion

气血辨证

Qi-Blood Syndrome Differentiation (*Qi*-Blood Pattern Identification)

气血辨证 [qì xuè biàn zhèng]

***qi*-blood syndrome differentiation; *qi*-blood pattern identification:** differentiation of syndromes or identification of patterns according to the state of *qi* and blood

气虚 [qì xū]

***qi* deficiency:** (1) a general term denoting the decline of *qi* activity manifested by shortness of breath, weak voice, lassitude, listlessness and sweating upon mild exertion, mostly caused by overfatigue or protracted illness; (2) term particularly denoting deficiency of lung *qi*; (3) abbreviation for *qi* deficiency syndrome (气虚证 [qì xū zhèng])

气虚证 [qì xū zhèng]

***qi* deficiency syndrome:** syndrome of insufficiency of genuine *qi* with diminished function of the internal organs, marked by shortness of breath, lassitude, listlessness, spontaneous sweating, pale tongue, and pulse of deficiency type

血虚 [xuè xū]

blood deficiency: a morbid condition characterized by insufficiency of blood to nourish organs, tissues and meridians, usually resulting from profuse bleeding or chronic hemorrhage, or impaired blood production due to diminished function of the internal organs, especially the spleen

血虚证 [xuè xū zhèng]

blood deficiency syndrome: syndrome marked by pale or sallow complexion, pale lips and nails, dizziness, dimmed vision, palpitation, numbness of extremities, and thready pulse

气血两虚 [qì xuè liǎng xū]

***qi*-blood dual deficiency:** (1) diminished supply of both *qi* and blood to the body, also called 气血两亏 [qì xuè liǎng kuī]; (2) abbreviation for *qi*-blood dual deficiency syndrome (气血两虚证 [qì xuè liǎng xū zhèng])

气血两亏 [qì xuè liǎng kuī]

***qi*-blood dual insufficiency,** same as *qi*-blood dual deficiency (气血两虚 [qì xuè liǎng xū])

气血两虚证 [qì xuè liǎng xū zhèng]

***qi*-blood dual deficiency syndrome:** a syndrome marked by listlessness, lack of strength, shortness of breath, pale or sallow complexion, dizziness, dimmed vision, pale lips and nails, palpitation, insomnia, pale tongue, and weak pulse

气郁 [qì yù]

***qi* depression:** (1) a morbid condition often caused by emotional depression involving liver *qi*; (2) abbreviation for *qi* depression syndrome (气郁证 [qì yù zhèng])

气郁证 [qì yù zhèng]

***qi* depression syndrome:** a syndrome marked by a feeling of distension in the chest, pain in the hypochondriac region, irritability, irascibility, anorexia, and menstrual disorders in women

气滞 [qì zhì]

***qi* stagnation:** (1) a pathological change characterized by impeded circulation of *qi* that leads to a local obstruction, manifested as distension or pain in the affected part; (2) abbreviation for *qi* stagnation syndrome

(气滞证 [qì zhì zhèng])

气滞证 [qì zhì zhèng]

***qi* stagnation syndrome:** a syndrome resulting from stagnation of *qi*, marked by thoracic, hypochondriac, epigastric and abdominal distention or pain, on and off, often ameliorated by sighing or belching

气滞血瘀 [qì zhì xuè yū]

(1) *qi* stagnation and blood stasis: coexistence of *qi* stagnation and blood stasis; **(2) *qi* stagnation with blood stasis:** a morbid condition in which long-standing stagnation of *qi* leads to blood stasis, marked by aggravation of local pain with tenderness, and even formation of mass

气滞血瘀证 [qì zhì xuè yū zhèng]

***qi*-stagnation blood-stasis syndrome:** a syndrome resulting from *qi* stagnation and blood stasis, marked by a scurrying or stabbing pain in the thoracic, hypochondriac, epigastric or abdominal region with or without mass formation, purple tongue or purple-spotted tongue, wiry and choppy pulse, also called 气血瘀滞证 [qì xuè yū zhì zhèng]

气血瘀滞证 [qì xuè yū zhì zhèng]

***qi*-blood-stagnation syndrome,** same as *qi*-stagnation blood-stasis syndrome (气滞血瘀证 [qì zhì xuè yū zhèng])

气虚血瘀 [qì xū xuè yū]

***qi* deficiency and blood stasis:** (1) a morbid condition characterized by coexistence of *qi* deficiency and blood stasis; (2) a morbid condition in which deficiency of *qi* leads to blood stasis

气虚血瘀证 [qì xū xuè yū zhèng]

syndrome of *qi* deficiency and blood stasis: a syndrome marked by manifestations of blood stasis such as stabbing pain fixed in location together with listlessness, lassitude, shortness of breath and sweating upon mild exertion showing *qi* deficiency

津液辨证

Body-fluid Syndrome Differentiation (Body-fluid Pattern Identification)

津液辨证 [jīn yè biàn zhèng]

body-fluid syndrome differentiation; body-fluid pattern identification: differentiation of syndromes or identification of patterns according to the condition of body fluids

津液亏虚证 [jīn yè kuī xū zhèng]

fluid insufficiency syndrome: a syndrome marked by dry mouth and throat, parched or cracked lips, thirst with desire to drink, oliguria, constipation, reddened tongue lacking moisture, and rapid thready weak pulse

脏腑津亏 [zàng fǔ jīn kuī]

fluid insufficiency of *zang-fu* organs: a general term for fluid insufficiency involving various *zang-fu* organs

肺津亏损 [fèi jīn kuī sǔn]

lung fluid consumption: a morbid condition characterized by insufficiency fluid in the lung

肺燥津伤证 [fèi zào jīn shāng zhèng]

lung fluid consumption syndrome: a syndrome marked by dryness of the nose and mouth, dry cough with hoarseness, and dry tongue coating

胃津亏损 [wèi jīn kuī sǔn]

stomach fluid consumption: a morbid condition characterized by insufficient fluid in the stomach

胃燥津亏证 [wèi zào jīn kuī zhèng]

stomach fluid insufficiency syndrome: a syndrome marked by dry lips and mouth, retching, constipation, emaciation, and absence of tongue coating

大肠津亏 [dà cháng jīn kuī]

large intestinal fluid insufficiency: a morbid condition characterized by insufficient fluid in the large intestine, often seen in the aged, postpartum women or at the late stage of a febrile disease

肠燥津亏证 [cháng zào jīn kuī zhèng]

large intestinal fluid insufficiency syndrome: a syndrome marked by constipation, dry throat and fidgetiness

津亏血燥 [jīn kuī xuè zào]

fluid insufficiency with concentrated blood: a morbid condition marked by withered skin, dry throat, thirst, oliguria, reddened tongue without saliva, thready and rapid pulse

津亏热结 [jīn kuī rè jié]

fluid insufficiency with retained heat: a morbid condition characterized by insufficiency of fluid with retention of heat in the interior

津亏热结证 [jīn kuī rè jié zhèng]

syndrome of fluid insufficiency with retained heat: a syndrome marked by fever, thirst, dry lips and tongue, oliguria, constipation, restlessness, reddened tongue with yellow coating, and rapid pulse

津亏火炽 [jīn kuī huǒ chì]

fluid insufficiency with exuberant fire: a morbid condition marked by fever, fidgetiness, insomnia, dry and sore throat, constipation, reddened tongue and thready, rapid pulse

饮证 [yǐn zhèng]

retained-fluid syndrome: abbreviation for syndrome of interior retention of water-fluid (水饮内停证 [shuǐ yǐn nèi tíng zhèng])

水饮内停证 [shuǐ yǐn nèi tíng zhèng]

interior retention of water-fluid syndrome: a syndrome marked by dizziness, thoracic and epigastric stuffy sensation, vomiting of clear fluid, slippery tongue coating, and wiry pulse

饮停心包证 [yǐn tíng xīn bāo zhèng]

retained fluid in pericardium syndrome: a syndrome marked by palpitation, orthopnea with fullness and stuffy sensation in the heart and chest, pale purplish tongue with white slippery coating, and hidden or weak pulse

饮停胸胁证 [yǐn tíng xiōng xié zhèng]

syndrome of retained fluid in the chest and hypochondrium: a syndrome marked by fullness and stuffy sensation in the chest, cough, dyspnea, white slippery tongue coating, and wiry and slippery pulse

寒饮内停证 [hán yǐn nèi tíng zhèng]

syndrome of interior retention of cold-fluid: a syndrome marked by aversion to cold with cool limbs, cough with frothy expectoration, or dizziness with palpitation and suffocating sensation, or epigastric stuffiness with vomiting of clear fluid, or costal and hypochondriac distention, plump tongue with white slippery coating, and wiry slippery pulse

寒饮停肺证 [hán yǐn tíng fèi zhèng]

syndrome of retention of cold-fluid in the lung: a syndrome marked by cough, dyspnea, wheezing or orthopnea, thin whitish sputum, white slippery tongue coating, and wiry pulse

寒饮停胃证 [hán yǐn tíng wèi zhèng]

syndrome of retention of cold-fluid in the stomach: a syndrome marked by epigastric distention with splashing sound in the stomach, vomiting of clear fluid, white slippery tongue coating, and wiry pulse, also called syndrome of stomach cold with retained fluid (胃寒饮停证 [wèi hán yǐn tíng zhèng])

胃寒饮停证 [wèi hán yǐn tíng zhèng]

syndrome of stomach cold with retained fluid, same as syndrome of retention of cold-fluid in the stomach (寒饮停胃证 [hán yǐn tíng wèi zhèng])

水停证 [shuǐ tíng zhèng]

water retention syndrome: a syndrome marked by edema and oliguria, or accompanied by ascites, pale plump tongue with white slippery coating, and soggy and relaxed pulse, also called water-*qi* syndrome or edema syndrome (水气证 [shuǐ qì zhèng])

水气证 [shuǐ qì zhèng]

water-*qi* syndrome; edema syndrome, same as water retention syndrome (水停证 [shuǐ tíng zhèng])

痰证 [tán zhèng]

phlegm syndrome: a general term for a group of syndromes marked by cough, dyspnea with profuse expectoration, or by nausea, vomiting and dizziness, or by formation of local round masses, also called (痰浊证[tán zhuó zhèng])

痰浊证 [tán zhuó zhèng]

phlegm-turbidity syndrome, same as phlegm syndrome (痰证 [tán zhèng])

风痰证 [fēng tán zhèng]

wind-phlegm syndrome: a syndrome marked by cough with frothy expectoration, stuffy sensation in the chest, dizziness, headache, or phlegmatic sounds in the throat, wry eye and mouth corner, white greasy tongue coating, and wiry and slippery pulse

寒痰证 [hán tán zhèng]

cold-phlegm syndrome: a syndrome marked by cough with whitish expectoration, dyspnea or wheezing, aversion to cold with cool limbs, white greasy tongue coating, and wiry slippery or tense pulse

湿痰证 [shī tán zhèng]

damp-phlegm syndrome: a syndrome marked by cough with profuse expectoration, heavy sensation of the limbs, stuffy feeling in the chest and stomach, reduced food intake, stickiness of the mouth, white greasy tongue coating, and wiry and slippery pulse

热痰证 [rè tán zhèng]

heat-phlegm syndrome: a syndrome marked by cough with yellowish expectoration, fever, thirst, reddened tongue with yellow greasy coating, and slippery and rapid pulse

燥痰证 [zào tán zhèng]

dryness-phlegm syndrome: a syndrome marked by cough with scanty sticky sputum difficult to spit out, or blood streaks in the sputum, chest pain with stuffy sensation, dry nose and mouth, tongue with scanty moisture but greasy coating, and choppy pulse

病因辨证

Disease-cause Syndrome Differentiation (Disease-cause Pattern Identification)

病因辨证 [bìng yīn biàn zhèng]

disease-cause syndrome differentiation; disease-cause pattern identification: analysis and differentiation of pathological conditions attributable to different kinds of causal factors for making diagnosis

审证求因 [shěn zhèng qiú yīn]

seeking the cause from symptoms: determining the cause of the disease according to the clinical manifestations

外风证 [wài fēng zhèng]

external wind syndrome: a general term for syndromes caused by exogenous pathogenic wind alone or together with pathogenic factors such as damp, heat, or pestilent toxin

风邪犯表证 [fēng xié fàn biǎo zhèng]

syndrome of wind pathogen invading the exterior: a syndrome marked by aversion to wind, fever, sweating, and floating pulse, sometimes accompanied by skin itching and edema, or by cough, sore throat and general aching, also called syndrome of external invasion of wind pathogen (风邪外袭证 [fēng xié wài xí zhèng])

风邪外袭证 [fēng xié wài xí zhèng]

syndrome of external invasion of wind pathogen, same as syndrome of wind pathogen invading the exterior (风邪犯表证 [fēng xié fàn biǎo zhèng])

风袭表疏证 [fēng xí biǎo shū zhèng]

syndrome of wind attack to the exterior: a synonym for exterior deficiency syndrome (表虚证 [biǎo xū zhèng])

风中经络证 [fēng zhòng jīng luò zhèng]

syndrome of wind hitting meridians: a syndrome marked by numbness and itching of the skin, or sudden onset of wry eye and skewed mouth, also called syndrome of wind pathogen attacking collateral meridians (风邪袭络证 [fēng xié xí luò zhèng])

风邪袭络证 [fēng xié xí luò zhèng]

syndrome of wind pathogen attacking collateral meridians, same as syndrome of wind hitting meridians (风中经络证 [fēng zhòng jīng luò zhèng])

风寒证 [fēng hán zhèng]

wind-cold syndrome: a general term for various syndromes caused by exogenous wind-cold

风寒表证 [fēng hán biǎo zhèng]

exterior wind-cold syndrome: a syndrome marked by aversion to cold with mild fever, no sweating, general aching, or congested nose with watery discharge, dyspnea, thin white tongue coating, and floating and tense pulse

风寒袭表证 [fēng hán xí biǎo zhèng]

syndrome of wind-cold attacking the exterior, same as exterior wind-cold syndrome (风寒表证 [fēng hán biǎo zhèng])

风寒袭肺证 [fēng hán xí fèi zhèng]

syndrome of wind-cold attacking the lung: a syndrome marked by aversion to cold, no sweating, cough, dyspnea, whitish expectoration, whitish tongue coating, and floating and tense pulse

风寒犯头证 [fēng hán fàn tóu zhèng]

syndrome of wind-cold invading the head: a syndrome marked by headache with pain in the nape and back, aggravated by wind and cold, thin white tongue coating, and floating and tense pulse

风寒袭络证 [fēng hán xí luò zhèng]

syndrome of wind-cold attacking collateral meridians: a synonym for syndrome of cold stagnating in meridians (寒滞经脉证 [hán zhì jīng mài zhèng])

风寒湿阻证 [fēng hán shī zǔ zhèng]

syndrome of obstruction by wind-cold-damp: a syndrome marked by joint pain, wandering or accompanied by heavy sensation

风热证 [fēng rè zhèng]

wind-heat syndrome: a general term for various syndromes caused by exogenous wind-heat

风热表证 [fēng rè biǎo zhèng]

wind-heat exterior syndrome: an exterior syndrome marked by fever with slight aversion to wind and cold, headache, somewhat thirst, or sore throat, reddened tongue tip and edges, yellowish thin tongue coating, rapid floating pulse

风热外袭证 [fēng rè wài xí zhèng]

syndrome of external invasion of wind-heat, synonymous with wind-heat syndrome (风热证 [fēng rè zhèng])

风热犯肺证 [fēng rè fàn fèi zhèng]

syndrome of wind-heat invading the lung: a syndrome marked by fever with mild aversion to wind and cold, general aching or sore throat, cough, dyspnea, reddened tip of the tongue with thin yellowish coating, rapid floating pulse

风热闭肺证 [fēng rè bì fèi zhèng]

syndrome of wind-heat blocking the lung: a syndrome marked by fever with aversion to wind, cough, dyspnea with coarse breath, pain and suffocating feeling in the chest, no sweating, reddened tongue, and rapid floating pulse

风热犯头证 [fēng rè fài tóu zhèng]

syndrome of wind-heat invading the head: a syndrome marked by headache with a distention sensation, fever or aversion to wind, thirst, flushing of face, reddened tongue tip and edges, thin and yellowish tongue coating, and rapid floating pulse

风热犯目证 [fēng rè fàn mù zhèng]

syndrome of wind-heat invading the eye: a syndrome marked by reddened and painful eye with excessive gum excretion and tears, fever, and aversion to wind

风湿证 [fēng shī zhèng]

wind-damp syndrome: an exterior syndrome marked by chills and fever, aching joints, heaviness in the head as if if were tightly bound, and white greasy tongue coating

风湿袭表证 [fēng shī xí biǎo zhèng]

syndrome of wind-damp attack to the exterior, same as wind-damp syndrome (风湿证 [fēng shī zhèng])

风湿外袭证 [fēng shī wài xí zhèng]

syndrome of external invasion of wind-damp, same as wind-damp syndrome (风湿证 [fēng shī zhèng])

风湿犯头证 [fēng shī fàn tóu zhèng]

syndrome of wind-damp invading the head: a syndrome marked by headache as if the head were tightly bound, slight aversion to wind and cold, heavy feeling in the body and limbs, stuffy sensation in the chest, anorexia, white slippery tongue coating, and soggy pulse

风燥袭表证 [fēng zào xí biǎo zhèng]

syndrome of wind-dryness attack to the exterior: a syndrome marked by mild fever, aversion to wind and cold, headache, no sweating, dry nose and throat, thirst, and floating pulse

实寒证 [shí hán zhèng]

excess-cold syndrome: a general term for syndromes caused by excessive cold pathogen

寒滞胃肠证 [hán zhì wèi cháng zhèng]

syndrome of cold stagnating in the stomach and intestines: a syndrome marked by severe epigastric and abdominal pain with cold sensation, alleviated by warmth, vomiting, watery diarrhea, aversion to cold with cool limbs, white tongue coating, and wiry tense pulse

寒滞心脉证 [hán zhì xīn mài zhèng]

syndrome of cold stagnating in the heart vessels: a syndrome marked by pectoral pain aggravated by cold and alleviated by warmth, white tongue coating, and sunken and slow or tense pulse

寒凝胞宫证 [hán níng bāo gōng zhèng]

syndrome of cold congealing in the uterus: a syndrome marked by cold and pain in the lower abdomen, dysmenorrhea or delayed periods with dark menstrual discharge, white tongue coating, and sunken and tense pulse

寒滞经脉证 [hán zhì jīng mài zhèng]

syndrome of cold stagnating in the meridians: a syndrome marked by aversion to cold, pain and cold feeling in the limbs with contracture or numbness and purple or pale discoloration of the skin, white tongue coating, and wiry and tense pulse

暑证 [shǔ zhèng]

summer-heat syndrome: a general term for fire- or heat-natured syndromes that only occur in the season of summer and are caused by summer-heat

暑湿袭表证 [shǔ shī xí biǎo zhèng]

syndrome of summer-damp attack to the exterior: a syndrome marked by fever, slight aversion to wind and cold, heavy sensation in the body, lassitude, thirst, reddened tongue with yellowish coating, and rapid soggy pulse

暑伤津气证 [shǔ shāng jīn qì zhèng]

syndrome of summer-heat damage to fluid and *qi*: a syndrome marked by fever, sweating, severe thirst, vexation, flushed face, lassitude, shortness of breath, scanty dark urine, reddened tongue with dry yellow coating, and big floating but weak pulse

暑闭气机证 [shǔ bì qì jī zhèng]

syndrome of summer-heat blocking *qi* activity: a syndrome marked by sudden fainting with fever, cold limbs, dyspnea, and trismus

暑热闭神证 [shǔ rè bì shén zhèng]

syndrome of summer-heat blocking mental activity: a syndrome marked by high fever, severe thirst, sudden fainting with loss of consciousness and trismus, sunken and hidden pulse

湿证 [shī zhèng]

damp syndrome: a general term for syndromes caused by pathogenic damp which may come from the external environment or may be derived from within the body owing to abnormal transportation and transformation of fluid

表湿证 [biǎo shī zhèng]

exterior damp syndrome, synonymous with wind-damp syndrome (风湿证 [fēng shī zhèng])

湿热蕴脾证 [shī rè yùn pí zhèng]

damp-heat accumulating in the spleen syndrome: a syndrome marked by abdominal distention, nausea, vomiting, anorexia, heavy sensation in the limbs, or jaundice, reddened tongue with yellow greasy coating, and rapid soggy pulse

湿热下注证 [shī rè xià zhù zhèng]

down-pouring damp-heat syndrome: a syndrome marked by frequent and painful urination, or yellow fetid discharge from the vagina, or ulceration of the leg with purulent discharge

外燥证 [wài zào zhèng]

external dryness syndrome: a general term for syndromes caused by climatic dryness commonly marked by dry skin, dry nose, mouth and throat

温燥证 [wēn zào zhèng]

warm-dryness syndrome: a syndrome marked by fever with slight aversion to wind and cold, dry cough with scanty expectoration, fidgetiness, thirst, dry skin, nose and throat, thin yellowish tongue coating, and rapid floating pulse

凉燥证 [liáng zào zhèng]

cool-dryness syndrome: a syndrome marked by more chills than fever, headache, no sweating, dry nose, mouth and throat, cough with scanty expectoration, thin and dry whitish tongue coating, and floating and tense pulse

燥邪犯肺证 [zào xié fàn fèi zhèng]

syndrome of dryness pathogen invading the lung: a syndrome marked by mild chills and fever, dry cough, no expectoration or scanty sputum with blood streaks, thirst, and dry tongue without moisture

燥干清窍证 [zào gān qīng qiào zhèng]

dry orifice syndrome: a syndrome marked by dry nose, mouth and eyes with lack of nasal mucus, saliva and tears

实火证 [shí huǒ zhèng]

excess-fire syndrome: a general term for syndromes marked by fever, thirst with desire for cold drinks, flushed face, blood-shot eyes, constipation, scanty dark urine, reddened tongue with yellow coating, and rapid or surging pulse

火毒证 [huǒ dú zhèng]

fire-toxin syndrome: a syndrome marked by local redness, swelling and burning pain, followed by abscess formation and accompanied by fever, thirst, reddened tongue with yellow coating, and rapid pulse

脓毒证 [nóng dú zhèng]

pus toxin syndrome: a syndrome marked by purulent discharge for an ulcerative lesion with stinking fetid smell, accompanied by fever, thirst, curdy and greasy tongue coating, and rapid slippery pulse

食积证 [shí jī zhèng]

food stagnancy syndrome: a syndrome in children marked by epigastric and abdominal distention, vomiting of sour matter, anorexia, offensive odor of stools, curdy and greasy tongue coating, also called syndrome of interior retention of milk (乳食内积证 [rǔ shí nèi jī zhèng])

乳食内积证 [rǔ shí nèi jī zhèng]

syndrome of interior retention of milk, same as food stagnancy syndrome (食积证 [shí jī zhèng])

虫积证 [chóng jī zhèng]

worm accumulation syndrome: a general term for syndromes caused by intestinal accumulation of parasitic worms, often marked by abdominal distention or pain, emaciation, lack of strength, and sallow complexion

疫毒证 [yì dú zhèng]

pestilential toxin syndrome: a general term for various syndromes caused by epidemic pathogens

脏腑辨证

Zang-Fu Organ Syndrome Differentiation (Organ Pattern Identification)

脏腑辨证 [zàng fǔ biàn zhèng]

***zang-fu* organ syndrome differentiation; organ pattern identification:** differentiation of syndromes or identification of patterns according to the pathological changes of *zang-fu* organs

心虚 [xīn xū]

heart insufficiency: a general term for deficiency conditions of the heart

心气虚 [xīn qì xū]

heart *qi* deficiency: a morbid condition resulting from insufficiency of heart *qi* with impaired blood-pumping function, chiefly manifested by palpitation, also called heart *qi* insufficiency (心气不足 [xīn qì bù zú])

心气不足 [xīn qì bù zú]

heart *qi* insufficiency, same as heart *qi* deficiency (心气虚 [xīn qì xū])

心气虚证 [xīn qì xū zhèng]

heart *qi* deficiency syndrome: syndrome of heart *qi* deficiency marked by palpitation, shortness of breath, listlessness, spontaneous sweating, pallor, pale tongue, and weak or irregular pulse

心阳虚 [xīn yáng xū]

heart yang deficiency: (1) a morbid condition resulting from advanced insufficiency of the heart *qi* with endogenous cold, also called decline of heart yang (心阳不振 [xīn yáng bù zhèn]); (2) an abbreviated term for heart yang deficiency syndrome (心阳虚证 [xīn yáng xū zhèng])

心阳不振 [xīn yáng bù zhèn]

decline of heart yang, synonymous with heart yang deficiency (心阳虚 [xīn yáng xū])

心阳虚证 [xīn yáng xū zhèng]

heart yang deficiency syndrome: syndrome of heart yang deficiency marked by palpitation, dyspnea, oppressive feeling in the chest, aversion to cold with cold limbs, bright pale complexion, dark lips and tongue with white coating, weak or irregular pulse

心血虚 [xīn xuè xū]

heart blood deficiency: (1) a morbid condition resulting from insufficient supply of nourishing blood to the heart with impairment of mental activities, also called 心血不足 [xīn xuè bù zú]; (2) an abbreviated name for heart blood deficiency syndrome (心血虚证 [xīn xuè xū zhèng])

心血不足 [xīn xuè bù zú]

heart blood insufficiency, same as heart blood deficiency (心血虚 [xīn xuè xū])

心血虚证 [xīn xuè xū zhèng]

heart blood deficiency syndrome: syndrome of heart blood deficiency marked by palpitation, dizziness, dream-disturbed sleep, forgetfulness, pale or sallow complexion, pale lips and tongue, and thready pulse

心阴虚 [xīn yīn xū]

heart yin deficiency: (1) a morbid condition resulting from consumption of heart yin with endogenous heat, also called heart yin insufficiency 心阴不足 [xīn yīn bù zú]; (2) an abbreviated name for heart yin deficiency syndrome (心阴虚证 [xīn yīn xū zhèng])

心阴不足 [xīn yīn bù zú]

heart yin insufficiency, same as heart yin deficiency (心阴虚 [xīn yīn xū])

心阴虚证 [xīn yīn xū zhèng]

heart yin deficiency syndrome: syndrome of deficient heart yin marked by mental irritability, palpitation, insomnia, low fever, night sweating, malar flush, thirst and thready rapid pulse

心火上炎 [xīn huǒ shàng yán]

flaring-up of heart fire: a morbid condition characterized by exuberant fire of the heart meridian which flares up to the mouth and tongue

心火上炎证 [xīn huǒ shàng yán zhèng]

up-flaring heart fire syndrome: syndrome of up-flaring fire from the heart meridian, marked by oral ulceration, mental irritability, insomnia, and red tip of the tongue

心火内炽 [xīn huǒ nèi chì]

internal flaming of heart fire: a morbid condition characterized by excessive heart fire causing mental disturbances, also called 心火内焚 [xīn huǒ nèi fén]

心火内焚 [xīn hoǔ nèi fén]

internal deflagration of heart fire, same as internal flaming of heart fire (心火内炽 [xīn huǒ nèi chì])

心火炽盛证 [xīn huǒ chì shèng zhèng]

heart fire flaming syndrome: a syndrome marked by fever, thirst, mental irritability, insomnia, palpitation, and in severe cases even delirium or mania

痰火扰心 [tán huǒ rǎo xīn]

phlegm-fire mental agitation: a morbid condition resulting from combined phlegm and fire which disturbs the heart (mind), chiefly manifested by mental disorders

痰火扰心证 [tán huǒ rǎo xīn zhèng]

phlegm-fire (mental) agitation syndrome: syndrome caused by phlegm-fire which disturbs the mind, marked by restlessness or raving madness accompanied by red tongue tip, yellow dense and greasy tongue coating, and slippery rapid pulse, also called 痰火扰神证 [tán huǒ rǎo shén zhèng]

痰火扰神证 [tán huǒ rǎo shén zhèng]

phlegm-fire (mental) agitation syndrome, same as 痰火扰心证 [tán huǒ rǎo xīn zhèng]

痰蒙心神 [tán méng xīn shén]

phlegm clouding of the mind: (1) a morbid condition caused by phlegm which clouds the mind, chiefly manifested by impairment of consciousness; (2) abbreviation for phlegm mental clouding syndrome (痰蒙心神证 [tán méng xīn shén zhèng])

痰迷心窍 [tán mí xīn qiào]

phlegm misting the heart orifices: a synonym for phlegm clouding of mind (痰蒙心神 [tán méng xīn shén])

痰蒙心神证 [tán méng xīn shén zhèng]

phlegm mental clouding syndrome: a syndrome marked by impairment of consciousness, psychotic depression, or even coma, accompanied with phlegmatic sound in the throat

水气凌心 [shuǐ qì líng xīn]

retained fluid attacking the heart: (1) a morbid condition caused by retained fluid which leads to disorder of the heart; (2) abbreviated name for syndrome of retained fluid attack heart (水气凌心证 [shuǐ qì líng xīn zhèng])

水气凌心证 [shuǐ qì líng xīn zhèng]

retained fluid attacking the heart syndrome: a syndrome marked by palpitation and shortness of breath associated with general edema

心脾两虚 [xīn pí liǎng xū]

heart-spleen dual deficiency: (1) a morbid condition characterized by deficiency of both heart blood and spleen *qi*; (2) abbreviated term for heart-spleen dual deficiency syndrome (心脾两虚证 [xīn pí liǎng xū zhèng])

心脾两虚证 [xīn pí liǎng xū zhèng]

heart-spleen dual deficiency syndrome: a syndrome marked by palpitation, amnesia, insomnia or dream-disturbed sleep, loss of appetite, abdominal distention, loose bowels, lassitude, sallow face and thready pulse

心肾不交 [xīn shèn bù jiāo]

heart-kidney disharmony: (1) a morbid condition characterized by breakdown of the normal physiological coordination between the heart and the kidney with excess of the heart yang and deficiency of the kidney yin; (2n abbreviated term for heart-kidney disharmony syndrome (心肾不

交证 [xīn shèn bù jiāo zhèng])

心肾不交证 [xīn shèn bù jiāo zhèng]

heart-kidney disharmony syndrome: a syndrome marked by fidgetiness, insomnia, palpitation, dizziness, tinnitus, aching of the lower back and knees, seminal emission, etc.

小肠实热 [xiǎo cháng shí rè]

excess heat in small intestine: (1) a morbid condition ascribed to shifting of the heart fire to the small intestine; (2) abbreviation for syndrome of excess heat in small intestine (小肠实热证 [xiǎo cháng shí rè zhèng])

小肠实热证 [xiǎo cháng shí rè zhèng]

syndrome of excess heat in small intestine: a syndrome marked by fidgetiness, oral ulceration, dark urine and burning pain upon urination, abdominal distension, yellow coating of the tongue, and rapid slippery pulse

肝阴虚 [gān yīn xū]

liver yin deficiency: a morbid condition attributed to lack of yin fluid for nourishing and moistening the liver, also called liver yin insufficiency (肝阴不足 [gān yīn bù zú])

肝阴不足 [gān yīn bù zú]

liver yin insufficiency, same as liver yin deficiency (肝阴虚 [gān yīn xū])

肝阴虚证 [gān yīn xū zhèng]

liver yin deficiency syndrome: a syndrome marked by dizziness, headache, blurred vision, dryness of the eyes, insomnia, thirst, dry throat, scanty tongue coating, and thready pulse

肝血虚 [gān xuè xū]

liver blood deficiency: a morbid condition characterized by insufficient blood supply to nourish the liver, also called 肝血不足 [gān xuè bù zú]

肝血不足 [gān xuè bù zú]

liver blood insufficiency, same as liver blood deficiency (肝血虚 [gān xuè xū])

肝血虚证 [gān xuè xū zhèng]

liver blood deficiency syndrome: a syndrome marked by sallow complexion, impaired vision, insomnia, deficient or absence of menstruation, pale tongue and lips

肝气虚 [gān qì xū]

liver *qi* deficiency: a morbid condition characterized by deficiency of *qi* resulting in impaired function of the liver in smoothing the flow of *qi*

肝气虚证 [gān qì xū zhèng]

liver *qi* deficiency syndrome: a syndrome marked by hypochondriac distention, emotional depression, fatigability, shortness of breath, dizziness, blurred vision, pale tongue, and weak pulse

肝寒 [gān hán]

liver cold: (1) a morbid condition characterized by cold due to insufficiency of liver yang, with symptoms such as depression, timidity, lassitude, cold limbs, deep and thready pulse; (2) stagnation of cold in the liver meridian (cf. 寒滞肝脉 [hán zhì gān mài])

肝寒证 [gān hán zhèng]

liver cold syndrome: an abbreviation for syndrome of cold stagnating in the liver meridian (寒滞肝脉 [hán zhì gān mài])

肝热 [gān rè]

liver heat: a general term for various heat syndromes of the liver such as liver fire, ascendant hyperactivity of liver yang

肝火 [gān huǒ]

liver fire: a morbid condition caused by emotional upset with retention of heat in the liver meridian

肝火证 [gān huǒ zhèng]

liver fire syndrome: an abbreviated name for liver fire flaming syndrome (肝火炽盛证 [gān huǒ chì shèng zhèng])

肝火炽盛 [gān huǒ chì shèng]

flaming of liver fire: (1) a morbid condition characterized by exuberant fire in the liver meridian that causes upward flow of *qi* and flaming of fire; (2) abbreviated term for liver fire flaming syndrome (肝火炽盛证 [gān huǒ chì shèng zhèng])

肝火炽盛证 [gān huǒ chì shèng zhèng]

liver fire flaming syndrome: a syndrome marked by hypochondriac pain, dryness and bitterness in the mouth, vomiting of bitter fluid, irritability, irascibility, insomnia or dream-disturbed sleep, flushing of the face, blood-shot eyes, constipation, dark urine, reddened tongue with yellow coating, and rapid wiry pulse

肝阳上亢 [gān yáng shàng kàng]

ascendant hyperactivity of liver yang: (1) a morbid condition that occurs when liver yin is insufficient to counterbalance yang, resulting in stirring of liver yang mainly involving the upper portion of the body; (2) abbreviated term for liver yang ascendant hyperactivity syndrome (肝阳上亢证 [gan yáng shàng kàng zhèng])

肝阳上亢证 [gān yáng shàng kàng zhèng]

liver yang ascendant hyperactivity syndrome: a syndrome marked by dizziness, headache, flushed face, blurred vision, tinnitus, bitter taste in the mouth and wiry pulse

肝阳亢盛 [gān yáng kàng shèng]

hyperactivity of liver yang, same as ascendant hyperactivity of liver yang (肝阳上亢 [gān yáng shàng kàng])

肝阳亢盛证 [gān yáng kàng shèng zhèng]

liver yang hyperactivity syndrome, same as liver yang ascendant hyperactivity syndrome (肝阳上亢证 [gān yáng shàng kàng zhèng]

肝火上炎 [gān huǒ shàng yán]

up-flaming of liver fire: a morbid condition in which fire is transformed from the depressed liver *qi* and flames up along the liver meridian, also called excess fire of the liver meridian (肝经实火 [gān jīng shí huǒ])

肝经实火 [gān jīng shí huǒ]

excessive fire of liver meridian, same as up-flaming of liver fire (肝火上炎 [gān huǒ shàng yán])

肝火上炎证 [gān huǒ shàng yán zhèng]

liver fire up-flaming syndrome: a syndrome marked by headache, dizziness, tinnitus with buzzing in the ears, impairment of hearing, blood-shot eyes, mental irritability, bitter taste in the mouth, yellow coating of the tongue, rapid wiry pulse, and in severe cases hematuria, hemoptysis or epistaxis

肝风内动 [gān fēng nèi dòng]

internal stirring of liver wind: a morbid condition characterized by arising of liver wind due to exuberant yang, intense heat-fire, or deficiency of yin-blood, often referred to simply as liver wind (肝风 [gān fēng])

肝风内动证 [gān fēng nèi dòng zhèng]

syndrome of liver wind stirring internally: a syndrome marked by convulsion, tremor or spasm

肝阳化风 [gān yáng huà fēng]

transformation of liver yang into wind: (1) a morbid condition of hyperactive liver yang that leads to the production of wind; (2) abbreviated term for liver yang transforming into wind syndrome (肝阳化风证 [gān yáng huà fēng zhèng])

肝阳化风证 [gān yáng huà fēng zhèng]

liver yang transforming into wind syndrome: a syndrome marked by dizziness with tendency to fall or even sudden attack of syncope, shaking of the head, tremor of limbs, irritability, irascibility, flushing of face, reddened tongue, and wiry pulse

热极生风 [rè jí shēng fēng]

extreme heat producing wind: (1) a morbid condition of extreme heat that produces wind; (2) abbreviation for extreme heat producing wind syndrome (热极生风证 [rè jí shēng fēng zhèng])

热极生风证 [rè jí shēng fēng zhèng]

extreme heat producing wind syndrome: a syndrome marked by high fever with restlessness, convulsions, opisthotonos, and impaired consciousness

阴虚动风 [yīn xū dòng fēng]

yin deficiency with stirring of wind: (1) a morbid condition of yin deficiency which stirs up endogenous wind; (2) abbreviated term for yin deficiency stirring wind syndrome (阴虚动风证 [yīn xū dòng fēng zhèng])

阴虚动风证 [yīn xū dòng fēng zhèng]

yin deficiency stirring wind syndrome: a syndrome marked by wriggling of extremities, accompanied by dizziness, tinnitus, malar flush, and dry reddened tongue

肝气郁结 [gān qì yù jié]

liver *qi* stagnation: (1) a morbid condition often caused by emotional depression, characterized by stagnation of liver *qi* with impaired function of smoothing the *qi* flow, usually abbreviated as liver stagnation 肝郁 [gān yù]; (2) abbreviated term for liver *qi* stagnation syndrome (肝气郁结证 [gān qì yù jié zhèng])

肝气郁结证 [gān qì yù jié zhèng]

liver *qi* stagnation syndrome: a syndrome marked by depression, frequent sighing, hypochondriac or lower abdominal distention or scurrying pain, in women distending pain of the breast and irregular menstruation, and wiry pulse, often abbreviated as liver stagnation syndrome (肝郁证 [gān yù zhèng])

肝郁 [gān yù]

liver stagnation: abbreviation for stagnation of liver *qi* (肝气郁结 [gān qì yù jié])

肝郁证 [gān yù zhèng]

liver stagnation syndrome: abbreviated term for liver *qi* stagnation syndrome (肝气郁结证 [gān qì yù jié zhèng])

肝气犯胃 [gān qì fàn wèi]

attack of the stomach by liver *qi*: (1) a morbid condition of the stomach due to invasion of hyperactive liver *qi*; (2) abbreviated term for liver *qi* attacking the stomach syndrome (肝气犯胃证 [gān qì fàn wèi zhèng])

肝气犯胃证 [gān qì fàn wèi zhèng]

liver *qi* attacking the stomach syndrome: a syndrome marked by dizziness, hypochondriac pain, irritability, epigastric distension and pain, anorexia, belching, nausea, vomiting, and taut pulse

肝胃不和 [gān wèi bù hé]

disharmony of liver and stomach, synonymous with attack of stomach by liver *qi* (肝气犯胃 [gān qì fàn wèi])

肝胃不和证 [gān wèi bù hé zhèng]

liver-stomach disharmony syndrome: a synonym for liver *qi* attacking the stomach syndrome (肝气犯胃证 [gān qì fàn wèi zhèng])

肝气犯脾 [gān qì fàn pí]

attack of the spleen by liver *qi*: (1) a morbid condition of the spleen due to invasion by hyperactive liver *qi*; (2) abbreviated term for liver *qi* attacking the spleen syndrome (肝气犯脾证 [gān qì fàn pí zhèng])

肝气犯脾证 [gān qì fàn pí zhèng]

liver *qi* attacking the spleen syndrome: a syndrome marked by dizziness, hypochondriac pain, irritability, anorexia, abdominal pain and distension, diarrhea, borborygmi, and wiry pulse

肝脾不和 [gān pí bù hé]

disharmony of the liver and spleen, synonymous with spleen attack by liver *qi* (肝气犯脾 [gān qì fàn pí])

肝脾不和证 [gān pí bù hé zhèng]

liver-spleen disharmony syndrome: a synonym for liver *qi* attacking the spleen syndrome (肝气犯脾证 [gān qì fàn pí zhèng])

肝郁脾虚 [gān yù pí xū]

liver stagnation and spleen insufficiency: (1) a morbid condition characterized by depressed liver activity of smoothing *qi* flow together with diminished transporting and transforming function of the spleen; (2) abbreviation for liver stagnation and spleen insufficiency syndrome (肝郁脾虚证 [gān yù pí xū zhèng])

肝郁脾虚证 [gān yù pí xū zhèng]

liver stagnation and spleen insufficiency syndrome: a syndrome marked by hypochondriac pain, abdominal distension, loose bowel, and lassitude

寒滞肝脉 [hán zhì gān mài]

stagnation of cold in liver meridian: (1) a morbid condition characterized by attack of pathogenic cold which stagnates in the liver meridian; (2) abbreviated term for cold stagnating in the liver meridian syndrome (寒滞肝脉证 [hán zhì gān mài zhèng])

寒滞肝脉证 [hán zhì gān mài zhèng]

cold stagnating in the liver meridian syndrome: a syndrome marked by spasmodic symptoms in the area related to the liver meridian, such as stretching pain with cold sensation in the lower abdomen and testicles

肝肾阴虚 [gān shèn yīn xū]

liver-kidney yin deficiency: (1) a morbid condition characterized by deficiency of yin fluid in the liver and kidney with harassment of endogenous heat; (2) abbreviation for liver-kidney yin deficiency syndrome (肝肾阴虚证 [gān shèn yīn xū zhèng])

肝肾阴虚证 [gān shèn yīn xū zhèng]

liver-kidney yin deficiency syndrome: a syndrome marked by dizziness, blurred vision, tinnitus, hypochondriac pain, aching of the loins and weakness of the knees and legs, malar flush, heat sensation in the palms and soles, red and dry tongue with scanty or no coating, and rapid thready pulse

胆气虚 [dǎn qì xū]

gallbladder *qi* deficiency: (1) a morbid condition characterized by insufficiency of gallbladder *qi* that causes mental uneasiness with a feeling of fear; (2) abbreviation for gallbladder *qi* deficiency syndrome (胆气虚证 [dǎn qì xū zhèng])

胆气虚证 [dǎn qì xū zhèng]

gallbladder *qi* deficiency syndrome: a syndrome marked by panic, suspicion, sighing, nervousness, irritability, lassitude, dizziness and insomnia

胆虚气劫 [dǎn xū qì jié]

gallbladder insufficiency with seizing of *qi*, same as gallbladder *qi* deficiency (胆气虚 [dǎn qì xū])

胆虚气劫证 [dǎn xū qì jié zhèng]

gallbladder insufficiency with seizing of *qi* syndrome, same as gallbladder *qi* deficiency syndrome (胆气虚证 [dǎn qì xū zhèng])

肝胆湿热 [gān dǎn shī rè]

damp-heat in the liver and gallbladder: (1) a morbid condition characterized by accumulation of damp-heat in the liver and gallbladder that interferes with their normal function in smoothing *qi* flow and bile excretion; (2) abbreviated term for liver-gallbladder damp-heat syndrome (肝胆湿热证 [gān dǎn shī rè zhèng])

肝胆湿热证 [gān dǎn shī rè zhèng]

liver-gallbladder damp-heat syndrome: a syndrome marked by fever and chills, jaundice, hypochondriac and abdominal pain, bitter taste in the mouth, nausea, and slippery and rapid pulse

胆热 [dǎn rè]

gallbladder heat: a morbid condition ascribed to attack on the gallbladder and gallbladder meridian by pathogenic heat

胆热证 [dǎn rè zhèng]

gallbladder heat syndrome: a syndrome marked by irritability, irascibility, hypochondriac distension, bitterness in the mouth or earache, tinnitus, insomnia, reddened tongue with yellow coating

胆火证 [dǎn huǒ zhèng]

gallbladder fire syndrome: a synonym for gallbladder heat syndrome (胆热证 [dǎn rè zhèng])

脾虚 [pí xū]

spleen insufficiency: a general term for deficiency conditions of the spleen

脾气虚 [pí qì xū]

spleen *qi* deficiency: (1) a morbid condition characterized by *qi* deficiency with impaired transforming and transporting function of the spleen, also called spleen *qi* insufficiency (脾气不足 [pī qì bù zú]); (2) abbreviated term for spleen *qi* deficiency syndrome (脾气虚证 [pí qì xū zhèng])

脾气不足 [pí qì bù zú]

spleen *qi* insufficiency, same as spleen *qi* deficiency (脾气虚 [pí qì xū])

脾气虚证 [pí qì xū zhèng]

spleen *qi* deficiency syndrome: a syndrome marked by dizziness, fatigue, sallow face, indigestion, abdominal distension, lassitude, anorexia, and loose bowels

脾阳虚 [pí yáng xū]

spleen yang deficiency: (1) a morbid condition characterized by decline of the spleen yang with diminished warming action, also called spleen yang insufficiency (脾阳不足 [pí yáng bù zú]); (2) abbreviated term for spleen yang deficiency syndrome (脾阳虚证 [pí yáng xū zhèng])

脾阳不足 [pí yáng bù zú]

spleen yang insufficiency, same as spleen yang deficiency (脾阳虚 [pí yáng xū])

脾阳虚证 [pí yáng xū zhèng]

spleen yang deficiency syndrome: a syndrome marked by cold limbs, cold and pain in the abdomen, anorexia, abdominal fullness, chronic diarrhea, lassitude, emaciation, and edema

脾胃虚寒 [pí wèi xū hán]

deficiency-cold of the spleen and stomach: a morbid condition characterized by decline of yang *qi* of the spleen and stomach with diminished warming and transporting activities, also known as 脾胃阳虚 [pí wèi yáng xū]

脾胃虚寒证 [pí wèi xū hán zhèng]

spleen-stomach deficiency-cold syndrome: a syndrome marked by cold and pains over the stomach, accompanied by anorexia, abdominal fullness, belching, vomiting thin fluid, chronic diarrhea, lassitude and cold limbs, also known as 脾胃阳虚证 [pí wèi yáng xū zhèng]

脾胃阳虚 [pí wèi yáng xū]

spleen-stomach yang deficiency, same as deficiency-cold of the spleen and stomach (脾胃虚寒 [pí wèi xū hán])

脾胃阳虚证 [pí wèi yáng xū zhèng]

spleen-stomach yang deficiency syndrome, same as spleen-stomach deficiency-cold syndrome (脾胃虚寒证 [pí wèi xū hán zhèng])

脾阴虚 [pí yīn xū]

spleen yin deficiency: (1) a morbid condition ascribed to deficiency of fluid in the spleen; (2) abbreviated term for spleen yin deficiency syndrome (脾阴虚证 [pí yīn xū zhèng])

脾阴虚证 [pí yīn xū zhèng]

spleen yin deficiency syndrome: a syndrome marked by anorexia, dryness of the lips and mouth, reddened tongue with scanty coating, and especially constipation with abdominal distention

脾虚湿困 [pí xū shī kùn]

spleen insufficiency with damp retention: (1) a morbid condition characterized by insufficiency of spleen *qi* leading to damp retention, which, in turn, further impairs the transporting and transforming function of the spleen; (2) abbreviated term for spleen insufficiency with damp retention syndrome (脾虚湿困证 [pí xū shī kùn zhèng])

脾虚湿困证 [pí xū shī kùn zhèng]

spleen insufficiency with damp retention syndrome: a syndrome marked by epigastric distension, poor appetite, borborygmi, diarrhea, nausea, thirst but no desire to drink, lassitude, and dense and slippery tongue coating

寒湿困脾 [hán shī kùn pí]

cold-damp disturbance of the spleen: (1) a morbid condition ascribed to the attack of cold-damp which impairs the function of the spleen; (2) abbreviation for cold-damp disturbance of the spleen syndrome (寒湿困脾证 [hán shī kùn pí zhèng])

寒湿困脾证 [hán shī kùn pí zhèng]

cold-damp disturbance of the spleen syndrome: a syndrome marked by epigastric and abdominal distention, stickiness and tastelessness in the mouth, nausea, loose bowels, heavy sensation in the head and body, or jaundice with dim yellow discoloration, pale plump tongue with white greasy coating, and soggy and relaxed pulse

湿困脾阳 [shī kùn pí yáng]

damp disturbance of spleen yang: a morbid condition characterized by invasion of damp which impairs the spleen yang. giving rise to clinical manifestations similar to cold-damp disturbance of the spleen (寒湿困脾 [hán shī kùn pí])

湿困脾阳证 [shī kùn pí yáng zhèng]

damp disturbance of spleen yang syndrome: a synonym for cold-damp disturbance of the spleen syndrome (寒湿困脾证 [hán shī kùn pí zhèng])

湿阻中焦 [shī zú zhōng jiāo]

damp retention in the middle energizer: a morbid condition referring to retention of pathogenic damp in the spleen and stomach

湿阻中焦证 [shī zú zhōng jiāo zhèng]

damp retention in the middle energizer syndrome: a syndrome marked by epigastric and abdominal distension, anorexia, lassitude, stickiness in the mouth, white thick greasy tongue coating and relaxed pulse

脾气下陷 [pí qì xià xiàn]

sinking of spleen *qi*: (1) a morbid condition characterized by weakness of the spleen with sinking of the middle *qi*, also known as 中气下陷 [zhōng qì xià xiàn] or 脾虚气陷 [pí xū qì xiàn]; (2) abbreviated term for spleen *qi* sinking syndrome (脾气下陷证 [pí qì xià xiàn zhèng])

脾气下陷证 [pí qì xià xiàn zhèng]

spleen *qi* sinking syndrome: a syndrome marked by bearing-down sensation in the epigastrium and abdomen, protracted diarrhea, even prolapse of the rectum or visceroptosis, also called 中气下陷证 [zhōng qì xià xiàn zhèng] or 脾虚气陷证 [pí xū qì xiàn zhèng]

中气下陷 [zhōng qì xià xiàn]

sinking of middle *qi*, same as sinking of spleen *qi* (脾气下陷 [pí qì xià xiàn])

中气下陷证 [zhōng qì xià xiàn zhèng]

middle *qi* sinking syndrome, same as spleen *qi* sinking syndrome (脾气下陷证 [pí qì xià xiàn zhèng])

脾虚气陷 [pí xū qì xiàn]

spleen insufficiency with sinking of *qi*, same as sinking of spleen *qi* (脾气下陷 [pí qì xià xiàn])

脾虚气陷证 [pí xū qì xiàn zhèng]

spleen insufficiency syndrome with sinking of *qi*, same as sinking of spleen *qi* (脾气下陷 [pí qì xià xiàn])

脾胃湿热 [pí wèi shī rè]

damp-heat in the spleen and stomach: (1) a morbid condition ascribed to accumulation of damp-heat which impairs the functions of the spleen and stomach, also known as 中焦湿热 [zhōng jiāo shī rè];

(2) abbreviated term for spleen-stomach damp-heat syndrome (脾胃湿热证 [pí wèi shī rè zhèng])

脾胃湿热证 [pí wèi shī rè zhèng]

spleen-stomach damp-heat syndrome: a syndrome marked by epigastric or abdominal distention, anorexia, nausea, vomiting, lassitude, heavy sensation of the body, or jaundice with bright yellow discoloration of the skin and the whites of the eyes, yellow dense and greasy tongue coating

中焦湿热 [zhōng jiāo shī rè]

damp-heat in the middle energizer, same as damp-heat in the spleen and stomach (脾胃湿热 [pí wèi shī rè])

中焦湿热证 [zhōng jiāo shī rè zhèng])

middle-energizer damp-heat syndrome, same as spleen-stomach damp-heat syndrome (脾胃湿热证 [pí wèi shī rè zhèng])

脾肺两虚 [pí fèi liǎng xū]

spleen-lung dual insufficiency: a morbid condition characterized by *qi* deficiency of both the spleen and the lung, also called spleen-lung *qi* deficiency (脾肺气虚 [pí fèi qì xū]); (2) abbreviated term for spleen-lung dual insufficiency syndrome (脾肺两虚证 [pí fèi liǎng xū zhèng])

脾肺两虚证 [pí fèi liǎng xū zhèng]

spleen-lung dual insufficiency syndrome: a syndrome marked by anorexia, loose stools, abdominal distension as well as dyspnea and productive cough

脾肺气虚 [pí fèi qì xū]

spleen-lung *qi* deficiency, same as spleen-lung dual insufficiency (脾肺两虚 [pí fèi liǎng xū])

脾肺气虚证 [pí fèi qì xū zhèng]

spleen-lung *qi* deficiency syndrome, same as spleen-lung dual insufficiency syndrome (脾肺两虚证 [pí fèi liǎng xū zhèng])

脾肾阳虚 [pí shèn yáng xū]

spleen-kidney yang deficiency: (1) a morbid condition characterized by insufficient yang-*qi* of the spleen and kidney with endogenous cold, also called deficiency-cold of the spleen and kidney (脾肾虚寒 [pí shèn xū h án]); (2) abbreviation for spleen-kidney yang deficiency syndrome (脾肾阳虚证 [pí shèn yáng xū zhèng])

脾肾阳虚证 [pí shèn yáng xū zhèng]

spleen-kidney yang deficiency syndrome: a syndrome marked by anasarca or chronic diarrhea before dawn together with aching of the loins, weakness of the knees and aversion to cold

脾肾虚寒 [pí shèn xū hán]

spleen-kidney deficiency-cold, synonymous with spleen-kidney yang deficiency (脾肾阳虚 [pí shèn yáng xū])

脾肾虚寒证 [pí shèn xū hán zhèng]

spleen-kidney deficiency-cold syndrome, synonymous with spleen-kidney yang deficiency syndrome (脾肾阳虚证 [pí shèn yáng xū zhèng])

胃虚 [wèi xū]

stomach insufficiency: a general term for deficiency conditions of the stomach

胃气虚 [wèi qì xū]

stomach *qi* deficiency: (1) a morbid condition characterized by weakness of the stomach *qi* with impairment of appetite and digestion; (2) abbreviation for stomach *qi* deficiency syndrome (胃气虚证 [wèi qì xū zhèng])

胃气虚证 [wèi qì xū zhèng]

stomach *qi* deficiency syndrome: a syndrome marked by dull epigastric pain relieved by pressure, anorexia, pale tongue, and weak pulse

胃阴虚 [wèi yīn xū]

stomach yin deficiency: (1) a morbid condition characterized by deficiency of fluid in the stomach impairing the harmonizing and descending activities, also called stomach yin insufficiency (胃阴不足 [wèi yīn bù zú]) (2) abbreviated term for stomach yin deficiency syndrome (胃阴虚证 [wèi yīn xū zhèng])

胃阴不足 [wèi yīn bù zú]

stomach yin insufficiency, same as stomach yin deficiency (胃阴虚 [wèi yīn xū])

胃阴虚证 [wèi yīn xū zhèng]

stomach yin deficiency syndrome: a syndrome marked by dryness in the mouth, thirst, anorexia, constipation, retching, and reddened furless tongue

胃阳虚 [wèi yáng xū]

stomach yang deficiency: (1) a morbid condition characterized by decline of yang-*qi* which fails to warm the stomach; (2) abbreviated term for stomach yang deficiency syndrome (胃阳虚证 [wèi yáng xū zhèng])

胃阳虚证 [wèi yáng xū zhèng]

stomach yang deficiency syndrome: continuous epigastric pain, ameliorated by warmth and pressure, reduced food intake, stuffy sensation in the stomach, aversion to cold with cold limbs, pale tongue with whitish coating, and deep, slow and weak pulse

胃寒 [wèi hán]

cold in the stomach: a morbid condition due to deficiency of stomach yang or caused by direct attack of pathogenic cold, the former being deficiency-cold of the stomach, and the latter excess-cold in the stomach

胃虚寒 [wèi xū hán]

deficiency-cold of the stomach: cf. cold in the stomach (胃寒 [wèi hán])

胃虚寒证 [wèi xū hán zhèng]

stomach deficiency-cold syndrome: a synonym for stomach yang deficiency syndrome (胃阳虚证 [wèi yáng xū zhèng])

胃实寒 [wèi shí hán]

excess-cold in the stomach: cf. cold in the stomach (胃寒 [wèi hán])

胃实寒证 [wèi shí hán zhèng]

stomach excess-cold syndrome: a synonym for syndrome of cold invading the stomach (寒邪犯胃证 [hán xié fàn wèi zhèng])

寒邪犯胃证 [hán xié fàn wèi zhèng]

cold invading the stomach syndrome: a syndrome marked by acute severe epigastric pain with cold sensation, vomiting of watery fluid, aversion to cold with cold limbs and whitish tongue coating

胃热 [wèi rè]

stomach heat: a morbid condition due to impairment of the stomach by pathogenic heat or caused by overeating of hot pungent food, mainly manifested as thirst, foul breath, hyperorexia, oliguria with dark urine, constipation, and even ulceration of the mouth or gingivitis, also called 胃中热 [wèi zhōng rè]

胃中热 [wèi zhōng rè]

heat in the stomach, same as stomach heat (胃热 [wèi rè])

胃热壅盛 [wèi rè yōng shèng]

intense stomach heat: (1) a morbid condition due to flaring up of stomach fire, marked by dire thirst and preference for cold drinks, foul breath, oral ulcer, toothache and gingivitis, also called 胃火炽盛 [wèi huǒ chì shèng] or 胃火上炎 [wèi huǒ shàng yán]; (2) accumulation of pathogenic heat in the stomach and intestine seen in cases of epidemic febrile disease, marked by high fever, constipation, abdominal pain, and even delirium (3) abbreviated term for intense stomach-heat syndrome (胃热壅盛证 [wèi rè yōng shèng zhèng])

胃热壅盛证 [wèi rè yōng shèng zhèng]

intense stomach-heat syndrome: a syndrome marked by dire thirst and preference for cold drinks, foul breath, oral ulcer, toothache and gingivitis

胃火 [wèi huǒ]

stomach fire: intense stomach heat or fire accumulated in the stomach

胃火证 [wèi huǒ zhèng]

stomach-fire syndrome: a syndrome marked by dire thirst and preference for cold drinks, foul breath, oral ulcer, toothache and gingivitis

胃火炽盛 [wèi huǒ chì shèng]

flaming stomach fire: cf. 胃热壅盛 [wèi huǒ yōng shèng]

胃火炽盛证 [wèi huǒ chì shèng zhèng]

flaming stomach fire syndrome, synonymous with intense stomach-heat syndrome 胃热壅盛证 [wèi rè yōng shèng zhèng]

胃火上炎 [wèi huǒ shàng yán]

flaring-up of stomach fire, synonymous with intense stomach heat (胃热壅盛 [wèi huǒ yōng shèng])

肺虚 [fèi xū]

lung insufficiency: a general term for deficiency conditions of the lung

肺气虚 [fèi qì xū]

lung *qi* deficiency: (1) a morbid condition characterized by diminished function of the lung in governing *qi* and defending the exogenous pathogens, also called 肺气不足 [fèi qì bù zú]; (2) abbreviation for lung *qi* deficiency syndrome (肺气虚证 [fèi qì xū zhèng])

肺气不足 [fèi qì bù zú]

lung *qi* insufficiency, same as lung *qi* deficiency (肺气虚 [fèi qì xū])

肺气虚证 [fèi qì xū zhèng]

lung *qi* deficiency syndrome: a syndrome marked by pale complexion, shortness of breath, feeble voice, intolerance of wind, and spontaneous sweating

肺阴虚 [fèi yīn xū]

lung yin deficiency: (1) a morbid condition characterized by insufficient lung yin with endogenous heat, also called 肺阴不足 [fèi yīn bù zú]; (2) abbreviation of lung yin deficiency syndrome (肺阴虚证 [fèi yīn xū zhèng])

肺阴不足 [fèi yīn bù zú]

lung yin insufficiency, same as lung yin deficiency (肺阴虚 [fèi yīn xū])

肺阴虚证 [fèi yīn xū zhèng]

lung yin deficiency syndrome: a syndrome marked by nonproductive cough, afternoon fever, night sweating, malar flush, dry throat, red and dry tongue, thready and rapid pulse

肺虚热证 [fèi xū rè zhèng]

lung deficiency-heat syndrome, synonymous with lung yin deficiency syndrome (肺阴虚证 [fèi yīn xū zhèng])

肺实 [fèi shí]

lung excessiveness: a general term for excess syndromes of the lung

风寒袭肺 [fēng hán xí fèi]

attack of wind-cold to the lung: a morbid condition characterized by attack of wind-cold which impairs the normal flow of lung *qi*

风寒袭肺证 [fēng hán xí fèi zhèng]

syndrome of wind-cold attacking the lung: a syndrome marked by chills, stuffy nose, sneezing, profuse watery nasal discharge, thin sputum, thin white tongue coating, and floating tense pulse

风寒束肺 [fēng hán shù fèi]

restraint of wind-cold on the lung, synonymous with attack of wind-cold to the the lung (风寒袭肺 [fēng hán xí fèi])

风寒束肺证 [fēng hán shù fèi zhèng]

wind-cold restraining the lung syndrome, synonymous with wind-cold attacking the lung syndrome (风寒袭肺证 [fēng hán xí fèi zhèng])

风热犯肺 [fēng hán fàn fèi]

attack of wind-heat to the lung: (1) a morbid condition characterized by attack of wind-heat to the lung and the superficies (2) abbreviated term for wind-heat attacking the lung syndrome (风热犯肺证 [fēng hán fàn fèi zhèng])

风热犯肺证 [fēng hán fàn fèi zhèng]

wind-heat attacking the lung syndrome: a syndrome marked by fever with mild chills, headache, sore throat, cough, reddened tip of the tongue with thin yellowish coating, and rapid floating pulse

痰湿阻肺 [tán shī zǔ fèi]

obstruction of the lung by phlegm-damp: (1) a morbid condition characterized by accumulation of phlegm-damp that obstructs the lung; (2) abbreviated term for phlegm-damp obstructing the lung syndrome (痰湿阻肺证 [tán shī zǔ fèi zhèng])

痰湿阻肺证 [tán shī zǔ fèi zhèng]

phlegm-damp obstructing the lung syndrome: a syndrome marked by cough with expectoration of copious whitish thin sputum, feeling of stuffiness in the chest, whitish greasy coating of the tongue, and soggy pulse

痰浊阻肺 [tán zhuó zǔ fèi]

obstruction of the lung by phlegm-turbidity, synonymous with obstruction of lung by phlegm-damp (痰湿阻肺 [tán shī zǔ fèi])

痰浊阻肺证 [tán zhuó zǔ fèi zhèng]

phlegm-turbidity obstructing the lung syndrome, synonymous with syndrome of phlegm-damp obstructing the lung (痰湿阻肺证 [tán shī zǔ fèi zhèng])

痰热闭肺 [tán rè bì fèi]

obstruction of the lung by phlegm-heat: (1) a morbid condition characterized by accumulation of phlegm-heat that obstructs the passage of lung *qi*; (2) abbreviated term for phlegm-heat obstructing the lung syndrome (痰热闭肺证 [tán rè bì fèi zhèng])

痰热闭肺证 [tán rè bì fèi zhèng]

phlegm-heat obstructing the lung syndrome: a syndrome marked by cough, dyspnea, expectoration of thick, yellow or blood-stained sputum, chest pain, reddened tongue with yellowish greasy coating, and rapid slippery pulse

肺热 [fèi rè]

lung heat: a general term for heat conditions of the lung

肺热炽盛 [fèi rè chì shèng]

intense lung heat: a morbid condition characterized by excessive pathogenic heat accumulated in the lung, also called accumulation of pathogenic heat in the lung 邪热壅肺 [xié rè yōng fèi]; (2) abbreviation for intense lung heat syndrome (肺热炽盛证 [fèi rè chì shèng zhèng])

肺热炽盛证 [fèi rè chì shèng zhèng]

intense lung heat syndrome: a syndrome marked by fever, thirst, cough, dyspnea or chest pain, constipation, dark urine, reddened tongue with yellow coating, also called accumulated pathogenic heat in the lung syndrome 邪热壅肺证 [xié rè yōng fèi zhèng]

邪热壅肺 [xié rè yōng fèi]

accumulation of pathogenic heat in lung, synonymous with intense lung heat (肺热炽盛 [fèi rè chì shèng])

邪热壅肺证 [xié rè yōng fèi zhèng]

accumulated pathogenic heat in the lung syndrome, synonymous with intense lung heat syndrome (肺热炽盛证 [fèi rè chì shèng zhèng])

肺火 [fèi huǒ]

lung fire: (1) a morbid condition referred to intense heat in the lung, either of deficiency type or of excess type; (2) abbreviation for lung fire syndrome (肺火证 [fèi huǒ zhèng])

肺火证 [fèi huǒ zhèng]

lung fire syndrome: a syndrome marked by fever, cough with yellow sputum, or hemoptysis

肺燥 [fèi zào]

lung dryness: a general term for dryness of the lung due to either deficiency of yin fluid or due to the attack of pathogenic factor of dryness, manifested by dry cough, dryness of the nasal cavity and pharynx, sore throat, thirst, hoarseness, hemoptysis, etc.

阴虚肺燥 [yīn xū fèi zào]

yin deficiency with lung dryness: (1) a morbid condition characterized by deficiency of yin fluid and dryness of the lung; (2) abbreviation for syndrome of yin deficiency with lung dryness (阴虚肺燥证 [yīn xū fèi zào zhèng])

阴虚肺燥证 [yīn xū fèi zào zhèng]

syndrome of yin deficiency with lung dryness: a syndrome marked by dry cough, sore throat, hoarseness, blood-stained sputum, reddened tongue with scanty coating, and rapid thready pulse

肺肾两虚 [fèi shèn liǎng xū]

insufficiency of both lung and kidney: a general term for deficiency conditions of both the lung and the kidney, such as deficiency of lung-kidney *qi* and deficiency of lung-kidney yin

肺肾阴虚 [fèi shèn yīn xū]

lung-kidney yin deficiency: (1) a morbid condition characterized by deficiency of yin fluid of the lung and kidney with harassment of endogenous heat; (2) abbreviation for lung-kidney yin deficiency syndrome (肺肾阴虚证 [fèi shèn yīn xū zhèng])

肺肾阴虚证 [fèi shèn yīn xū zhèng]

lung-kidney yin deficiency syndrome: a syndrome marked by dry cough, shortness of breath, dry throat, afternoon fever, lumbago, night sweats, and nocturnal emission

肺肾气虚 [fèi shèn qì xū]

lung-kidney *qi* deficiency: (1) a morbid condition characterized by dual deficiency of lung *qi* and kidney *qi*; (2) abbreviation for lung-kidney *qi* deficiency syndrome (肺肾气虚证 [fèi shèn qì xū zhèng])

肺肾气虚证 [fèi shèn qì xū zhèng]

lung-kidney *qi* deficiency syndrome: a syndrome marked by dyspnea, asthma, shortness of breath, spontaneous sweating, and cough with profuse sputum

肺肾阳虚 [fèi shèn yáng xū]

lung-kidney yang deficiency: (1) a morbid condition characterized by decline of kidney yang with flooding of cold-water into the lung; (2) abbreviation for lung-kidney yang deficiency syndrome (肺肾阳虚证 [fèi shèn yáng xū zhèng])

肺肾阳虚证 [fèi shèn yáng xū zhèng]

lung-kidney yang deficiency syndrome: a syndrome marked by cough, asthma, profuse white thin sputum, and whitish slippery tongue coating

水寒射肺 [shuǐ hán shè fèi]

water-cold flooding the lung: a synonym for lung-kidney yang deficiency (肺肾阳虚 [fèi shèn yáng xū])

水寒射肺证 [shuǐ hán shè fèi zhèng]

water-cold flooding the lung syndrome: a synonym for lung-kidney yang deficiency syndrome (肺肾阳虚证 [fèi shèn yáng xū zhèng])

大肠虚寒 [dà cháng xū hán]

deficiency-cold of the large intestine: (1) a morbid condition characterized by diarrhea of deficiency-cold type; (2) abbreviated term for large intestinal deficiency-cold syndrome (大肠虚寒证 [dà cháng xū hán zhèng])

大肠虚寒证 [dà cháng xū hán zhèng]

large intestinal deficiency-cold syndrome: a syndrome marked by diarrhea with watery stool, intolerance of cold, cold limbs, dull pain and cold feeling in the abdomen, pale tongue with white moistened coating

大肠寒结 [dà cháng hán jié]

cold retention in the large intestine: (1) a morbid condition characterized by retention of cold in the interior with constipation; (2) abbreviated term for large intestinal cold retention syndrome (大肠寒结证 [dà cháng hán jié zhèng])

大肠寒结证 [dà cháng hán jié zhèng]

large intestinal cold retention syndrome: a syndrome marked by constipation with dull pain and cold feeling in the abdomen, and pale tongue with white moistened coating

大肠热结 [dà cháng rè jié]

heat retention in the large intestine: (1) a morbid condition characterized by exuberant heat in the large intestine that causes dryness and constipation, also called heat retention with intestinal dryness (热结肠燥 [rè jié cháng zào]); (2) abbreviation for large intestinal heat retention syndrome (大肠热结证 [dà cháng rè jié zhèng])

大肠热结证 [dà cháng rè jié zhèng]

large intestinal heat retention syndrome: a syndrome marked by constipation with abdominal pain and tenderness, yellow and dry coating of the tongue, deep and forceful pulse, also called syndrome of heat retention with intestinal dryness (热结肠燥证 [rè jié cháng zào zhèng])

热结肠燥 [rè jié cháng zào]

heat retention with intestinal dryness, same as heat retention in the large intestine (大肠热结 [dà cháng rè jié])

热结肠燥证 [rè jié cháng zào zhèng]

heat retention with intestinal dryness syndrome, same as large intestinal heat retention syndrome (大肠热结证 [dà cháng rè jié zhèng])

大肠液亏 [dà cháng yè kuī]

large intestinal fluid deficiency: (1) a morbid condition ascribed to insufficient fluid in the large intestine; (2) abbreviation of large intestinal fluid deficiency syndrome (大肠液亏证 [dà cháng yè kuī zhèng])

大肠液亏证 [dà cháng yè kuī zhèng]

large intestinal fluid deficiency syndrome: a syndrome marked by constipation or difficulty in defecation accompanied by dry throat, and red tongue with scanty coating

大肠湿热 [dà cháng shī rè]

large intestinal damp-heat: (1) a morbid condition characterized by accumulation of damp-heat in the large intestine; (2) abbreviation of large intestinal damp-heat syndrome (大肠湿热证 [dà cháng shī rè zhèng])

大肠湿热证 [dà cháng shī rè zhèng]

large intestinal damp-heat syndrome: a syndrome marked by discharge of purulent and bloody stools, abdominal pain, tenesmus, scanty dark urine, yellow and greasy tongue coating, and slippery and rapid pulse

肾虚 [shèn xū]

kidney insufficiency: a general term for deficiency conditions of the kidney

肾亏 [shèn kuī]

kidney consumption, synonymous with kidney insufficiency 肾虚 [shèn xū]

肾气虚 [shèn qì xū]

kidney *qi* deficiency: (1) a morbid condition characterized by weakness of the kidney function in managing growth, development, reproduction, water metabolism, etc.; (2) abbreviation of kidney *qi* deficiency syndrome (肾气虚证 [shèn qì xū zhèng])

肾气虚证 [shèn qì xū zhèng]

kidney *qi* deficiency syndrome: a syndrome marked by dizziness, forgetfulness, tinnitus, backache, hyposexuality, and weak pulse

肾气不固 [shèn qì bù gù]

insecurity of kidney *qi*: (1) a morbid condition characterized by diminished storing and astringing function of the kidney, also called 下元不固 [xiàyuán bù gù]; (2) abbreviated term for kidney *qi* insecurity syndrome (肾气不固证 [shèn qì bù gù zhèng])

下元不固 [xià yuán bù gù]

insecurity of the lower origin: a synonym for insecurity of kidney *qi* (肾气不固 [shèn qì bù gù])

脬气不固 [pāo qì bù gù]

insecurity of bladder *qi*: a morbid condition marked by loss of control of urination, such as enuresis and incontinence of urine

肾气不固证 [shèn qì bù gù zhèng]

kidney *qi* insecurity syndrome: a syndrome marked by frequent urination, dribbling of urine after voiding, incontinence of urine or feces, nocturnal emission or premature ejaculation in males, continuous dribbling of menstrual discharge or liability to abortion in females, aching back and knees, and weak pulse

肾阴虚 [shèn yīn xū]

kidney yin deficiency: (1) a morbid condition caused by consumption of fluid and essence of the kidney in chronic diseases or due to intemperance in sexual life, also called 肾阴不足 [shèn yīn bù zú], 真阴不足 [zhēn yīn bù zú], 肾水不足 [shèn shuǐ bù zú], 下元亏损 [xià yuán kuī sǔn]; (2) abbreviation for kidney yin deficiency syndrome (肾阴虚证 [shèn yīn xū zhèng])

肾阴不足 [shèn yīn bù zú]

kidney yin insufficiency, same as kidney yin deficiency (肾阴虚 [shèn yīn xū])

真阴不足 [zhēn yīn bù zú]

insufficiency of genuine yin, same as kidney yin deficiency (肾阴虚 [shèn yīn xū])

肾水不足 [shèn shuǐ bù zú]

kidney water insufficiency, same as kidney yin deficiency (肾阴虚 [shèn yīn xū])

下元亏损 [xià yuán kuī sǔn]

consumption of the lower origin, same as kidney yin deficiency (肾阴虚 [shèn yīn xū])

肾阴虚证 [shèn yīn xū zhèng]

kidney yin deficiency syndrome: a syndrome marked by lumbago, lassitude, dizziness, tinnitus, nocturnal emission in men and oligmenorrhea in women, emaciation, dry throat, thirst, flushed cheeks, hot sensation in the palms and soles, afternoon fever, night sweating, reddened tongue with little or no coating, thready and rapid pulse, also called 真元亏虚证 [zhēn yuán kuī xū zhèng] or 肾水亏虚证 [shèn shuǐ kuī xū zhèng]

真元亏虚证 [zhēn yuán kuī xū zhèng]

genuine origin consumption syndrome, same as kidney yin deficiency syndrome (肾阴虚证 [shèn yīn xū zhèng])

肾水亏虚证 [shèn shuǐ kuī xū zhèng]

kidney-water consumption syndrome, same as kidney yin deficiency syndrome (肾阴虚证 [shèn yīn xū zhèng])

精髓空虚 [jīng suí kōng xū]

emptiness of essence-marrow: a morbid condition ascribed to kidney insufficiency with deprivation of essence and marrow, usually manifested by dizziness, amnesia, poor intelligence, and even dementia

肾阳虚 [shèn yáng xū]

kidney yang deficiency: (1) a morbid condition characterized by insufficiency of kidney yang with diminished warming function, also called 肾阳不足 [shèn yáng bù zú]; (2) abbreviation of kidney yang deficiency syndrome (肾阳虚证 [shèn yáng xū zhèng])

肾阳不足 [shèn yáng bù zú]

kidney yang insufficiency, same as kidney yang deficiency (肾阳虚 [shèn yáng xū])

元阳亏虚 [yuán yáng kuī xū]

consumption of original yang, same as 肾阳虚 [shèn yáng xū]

肾阳虚证 [shèn yáng xū zhèng]

kidney yang deficiency syndrome: a syndrome marked by aversion to cold, cold limbs, listlessness, weakness and soreness of the loins and knees, seminal emission or impotence in men and frigidity or infertility in women, nocturia, whitish tongue coating and weak pulse at the cubit

肾阳衰微 [shèn yáng shuāi wēi]

failure of kidney yang: severe case of kidney yang deficiency (cf. 肾阳虚 [shèn yáng xū])

肾火偏亢 [shèn huǒ piān kàng]

exuberance of kidney fire: relative excess of kidney fire due to deficiency of kidney yin, marked by hyperaphrodisia, insomnia and dream-disturbed sleep

命门火旺 [mìng mén huǒ wàng]

intense fire of the life gate, same as exuberance of kidney fire (肾火偏亢 [shèn huǒ piān kàng])

肾虚水泛 [shèn xū shuǐ fàn]

kidney insufficiency with edema: a morbid condition characterized by deficiency of kidney *qi* with impaired water metabolism and resultant flooding of retained fluid

肾虚水泛证 [shèn xū shuǐ fàn zhèng]

syndrome of kidney insufficiency with edema: a syndrome marked by edema, particularly of the lower extremities, accompanied by oliguria, tinnitus, aching of the back and knees, pale tongue with whitish slippery coating, and weak pulse

肾不纳气 [shèn bù nà qì]

failure of the kidney to receive air: (1) a morbid condition in which deficiency of the kidney *qi* leads to dyspnea with prolonged expiration; (2) abbreviated term for kidney failure in receiving air syndrome (肾不纳气证 [shèn bù nà qì zhèng])

肾不纳气证 [shèn bù nà qì zhèng]

kidney failure in receiving air syndrome: a syndrome marked by dyspnea with prolonged exhalation, asthenic cough, and feeble voice

热结膀胱 [rè jié páng guāng]

heat retention in the bladder: a morbid condition in which the pathogenic factor of an acute febrile disease is transformed into heat and accumulated in the urinary bladder

热结膀胱证 [rè jié páng guāng zhèng]

bladder heat retention syndrome: a syndrome marked by distension and fullness of the lower abdomen, stranguria, frequent urination, and fever without chills

膀胱虚寒 [páng guāng xū hán]

deficiency-cold of the bladder: a morbid condition characterized by impaired activities of the urinary bladder with cold manifestations due to consumption of kidney yang

膀胱虚寒证 [páng guāng xū hán zhèng]

bladder deficiency-cold syndrome: a syndrome marked by frequent urination, incontinence or dribbling of urine, cold feeling in the lower abdomen, whitish moist tongue coating, and weak pulse

膀胱湿热 [páng guāng shī rè]

damp-heat in the bladder: (1) a morbid condition ascribed to the accumulation of damp-heat in the urinary bladder; (2) abbreviated term for bladder damp-heat syndrome (膀胱湿热证 [páng guāng shī rè zhèng])

膀胱湿热证 [páng guāng shī rè zhèng]

bladder damp-heat syndrome: a syndrome marked by frequency and urgency of urination, stranguria, turbid urine or hematuria, reddened tongue with yellow greasy coating, and rapid pulse

三焦虚寒 [sān jiāo xū hán]

deficiency-cold of the triple energizer: deficiency-cold conditions occurring simultaneously in the upper, middle and lower energizers

上焦虚寒 [shàng jiāo xū hán]

deficiency-cold of the upper energizer: deficiency-cold conditions of the heart and lung with symptoms such as listlessness and shortness of breath

中焦虚寒 [zhōng jiāo xū hán]

deficiency-cold of the middle energizer: deficiency-cold conditions of the spleen and stomach with symptoms such as diarrhea, abdominal pain and distension, also known as 脾胃虚寒 [pí wèi xū hán]

下焦虚寒 [xià jiāo xū hán]

deficiency-cold of the lower energizer: deficiency-cold conditions of the liver, kidney, intestines and urinary bladder with symptoms such as chronic diarrhea, incontinence of urine, and edema

三焦实热 [sān jiāo shí rè]

excess-heat in triple energizer: (1) heat in the triple energizer of excess type; (2) febrile disease with the pathogen penetrating into the *qi* system

上焦实热 [shàng jiāo shí rè]

excess-heat in upper energizer: excessive heat syndrome of the heart and lung with symptoms such as asthma, stuffiness and fullness in the chest

中焦实热 [zhōng jiāo shí rè]

excess-heat in middle energizer: excess-heat syndrome of the spleen and stomach with symptoms such as abdominal distension with nausea and constipation

下焦实热 [xià jiāo shí rè]

excess-heat in lower energizer: excess-heat syndrome of the urinary bladder and large intestine with the symptoms such as hematuria, burning sensation upon urination, or passage of purulent bloody stools

冲任失调 [chōng rèn shī tiáo]

disorder of thoroughfare and conception vessels: a morbid condition characterized by disordered function of the thoroughfare and conception vessels

冲任失调证 [chōng rèn shī tiáo zhèng]

thoroughfare-conception-vessel disorder syndrome: a syndrome marked by irregular menstruation and lower abdominal distention and pain

冲任不固 [chōng rèn bù gù]

insecurity of thoroughfare and conception vessels: a syndrome marked by continuous dribbling of menstrual discharge, profuse uterine bleeding or liability to abortion

带脉病证 [dài mài bìng zhèng]

belt vessel syndrome: a syndrome marked by pain around the waist, weakness of the lower limbs, abnormal menstruation or leukorrhea

阴跷脉病证 [yīn qiāo mài bìng zhèng]

yin-heel vessel syndrome: a syndrome marked by redness and pain of the eyes, muscular disability, lower abdominal pain, testicular pain in men and metrostaxis in women

阳跷脉病证 [yáng qiāo mài bìng zhèng]

yang-heel vessel syndrome: a syndrome mainly marked by insomnia

阴维脉病证 [yīn wéi mài bìng zhèng]

yin-link vessel syndrome: a syndrome marked by chest pain, hypochondriac distension, lumbar pain in men and vaginal pain in women

阳维脉病证 [yáng wéi mài bìng zhèng]

yang-link vessel syndrome: a syndrome mainly marked by chills and fever accompanied by dizziness

治疗学 THERAPEUTICS

治则 Principles of Treatment

辨证施治 [piàn zhèng shī zhì]

syndrome differentiation and treatment; pattern identification and treatment: diagnosis and treatment based on overall analysis of symptoms and signs, including the cause, nature and location of the illness and the patient's physical condition, according to traditional Chinese medical theories, also known as 辨证论治 [biàn zhèng lùn zhì]

辨证论治 [biàn zhèng lùn zhì]

synonymous with 辨证施治 [biàn zhèng shī zhì]

审因施治 [shěn yīn shī zhì]

cause determination and treatment: diagnosis and treatment based on determination of the cause of the illness

审因论治 [shěn yīn lùn zhì]

synonymous with 审因施治 [shěn yīn shī zhì]

整体观念 [zhěng tǐ guān niàn]

holistic conception: viewing of the various parts of the human body as an organic whole, closely related to each other and to the external environment

因人制宜 [yīn rén zhì yí]

suited to person: a principle of treatment that the patient should be treated in accordance with his or her age, constitution, mental attitude and life style

因时、因地、因人制宜 [yīn shí、yīn dì、yīn rén zhì yí]

suited to time, place and person: a comprehensive principle of treatment based on the correspondence between man and the universe that treatment should be determined with an overall consideration of the seasonal, geographical and personal conditions

同病异治 [tóng bìng yì zhì]

different treatments for the same disease: a therapeutic principle of applying different methods of treatment to the same kind of disease in the light of different physical reactions and clinical manifestations (i.e., different syndromes)

异病同治 [yì bìng tóng zhì]

same treatment for different diseases: a therapeutic principle of applying the same method of treatment to patients with different kinds of diseases if they are alike in clinical manifestations and pathogenesis (i.e., with the same syndrome)

治病求本 [zhì bìng qiú běn]

treating disease from the root: the guiding principle of treatment that the fundamental cause of a disease should be dealt with

标 [biāo]

tip; the incidental: that referring to (1) manifestation of a disease in relation to its cause; (2) pathogenic factor in relation to body resistance; (3) complication or relapse of a disease in relation to its primary onset; (4) disease in the exterior in relation to that in the interior

本 [běn]

root; the fundamental: that referring to (1) cause of a disease in relation to its manifestations; (2) body resistance in relation to pathogenic factors; (3) primary onset of a disease in relation to its complications; (4) disease in the interior in relation to that in the exterior

治本 [zhì běn]

treating the fundamental: treating the cause of a disease

治标 [zhì biāo]

treating the incidental: treating the manifestations of a disease

标本兼[同]治 [biāo běn jiān/tóng zhì]

treating the incidental and fundamental simultaneously: a therapeutic principle applied to cases of severe illness with marked symptoms or complications

治未病 [zhì wèi bìng]

preventive treatment: (1) prevention of disease; (2) early treatment for prevention of complications

扶正祛邪 [fú zhèng qù xié]

supporting the healthy and eliminating the evil: two general principles of treatment — to strengthen the patient's resistance and to dispel the invading pathogenic factors, which can be applied separately or in combination according to the particular condition of the case

扶正兼祛邪 [fú zhèng jiān qù xié]

supporting the healthy with elimination of the evil: a principle of treatment that strengthening of healthy *qi* is primary and dispelling of the pathogenic factors is auxiliary, indicated for complicated cases of deficiency and excess with predominance of healthy *qi* deficiency

祛邪兼扶正 [qù xié jiān fú zhèng]

dispelling the evil with support for the healthy: a principle of treatment that elimination of the pathogenic factors is primary and strengthening of healthy *qi* is auxiliary, indicated for complicated cases of deficiency and excess with predominance of excess of pathogenic factors

扶正固本 [fú zhèng gù běn]

supporting the healthy and strengthening the root: (1) reinforcing the body resistance and improving the constitution; (2) restoring the normal functioning of the body to improve the constitution

扶正培本 [fú zhèng péi běn]

same as 扶正固本 [fú zhèng gù běn]

攻补兼施 [gōng bǔ jiān shī]

simultaneous attack and reinforcement: a principle of treatment with attacking and reinforcing methods used in combination, suitable for patients with a weak constitution suffering from an excess syndrome

先攻后补 [xiān gōng hòu bǔ]

attack followed by reinforcement: a principle of treatment indicated in cases where, although the healthy *qi* is insufficient, excess of pathogenic factors predominates and combined use of reinforcement therapy may aggravate the disease

先补后攻 [xiān bǔ hòu gōng]

reinforcement followed by attack: a principle of treatment marked by reinforcing first and then attacking, indicated for a debilitated patient who is incapable of withstanding the required attack therapy

寓攻于补 [yù gōng yú bǔ]

attacking for reinforcing: one of the therapeutic principles for a complicated case of deficiency and excess that reinforcing therapy is applied for the purpose of eliminating the pathogenic factors

寓补于攻 [yù bǔ yú gōng]

reinforcing for attacking: one of the therapeutic principles for a complicated case of deficiency and excess that attacking therapy is applied for the purpose of reinforcing healthy *qi*

正治 [zhèng zhì]

routine treatment: use of medicines opposite in nature to the disease, e.g., treating heat syndrome with medicines cold in nature

反治 [fǎn zhì]

contrary treatment: use of medicines similar in nature to the disease, e.g., treating pseudo-heat syndrome with medicines hot in nature

逆治 [nì zhì]

treatment in the same direction, same as 正治 [zhèng zhì]

从治 [cóng zhì]

treatment in the opposite direction, same as 反治 [fǎn zhì]

反佐 [fǎn zuǒ]

use of corrigents: use of drugs with property opposite to that of the principal ingredient in order to favorably modify the action of the latter which might be too powerful or harsh

阴病治阳 [yīn bìng zhì yáng]

treating yang for yin diseases: (1) Since chronic diseases of cold nature (pertaining to yin) are apt to damage yang, it is necessary to invigorate yang in the treatment. (2) Diseases with symptoms of the yin meridians are often treated by needling the points on the yang meridians, e.g., needling *dazhu* (BL11) and *fengmen* (BL12) (points of foot *taiyang* meridian) to treat cough after catching cold, a manifestation of pathological changes in the lung meridian of hand *taiyin* .

阳病治阴 [yáng bìng zhì yīn]

treating yin for yang diseases: (1) A febrile disease (pertaining to yang) is apt to injure yin (vital essence and fluid) and should be treated with the method of replenishing yin in protracted cases. (2) Diseases with symptoms of the yang meridians may be treated by needling the points of the yin meridians, e.g., needling *neiguan* (PC6) (a point of hand *jueyin* meridian) to treat vomiting, a manifestation of pathological changes in the stomach meridian of foot *yangming*.

上病下取，下病上取 [shàng bìng xià qǔ, xià bìng shàng qǔ]

treating the lower for the upper, and treating the upper for the lower: (1) In acupuncture, the points on the lower part of the body are needled when the symptoms appear in the upper part, and vice versa, e.g., needling *taichong* (LR3) on the foot to treat dizziness, needling *baihui* (GV20) on the top of the head to treat prolapse of the rectum. (2) In medication, drugs acting on the lower part of the body are often administered while the symptoms appear in the upper part, and vice versa, e.g., using rhubarb to induce catharsis for treating dizziness due to excessive fire, and using drugs to clear up the lung for inducing diuresis.

左病右取，右病左取 [zuǒ bìng yòu qǔ, yòu bìng zuǒ qǔ]

treating disease of the left with points on the right, and vice versa: treating disease in one side of the body by needling points on the opposite side

寒因寒用 [hán yīn hán yòng]

using cold for cold: treating pseudo-cold symptoms with drugs cool or cold in property

热因热用 [rè yīn rè yòng]

using heat for heat: treating pseudo-heat symptoms with drugs warm or hot in property

塞因塞用 [sāi yīn sāi yòng]

filling for the stuffed: treating a stuffed condition such as abdominal distension or constipation with tonics if it is caused by insufficient functioning of the spleen

通因通用 [tōng yīn tōng yòng]

opening for the opened: an unusual treatment, e.g., purgation in treating diarrhea caused by food stagnation

常用引文 Commonly Used Citations

治病必求其本。[zhì bìng bì qiú qí běn]

Disease should be treated from its root.

治标不如治本。[zhì biāo bù rú zhì běn]

Radical treatment is better than symptomatic relief.

急则治标。[jí zé zhì biāo]

In emergency cases treat the acute symptoms.

缓则治本。[huǎn zé zhì běn]

In non-acute cases treat the root of the disease.

上工治未病。[shàng gōng zhì wèi bìng]

A good doctor treats a disease before it occurs. Preventive treatment is better than curative treatment.

治寒以热。[zhì hán yǐ rè]

Treat cold with heat.

治热以寒。[zhì rè yǐ hán]

Treat heat with cold.

实则泻之。[shí zé xiè zhī]

Excess is treated by purgation or reduction.

虚则补之。[xū zé bǔ zhī]

Deficiency is treated by reinforcement or tonification.

寒者热之。[hán zhě rè zhī]

Treat cold with heat.

热者寒之。[rè zhě hán zhī]

Treat heat with cold.

客者除之。[kè zhě chú zhī]

Remove what is intruding.

逸者行之。[yì zhě xíng zhī]

Activate what flows sluggishly.

留者攻之。[liú zhě gōng zhī]

Attack what is lingering.

燥者濡之。[zào zhě rú zhī]

Moisten what is dried.

急者缓之。[jí zhě huǎn zhī]

Relieve what goes into spasm.

散者收之。[sàn zhě shōu zhī]

Consolidate what has come loose.

劳者温之。[láo zhě wēn zhī]

Give warming tonics to the debilitated.

坚者削之。[jiān zhě xiāo zhī]

Disintegrate what has turned into a hard mass.

结者散之。[jié zhě sàn zhī]

Resolve what is bound together.

下者举之。[xià zhě jǔ zhī]

Lift what prolapses.

高者抑之。[gāo zhě yì zhī]

Suppress what goes perversely upward.

惊者平之。[jīng zhě píng zhī]

Calm the one who takes fright.

微者逆之。[wēi zhě nì zhī]

Treat mild and simple cases with drugs opposite in nature to the

disease. For example, cold syndrome should be treated with drugs warm or hot in nature, and heat syndrome with drugs cool or cold in nature.

甚者从之。[shè zhě cóng zhī]

Treat complicated cases with drugs similar in nature to the pseudo-symptoms. For example, in treating a febrile case with pseudo-cold symptoms, drugs of cold nature should be used.

木郁达之。[mù yù dá zhī]

Mollify the liver (wood) if it is depressed.

火郁发之。[huǒ yù fā zhī]

Expel the fire if it is accumulated.

土郁夺之。[tǔ yù duó zhī]

Remove the damp if it is accumulated in the spleen (earth).

金郁泻之。[jīn yù xiè zhī]

Purge the lung (metal) if it is obstructed.

水郁折之。[shuǐ yù zhé zhī]

Drain water if it is retained.

形不足者温之以气。[xīng bù zú zhě wēn zhī yǐ qì]

Treat patients with a flabby appearance with warming drugs to reinforce *qi*.

精不足者补之以味。[jīng bù zú zhě bǔ zhī yǐ wèi]

Treat patients deficient in essence with a nutritious diet or drugs rich in flavor.

其高者因而越之。[qí gāo zhě yīn ér yuè zhī]

Troubles in the upper portion may be treated by emesis.

其下者引而竭之。[qí xià zhě yǐn ér xiē zhī]

Troubles in the lower portion may be treated by diuresis or purgation.

壮水之主，以制阳光。[zhuàng shuǐ zhī zhǔ, yǐ zhì yáng guāng]

Enrich the governor of water to restrain the brilliance of yang: When exuberance of yang is caused by deficiency of yin, it should be treated by replenishing yin instead of suppressing yang directly.

益火之源，以消阴翳。[yì huǒ zhī yuán, yǐ xiāo yīn yì]

Reinforce the source of fire to disperse the shroud of yin. For example, warming tonics to invigorate the life gate fire are used to treat general debility with aversion to cold, aching and creeping chill in the back, impotence, and frequent urination at night.

虚者补其母，实者泻其子。[xū zhě bǔ qí mǔ, shí zhě xiè qí zǐ]

In insufficiency, tonify the "mother" organ; in excessiveness, purge the "child" organ. For example, insufficiency of the liver is usually treated by tonifying the kidney, while excessiveness of the liver may be treated by dispelling fire from the heart.

无犯胃气。[wú fàn wèi qì]

Medication should not impair stomach *qi*.

有胃气则生，无胃气则死。[yǒu wèi qì zé shēng, wú wèi qì zé sǐ]

So long as stomach *qi* remains, there is hope of life, otherwise death will occur.

治法 Methods of Treatment

三法 [sān fǎ]

three principal therapeutic methods: diaphoresis, emesis and purgation

八法 [bā fǎ]

eight principal therapeutic methods: diaphoresis, emesis, purgation, mediation, warming, heat reduction, tonification, and resolution

汗法 [hàn fǎ]

diaphoretic therapy: one of the eight principal therapeutic methods used for relieving exterior syndromes, also called exterior-releasing therapy (解表法 [jiě biǎo fǎ])

解表法 [jiě biǎo fǎ]

exterior-releasing therapy: a general term for dispelling pathogenic factors from the exterior of the body, commonly used in the treatment of exterior syndromes

辛温解表 [xīn wēn jiě biǎo]

releasing the exterior with pungent-warm: method for treating wind-cold exterior syndrome by using drugs pungent in flavor and warm in nature

辛凉解表 [xīn liáng jiě biǎo]

releasing the exterior with pungent-cool: method for treating wind-heat exterior syndrome by using drugs pungent in flavor and cool in nature

辛凉清热 [xīn liáng qīng rè]

clearing heat with pungent-cool: method of using drugs pungent in flavor and cool in nature to release the exterior and clear heat for treating a febrile disease at both the defense and *qi* levels, also known as releasing the exterior and clear heat (解表清热 [jiě biǎo qīng rè])

解表清热 [jiě biǎo qīng rè]

releasing the exterior and clearing heat, synonymous with clearing heat with pungent-cool (辛凉清热 [xīn liáng qīng rè])

疏散风热 [shū sàn fēng rè]

dispersing wind-heat, synonymous with releasing the exterior with pungent-cool (辛凉解表 [xīn liáng jiě biǎo])

发汗解表 [fā hàn jiě biǎo]

inducing diaphoresis to release the exterior: method for treating exterior syndromes by using diaphoretics

解表清肺 [jiě biǎo qīng fèi]

releasing the exterior and clearing the lung: method of treating attack of wind-heat to the lung

解肌 [jiě jī]

releasing muscles: a general term for dispelling pathogenic factors from the superficial muscles

解肌清热 [jiě jī qīng rè]

releasing muscles and clearing heat: method of treating heat accumulated in the superficial muscles

解肌发表 [jiě jī fā biǎo]

releasing muscles to relieve exterior: method of dispelling pathogenic factors from the superficial muscles and other exterior parts of the body

解肌透疹 [jiě jī tòu zhěn]

releasing muscles to promote eruption: method of dispersing pathogens in the superficial muscles to promote skin eruption, chiefly used in the treatment of measles and rubella

解毒透疹 [jiě dú tòu zhě]

removing toxins to promote eruption: method of applying toxin-removing and pathogen-dispelling treatment to promote skin eruption in the treatment of measles and rubella

疏风 [shū fēng]

dispersing wind: a general term for relieving exogenous wind syndromes

疏风散寒 [shū fēng sàn hán]

dispersing wind-cold: method of using drugs pungent in flavor and warm in nature in the treatment of an exterior syndrome of wind-cold

疏风解表 [shū fēng jiě biǎo]

dispersing wind and releasing the exterior: method of treating an exterior syndrome caused by exogenous pathogenic wind

疏风清热 [shū fēng qīng rè]

dispersing wind and clearing heat: method often used for treating attack of wind-heat to the exterior or stagnation of wind-heat in the superficial muscles

疏风泄热 [shū fēng xiè rè]

dispersing wind and removing heat, same as dispersing wind and clearing heat (疏风清热 [shū fēng qīng rè])

疏风清肺 [shū fēng qīng fèi]

dispersing wind and clearing the lung: method of dispelling wind and heat from the lung meridian

疏风透疹 [shū fēng tòu zhěn]

dispersing wind to promote eruption: method of using wind-dispersing treatment to promote eruption in cases of measles and rubella, also called releasing the exterior to promote eruption (解表透疹 [jiě biǎo tòu zhěn])

解表透疹 [jiě biǎo tòu zhě]

releasing the exterior to promote eruption, synonymous with dispersing wind to promote eruption (疏风透疹 [shū fēng tòu zhěn])

疏风宣肺 [shū fēng xuān fèi]

dispersing wind and ventilating the lung: method for treating attack on the lung by pathogenic wind

疏风和营 [shū fēng hé yíng]

dispersing wind and harmonizing the nutrient (system): method for treating disharmony between the nutrient and defensive systems caused by attack of pathogenic wind to the exterior of the body

疏风止痒 [shū fēng zhǐ yǎng]

dispersing wind to relieve itching: wind-dispersing treatment to relieve itching caused by wind-toxin

祛风 [qù fēng]

dispelling wind: method of expelling pathogenic wind from the body surface, meridians, muscles and joints, used for treating external contraction at the early stage with exterior syndrome, and also for rheumatic or rheumatoid arthritis

祛风解表 [qù fēng jiě biǎo]

dispelling wind and releasing the exterior: method of dispelling wind from the body surface in the treatment of exterior syndrome caused by exogenous wind

祛风散寒 [qù fēng sàn há]

dispelling wind and dispersing cold: a common method of treating exterior syndrome of wind-cold, also known as dispersing wind-cold (疏风散寒 [shū fēng sàn hán])

祛风清热 [qù fēng qīng rè]

dispelling wind and clearing heat: a common method of treating exterior syndrome of wind-heat, also known as dispersing wind and clearing heat (疏风清热 [shū fēng qīng rè])

祛风除湿 [qù fēng chū shī]

dispelling wind and removing dampness: method of treating wind-damp contraction such as rheumatism

祛风化痰 [qù fēng huà tán]

dispelling wind and resolving phlegm: therapeutic method for treating wind-phlegm syndrome

祛风止痛 [qù fēng zhǐ tòng]

dispelling wind to relieve pain: wind-dispelling treatment to relieve pain caused by attack of pathogenic wind

祛风除湿止痛 [qù fēng chú shī zhǐ tòng]

dispelling wind and removing dampness to relieve pain: a common method of treating painful conditions caused by wind-damp, e.g., rheumatic pains

祛风解痉 [qù fēng jiě jìng]

dispelling wind and relieving spasm: method of treating pathogenic wind attacking the meridians

祛风通络 [qù fēng tōng luò]

dispelling wind and unblocking collateral meridians: method of treating pathogenic wind attack on collateral meridians

祛风止痒 [qù fēng zhǐ yǎng]

dispelling wind to relieve itching, same as dispersing wind to relieve itching (疏风止痒 [shū fēng zhǐ yǎng])

祛风行水 [qù fēng xíng shuǐ]

dispelling wind and promoting diuresis: treatment for wind-edema

养血祛风 [yǎng xuè qù fēng]

nourishing blood and dispelling wind: treatment for attack of wind in blood deficiency

宣肺 [xuān fèi]

ventilating the lung: method of treating affection of the lung by exogenous pathogens that leads to such functional disturbances as cough, dyspnea or edema

宣肺化痰 [xuān fèi huà tán]

ventilating the lung and resolving phlegm: method of treating accumulation of turbid-phlegm in the lung by expelling the phlegm

宣肺化饮 [xuān fèi huà yǐn]

ventilating the lung and resolve retained fluid: method of removing fluid and phlegm to treat retained fluid in the lung

宣肺止咳 [xuān fèi zhǐ ké]

ventilating the lung to relieve cough: treatment of regulating *qi* to facilitate free movement of air in the lung for relieving cough

宣肺平喘 [xuān fèi píng chuǎn]

ventilating the lung to relieve dyspnea: treatment of regulating *qi* to facilitate free movement of air in the lung for relieving dyspnea

宣肺止咳平喘 [xuān fèi zhǐ ké píng chuǎn]

ventilating the lung to relieve cough and dyspnea: treatment for cough and dyspnea by facilitating free movement of air in the lung

宣肺降气 [xuān fèi jiàng qì]

ventilating the lung and directing *qi* downward: method of treating impairment of the dispersing and descending function of the lung caused by pathogenic factors

透表 [tòu biǎo]

expelling through the exterior: therapy expelling pathogenic factors from the body in the treatment of acute febrile disease at the early stage with exterior syndrome of wind-heat

透表清热 [tòu biǎo qīng rè]

expelling through the exterior and clearing heat: method combining use of exterior-releasing and heat-clearing treatments to relieve a syndrome involving both the defense and *qi* systems

透疹 [tòu zhěn]

promoting eruption: therapy for measles and rubella by using pungent and cool-natured drugs with the effect of expelling pathogens from the exterior part of the body through skin eruption in order to prevent complications

透斑 [tòu bān]

driving rash out: therapy for acute febrile disease with indistinct maculation by applying drugs to expel heat from the blood

透邪 [tòu xié]

driving pathogens out: method of driving pathogens out of the body, usually used in the treatment of an exterior syndrome, also known as 达邪 ([dá xié])

达邪 [dá xié]

expelling pathogens, synonymous with driving pathogens out (透邪 [tòu xié])

透泄 [tòu xiè]

expelling from the exterior and removing from the interior: therapeutic method of using drugs pungent in flavor and cool in nature to eliminate pathogenic heat from the exterior portion of the body, together with drugs bitter in taste and cold in nature to remove pathogenic heat of the interior

调和营卫 [tiáo hé yíng wèi]

regulating nutrient and defensive *qi*: therapy to relieve exterior syndrome associated with spontaneous sweating

开鬼门 [kāi guǐ mén]

opening the "devil's gates" (pores): therapeutic method to induce perspiration

发汗禁例 [fā hàn jìn lì]

contraindications of diaphoresis: cases in which diaphoresis is contraindicated, such as heat due to deficiency of yin, external cold due to deficiency of yang, and hemorrhagic diseases

辛开苦泄 [xīn kāi kǔ xiè]

dispersion with pungent and purgation with bitter: (1) therapeutic method of administering pungent drugs to disperse pathogenic factors from the exterior together with bitter drugs to relieve interior heat; (2) therapeutic method of using pungent drugs to remove phlegm-dampness in the chest and bitter drugs to remove damp-heat

开泄 [kāi xiè]

dispersion and purgation: abbreviation of 辛开苦泄 [xīn kāi kǔ xiè]

扶正解表 [fú zhèng jiě biǎo]

supporting the normal and relieving the exterior: therapeutic method of combined use of exterior-releasing drugs and tonics to treat exterior syndrome occurring in a deficiency condition

滋阴解表 [zī yīn jiě biǎo]

enriching yin and releasing the exterior: therapeutic method of using both yin-tonifying and exterior-releasing drugs to expel exogenous pathogenic factors from the exterior portion of the body with yin deficiency

养阴解表 [yǎng yīn jiě biǎo]

nourishing yin and releasing the exterior, same as enriching yin and releasing the exterior (滋阴解表 [zī yīn jiě biǎo])

助阳解表 [zhù yáng jiě biǎo]

reinforcing yang and releasing the exterior: therapeutic method of using both yang-tonifying and exterior-releasing drugs to expel exogenous pathogenic factors from the exterior portion of the body with yang deficiency

益气解表 [yì qì jiě biǎo]

strengthening *qi* and releasing the exterior: therapeutic method of using both *qi*-tonifying and exterior-releasing drugs to expel exogenous pathogenic factors from the exterior portion of the body with *qi* deficiency

养血解表 [yǎng xuè jiě biǎo]

nourishing blood and releasing the exterior: therapeutic method of using both blood-tonifying and exterior-releasing drugs to expel exogenous pathogenic factors from the exterior portion of the body with blood deficiency

化饮解表 [huà yǐn jiě biǎo]

resolving retained fluid and releasing the exterior: method for treating a complex syndrome of wind-cold in the exterior and retained fluid in the interior

表里双解 [biǎo lǐ shuāng jiě]

relieving both the exterior and interior: treatment entailing dispelling pathogenic factors from both the exterior and the interior, indicated for a disease involving both the exterior and interior of the body

逆流挽舟 [nì liú wǎn zhōu]

"rowing upstream": a term metaphorically referring to the treatment of dysentery at its initial stage with exterior syndrome by using exterior-releasing and damp-expelling drugs to drive the pathogen outward, i.e., in the opposite direction to the inward penetration of the pathogen

清法 [qīng fǎ]

(heat-)clearing therapy: one of the eight principal therapeutic methods by administering medicines of cool or cold nature to treat fire or heat syndromes, also called 清热法 [qīng rè fǎ]

清热法 [qīng rè fǎ]

heat-clearing therapy: a general term for therapeutic methods for treating various kinds of heat syndromes, also abbreviated as clearing therapy (清法 [qīng fǎ])

苦寒清热 [kǔ hán qīng rè]

clearing heat with bitter-cold: a common therapeutic method for relieving internal heat by using drugs bitter in taste and cold in nature, also called purging heat with bitter-cold (苦寒泄热 [kǔ hán xiè rè])

苦寒泄热 [kǔ hán xiè rè]

purging heat with bitter-cold: another term for clearing heat with bitter-cold (苦寒清热 [kǔ hán qīng rè])

苦寒清气 [kǔ hán qīng qì]

clearing *qi* with bitter-cold: method of clearing heat from the *qi* system with drugs bitter in taste and cold in nature, usually used in the treatment of acute febrile diseases at the *qi* stage

清热生津 [qīng rè shēng jīn]

clearing heat and promoting fluid production: therapeutic method of using sweet-cool heat-clearing drugs together with fluid-production promoting drugs for treating fire or heat syndromes with damage to body fluids

除烦止渴 [chú fán zhǐ kě]

relieving restlessness and thirst: therapeutic method of relieving vexing thirst in cases of heat syndromes

清热解毒 [qīng rè jiě dú]

clearing heat and removing toxins: a common method of treating acute infectious diseases and pyogenic inflammations by using heat-clearing and toxin-resolving drugs

清热泻火 [qīng rè xiè huǒ]

clearing heat and purging fire: method of treating exuberant fire and heat

清热祛湿 [qīng rè qù shī]

clearing heat and dispelling damp: therapeutic method of using heat-clearing drugs together with damp-dispelling drugs for treating accumulation of damp-heat

清热除湿 [qīng rè chú shī]

clearing heat and removing damp, same as clearing heat and dispelling damp (清热祛湿 [qīng rè qù shī])

清热利湿 [qīng rè lì shī]

clearing heat and draining damp: method of clearing heat and removing damp through diuresis to treat accumulation of damp-heat in the lower energizer by using heat-clearing drugs together with diuretics

清热燥湿 [qīng rè zào shī]

clearing heat and drying dampness: therapeutic method for relieving accumulation of damp-heat

清热消食 [qīng rè xiāo shí]

clearing heat and promoting digestion: method of combined use of hear-clearing drugs and digestants to treat food stagnation with stomach heat

清热导滞 [qīng rè dǎo zhì]

clearing heat and relieving (food) stagnation: method of using heat-clearing drugs and digestants to treat food stagnation with stomach heat or undigested food retained in the stomach and intestines

清热明目 [qīng rè míng mù]

clearing heat to improve vision: method of treating eye diseases of heat nature by using heat-clearing, fire-purging and toxin-resolving drugs

清热和胃 [qīng rè hé wèi]

clearing heat and harmonizing the stomach: method of treating exuberance of stomach fire

清热和中 [qīng rè hé zhōng]

clearing heat and harmonizing the middle, same as clearing heat and harmonizing the stomach (清热和胃 [qīng rè hé wèi])

清热止呕 [qīng rè zhǐ ǒu]

clearing heat to stop vomiting: method of treating vomiting caused by exuberant heat in the stomach

清热止泻 [qīng rè zhǐ xiè]

clearing heat to stop diarrhea: method of treating diarrhea due to retention of heat in the intestines

清热止痢 [qīng rè zhǐ lì]

clearing heat to relieve dysentery: method of treating dysentery due to retention of heat in the intestines

清热止血 [qīng rè zhǐ xuè]

clearing heat to stop bleeding: method of using heat-clearing and blood-cooling hemostatics to treat bleeding

清热解暑 [qīng rè jiě shǔ]

clearing summer-heat: the basic method for treating summer heat

清暑热 [qīng shǔ rè]

same as **清热解暑** [qīng rè jiě shǔ]

祛暑化湿 [qù shǔ huà shī]

eliminating summer-heat and resolving dampness: method of combined use of summer-heat-clearing drugs and damp-resolving drugs for treating summer dampness syndrome

清暑化湿 [qīng shǔ huà shī]

same as 祛暑化湿 [qù shǔ huà shī]

清暑利湿 [qīng shǔ lì shī]

clearing summer-heat and removing dampness: the basic method for treating summer damp

清营 [qīng yíng]

clearing the nutrient (of heat): a common method of treating acute febrile disease involving the nutrient (*ying*) system or at the *ying* stage

清营泄热 [qīng yíng xiè rè]

clearing the nutrient and purging heat, same as clearing the nutrient of heat (清营 [qīng yíng])

清营透疹 [qīng yíng tòu zhěn]

clearing the nutrient and driving eruptions out: a combined method of clearing the nutrient of heat and promoting eruptions for treating pathogenic heat entering the nutrient system

清热凉血 [qīng rè liáng xuè]

clearing heat and cooling the blood: method of removing heat from the blood for treating acute febrile diseases and other diseases with exuberant heat in the blood, also abbreviated as cooling the blood (凉血 [liáng xuè])

凉血 [liáng xuè]

cooling the blood: abbreviation for clearing heat and cooling the blood

(清热凉血 [qīng rè liáng xuè])

凉血解毒 [liáng xuè jiě dú]

cooling the blood and removing toxins: method of removing heat-toxin from the blood for treating infections with the toxins in the nutrient and blood systems

清热开窍 [qīng rè kāi qiào]

clearing heat to cause resuscitation: method of treating impaired consciousness in cases of acute febrile diseases

清脏腑热 [qīng zàng fǔ rè]

clearing *zang-fu* organ heat: a general term for clearing heat from *zang-fu* organs

清肝 [qīng gān]

clearing the liver: method of clearing the liver of heat or fire

清肝泻火 [qīng gāng xiè huǒ]

clearing the liver and purging fire: method of treating excessive fire in the liver, also abbreviated as 泻肝 [xiè gān], or known as 清肝火 [qīng gān huǒ]

泻肝 [xiè gān]

purging the liver: abbreviation for clearing the liver and purging fire (清肝泻火 [qīng gān xiè huǒ])

清肝火 [qīng gān huǒ]

clearing liver fire: synonym for clearing the liver and purging fire (清肝泻火 [qīng gān xiè huǒ])

清肝明目 [qīng gān míng mù]

clearing the liver to improve vision: synonym for clearing heat to improve vision (清热明目 [qīng rè míng mù])

清心 [qīng xīn]

clearing the heart: method of clearing exuberant heat or fire from the heart or pericardium

清心火 [qīn xīn huǒ]

clearing heart fire: method of clearing the heart of pathogenic fire

清心泻火 [qīng xīn xiè huǒ]

clearing the heart and purging fire: method of treating exuberant heart fire

清心安神 [qīng xīn ān shén]

clearing the heart and calming the mind: method of clearing the heart fire and inducing tranquilization for treating mental disturbance caused by heat

清心开窍 [qīn xīn kāi qiào]

clearing the heart to restore consciousness: method of treating exuberant heat or fire in the heart with impaired consciousness

泻心火 [xiè xīn huǒ]

purging heart fire: method of treating exuberant fire in the heart

泻心 [xiè xīn]

purging the heart: method of treating excessive heat or pathogenic fire in the heart and stomach

清肺热 [qīng fèi rè]

clearing lung heat: method of treating excessive heat in the lung, also known as clearing the lung (清肺 [qīng fèi])

清肺火 [qīng fèi huǒ]

clearing lung fire: method of treating exuberant fire in the lung, also known as clearing the lung (清肺 [qīng fèi])

清肺 [qīng fèi]

clearing the lung, same as clearing lung heat (清肺热 [qīng fèi rè]) or clearing lung fire (清肺火 [qīng fèi huǒ])

清肺润燥 [qīng fèi rùn zào]

clearing the lung and moistening dryness: method of treating dryness-heat in the lung

清肺化痰 [qīng fèi huà tán]

clearing the lung and resolving phlegm: method of treating heat-phlegm in the lung

清肺止咳 [qīng fèi zhǐ ké]

clearing the lung to relieve cough: method of treating cough due to exuberant heat in the lung

清肺止喘 [qīng fèi zhǐ chuǎn]

clearing the lung to relieve dyspnea: method of treating dyspnea due to exuberant heat in the lung

清肺利咽 [qīng fèi lì yān]

clearing the lung to soothe the throat: method of treating sore throat due to exuberant heat in the lung

清热泻肺 [qīng rè xiè fèi]

clearing heat and purging the lung: method of treating exuberant lung heat, also abbreviated as purging the lung (泻肺 [xiè fèi])

泻肺 [xiè fèi]

purging the lung: abbreviation for clearing heat and purging the lung (清热泻肺 [qīng rè xiè fèi])

泻肺平喘 [xiè fèi píng chuǎn]

purging the lung to relieve dyspnea: method of treating dyspnea caused by accumulation of pathogens in the lung

清胃热 [qīng wèi rè]

clearing stomach heat: method of treating excessive heat in the stomach, also known as clearing the stomach and purging heat 清胃泄热 [qīng wèi xiè rè], and abbreviated as clearing the stomach (清胃 [qīng wèi]

清胃火 [qīng wèi huǒ]

clearing stomach fire: method of treating exuberant fire in the stomach, also known as clearing the stomach and purging fire 清胃泄火 [qīng wèi xiè huǒ], and abbreviated as clearing the stomach (清胃 [qīng wèi])

清胃泄热 [qīng wèi xiè rè]

clearing the stomach and purging heat, synonymous with clearing stomach heat (清胃热 [qīng wèi rè])

清胃泄火 [qīng wèi xiè huǒ]

clearing the stomach and purging fire, synonymous with clearing stomach fire (清胃火 [qīng wèi huǒ]

清胃 [qīng wèi]

clearing the stomach: abbreviation for clearing the stomach and purging heat 清胃泄热 [qīng wèi xiè rè] or clearing the stomach and purging fire 清胃泄火 [qīng wèi xiè huǒ]

清肠止泻 [qīng cháng zhǐ xiè]

clearing the intestines to stop diarrhea, same as clearing heat to stop diarrhea (清热止泻 [qīng cháng zhǐ xiè])

清肠止痢 [qīng cháng zhǐ lì]

clearing the intestine to relieve dysentery, same as clearing heat to relieve dysentery (清热止痢 [qīng rè zhǐ lì])

清肠润燥 [qīng cháng rùn zào]

clearing the intestine and moistening dryness: method of treating constipation due to excessive heat in the intestine

清相火 [qīng xiāng huǒ]

clearing ministerial fire, synonymous with 清泄相火 [qīng xiè xiàng huǒ]

清泄相火 [qīng xiè xiàng huǒ]

clearing and purging ministerial fire: method of treating preponderance of ministerial fire

凉血散瘀 [liáng xuè sàn hán]

cooling the blood and dissipating stasis: method for treating blood heat with blood stasis

凉血止痢 [liáng xuè zhǐ lì]

cooling the blood and relieving dysentery: method of treating dysentery with bloody stools caused by blood heat

凉血止血 [liáng xuè zhǐ xuè]

cooling the blood to stop bleeding: method of using blood-cooling hemostatics to treat bleeding caused by blood heat

下法 [xià fǎ]

purgative therapy: one of the eight principal therapeutic methods used to relieve constipation, remove stagnation of food or blood, and expel internal heat and excessive fluid through the bowels, also known as purgation (泻下 [xiè xià], 攻下 [gōng xià], and 通下 [tōng xià])

泻下 [xiè xià]

purgation, synonymous with purgation therapy (下法 [xià fǎ])

攻下 [gōng xià]

purgation, same as 泻下 [xiè xià]

通下 [tōng xià]

purgation, same as 泻下 [xiè xià]

通里 [tōng lǐ]

unblocking the interior: another expression for purgation therapy (下法 [xià fǎ])

寒下 [hán xià]

cold purgation: method of inducing purgation with drugs cold in nature to treat excessive heat in the interior manifested as constipation and abdominal distention with fever and thirst, as occurring in damp-heat dysentery, stagnation of undigested food, and retention of water

温下 [wēn xià]

warm purgation: method of inducing purgation with drugs warm in nature to treat stagnation of food or accumulation of pathogenic factors marked by a cold syndrome, e.g., constipation and abdominal pain with cold extremities and white tongue coating

温下寒积 [wēn xià hán jī]

warm-purgation of cold accumulation: method of administering warming drugs with cathartics for treating constipation due to cold congealing in cases of yang deficiency

缓下 [huǎn xià]

laxation: therapeutic method with mild action to relieve constipation

润下 [rùn xià]

lubricant laxation: method of inducing laxation with lubricants for the treatment of constipation due to intestinal dryness

峻下 [jùn xià]

drastic purgation: therapeutic method with drastic action to cause purgation

急下存阴 [jí xià cún yīn]

timely purgation to preserve yin: therapeutic method for persistent high fever and impairment of body fluid by administering drastic cathartics to purge excessive heat to prevent further loss of fluid, also known as timely purgation to preserve fluid (急下存津 [jí xià cún jīn])

急下存津 [jī xià cún jīn]

timely purgation to preserve fluid, same as timely purgation to preserve yin (急下存阴 [jí xià cún yīn])

增液通下 [zēng yè tōng xià]

increasing fluid to induce laxation, synonymous with moistening the intestines to loose the bowels (润肠通便 [rùn cháng tōng biàn])

润肠通便 [rùn cháng tōng biàn]

moistening the intestines to loose the bowels: treatment for constipation due to intestinal dryness

通腑泄热 [tōng fǔ xiè rè]

unblocking the bowels and purging heat: therapeutic method of removing internal heat by catharsis, also abbreviated as unblocking and purging (通泄 [tōng xiè])

通泄 [tōng xiè]

unblocking and purging: abbreviation for unblocking the bowels and purging heat (通腑泄热 [tōng fǔ xiè rè])

逐水 [zhú shuǐ]

hydrogogue therapy: therapeutic method of producing a watery discharge, especially from the bowels

泻下逐水 [xiè xià zhú shuǐ]

driving out water by catharsis: method of eliminating water retention by using hydrogogues

攻逐水饮 [gōng zhú shuǐ yǐn]

driving out retained water, synonymous with driving out water by catharsis 泻下逐水 [xiè xià zhú shuǐ]

泻水逐饮 [xiè shuǐ zhú yǐn]

same as 攻逐水饮 [gōng zhú shuǐ yǐn]

泻下逐饮 [xiè xià zhú yǐn]

expelling retained fluid by catharsis: method of treating retained fluid by catharsis

轻下 [qīng xià]

mild purgation: method of causing bowel movement with mild laxative drugs

釜底抽薪 [fǔ dǐ chōu xīn]

"taking away firewood from under the cauldron": metaphorical expression for the method of clearing heat or fire by purgation

去菀陈莝 [qù yù chén cuò]

eliminating the stale and the stagnant: an ancient term for the elimination of retained water and stagnant blood

攻下逐瘀 [gōng xià zhú yū]

eliminating stagnant blood by catharsis: method of using purgatives together with stasis-resolving drugs for treating blood stasis

先攻后补 [xiān gōng hòu bǔ]

elimination before tonification: therapy of attacking the pathogenic factors first and then administering tonics for recuperation

先补后攻 [xiān bǔ hòu gōng]

tonification before elimination: therapy administering tonics to improve the patient's general condition first and then driving the pathogenic factors out

攻补兼施 [gōng bǔ jiān shī]

elimination and tonification in combination: therapy to strengthen the body resistance and eliminate pathogenic factors simultaneously

误下 [wù xià]

erroneous administration of purgatives: administration of purgatives in cases in which purgation is contraindicated

和法 [hé fǎ]

harmonization: therapy involving the administering of drugs with regulatory or intermediary action to restore normal correlation between the internal organs or eliminate pathogenic factors from the part between the exterior and interior of the body, also known as harmonizing therapy (和解法 [hé jiě fǎ])

和解法 [hé jiě fǎ]

harmonizing therapy, same as harmonization (和法 [hé fǎ])

和解表里 [hé jiě biǎo lǐ]

harmonizing the exterior and interior: method of treating mild cases of dual exterior-interior syndrome

和解少阳 [hé jiě shào yáng]

harmonizing *shaoyang* meridian: method of treating *shaoyang* disease (cf. 少阳病 [shào yáng bìng]) by administering medicines to combat pathogenic factors lingering at *shaoyang* meridian and at the same time to strengthen the body resistance

开达膜[募]原 [kāi dá mò/mù yuán]

dredging the pleuro-diaphragmatic space: method of treating a disease which is believed to be located in the pleuro-diaphragmatic space with irregular spells of alternate fever and chills occurring one to three times a day, accompanied by tightness in the chest, nausea, headache, irritability, and taut and rapid pulse

和胃 [hé wèi]

harmonizing the stomach: method for treating dysfunction of the stomach with such symptoms as epigastric distension and distress, anorexia, belching, or nausea, also known as harmonizing the middle (和中 [hé zhōng])

和中 [hé zhōng]

harmonizing the middle: another name for harmonizing the stomach (和胃 [hé wèi])

理中 [lǐ zhōng]

regulating the middle: method to regulate the spleen and stomach in deficiency-cold conditions

理气和胃 [lǐ qì hé wèi]

regulating *qi* and harmonizing the stomach: method of regulating *qi* and removing stagnation to restore the normal function of the stomach, indicated in the treatment of stomach-qi stagnation

调和脾胃 [tiáo hé pí wèi]

harmonizing the spleen and stomach: method of treating disharmony of the spleen and stomach by regulating their *qi* activity

调和肝胃 [tiáo hé gān wèi]

harmonizing the liver and stomach: method of soothing the liver and harmonizing the stomach to treat dysfunction of the stomach caused by perverted flow of the liver *qi*

调和肝脾 [tiáo hé gān pí]

harmonizing the liver and spleen: method of soothing the liver, invigorating the spleen and regulating the *qi* activity to treat liver *qi* stagnation with spleen insufficiency

交通心肾 [jiāo tōng xīn shèn]

coordinating the heart and kidney: therapy of treating pathological changes due to breakdown of the normal coordination between the heart and the kidney by nourishing kidney yin, astringing kidney yang, reducing heart fire and calming the mind

调和气血 [tiāo hé qì xuè]

harmonizing *qi* and blood: method of using *qi*-regulating and blood-activating drugs to treat disharmony of *qi* and blood

调理气血 [tiáo lǐ qì xuè]

regulating *qi* and blood, same as hormonizing *qi* and blood (调和气血 [tiāo hé qì xuè])

理气和血 [lǐ qì hé xuè]

regulating *qi* and harmonizing blood, synonymous with harmonizing *qi* and blood (调和气血 [tiáo hé qì xuè])

和血熄风 [hé xuè xī fēng]

harmonizing blood to extinguish wind: method of tonifying liver blood to treat wind syndrome of blood deficiency stirring wind, also known as nourishing blood to extinguish wind (养血熄风 [yǎng xuè xī fēng])

养血熄风 [yǎng xuè xī fēng]

nourishing blood to extinguish wind, synonymous with harmonizing blood to extinguish wind (和血熄风 [hé xuè xī fēng])

和血调经 [hé xuè tiáo jīng]

harmonizing blood to regulate menstruation: method of activating blood and regulating *qi* to treat menstrual disorders due to disharmony of *qi* and blood

和血安胎 [hé xuè ān tāi]

harmonizing blood to prevent abortion: method of activating blood and regulating *qi* to prevent abortion caused by disharmony of *qi* and blood

和血止痛 [hé xuè zhǐ tòng]

harmonizing blood to alleviate pain: method of relieving pain by normalizing the blood flow

和营止痛 [hé yíng zhǐ tòng]

harmonizing nutrients to alleviate pain: method of regulating the nutrient and blood to relieve pain due to disturbed nutrient-blood flow

和营活血 [hé yíng huó xuè]

harmonizing nutrients and activating blood: therapeutic method of using blood-tonifying and nutrient-harmonizing drugs together with blood-activating and stasis-resolving drugs to treat blood deficiency complicated by blood stasis

和营生新 [hé yíng shēng xīn]

harmonizing nutrients to promote regeneration: method of regulating the nutrient and blood and facilitating blood flow to promote blood and tissue regeneration for treating unhealed wounds

温法 [wēn fǎ]

warming therapy: one of the eight principal therapeutic methods in which warming drugs are used for treating cold syndromes, also known as cold-dispelling therapy (祛寒法 [qù hán fǎ])

祛寒法 [qù hán fǎ]

cold-dispelling therapy: therapy to dispel internal cold by administering warming drugs, also called warming therapy (温法 [wēn fǎ])

温里 [wēn lǐ]

warming the interior: a general term for the methods of treating interior-cold syndromes

温肝 [wēn gān]

warming the liver: method for treating pain with cold sensation in the lower abdomen along the liver meridian

温心阳 [wēn xīn yáng]

warming heart yang: method for treating yang deficiency of the heart

回阳救逆 [huí yáng jiù nì]

restoring yang from collapse: method of treating yang exhaustion with cold limbs (collapse)

回阳 [huí yáng]

restoring yang, synonymous with restoring yang from collapse (回阳救逆 [huí yáng jiù nì])

救脱 [jiù tuō]

saving from collapse: emergency treatment for collapse

通阳 [tōng yáng]

unblocking yang: method of normalizing the flow of yang-*qi* by using drugs warm or hot in nature to remove obstruction of yang-*qi* caused by accumulation of cold-dampness, phlegm and stagnant blood

宣痹通阳 [xuān bì tōng yáng]

removing impediment and unblocking yang: method of removing impediment to normalize the flow of yang-*qi*, as in the treatment of angina pectoris

通脉 [tōng mài]

invigorating the pulse: method of stimulating the pulse-beat by warming up and restoring the normal flow of yang-*qi*

温中 [wēn zhōng]

warming the middle: method of treating yang deficiency of the spleen and stomach by dispelling cold and harmonizing the middle energizer with warming tonics

温脾 [wēn pí]

warming the spleen: method of treating deficiency-cold of the spleen by using warming tonics, also known as warming the middle (温中 [wēn zhōng])

温胃 [wēn wèi]

warming the stomach: method of treating stomach cold by using drugs warm or hot in nature

温中祛寒 [wēn zhōng qù hán]

warming the middle and dispelling cold: method of using drugs warm or hot in nature to treat deficiency-cold of the middle energizer (i.e., the spleen and stomach), also called warming the middle and dispersing cold (温中散寒 [wēn zhōng sàn hán])

温中散寒 [wen zhōng sàn hán]

warming the middle and dispersing cold, same as warming the middle and dispelling cold (温中祛寒 [wēn zhōng qù hán])

温中行气 [wēn zhōng xíng qì]

warming the middle and moving *qi*: method of treating abdominal distention or pain due to cold in the spleen and stomach with *qi* stagnation

温中和胃 [wēn zhōng hé wèi]

warming the middle and harmonizing the stomach: method of warming yang and invigorating the stomach for the treatment of stomach yang deficiency

温补胃阳 [wēn bǔ wèi yang]

warming and tonifying stomach yang, synonymous with warming the middle and harmonizing stomach (温中和胃 [wēn zhōng hé wèi])

温胃降逆 [wēn wèi jiàng nì]

warming the stomach to check upward perversion of *qi*: method of treating vomiting, retching or hiccups due to deficiency-cold of the stomach

温胃止呕 [wēn wèi zhǐ ǒu]

warming the stomach to stop vomiting: method of treating vomiting due to cold in the stomach, also called warming the middle to stop vomiting (温中止呕 [wēn zhōng zhǐ ǒu] or 温中止吐 [wēn zhōng zhǐ tù])

温中止呕 [wēn zhōng zhǐ ǒu]

warming the middle to stop vomiting, synonymous with warming the stomach to stop vomiting (温胃止呕 [wēn wèi zhǐ ǒu])

温中止泻 [wēn zhōng zhǐ xiè]

warming the middle to stop diarrhea: method of treating diarrhea due to deficiency-cold of the spleen

温中止痛 [wēn zhōng zhǐ tòng]

warming the middle to alleviate pain: method of treating abdominal pain due to deficiency-cold of the spleen and stomach

温肺 [wēn fèi]

warming the lung: method of treating deficiency-cold of the lung with warming tonics

温肺化痰 [wēn fèi huà tán]

warming the lung and resolving phlegm: method of treating accumulation of cold-phlegm in the lung

温肺化饮 [wēn fèi huà yǐn]

warming the lung and resolve retained fluid: method of treating retention of cold fluid in the lung by using warming and fluid-resolving drugs

温肾 [wēn shèn]

warming the kidney: method of invigorating kidney yang by using warming tonics, also known as warming kidney yang (温肾阳 [wēn shèn yáng])

温肾阳 [wēn shèn yáng]

warming kidney yang, same as warming the kidney (温肾 [wēn shèn])

温补肾阳 [wēn bǔ shèn yáng]

warming and tonifying kidney yang: therapeutic method of warming yang and tonifying the kidney for treating kidney yang deficiency

温肾纳气 [wēn shèn nà qì]

warming the kidney to improve respiration: method of warming kidney yang for improving the respiration, particularly for relieving dyspnea in cases of chronic asthma

纳气平喘 [nà qì píng chuàn]

improving respiration to relieve asthma: method of relieving dyspnea by improving the kidney's function in reception of *qi*

温肾缩尿 [wēn shèn suō niào]

warming the kidney to reduce urination: method of treating frequent micturition or enuresis by using warming tonics for the kidney

温肾止泻 [wēn shèn zhǐ xiè]

warming the kidney to stop diarrhea: therapeutic method of using kidney-warming tonics to relieve chronic diarrhea caused by kidney yang deficiency

温肾壮阳 [wēn shèn zhuàng yáng]

warming the kidney to invigorate yang: therapeutic method promoting virility in the treatment of sexual impotence

温肾健脾 [wēn shèn jiàn pí]

warming the kidney to invigorate the spleen: treatment for kidney yang deficiency involving the spleen

温补脾肾 [wēn bǔ pí shèn]

warming and tonifying the spleen and kidney: treatment for yang deficiency of the spleen and kidney

温经祛寒 [wēn jīng qù hán]

warming the meridians and dispelling cold: method of treating joint pains and menstrual complaints due to cold congealing in the meridians, also known as warming the meridians and dispersing cold (温经散寒 [wēn jīng sàn hán])

温经散寒 [wēn jīng sàn hán]

warming the meridians and dispersing cold, synonymous with warming the meridians and expelling cold (温经祛寒 [wēn jīng qù hán])

温经通阳 [wēn jīng tōng yáng]

warming meridian and unblocking yang: method for treating stagnation of cold in the meridians

温经回阳 [wēn jīng huí yáng]

warming meridian and restoring yang: method of treating impending collapse by warming and tonifying yang *qi* in the meridians

温经暖宫 [wēn jīng nuǎn gōng]

warming meridian and heating the uterus: therapeutic method used for treating cold congealing in the uterus

温经通络 [wēn jīng tōng luò]

warming and unblocking the meridians: therapeutic method of using warming drugs to free the flow of *qi* and blood in the meridians for relieving cold stagnation

温经活血 [wēn jīng huó xuè]

warming the meridians and activating blood: thereapeutic method of combining the use of meridian-warming and blood-activating drugs for treating cold congealing in the meridians with sluggish blood flow

温经止痛 [wēn jīng zhǐ tòng]

warming the meridians to alleviate pain: therapeutic method for relieving pain caused by cold stagnation in the meridians

甘温除热 [gān wēn chú rè]

relieving fever with sweet-warm: method of using drugs sweet in taste and warm in nature to treat fever caused by deficiency of *qi*

温里散寒 [wēn lǐ sàn hán]

warming the interior and dispersing cold: therapeutic treatment for interior-cold syndromes

温里祛寒 [wēn lǐ qù hán]

warming the interior and dispelling cold, synonymous with warming the interior and dispersing cold (温里散寒 [wēn lǐ sàn hán])

苦温平燥 [kǔ wēn píng zào]

relieving dryness with bitter-warm: method for treating exterior syndrome due to cold and dryness by using drugs bitter in taste and warm in nature

补法 [bǔ fǎ]

(1) tonification; tonic therapy: a general term for the methods of treating various deficiency syndromes by using tonics, one of the eight principal therapeutic methods; **(2) reinforcement:** reinforcing method in acupuncture

补气 [bǔ qì]

tonifying *qi*: therapy for *qi* deficiency, also known as replenishing *qi* (益气 [yi qi])

益气 [yì qì]

replenishing *qi*, synonymous with tonifying *qi* (补气 [bǔ qì])

补气固表 [bǔ qì gù biǎo]

replenishing *qi* to strengthen superficies: method used in treating spontaneous sweating and aversion to wind due to superficial *qi* deficiency

补益心气 [bǔ yì xīn qì]

reinforcing heart *qi*: method for treating deficiency of heart *qi*

补心益气 [bǔ xīn yì qì]

tonifying the heart and replenishing *qi*, same as reinforcing heart *qi* (补益心气 [bǔ yì xīn qì])

健脾 [jiàn pí]

invigorating the spleen: method of invigorating the transporting and transforming functions of the spleen

补脾 [bǔ pí]

reinforcing the spleen: method for treating diminished functional activities of the spleen by administering tonics, also known as 培土 [péi tǔ]

培土 [péi tǔ]

banking up earth, synonymous with reinforcing the spleen (补脾 [bǔ pí])

运脾 [yùn pí]

activating the spleen: method chiefly involving administering drugs to dispel dampness together with tonics for activating functioning of the spleen to treat accumulation of dampness in the spleen marked by indigestion with nausea, abdominal distention, diarrhea, white greasy coating of the tongue, and soft pulse

醒脾 [xǐng pí]

enlivening the spleen: method by using tonics to treat dyspepsia due to diminished function of the spleen marked by anorexia, dull abdominal pain, loose bowels, pale tongue and feeble pulse

健脾和胃 [jiàn pí hé wèi]

invigorating the spleen and harmonizing the stomach: method of treating diminished function of the spleen and stomach by administering tonics and stomachics

健脾消食 [jiàn pí xiāo shí]

invigorating the spleen to promote digestion: method of treating indigestion due to spleen insufficiency

健脾化湿 [jiàn pí huà shī]

invigorating the spleen to resolve dampness: method chiefly involving using tonics to treat stagnancy of dampness due to spleen insufficiency

健脾利湿 [jiàn pí lì shī]

invigorating the spleen and removing dampness through diuresis: method of using spleen tonics with diuretics to treat spleen insufficiency with damp retention or damp disturbance of the spleen

健脾利水 [jiàn pí lì shuǐ]

invigorating the spleen and removing edema through diuresis: combined use of spleen *qi* tonics and diuretics for treating spleen insufficiency with edema

健脾化痰 [jiàn pí huà tán]

invigorating the spleen to resolve phlegm: method chiefly involving using tonics to treat retention of phlegm due to spleen insufficiency

健脾止泻 [jiàn pí zhǐ xiè]

invigorating the spleen to arrest diarrhea: treatment for chronic diarrhea due to spleen insufficiency

健脾补肺 [jiàn pí bǔ fèi]

invigorating the spleen and tonifying the lung: a treatment for insufficiency of the spleen and lung

健脾益气 [jiàn pí yì qì]

invigorating the spleen and replenishing *qi*: method of treating spleen *qi* deficiency, also known as tonifying the spleen and replenishing *qi* (补脾益气 [bǔ pí yì qì])

补脾益气 [bǔ pí yì qì]

tonifying the spleen and replenishing *qi*, synonymous with invigorating the spleen and replenishing *qi* (健脾益气 [jiàn pí yì qì])

补益中气 [bǔ yì zhōng qì]

replenishing the middle *qi*: method of replenishing *qi*, invigorating the spleen and harmonizing the stomach, used for treating *qi* deficiency of the spleen and stomach, also called tonifying the middle and replenishing *qi* (补中益气 [bǔ zhōng yì qì])

补中益气 [bǔ zhōng yì qì]

tonifying the middle and replenishing *qi*, synonymous with tonifying the spleen and replenishing *qi* (补脾益气 [bǔ pí yì qì])

温补脾胃 [wēn bǔ pí wèi]

warming and tonifying the spleen and stomach: treatment for yang deficiency of the spleen and stomach

健胃 [jiàn wèi]

invigorating the stomach: method of invigorating the stomach function to promote digestion

开胃 [kāi wèi]

improving appetite: method of stimulating the desire for food

健胃止呕 [jiàn wèi zhǐ ǒu]

invigorating the stomach to stop vomiting: method of arresting vomiting by using stomachics

升提中气 [shēng tí zhōng qì]

elevating the middle *qi*: method of invigorating the function of the spleen in sending *qi* and nutrients upward for treating chronic diarrhea, visceroptosis and prolapse of the rectum and uterus

升举中气 [shēng jǔ zhōng qì]

raising the middle *qi*, same as 升提中气 [shēng tí zhōng qì]

升阳举陷 [shēng yáng jǔ xiàn]

elevating yang to cure drooping: method of treating spleen insufficiency with drooping symptoms such as protracted diarrhea, prolapse of the rectum, and prolapse of the uterus, also abbreviated as elevating yang (升阳 [shēng yáng])

升阳 [shēng yáng]

elevating yang: abbreviation for elevating yang to cure drooping (升阳举陷 [shēng yáng jǔ xiàn])

补脾益肺 [bǔ pí yì fèi]

tonifying the spleen to replenish the lung: method of treating chronic consumptive diseases of the lung by tonifying the spleen, also known as 培土生金 [péi tǔ shēng jīn]

培土生金 [péi tǔ shēng jīn]

banking up earth to benefit metal: expression for tonifying the spleen to replenish the lung (补脾益肺 [bǔ pí yì fèi])

培土抑木 [péi tǔ yì mù]

banking up earth to check wood: method of treating dysfunction of the spleen due to stagnation of the liver *qi*

补肺 [bǔ fèi]

tonifying the lung: a general term for the methods of using tonics to treat deficiency syndromes of the lung

补益肺气 [bǔ yì fèi qì]

replenishing lung *qi*: method of treating lung *qi* deficiency

补肺益气 [bǔ fèi yì qì]

tonifying the lung and replenishing *qi*, synonymous with replenishing lung *qi* (补益肺气 [bǔ yì fèi qì])

补血 [bǔ xuè]

tonifying the blood: method of treating deficiency of blood with blood tonics, also called nourishing the blood (养血 [yǎng xuè])

养血 [yǎng xuè]

nourishing the blood, synonymous with tonifying the blood (补血 [bǔ xuè])

补气生血 [bǔ qì shēng xuè]

tonifying *qi* and generating blood: therapeutic method of treating deficiency of both *qi* and blood primarily due to *qi* deficiency

补养心血 [bǔ yǎng xīn xuè]

nourishing heart blood: method of treating deficiency of heart blood with giddiness, pallor, palpitation, insomnia, and forgetfulness

补益心脾 [bǔ yì xīn pí]

tonifying the heart and spleen: method of treating deficiency of both the heart blood and spleen *qi*

补益气血 [bǔ yì qì xuè]

tonifying *qi* and blood: therapeutic method for deficiency of both *qi* and blood

补气养血 [bǔ qì yǎng xuè]

tonifying *qi* and nourishing blood, same as tonifying *qi* and blood (补益气血 [bǔ yì qì xuè])

补阴 [bǔ yīn]

tonifying yin: general method of treating yin deficiency by administering tonics, also called 养阴 [yǎng yīn], 滋阴 [zī yīn], 育阴 [yù yīn], or 益阴 [yì yīn]

养阴 [yǎng yīn]

nourishing yin, same as tonifying yin (补阴 [bǔ yīn])

滋阴 [zī yīn]

replenishing yin, same as tonifying yin (补阴 [bǔ yīn])

育阴 [yù yīn]

fostering yin, same as tonifying yin (补阴 [bǔ yīn])

益阴 [yì yīn]

supplementing yin, same as tonifying yin (补阴 [bǔ yīn])

酸甘化阴 [suān gān huà yīn]

transformation of sour-sweet into yin: method of replenishing yin with drugs sour and sweet in taste

补肝阴 [bǔ gān yīn]

tonifying liver yin: method of treating liver yin deficiency

养肝阴 [yǎng gān yīn]

nourishing liver yin, synonymous with 补肝阴 [bǔ gān yīn]

滋养肝肾 [zī yǎng gān shèn]

nourishing the liver and kidney: (1) method of reinforcing the liver yin by replenishing the kidney essence; (2) method of using tonics to treat yin deficiency of both the liver and the kidney, also called tonifying the liver and kidney (补益肝肾 [bǔ yì gān shèn])

补益肝肾 [bǔ yì gān shèn]

tonifying the liver and kidney, same as nourishing the liver and kidney (滋养肝肾 [zī yǎng gān shèn])

补养心阴 [bǔ yǎng xīn yīn]

nourishing heart yin: method of treating heart yin deficiency marked by palpitation, insomnia or dream-disturbed sleep, also abbreviated as nourishing the heart (养心 [yǎng xīn])

补心阴 [bǔ xīn yīn]

tonifying heart yin, synonymous with 补养心阴 [bǔ yǎng xīn yīn]

养心阴 [yǎng xīn yīn]

same as 补养心阴 [bǔ yǎng xīn yīn]

养心 [yǎng xīn]

nourishing the heart: abbreviation for nourishing heart yin (补养心阴 [bǔ yǎng xīn yīn])

滋养胃阴 [zī yǎng wèi yīn]

replenishing stomach yin: method involving using tonics to treat stomach yin deficiency, also abbreviated as 养胃 [yǎng wèi]

养胃阴 [yǎng wèi yīn]

nourishing stomach yin, synonymous with replenishing stomach yin (滋养胃阴 [zī yǎng wèi yīn])

补胃阴 [bǔ wèi yīn]

tonifying stomach yin, synonymous with replenishing stomach yin (滋养胃阴 [zī yǎng wèi yīn])

养胃 [yǎng wèi]

nourishing the stomach: abbreviation for nourishing stomach yin (滋养胃阴 [zī yǎng wèi yīn])

养胃生津 [yǎng wèi shēng jīn]

nourishing the stomach to produce fluid: method of treating deficiency of stomach yin-fluid

补养肺阴 [bǔ yǎng fèi yīn]

replenishing lung yin: method of using tonics to treat lung yin deficiency marked by dry throat and nonproductive cough

补肺阴 [bǔ fèi yīn]

tonifying lung yin, synonymous with replenishing lung yin 补养肺阴 [bǔ yǎng fèi yīn]

养肺阴 [yǎng fèi yīn]

nourishing lung yin, synonymous with replenishing lung yin 补养肺阴 [bǔ yǎng fèi yīn]

滋阴润肺 [zī yīn rùn fèi]

replenishing yin to moisten the lung: method of treating dryness of the lung by administering yin tonics

滋补肺肾 [zī bǔ fèi shèn]

nourishing the lung and kidney: method of treating yin deficiency of both the lung and the kidney

补肾 [bǔ shèn]

tonifying the kidney: a general term for treating deficiency syndromes of the kidney

补益肾气 [bǔ yì shèn qì]

replenishing kidney *qi*: method for treating kidney *qi* deficiency, also known as tonifying the kidney and replenishing *qi* (补肾益气 [bǔ shèn yì qì])

补肾益气 [bǔ shèn yì qì]

tonifying the kidney and replenishing *qi*, synonymous with replenishing kidney *qi* (补益肾气 [bǔ yì shèn qì])

滋补肾阴 [zī bǔ shèn yīn]

replenishing kidney yin: method of treating kidney yin deficiency, also abbreviated as replenishing the kidney (滋肾 [zī shèn])

补肾阴 [bǔ shèn yīn]

tonifying kidney yin, synonymous with replenishing kidney yin (滋补肾阴 [zī bǔ shèn yīn])

滋肾阴 [zī shèn yīn]

nourishing kidney yin, synonymous with replenishing kidney yin (滋补肾阴 [zī bǔ shè yīn])

滋肾 [zī shèn]

replenishing the kidney: abbreviation for replenishing kidney yin (滋补肾阴 [zī bǔ shèn yīn])

补肾固精 [bǔ shèn gù jīng]

tonifying the kidney to arrest emission: method of treating kidney insufficiency with seminal emission or spermatorrhea

滋阴补血 [zī yīn bǔ xuè]

nourishing yin and tonifying the blood: method of using yin tonics together with blood tonics for treating yin-blood deficiency

滋阴润燥 [zī yī rùn zào]

replenishing yin to moisten dryness: method of nourishing yin, clearing heat and promoting fluid production for treating yin deficiency with internal dryness

滋阴利水 [zī yīn lì shuǐ]

nourishing yin and promoting diuresis: method of using yin-nourishing drugs combined with diuretics to treat edema complicated with yin deficiency

滋阴清热 [zī yīn qīng rè]

nourishing yin and clearing heat: method of treating yin deficiency with endogenous heat

滋阴降火 [zī yīn jiàng huǒ]

nourishing yin and reducing fire: method of treating yin deficiency with exuberant fire

滋阴凉血 [zī yīn liáng xuè]

nourishing yin and cooling blood: method of combined use of yin-nourishing and blood-cooling drugs to treat syndromes of blood heat with damage to yin or yin deficiency with blood heat

滋阴抑阳 [zī yīn yì yáng]

nourishing yin to suppress yang: therapeutic method of supplementing yin fluid to suppress excessive yang *qi* for treating yin deficiency with exuberant yang

壮水制阳 [zhuàng shuǐ zhì yang]

supplementing water to inhibit yang, synonymous with 滋阴抑阳 [zī yīn yì yáng]

补阳 [bǔ yáng]

tonifying yang: a general term for the methods of treating yang deficiency of the heart, spleen and kidney with tonics, also called supporting yang (扶阳 [fú yáng] or 助阳 [zhù yáng])

扶阳 [fú yāng]

supporting yang, synonymous with tonifying yang (补阳 [bǔ yáng])

助阳 [zhù yáng]

supporting yang, synonymous with tonifying yang (补阳 [bǔ yáng])

壮阳 [zhuàng yáng]

invigorating yang, synonymous with tonifying yang (补阳 [bǔ yáng]), especially referring to promotion of virility in the treatment of sexual impotence

补火壮阳 [bǔ huǒ zhuàng yáng]

supplementing fire and invigorating yang: therapeutic method of invigorating yang by supplementing the fire of the life gate

补肾助阳 [bǔ shèn zhù yáng]

tonifying the kidney and supporting yang: method of treating kidney yang deficiency

温补命门 [wēn bǔ mìng mén]

warming and tonifying the life gate: method of invigorating vital function of the kidney with warming tonics, used in the treatment of declining fire of the life gate manifested by aversion to cold, chronic diarrhea before dawn or sexual impotence

引火归原 [yǐn huǒ guī yuán]

conducting fire back to its origin: therapeutic method of leading the ascending fire down to the kidney, used in the treatment of declining fire of the life gate with floating of asthenic yang

补肾纳气 [bǔ shèn nà qì]

tonifying the kidney to improve inspiration: method of using kidney tonics to treat dyspnea and cough due to *qi* deficiency of the lung and kidney, also called tonifying the kidney and reinforcing the lung (补肾益肺 [bǔ shèn yì fèi])

补肾益肺 [bǔ shèn yì fèi]

tonifying the kidney and reinforcing the lung: synonym for tonifying the kidney to improve inspiration (补肾纳气 [bǔ shèn nà qì])

补火生土 [bǔ huǒ shēng tǔ]

reinforcing fire to produce earth: method of administering kidney yang-strengthening tonics to warm and tonify the spleen for treating spleen deficiency-cold syndrome

补肾健骨 [bǔ shèn jiàn gǔ]

tonifying the kidney to strengthen the bones: method of treating weakness of bones by using kidney tonics

强筋健骨 [qiáng jīn jiàn gǔ]

strengthening the muscles and bones: treatment indicated for weak muscles and bones in those with debility or after injury

消法 [xiāo fǎ]

resolution; resolving method: one of the eight principal therapeutic methods for removing retained food and mass due to stagnation of *qi* and blood with digestants or resolvents

消食化滞 [xiāo shí huà zhí]

promoting digestion and resolving (food) stagnation, synonymous with 消食导滞 [xiāo shí dǎo zhì]

消食导滞 [xiāo shí dǎo zhì]

promoting digestion and removing (food) stagnancy: method of curing dyspepsia caused by improper diet or overeating with digestants and laxatives, also abbreviated as 消导 [xiāo dǎo]

消导 [xiāo dǎo]

abbreviation for 消食导滞 [xiāo shí dǎo zhì]

消食和胃 [xiāo shí hé wèi]

promoting digestion to harmonize the stomach: therapeutic method of harmonizing the stomach by promoting digestion and treating food stagnation in the stomach and intestines

消积 [xiāo jī]

relieving accumulation: therapeutic method that can relieve accumulation of *qi* or undigested food

消积除胀 [xiāo jī chú zhàng]

removing accumulation and relieving distension: therapeutic method of relieving epigastric or abdominal distension caused by stagnation of *qi* or accumulation of undigested food, also known as 消食下气 [xiāo shí xià qì]

消食下气 [xiāo shí xià qì]

promoting digestion and relieving distension, synonymous with removing accumulation and relieving distension 消积除胀 [xiāo jī chú zhàng]

消痞 [xiāo pǐ]

(1) disintegrating mass: therapeutic method for removing mass in the hypochondriac region; **(2) relieving stuffiness:** method for treating stuffiness in the chest and epigastrium caused by stagnancy of phlegm and food

消胀 [xiāo zhàng]

relieving distension: method for treating abdominal distension and flatulence

消肿 [xiāo zhǒng]

relieving swelling: therapeutic method that induces detumescence or promotes subsidence of swelling

消肿退红 [xiāo zhǒng tuì hóng]

relieving swelling and redness: method of treating inflammation with local swelling and redness

理气 [lǐ qì]

regulating *qi*: a general term for treating disordered flow of *qi*

行气 [xíng qì]

moving *qi*: method of relieving stagnation of *qi*, also called 利气 [lì qì] or 通气 [tōng qì]

利气 [lì qì]

same as 行气 [xīng qì]

通气 [tōng qì]

same as 行气 [xíng qì]

理气止痛 [lǐ qì zhǐ tòng]

regulating *qi* to alleviate pain: treatment for pain attributed to *qi* stagnation

行气止痛 [xíng qì zhǐ tòng]

moving *qi* to alleviated pain, synonymous with regulating *qi* to alleviate pain (理气止痛 [lǐ qì zhǐ tòng])

行气宽胸 [xíng qì kuān xiōng]

moving *qi* to soothe the chest: therapeutic method of relieving stuffiness of the chest by promoting the flow of *qi*

行气宽中 [xíng qì kuān zhōng]

moving *qi* to soothe the middle: method of promoting the flow of *qi* to alleviate stagnancy in the spleen and stomach, also known as 行气消痞 [xíng qì xiāo pǐ]

行气化痰 [xíng qì huà tán]

moving *qi* and resolving phlegm: method of combined use of *qi*-regulating drugs and phlegm-resolving drugs for treating syndrome of *qi* stagnation with phlegm congealing

理气化痰 [lǐ qì huà tán]

regulating *qi* and resolving phlegm, same as moving *qi* and resolving phlegm (行气化痰 [xíng qì huà tán])

降气化痰 [jiàng qì huà tán]

directing *qi* downward and resolving phlegm: method of combined use of *qi*-descending drugs and phlegm-resolving drugs for treating reversed flow of *qi* due to phlegm obstruction

理气健脾 [lǐ qì jiàn pí]

regulating *qi* and invigorating the spleen: treatment for diminished transporting function of the spleen in syndromes of spleen *qi* stagnation, spleen *qi* deficiency, and spleen insufficiency with *qi* stagnation

行气消痞 [xíng qì xiāo pǐ]

moving *qi* to relieve stuffiness, synonymous with moving *qi* to soothe the middle (行气宽中 [xíng qì kuān zhōng])

理气消痞 [lǐ qì xiāo pǐ]

regulating *qi* to relieve stuffiness, same as moving *qi* to relieve stuffiness (行气消痞 [xíng qì xiāo pǐ])

行气活血 [xíng qì huó xuè]

moving *qi* and activating the blood: therapeutic method for relieving *qi* stagnation with blood stasis, also called regulating *qi* and activating blood (理气活血 [lǐ qì huó xuè])

理气活血 [lǐ qì huó xuè]

regulating *qi* and activating the blood, same as moving *qi* and activating blood (行气活血 [xíng qì huó xuè])

行气通络 [xíng qì tōng luò]

moving *qi* to unblock collaterals: therapeutic method for relieving obstruction of collaterals by stagnant *qi*

顺气 [shùn qì]

arranging *qi*: method of putting the flow of *qi* in its normal direction, synonymous with checking upward perversion of *qi* (降逆下气 [jiàng nì xià qì])

宽胸 [kuān xiōng]

soothing the chest: measure to relieve chest stuffiness

宽胸散结 [kuān xiōng sàng jié]

soothing the chest and removing stagnation: treatment for angina pectoris with stuffy sensation in the chest

宽中散结 [kuān zhōng sàn jié]

soothing the middle and dissipating stagnation: therapeutic method for relieving stagnation in the middle energizer

降逆下气 [jiàng nì xià qì]

checking upward perversion of *qi*: method of treating upward perverted flow of *qi* in the lung and stomach manifested as cough, asthma, hiccuping or vomiting, also abbreviated as 降气 [jiàng qì] or 下气 [xià qì]

降气 [jiàng qì]

directing *qi* downward, synonymous with checking upward perversion of *qi* (降逆下气 [jiàng nì xià qì])

下气 [xià qì]

abbreviation for checking upward perversion of *qi* (降逆下气 [jiàng nì xià qì])

降气平喘 [jiàng qì píng chuǎn]

directing *qi* downward to relieve asthma: treatment for asthma, also called 降逆平喘 [jiàng nì píng chuǎn]

降逆平喘 [jiàng nì píng chuǎn]

checking upward perversion of *qi* to relieve asthma, same as directing *qi* downward to relieve asthma (降气平喘 [jiàng qì píng chuǎn])

降逆止呕 [jiàng nì zhǐ ǒu]

checking upward perversion of *qi* to stop vomiting: method of moving *qi* and harmonizing the stomach to treat vomiting

降逆止呃 [jiàng nì zhǐ è]

checking upward perversion of *qi* to stop hiccuping: treatment for hiccuping

降气止呃 [jiàng qì zhǐ è]

directing *qi* downward to stop hiccuping, same as checking upward perversion of *qi* to stop hiccuping (降逆止呃 [jiàng nì zhǐ è])

调气 [tiáo qì]

adjusting *qi*: (1) regulating the *qi* flowing in the meridians; (2) adjusting the flow of *qi* in order to guarantee a smooth normal circulation, a term for promoting natural flow of *qi* in general, and keeping it going downwards in particular

破气 [pò qì]

breaking stagnant *qi*: drastic measure to relieve stagnation of *qi*

疏肝 [shū gān]

soothing the liver: method of restoring the normal functioning of a depressed liver

疏肝养血 [shū gān yǎng xuè]

soothing the liver and nourishing the blood: therapeutic method with combined use of liver-soothing drugs and blood-nourishing drugs for treating liver depression with blood deficiency

疏肝理气 [shū gān lǐ qì]

soothing the liver and regulating *qi*: treatment for liver *qi* depression syndrome, also known as soothing the liver and relieving depression (疏

肝解郁 [shū gān jiě yù])

疏肝解郁 [shū gān jiě yù]

soothing the liver and relieving depression, synonymous with soothing the liver and regulating *qi* (疏肝理气 [shū gān lǐ qì])

疏肝和胃 [shū gān hé wèi]

soothing the liver and harmonizing the stomach: method of regulating the *qi* activity of the liver and stomach for treating liver-stomach *qi* stagnation and liver-stomach disharmony

疏肝理脾 [shū gān lǐ pí]

soothing the liver and regulating the spleen: method of regulating the activities of the liver and spleen to restore their normal coordination for treating liver stagnation with spleen insufficiency

疏肝和脾 [shū gān hé pí]

soothing the liver and harmonizing the spleen, synonymous with 疏肝理脾 [shū gān lǐ pí]

疏肝健脾 [shū gān jiàn pí]

soothing the liver and invigorating the spleen: method of regulating liver *qi* and strengthening spleen *qi* to harmonize the liver and spleen for treating depressed liver with spleen insufficiency

理气解郁 [lǐ qì jiě yù]

regulating *qi* and relieving depression: treatment for *qi* depression syndrome

理气导滞 [lǐ qì dǎo zhì]

regulating *qi* and removing stagnation: general method for treating *qi* stagnation syndrome

理气消胀 [lǐ qì xiāo zhàng]

regulating *qi* to relieve distension: method of treating abdominal distension caused by *qi* stagnation

理气化湿 [lǐ qì huà shī]

regulating *qi* and resolving dampness: method of using *qi*-regulating drugs together with damp-resolving aromatics to treat damp retention with *qi* stagnation

理气化瘀 [lǐ qì huà yū]

regulating the flow of *qi* to remove blood stasis: method of using *qi*-regulating drugs together with stasis-resolving drugs to treat syndrome of *qi* stagnation and blood stasis

理气止痛 [lǐ qì zhǐ tòng]

regulating the *qi* to alleviate pain: method of treating painful conditions due to *qi* stagnation

理气通经 [lǐ qì tōng jīng]

regulating *qi* to promote menstrual discharge: treatment for amenorrhea due to *qi* stagnation

理气安胎 [lǐ qì ān tāi]

regulating *qi* to quiet the fetus: method of preventing abortion due to *qi* stagnation

理血 [lǐ xuè]

regulating blood: a collective term for various methods to treat blood disorders, including tonify blood, remove heat from blood, promote blood flow as well as resolve stasis and stop bleeding

活血 [huó xuè]

activating blood: a general term for promoting blood flow in the treatment of blood stasis

活血行气 [huó xuè xíng qì]

activating blood and moving *qi*: method of treating blood stasis with *qi* stagnation

活血化瘀 [huó xuè huà yū]

activating blood and resolving stasis: a general term for various methods with blood-activating and stasis-resolving effect indicated in the treatment of blood stasis

活血祛瘀 [huó xuè qù yū]

activating blood and dispelling stasis, synonymous with activating the blood and resolve stasis (活血化瘀 [huó xuè huà yū])

活血调经 [huó xuè tiáo jīng]

activating blood to regulate menstruation: method of activating blood and regulating *qi* to treat irregular menstruation due to disharmony of *qi* and blood

活血通经 [huó xuè tōng jīng]

activating blood to stimulate menstruation: method of using blood-activating drugs to treat amenorrhea

活血通络 [huó xuè tōng luò]

activating blood to unblock collaterals: method of using blood-activating drugs to treat blood stasis in collateral meridians

活血止痛 [huó xuè zhǐ tòng]

activating blood to alleviate pain: method for treating painful conditions caused by blood stasis

祛瘀活血 [qù yū huó xuè]

removing stasis to activate blood: method of promoting blood circulation by eliminating stasis

祛瘀消肿 [qù yū xiāo zhǒng]

removing stasis to relieve swelling: treatment for hematoma and the like

祛瘀通络 [qù yū tōng luò]

removing stasis to unblock collaterals: method of treating obstruction of the collateral meridians by stagnant blood

祛瘀生新 [qù yū shēng xīn]

removing stasis to promote regeneration: therapeutic method of activating blood and remove stasis to promote blood regeneration for treating blood stasis complicated with blood deficiency

破血祛瘀 [pò xuè qù yū]

breaking stagnant blood: treatment for blood stasis with drastic drugs, also abbreviated as breaking blood 破血 [pò xuè] or breaking stagnancy 破瘀 [pò yū]

破血逐瘀 [pò xuè zhú yū]

breaking and expelling blood stasis, synonymous with breaking stagnant blood (破血祛瘀 [pò xuè qù yū])

破血 [pò xuè]

breaking blood: abbreviation for breaking stagnant blood (破血祛瘀 [pò xuè qù yū])

破瘀 [pò yū]

breaking stagnancy: abbreviation for breaking stagnant blood (破血祛瘀 [pò xuè qù yū])

破瘀消癥 [pò yū xiāo zhēng]

breaking stagnancy and eliminating masses: method of using blood-activating and stasis-removing drugs to eliminate stagnant blood and masses in the abdomen

破瘀生新 [pò yū shēng xīn]

breaking stagnancy and promoting regeneration: method of using drastic stasis-removing agents to eliminate stagnant blood and promote tissue regeneration

舒筋通络 [shū jīn tōng luò]

soothing tendons and unblocking collaterals: measure for treating blockage of meridian *qi* with muscle contraction

舒筋活络 [shū jīn huó luò]

soothing tendons and activating collaterals, synonymous with soothing tendons and unblocking collaterals (舒筋通络 [shū jīn tōng luò])

舒筋和络 [shū jīn hé luò]

soothing tendons and harmonizing collaterals, synonymous with soothing tendons and unblocking collaterals (舒筋通络 [shū jīn tōng luò])

舒筋止痛 [shū jīn zhǐ tòng]

soothing tendons to relieve pain: measure for treating painful conditions caused by muscle contraction

止血 [zhǐ xuè]

stopping bleeding; hemostasis: a general term for checking the escape of blood from vessels

清热止血 [qīng rè zhǐ xuè]

clearing heat to stop bleeding: method of using heat-clearing hemostatics to treat bleeding due to exuberant heat

凉血止血 [liáng xuè zhǐ xuè]

cooling blood to stop bleeding: method of using blood-cooling hemostatics to treat bleeding due to heat in the blood

补气摄血 [bǔ qì shè xuè]

replenishing *qi* to arrest bleeding: method of using *qi* tonics to treat chronic hemorrhage due to *qi* deficiency

补气止血 [bǔ qì zhǐ xuè]

replenishing *qi* to stop bleeding, same as replenishing *qi* to arrest bleeding (补气摄血 [bǔ qì shè xuè])

祛瘀止血 [qù yū zhǐ xuè]

removing stasis to stop bleeding: method of treating bleeding related to blood stasis

祛痰 [wù tán]

dispelling phlegm: a general term for measures for treating phlegm syndromes

化痰 [huà tán]

resolving phlegm: one of the measures to dispel phlegm in which the phlegm is disintegrated and dissolved

温化寒痰 [wēn huà hán tán]

warming and resolving cold phlegm: method of warming yang, dispelling cold and resolving phlegm for treating cold phlegm syndrome

清化热痰 [qīng huà rè tán]

clearing and resolving heat-phlegm: method of clearing heat and resolving phlegm for treating heat-phlegm syndrome

清热化痰 [qīng rè huà tán]

clearing heat and resolving phlegm: method of combined use of heat-clearing and phlegm-dispelling drugs to treat heat-phlegm syndrome

润肺化痰 [rùn fèi huà tán]

moistening the lung and resolving phlegm: treatment for dryness-phlegm affection of the lung

润燥化痰 rùn zào huà tán]

moistening dryness and resolving phlegm, synonymous with moisten the lung and resolve phlegm (润肺化痰 [rùn fèi huà tán])

润化燥痰 [rùn huà zào tán]

moistening and resolving dry phlegm, same as moistening dryness and resolving phlegm (润燥化痰 [rùn zào huà tán])

燥湿化痰 [zào shī huà tán]

drying dampness and resolving phlegm: treatment for damp-phlegm syndromes

祛寒化痰 [qù hán huà tán]

dispelling cold and resolving phlegm: method of combined use of cold-dispersing and phlegm-dispelling drugs for the treatment of cold-phlegm syndrome

治风化痰 [zhì fēng huà tán]

relieving wind and resolving phlegm: method of combined use of wind-dispersing and phlegm-dispelling drugs for the treatment of wind-phlegm syndrome

息风化痰 [xī fēng huà tán]

extinguishing wind and resolving phlegm: method of treating wind-phlegm syndrome by combined use of wind-extinguishing and phlegm-resolving drugs

涤痰 [dí tán]

flushing phlegm away: method of expelling phlegm with drastic expectorants for treating stubborn phlegm syndromes

豁痰 [huò tán]

scrubbing phlegm: method of eliminating phlegm for resuscitation used in treating impaired consciousness, e.g., loss of consciousness in cases of apoplexy

祛湿 [qù shī]

dispelling dampness: a general term for various measures to treat damp syndromes, including resolving dampness by using aromatics, eliminating dampness by using drugs bitter in taste and cold in nature, and removing dampness through diuresis

化湿 [huà shī]

resolving dampness: one of the measures to dispel dampness, especially that lodging in the upper energizer or exterior portion of the body by using aromatics

芳香化湿 [fāng xiāng huà shī]

resolving dampness with aromatics: method of using aromatics to treat damp syndromes

芳香化浊 [fāng xiāng huà zhuó]

resolving turbidity with aromatics: method of using aromatics to treat damp-turbidity syndromes

清热化湿 [qīng rè huà shī]

clearing heat and resolving dampness: method of treating damp-heat in the upper or middle portions of the body by using heat-clearing and damp-resolving drugs

燥湿 [zào shī]

drying dampness: one of the measures to dispel dampness, especially that lodging in the middle energizer (spleen and stomach) by using drugs bitter in taste

苦温燥湿 [kǔ wēn zào shī]

drying dampness with bitter-warm: method of treating cold-damp syndrome by using drugs bitter in taste and warm in nature

苦寒燥湿 [kǔ hán zào shī]

drying dampness with bitter-cold: method of treating damp-heat syndrome by using drugs bitter in taste and cold in nature

燥湿健脾 [zào shī jiàn pí]

drying dampness to invigorate the spleen: therapeutic method of administering pungent drying drugs to eliminate dampness for the purpose of invigorating the spleen, indicated in the treatment of damp disturbing the spleen

利湿 [lì shī]

draining damp: measure for dispelling dampness, especially that lodging in the lower energizer by using diuretics

利尿 [lì niào]

inducing diuresis: measure for increasing urine excretion

利水 [lì shuǐ]

same as 利尿 [lì niào]

清热利湿 [qīng rè lì shī]

clearing heat and draining damp: method of clearing heat and removing damp through diuresis to treat accumulation of damp-heat in the lower portion of the body by using heat-clearing drugs together with diuretics

淡渗利湿 [dàn shèn lì shī]

draining damp with bland diuretics: one of the common measures to treat diarrhea with watery stools, and edema with oliguria, also abbreviated as 渗湿 [shèn shī]

淡渗祛湿 [dàn shèn qù shī]

expelling damp with bland drugs, synonymous with 淡渗利湿 [dàn shèn lì shī]

渗湿 [shèn shī]

straining off dampness: abbreviated synonym for draining dampness with bland diuretics (淡渗利湿 [dàn shèn lì shī])

利水渗湿 [lì shuǐ shèn shī]

inducing diuresis to drain dampness: therapeutic method for getting rid of dampness by using diuretics

利水消肿 [lì shuǐ xiāo zhǒng]

inducing diuresis to alleviate edema: method of treating edema by using diuretics

温阳利湿 [wēn yáng lì shī]

warming yang to drain damp: method of removing dampness by administering warming drugs together with diuretics, usually used in treating cold-damp syndrome

温阳利水 [wēn yáng lì shuǐ]

warming yang to induce diuresis: one of the measures for treating water retention due to yang deficiency of the spleen and kidney by using yang-invigorating drugs and diuretics

温阳行水 [wēn yáng xíng shuǐ]

warming yang and promoting diuresis, same as 温阳利水 [wēn yáng lì shuǐ]

温肾利水 [wēn shèn lì shuǐ]

warming the kidney to induce diuresis: method of treating edema due to kidney yang deficiency

利小便，实大便 [lì xiǎo biàn, shí dà biàn]

treating diarrhea with diuretics

洁净府 [jìng jíng fǔ]

"cleaning the bladder": an ancient term for the treatment of edema by inducing diuresis

固涩 [gù sè]

inducing astringency; arresting discharges: therapy involving administering styptic or astringent agents for treating spontaneous sweating, seminal emission, chronic diarrhea, or hemorrhage, also called 收涩 [shōu sè]

收涩 [shōu sè]

causing contraction and arresting discharge, same as 固涩 [gù sè]

敛汗 [liǎn hàn]

arresting sweating: method of treating excessive or abnormal sweating

止汗 [zhǐ hàn]

suppressing sweating, same as 敛汗 [liǎn hàn]

敛汗固表 [liǎn hàn gù biǎo]

arresting sweating and strengthening the superficies: method for treating defensive *qi* deficiency with spontaneous sweating, also called 固表止汗 [gù biǎo zhǐ hàn]

固表止汗 [gù biǎo zhǐ hàn]

strengthening the superficies to arrest sweating, synonymous with arresting sweating and strengthening the superficies (敛汗固表 [liǎn hàn gù biǎo])

敛汗固脱 [liǎn hàn gù tuō]

arresting sweating to prevent collapse: method of strengthening the superficies and arresting sweating used in the treatment of incessant profuse sweating with impending collapse

敛肺 [liǎn fèi]

astringing the lung: method of treating deficiency syndromes of the lung with chronic persistent cough by administering astringents and tonics

敛肺止咳 [liàn fèi zhǐ ké]

astringing the lung to stop coughing: method of using astringents to treat persistent unproductive cough due to lung insufficiency

敛肺平喘 [liǎn fèi píng chuǎn]

astringing the lung to relieve dyspnea: method of using astringents to treat dyspnea due to lung insufficiency

敛气 [liǎn qì]

astringing *qi*: method of administering astringents to treat consumption of *qi*

敛阴 [liǎn yīn]

astringing yin: method of administering astringents to replenish and preserve yin fluid for treating consumption of yin

固精 [gù jīng]

arresting emission: abbreviation for strengthening the kidney to arrest emission (固肾涩精 [gù shèn sè jīng])

涩精 [sè jīng]

checking emission, same as arrest emission (固精 [gù jīng])

固肾 [gù shèn]

strengthening the kidney: therapeutic method for treating insecurity of kidney *qi*

固肾涩精 [gù shèn sè jīng]

strengthening the kidney to arrest emission: method of treating seminal emission due to insecurity of kidney *qi* by using kidney tonics with astringents

固肾缩尿 [gù shèn suō niào]

strengthening the kidney to reduce urination: method of treating frequent urination or enuresis due to kidney *qi* insufficiency

固经止血 [gù jīng zhǐ xuè]

astringing menstruation and checking bleeding: treatment for excessive menstrual discharge

固崩止血 [gù bēng zhǐ xuè]

arresting blood flooding: treatment for profuse uterine bleeding

固冲止血 [gù chōng zhǐ xuè]

astringing thoroughfare vessel to check bleeding: method of astringing the thoroughfare and conception vessels to treat abnormal uterine bleeding or excessive menstrual flow

固肾止带 [gù shèn zhǐ dài]

strengthening the kidney to check leukorrhagia: treatment for excessive leukorrhea due to kidney insufficiency

涩精止遗 [sè jīng zhǐ yí]

astringing semen and checking emission: a treatment for seminal emission or spermatorrhea with astringents

固崩止带 [gù bēng zhǐ dài]

arresting metrorrhagia and leukorrhagia: astringing method for treating abnormal uterine bleeding or excessive leukorrhea

涩肠止泻 [sè cháng zhǐ xiè]

astringing the intestines to check diarrhea: method of treating chronic diarrhea with astringents

涩肠止痢 [sè cháng zhǐ lì]

astringing the intestines to check dysentery: method of treating chronic dysentery with astringents

固冲止带 [gù chōng zhǐ dài]

strengthening the thoroughfare vessel and stopping leukorrhagia: method of treating leukorrhagia due to kidney insufficiency with insecurity of the thoroughfare and conception vessels

润燥 [rùn zào]

moistening (dryness): a general term for measures to relieve dryness

甘寒润燥 [gān hán rùn zào]

moistening (dryness) with sweet-cold: method of treating deficiency of fluid in the lung and kidney by administering sweet-tasted and cold natured drugs

养阴润燥 [yǎng yīn rùn zào]

nourishing yin to moisten dryness: method of treating yin deficiency with endogenous dryness

养血润燥 [yǎng xuè rùn zào]

nourishing blood to moisten dryness: method of treating blood deficiency with endogenous dryness

养血润肠 [yǎng xuè rùn cháng]

nourishing blood to moisten the intestine: method of treating constipation due to blood deficiency with dryness of the intestine

润肠通便 [rùn cháng tōng biàn]

moistening the intestine to loose the bowels: method of combined use of moistening drugs together with laxatives to relieve constipation due to intestinal dryness

润肺 [rùn fèi]

moistening the lung: therapy involving using medicines with moistening action to relieve dryness syndrome of the lung

养阴润肺 [yǎng yīn rùn fèi]

nourishing yin to moisten the lung: method of treating dryness syndrome of the lung due to yin deficiency

润肺生津 [rùn fèi shēng jīn]

moistening the lung and producing fluid: method of treating lung yin deficiency with dryness

润肺止咳 [rùn fèi zhǐ ké]

moistening the lung to relieve cough: treatment for cough due to lung yin deficiency with dryness

止咳化痰 [zhǐ ké huà tán]

checking cough and resolving phlegm: method of symptomatic relief of cough with expectoration

甘寒生津 [gān hán shēng jīn]

producing fluid with sweet-cold: method of replenishing body fluid with drugs sweet in taste and cold in nature

益气生津 [yì qì shēng jīn]

replenishing *qi* and producing fluid: method of administering tonics to treat a prostrated state with deficiency of *qi* and fluid after profuse sweating

安神 [ān shén]

calming the mind: a general term for tranquilizing measures

安神定志 [ān shén dìng zhì]

calming and stabilizing the mind: method of treating palpitations and insomnia due to heart insufficiency

益气安神 [yì qì ān shén]

replenishing *qi* to calm the mind: method of treating palpitations, insomnia and forgetfulness due to heart *qi* deficiency

益肾宁神 [yì shèn níng shén]

replenishing the kidney to calm the mind: method of treating palpitations and insomnia caused by frightening or disharmony between the heart and kidney

补肾安神 [bǔ shèn ān shén]

tonifying the kidney to calm the mind, same as replenishing the kidney to calm the mind (益肾宁神 [yì shèn níng shén])

养心安神 [yǎng xīn ān shén]

nourishing the heart to calm the mind: method of using heart-blood tonics and tranquilizing drugs to treat palpitations, insomnia, dream-disturbed sleep and forgetfulness due to heart insufficiency

镇惊安神 [zhèn jīng ān shén]

settling fright and calming the mind: therapeutic method involving the use of settling tranquilizers to relieve mental uneasiness caused by fright

镇心安神 [zhèn xīn ān shén]

settling the heart and calming the mind, same as settling fright and calming the mind 镇惊安神 [zhèn jīng ān shén]

镇惊 [zhèn jīng]

settling fright, abbreviation for settling fright and calming the mind 镇惊安神 [zhèn jīng ān shén]

重镇安神 [zhòng zhèn ān shén]

calming the mind with heavy settling (drugs): method of treating insomnia and excitement due to exuberant heart yang

镇静安神 [zhèn jìng ān shén]

inducing sedation and calming the mind, synonymous with 重镇安神 [zhòng zhèn ān shén]

潜阳 [qiǎn yáng]

subduing yang: method of checking exuberant yang by administering weighty agents to treat adverse upsurge of liver yang due to deficiency of yin

潜阳熄风 [qiǎn yáng xī fēng]

subduing yang and extinguishing wind: therapeutic method of transformation liver yang into wind

滋阴潜阳 [zī yīn qiǎn yáng]

nourishing yin and subduing yang: method of treating exuberance of liver yang due to yin deficiency by using yang-suppressing and yin-nourishing drugs in combination

柔肝 [róu gān]

emolliating the liver: method of treating liver yin deficiency or liver blood insufficiency, also called nourishing the liver (养肝 [yǎng gān])

养肝 [yǎng gān]

nourishing the liver: therapeutic method of nourishing liver yin or blood, synonymous with emolliating the liver (柔肝 [róu gān])

养血柔肝 [yǎng xuè róu gān]

nourishing blood and emolliating the liver: therapeutic method of nourishing liver blood

平肝 [píng gān]

pacifying the liver: a general term for methods of treating hyperactivity of the liver

平肝潜阳 [píng gān qiǎn yáng]

pacifying the liver and subduing yang: method of treating hyperactivity of the liver by administering heavy agents such as shells, metals or minerals, also called settling the liver and subduing yang (镇肝潜阳 [zhèn gān qiǎn yáng])

镇肝潜阳 [zhèn gān qiǎn yáng]

settling the liver and subduing yang, synonymous with pacifying the liver and subduing yang (平肝潜阳 [píng gān qiǎn yáng])

镇潜 [zhèn qiǎn]

settling and subduing: abbreviation for settling the liver and subduing yang (镇肝潜阳 [zhèn gān qiǎn yáng])

息[熄]风 [xī fēng]

extinguishing wind: method of administering sedatives to relieve endogenous wind syndrome, indicated in the treatment of vertigo, tremor, convulsion, epilepsy, etc.

熄风解痉 [xī fēng jiě jìng]

extinguishing wind and relieving spasm: method of relieving involuntary muscle contractions in syndrome of internal stirring of liver wind

息风定痉 [xī fēng dìng jìng]

extinguishing wind and arresting spasm, synonymous with 息风解痉 [xī fēng jiě jìng]

熄风定痫 [xī fēng dìng xián]

extinguishing wind and arresting epilepsy: treatment for epilepsy caused by wind-phlegm

滋阴熄风 [zī yīng xī fēng]

nourishing yin to extinguish wind: method of treating endogenous wind due to serious impairment of yin fluid at the late stage of a febrile disease

平肝熄风 [píng gān xī fēng]

pacifying the liver to extinguish wind: method of treating endogenous wind caused by hyperactivity of the liver

清热熄风 [qīng rè xī fēng]

clearing heat to extinguish wind: method of treating convulsions due to high fever

养血熄风 [yǎng xuè xī fēng]

nourishing blood to extinguish wind: method of treating endogenous wind caused by blood deficiency, with such symptoms as dizziness or involuntary movement of the limbs

开窍 [kāi qiào]

inducing resuscitation: therapeutic method of bringing an unconscious person back to consciousness, also called 醒神 [xǐng shén]

醒神 [xǐng shén]

arousing from unconsciousness, synonymous with inducing resuscitation (开窍 [kāi qiào])

芳香开窍 [fāng xiāng kāi qiào]

inducing resuscitation with aromatics: emergency treatment for loss of consciousness in cases of apoplexy, epilepsy or high fever involving administering aromatic drugs

涤痰开窍 [dí tán kāi qiào]

flushing phlegm away to induce resuscitation: method of treating impairment of consciousness in cases of apoplexy or psychosis

清热化痰开窍 [qīng rè huà tán kāi qiào]

clearing heat and resolving phlegm to restore consciousness: method of relieving convulsions and coma due to high fever by administering heat-clearing and phlegm-resolving drugs

豁痰醒脑 [huò tán xǐng nǎo]

scrubbing phlegm to arouse the brain: method of eliminating phlegm for resuscitation used in treating loss of consciousness

吐法 [tǔ fǎ]

emetic method; emesis: one of the eight principal therapeutic methods used to expel noxious substances (such as retained phlegm, undigested food or toxic substances) by using emetics or mechanical stimulation to induce vomiting

探吐 [tàn tǔ]

mechanical induction of vomiting: method of inducing vomiting with mechanical stimulation of the soft palate or throat

涌吐禁例 [yǒng tǔ jìn lì]

contraindications for emesis: conditions that make emetic therapy inadvisable, e.g., insufficiency of the spleen and stomach, hemorrhagic diseases, old age, and debility

止痛 [zhǐ tòng]

alleviating pain: any therapeutic measure that can give relief from pain

止痒 [zhǐ yǎng]

relieving itching: any therapeutic measure that has an antipruritic effect

燥湿止痒 [zào shī zhǐ yǎng]

drying dampness and relieving itching: therapeutic method for removing exudate and alleviating itching, as used in the treatment of eczema

润燥止痒 [zào shī zhǐ yǎng]

moistening dryness to relieve itching: therapeutic method of tonify blood, nourishing yin, dispelling wind and moistening dryness for relieving itching in cases of blood deficiency with wind-dryness

止呕 [zhǐ ǒu]

arresting vomiting: any therapeutic measure that has an anti-emetic effect

止呃 [zhǐ è]

stopping hiccups: any therapeutic measure that can give relief in cases of of hiccups

止渴 [zhǐ kě]

quenching thirst: any therapeutic measure that has an antidiptic effect

止晕 [zhǐ yūn]

relieving fainting: any therapeutic method that can give relief of in cases of dizziness, vertigo, and even fainting

止痉 [zhǐ jìng]

relieving spasm: any therapeutic measure that relieves spasm

止遗尿 [zhǐ yí niào]

arresting enuresis: method of checking involuntary discharge of urine

安胎 [ān tāi]

preventing miscarriage: preventive and therapeutic measure for threatened miscarriage and habitual abortion

催生 [cuī shēng]

expediting child delivery: method of speeding up child delivery by strengthening the parturient's *qi*

催乳 [cuī rǔ]

stimulating lactation: method of starting or promoting the secretion and yielding of mammary milk

通乳 [tōng rǔ]

freeing milk flow: method of treating galactostasis

下乳 [xià rǔ]

promoting lactation: method of treating lack of lactation

回乳 [huí rǔ]

terminating lactation: method of bringing lactation to a halt

通经 [tōng jīng]

(1) stimulating menstrual discharge: any method that can stimulate menstruation in the treatment of amenorrhea; **(2) removing obstruction in meridians**

通经活络 [tōng jīng huó luò]

unblocking meridians and activating collaterals: therapeutic method of removing obstruction in the meridian system

通利血脉 [tōng lì xuè mài]

promoting blood circulation: therapeutic method of improving circulation in blood vessels

通络止痛 [tōng luò zhǐ tòng]

unblocking collaterals to alleviate pain: method of treating painful conditions caused by blockage in collateral meridians

通经止痛 [tōng jīng zhǐ tòng]

unblocking meridians to alleviate pain: method of treating painful conditions caused by blockage of meridian *qi*

调经 [tiáo jīng]

regulating menstruation: a general term referring to methods of treating irregular menstruation

通淋 [tōng lín]

relieving stranguria: any therapeutic method that is effective for treating stranguria

通利关节 [tōng lì guān jié]

easing joint movement: therapeutic method effective for relieving arthralgia and improving joint movement

退黄 [tuì huáng]

relieving jaundice: therapeutic method effective for treating jaundice

内消 [nèi xiāo]

elimination from within: therapeutic method of curing a sore before it undergoes suppuration by oral administration of antiphlogistics

内托 [nèi tuō]

expulsion from within: therapeutic method of administering tonics to promote pus discharge, also called 托法 [tuō fǎ]

托法 [tuō fǎ]

expulsion method, synonymous with expulsion from within (内托 [nèi tuō])

托毒 [tuō dú]

expelling toxins: method of expelling toxins from within in the treatment of boils and sores

托疮 [tuō chuāng]

promoting pus discharge: method of expelling pus in the treatment of boils, sores and abscess

排脓 [pái nóng]

draining pus: method of promoting pus discharge

清热排脓 [qīng rè pái nóng]

clearing heat and evacuating pus: therapeutic method of removing heat toxins and draining pus from an abscess

排脓消肿 [pái nóng xiāo zhǒng]

evacuating pus and eliminating swelling: method for treating abscess in external diseases

排脓托毒 [pái nóng tuō dú]

evacuating pus and expelling toxins: therapeutic method of evacuating pus and expelling toxins from the body

托里排脓 [tuō lǐ pái nóng]

evacuating pus from within: method of using tonics to expel toxins from within for the evacuation of pus

拔毒 [bá dú]

drawing out toxins: therapeutic method to remove toxins from inflammatory lesions

去火毒 [qù huǒ dú]

removing fire toxins: method of treating inflammatory external diseases

提脓拔毒 [tí nóng bá dú]

drawing out pus and toxins: method used in the treatment of inflammatory external diseases

化腐 [huà fǔ]

resolving putridity: therapeutic method for treating external diseases, especially wounds and sores

去腐肉 [qù fǔ ròu]

removing necrotic tissue: therapeutic method for treating external diseases, especially wounds and sores

蚀疮去腐 [shí chuāng qù fǔ]

corroding wounds and removing putridity

生肌 [shēn jī]

(1) promoting tissue regeneration; (2) promoting granulation

生肌敛疮 [shēng jī liǎn chuāng]

promoting tissue regeneration and wound healing: therapeutic method of promoting the healing of wounds or ulcer on the body surface

攻溃 [gōng kuì]

promoting suppuration: method of treating ulcers and boils by administering suppuratia

攻毒 [gōng dú]

counteracting toxins: removal of toxic properties from a poison

以毒攻毒 [yǐ dú gōng dú]

combating poison with poison: any measure to treat malignant or poisoning diseases with poisonous drugs, e.g., chaulmoogra for leprosy, gamboge for carbuncles

解毒 [jiě dú]

removing toxin; detoxication: (1) measure to lessen the virulence of pathogenic organism, as in the treatment of pyogenic inflammation; (2) method of neutralizing the toxic property of poisons, e.g., venom

解酒毒 [jǐ jiǔ dú]

removing alcoholic toxins: therapeutic method of relieving alcoholism

解毒消肿 [jiě dú xiāo zhǒng]

removing toxins and promoting subsidence of swelling: therapeutic method for treating abscesses and sores

消痈散结 [xiāo yōng sàn jié]

dispersing abscesses and dissipating nodulation: therapeutic method of dissolving abscesses before suppuration

消痈散疖 [xiāo yōng sàn jiē]

dispersing abscesses and dissipating boils: therapeutic method of dissolving abscesses and sores before suppuration

消肿止痛 [xiāo zhǒng zhǐ tòng]

dispersing swelling to alleviate pain: therapeutic method of dispersing inflammatory swelling for the purpose of relieving pain

止血行瘀 [zhǐ xuè xíng yū]

arresting bleeding and removing ecchymosis: therapeutic method of treating traumatic injuries

止血敛疮 [zhǐ xuè liǎn chuāng]

arresting bleeding and closing sores: method of treating sores

止血收口 [zhǐ xuè shōu kǒu]

arresting bleeding and closing cut: method for treating incisions

通鼻 [tōng bí]

unblocking the nose: any therapeutic method that relieves nasal obstruction

通鼻窍 [tōng bí qiào]

relieving stuffy nose, synonymous with unblocking nose (通鼻 [tōng bí])

利咽 [lì yān]

relieving sore throat: any therapeutic method that relieves a sore throat

消骨鲠 [xiāo gǔ gěng]

dissolving fish bone: therapeutic method for treating fish bone stuck in the throat or esophagus

乌须发 [wū xū fà]

blackening the hair and beard: therapeutic method for treating premature graying of the hair and beard

明目 [míng mù]

improving the eyesight: any therapeutic method that can ameliorate impairment of vision

退翳明目 [tuì yì míng mù]

removing nebula to improve vision: method of treating nebula

退目翳 [tuì mù yì]

removing nebula, synonymous with 退翳明目 [tuì yì míng mù]

聪耳 [cōng ěr]

improving the hearing; improving auditory acuity: method of treating impaired hearing

截疟 [jié nüè]

checking malaria: method of treating malaria

安蛔 [ān huí]

quieting ascaris: method of treating ascariasis, usually for relieving abdominal pain or biliary colic

安蛔定痛 [ān huí dìng tòng]

quieting ascaris to relieve pain: method of treating abdominal pain due to intestinal or biliary ascariasis

驱虫 [qū chóng]

expelling worms: method of treating intestinal parasites

驱虫消积 [qū chóng xiāo jī]

expelling intestinal worms and removing stagnancy: therapeutic method for expelling stagnation of intestinal parasites, especially ascarids

杀虫 [shā chóng]

killing worms: treatment for destroying intestinal parasites

化石 [huà shí]

dissolving calculi: therapeutic method of treating biliary or urinary calculi by dissolution

排石 [pái shí]

expelling calculi: method of treating biliary or urinary calculi by expulsion from the biliary duct or urinary tract

外治 [wài zhì]

external treatment: any treatment applied to the body surface or given from outside but not oral medication, also called 外治法 [wài zhì fǎ]

外治法 [wài zhì fǎ]

external therapy, same as external treatment (外治 [wài zhì])

外敷 [wài fū]

external application, also abbreviated as 敷 [fū]

敷 [fū]

abbreviation for 外敷 [wài fū]

罨 [yǎn]

compression: a therapeutic measure involving local application of a folded towel or cloth soaked in hot or cold water or medical solution

冷罨 [lěng yǎn]

cold compression: a therapeutic measure involving local application of a folded towel or cloth soaked in cold water

热罨 [rè yǎn]

hot compression: a therapeutic measure involving local application of a folded towel or cloth soaked in hot water

熨法 [yùn fǎ]

hot compression with rubbing: a therapeutic measure involving pressing and rubbing the diseased area with hot medical substances wrapped in cloth

熏蒸 [xūn zhēng]

fuming and steaming: therapy involving fumes from a burning roll of medicated paper or vapor from boiling medicinal ingredients

吸入 [xī rù]

inhalation: treatment of a disease by inhaling fumes or vapor

热烘 [rè hōng]

warming over a fire: therapeutic method involving heating the diseased area after applying medical ointment, indicated in the treatment of skin diseases with dryness and itching, such as tinea manuum, chronic eczema and neurodermatitis

烙法 [lào fǎ]

cauterization: application of a searing iron to destroy diseased tissue

溻浴 [tā yù]

medicated immersion: therapeutic method involving immersing a certain part of the body or the whole body in medicated solution

膏摩 [gāo mó]

rubbing with ointment: method of treating arthralgia or skin diseases

发泡 [fā pào]

vesiculation: skin stimulation with drugs to cause blister formation as therapeutic method

点眼 [diǎn yǎn]

eye dropping: therapeutic method of dropping medicated solution into the conjunctival sac

搐鼻 [chù bí]

insufflating into the nose: inhaling powdered medicine into the nostrils

含漱 [hán shù]

gargling: method of treatment involving holding a liquid in the mouth and throat and agitating it with air from the lung, also called 漱涤 [shù dí]

漱涤 [shù dí]

washing by gargling, same as gargling (含漱 [hán shù])

吹药 [chuī yào]

insufflation into the throat: blowing powdered medicine into the throat or inner part of the mouth for therapeutic purposes

扑粉 [pū fěn]

application of medicinal powder

导便 [dǎo biàn]

inducing defecation: method of opening the bowels involving an enema or suppository, also called 导法 [dǎo fǎ]

导法 [dǎo fǎ]

same as 导便 [dǎo biàn]

塞法 [sāi fǎ]

insertion method: therapeutic method involving inserting medicinal powder packed in cotton or gauze or suppositories into the nostrils, vagina or rectum

枯痔法 [kū zhì fǎ]

necrotizing therapy for hemorrhoids: method to curing hemorrhoids involving local application and injection of necrotizing agents

挂线疗法 [guà xiàn liáo fǎ]

ligation therapy: method of treating anal fistula by ligation with medicated silk thread or a rubber band to necrotize and remove it gradually

熏洗疗法 [xūn xǐ liáo fǎ]

fuming-washing therapy: therapeutic method involving fuming the diseased area with the vapor of a boiling decoction and then washing the area with the decoction

拔罐疗法 [bá guàn liáo fǎ]

cupping therapy: therapeutic method using a vacuumized cup or small jar sucked on the skin to cause local congestion

膏摩疗法 [gāo mó liáo fǎ]

massage therapy with ointment: a massage therapy in which medicated ointment is applied to the area to be treated before manipulation

食疗 [shí liáo]

diet therapy: therapeutic use of diet and food based on the tastes and actions of different foodstuffs, also called 食治 [shí zhì]

食治 [shí zhì]

same as 食疗 [shí liáo]

中药学 Chinese Pharmaceutics

中药 Chinese Medicinals

中药学 [zhōng yào xué]

Chinese pharmaceutics: the branch of health sciences dealing with the preparation, dispensing, and proper utilization of Chinese drugs

本草 [běn cǎo]

materia medica: traditional name for Chinese pharmaceutics

中药 [zhōng yào]

Chinese medicinals, Chinese drugs, usually referring to those recorded in Chinese materia medica

草药 [cǎo yào]

herbal drugs, medicinal herbs, usually referring to those not recorded in Chinese materia medica or only used in folk medicine. A clear-cut differentiation between medicinal herbs in folk medicine and regular traditional drugs is difficult to make, and so they are usually called 中草药 [zhōng cǎo yào] or Chinese traditional and herbal drugs in combination.

中草药 [zhōng cǎo yào]

Chinese herbal drugs: cf. Chinese drugs (中药 [zhōng yào]) and herbal drugs (草药 [cǎo yào])

药材 [yào cái]

medicinal substance, medicinal material: crude natural drug for processing

药材炮制 [yào cái páo zhì]

processing of medicinal substances: Crude drugs are treated by cleansing, cutting, soaking, drying, calcining, baking, steaming, simmering, carbonizing, roasting, etc., for fulfilling the therapeutic, dispensing or manufacturing requirements and assuring the safety and efficacy of drugs.

炮制 [páo zhì]

drug processing: treating of an individual herb or medicinal substance before its medical use

炮炙 [páo zhì]

processing (of drug): a term synonymous with 炮制 [páo zhì], but literally limited to processing with heat

修治 [xiū zhì]

(1) drug processing: an ancient term for 炮制 [páo zhì]; **(2) primary processing:** the elementary procedures of preparing a medicinal herb, including purification, crushing, cutting into slices, etc.

修事 [xiū shì]

an ancient term for drug processing (炮制 [páo zhì])

水制 [shuǐ zhì]

water processing: processing by utilizing water, including washing, bleaching, soaking, refining with water, etc.

火制 [huǒ zhì]

fire processing: processing by utilizing heat or fire, including stir-baking, baking, calcining, etc.

水火共制 [shuǐ huǒ gòng zhì]

water-fire processing: processing by utilizing water and heat or fire, including simmering, steaming, blanching, quenching, etc.

洗 [xǐ]

wash: cleanse by immersing in or applying water

泡 [pào]

macerate: immerse drugs in water to soften them before peeling or cutting

水飞 [shuǐ fēi]

elutriate, refine with water: remove impurities from a powdered drug and at the same time obtain finer powder by mixing it with water in a tank and allowing the supernatant turbid fluid to settle in another tank, and then collecting the deposit

煅 [duàn]

calcine: burn a drug on a fire to make it crispy

煅淬 [duàn cuì]

calcine and quench: calcine the drug until it is red-hot, and then dip it quickly into a specified liquid to make it crispy

制炭 [zhì tàn]

carbonize: heat a vegetable drug in an air-tight container or by stir-baking it over a strong fire till its outer part is charred while its inner part becomes yellowish-brown, so that its original property is retained

烘焙 [hōng bèi]

bake: dry a medical substance over a slow fire

煨 [wèi]

roast (in hot ashes): bake a drug wrapped in wet paper or coated with dough in hot ashes till the paper or coat turns black

炒 [chǎo]

stir-bake: bake a drug in a pan, with constant stirring

清炒 [qīng chǎo]

stir-bake (without adjuvant): bake a drug in a pan, with constant stirring and without adding any adjuvant

加辅料炒 [jiā fǔ liào chǎo]

stir-bake with adjuvant: bake a drug in a pan with constant stirring together with earth, bran, or rice as an adjuvant

微炒 [wēi chǎo]

stir-bake to just dry: bake a drug in a pan over a slow fire, with constant stirring, to make it dry

炒爆 [chǎo bào]

stir-bake to cracking: bake a drug (usually seeds) in a pan, with constant stirring, till it cracks

炒黄 [chǎo huáng]

stir-bake to yellow: bake a drug in a pan, with constant stirring, till it turns yellow and gives off a scent

炒焦 [chǎo jiāo]

stir-bake to brown: bake a drug in a pan, with constant stirring, till it turns brown

炒炭 [chǎo tàn]

stir-bake to charcoal: bake a drug in a pan, with constant stirring, till it partly turns to charcoal

炮 [páo]

stir-bake at a high temperature: prepare a drug by baking with stirring (usually together with hot sand) at a high temperature for a short while so as to reduce its violent action

炙 [zhì]

stir-bake with fluid adjuvant: bake, with stirring, a drug together with wine, vinegar, salt water, honey, or ginger juice, until the latter is infiltrated into the drug.

蒸 [zhēng]

steam: prepare a drug or a drug thoroughly mixed with a fluid adjuvant by steaming in a suitable container

炖 [dùn]

simmer in a bath: put a drug and fluid adjuvant into an airtight container, and heat it in a water bath or with steam until the fluid adjuvant has been absorbed

熬 [áo]

stew: boil slowly and gently for concentration

煮 [zhǔ]

boil: heat a drug together with water or fluid adjuvant

潬 [dàn]

blanch (in water): put certain seeds in boiling water, stir for a short time until the shrunken testa are extended, transfer the seeds to cold water and remove the testa

淬 [cuì]

quench: cool a red-hot substance rapidly by placing it in water in order to make it crispy

烧存性 [shāo cún xìng]

burn with the original property retained: burn a vegetable drug till its outer part is charred while its inner part becomes yellowish-brown, so that its original property is retained

去油 [qù yóu]

defat: remove fat or oil from drugs (such as croton seed) to reduce their toxicity.

去火毒 [qù hǒu dú]

remove fire toxin: eliminate the irritating quality of a newly prepared plaster base by placing it in a shady and cool place or in water for a period of time before using it

制霜 [zhì shuāng]

make into frost: make the defatted herbs (usually seeds) into frost-like powder or re-crystallize the mineral substances into fine particles

药味 [yào wèi]

(1) medicinal ingredients (in a prescription)**: (2) taste or flavor of a drug**, representing the basic action of a drug

气味 [qì wèi]

property and flavor: the property and flavor of a drug that represent the main effects of the drug

性味 [xìng wèi]

same as 气味 [qì wèi]

药性 [yào xìng]

drug properties: the basic properties of a drug, including its nature, taste, meridian tropism, acting direction, and toxicity

四性 [sì xìng]

four properties: the basic properties of drugs, i.e., cold, hot, warm and cool, classified according to their therapeutic effects, e.g., drugs effective for treating heat syndromes being endowed with cold or cool property, while those effective for cold syndromes, with warm or hot property

四气 [sì qì]

four natures: the basic natures of drugs, same as the four properties (四性 [sì xìng])

五味 [wǔ wèi]

five tastes (flavors): the taste of a drug — pungent, sweet, sour, bitter or salty, and sometimes tasteless in addition, representing the basic action of the drug, e.g., most drugs with a dispersing action being pungent, astringents being sour, and tonics being sweet

归经 [guī jīng]

meridian tropism: classification of drugs according to the meridian(s) on which their therapeutic action is manifested, e.g., *Radix Platycodi, Flos Farfarae* and *Radix Asteris* being grouped under the lung meridian owing to their antitussive effect in cases of lung diseases

升降浮沉 [shēng jiàng fú chén]

ascending, descending, floating and sinking: direction of the action of drugs. The ascending and floating drugs have an upward and outward effect, and are used for activating vitality, inducing sweating and dispelling cold, while the descending and sinking drugs, having a downward and inward effect, are used for tranquillizing, causing contraction, relieving cough, arresting emesis, and promoting diuresis or purgation.

大毒、常毒、小毒、无毒 [dà dú、cháng dú、xiǎo dú、wú dú]

extremely poisonous, moderately poisonous, slightly poisonous and

non-poisonous drugs: classification of drugs according to their toxicity.

三品 [sān pǐn]

three grades of drugs: an ancient classification of drugs chiefly based on their toxicity:

上品 [shàng pǐn]

high-grade drug: a drug that is non-toxic, possesses a rejuvenating effect and can be taken frequently and for a long period of time without harm.

中品 [zhōng pǐn]

medium-grade drug: a drug that has no or only slight toxic effect and is effective for treating diseases or deficiency

下品 [xià pǐn]

low-grade drug: a drug that is effective for expelling pathogens, but is toxic and should not be taken for a long period of time.

五味所入 [wǔ wèi suǒ rù]

what the different tastes act on: an ancient hypothesis in Chinese pharmacology based upon the theory of the five elements that drugs of different tastes act on different viscera selectively

剂量 [jì liàng]

dosage: the measured quantity of a drug to be taken

剂型 [jì xíng]

preparation form; dosage form: form of a prepared medicine

丸 [wán]

pill: a solid globular mass, coated or uncoated, made of finely powdered drugs with a suitable excipient or binder

水丸 [shuǐ wán]

watered pill: a small globular medicated mass, in which water is used as a binder

蜜丸 [mì wán]

honeyed pill: a globular medicated mass, in which processed honey is used as a binder

糊丸 [hú wán]

pasted pill: a small globular medicated mass, in which rice-paste or flour-paste is used as a binder

浓缩丸 [nóng suō wán]

concentrated pill: a small globular medicated mass, in which part of the drug is made into extract and used as a binder

微丸 [wēi wán]

minute pill: a very small globular medicated mass with a diameter less than 2.5 mm.

散 [sǎn]

powder: a medicated preparation in the form of discrete fine particles, for internal administration or topical application.

膏 [gāo]

a general term for soft extract, ointment and adhesive plaster

煎膏 [jiān gāo]

soft extract: a medicated preparation for oral administration, usually made by concentrating a decoction to a syrupy consistency with the addition of sugar or honey, also known as 膏滋 [gāo zī]

膏滋 [gāo zī]

another name for soft extract (煎膏 [jiān gāo])

软膏 [ruǎn gāo]

ointment: an unguent for application to the skin

乳膏 [rǔ gāo]

cream: ointment with an emulsifying base

膏药 [gāo yào]

adhesive plaster: a medicated dressing that consists of a film (as of cloth or paper) spread with a medicated substance

丹 [dān]

pellet: a medicated preparation in the form of small particles, usually made from minerals by sublimation for topical application, but some also for internal administration

露 [lù]

distillate: a liquid product of herbal medicine, usually aromatic, condensed from vapor during distillation

锭 [dìng]

pastil; lozenge: ingot-shaped tablet of medicine, prepared according to a specified method and used internally or externally.

药酒 [yào jiǔ]

medicinal wine: wine or spirit in which medicinal ingredients have been steeped

汤药 [tāng yào]

(medicinal) decoction: a liquid medicine prepared by boiling the ingredients in water, and taken after the dregs are removed

汤剂 [tāng jì]

decoction, same as 汤药 [tāng yào]

饮 [yǐn]

cold decoction: decoction to be taken cold

饮片 [yǐn piàn]

medicinal slices: herbs in small pieces or slices, mostly after appropriate processing

药面 [yào miàn]

medicinal powder: drug made into powder

茶 [chá]

(medicinal) tea: drug in coarse powder from or made into small cakes, taken as tea after being infused with boiling water or boiled in water

曲 [qū]

leaven: powdered drug mixed with wheat flour and beaten into cakes for fermentation, usually used as a stomachic

胶 [jiāo]

glue: solid lumps for internal administration after melting, prepared by extracting substance from animal skin, bone, shell or horn with water, concentrating the liquid to a thick gelatinoid consistency, drying and cutting into lumps

片 [piàn]

tablet: small, flattened pellet of compressed powdered medicine or extract of medicine with starch as a formative agent

冲剂 [chōng jì]

(medicinal) granules: granules made of drug extract, usually with sugar as a corrigent, to be dissolved in boiling water before being taken

冲服剂 [chōng fú jì]

same as 冲剂 [chōng jì]

溶化 [róng huà]

dissolve: dissolve a drug in water or a decoction before taking

烊化 [yáng huà]

melt: melt a drug (such as honey or ass-hide glue) in hot water or a decoction before taking

煎药法 [jiān yào fǎ]

method of making a decoction: The usual process is to mix the ingredients with an adequate amount of water, boil them for a certain period of time and remove the dregs from the liquid before taking.

文火 [wén huǒ]

slow fire: fire used for making decoctions which need a longer period of boiling, such as tonics

武火 [wǔ huǒ]

fierce fire: fire used for making decoctions which only allows a short period of boiling, such as pungent diaphoretics

先煎 [xiān jiān]

to be decocted first: While making a decoction, certain drugs (chiefly minerals and shells with active constituents difficult to be extracted) should be boiled before other ingredients are added.

后下 [hòu xià]

to be decocted later: Drugs with active constituents ready to diffuse or evaporate should be added when the decocting is nearly done.

包煎 [bāo jiān]

to be decocted with wrapping; wrap-decoct: Downy or powdered drugs or drugs containing much mucilage are usually wrapped with a piece of cloth or gauze when the decoction is made.

另煎 [lìng jiān]

to be decocted separately: Some expensive drugs, e.g., ginseng, should be decocted separately in order to avoid absorption of the extract by the dregs of other ingredients

单煎 [dān jiān]

to be decocted alone: a synonym for "to be decocted separately" (另煎 [lìng jiān])

服药法 [fú yào fǎ]

method of taking medicines

冲服 [chōng fú]

to be taken infused: take medicine (usually aromatics or powders) after pouring hot water or hot decoction of other drugs over it, with stirring

调服 [tiáo fú]

to be taken after mixing: take medicinal powder after mixing it with liquid such as a portion of hot decoction of other drugs, water, wine, etc.

吞服 [tūn fú]

to be swallowed

送服 [sòng fú]

to be taken with fluid: (pills or powder) to be swallowed together with warm water in most cases, dilute decoction of fresh ginger for warming drugs, mint solution for heat-clearing drugs, diluted salt water for tonics, etc.

噙化 [qín huà]

to be melted in the mouth: (pills or pastilles) to be melted in the mouth and then swallowed or spat out

食远服 [shí yuǎn fú]

to be taken midway between meals

临睡前服 [lín shuì qián fú]

to be taken before bedtime

空腹服 [kōng fù fú]

to be taken on an empty stomach: to be taken in the morning before breakfast

顿服 [dùn fú]

to be taken in one single dose

频服 [pín fú]

to be taken frequently: (decoction) to be taken in small portions at frequent intervals

温服 [wēn fú]

to be taken warm

热服 [rè fú]

to be taken hot: A decoction with ingredients hot in property for treating a cold syndrome may give better results if it is taken hot.

冷服 [lěng fú]

to be taken cold: A decoction with ingredients cold in nature for treating a heat syndrome may give better results if is taken cold

妊娠禁忌药 [rèn shēn jìn jì yào]

contraindications during pregnancy: drugs whose administration is prohibited during pregnancy

服药食忌 [fú yào shí jì]

dietary prohibitions during medication: species of food that are not allowed to be taken during the drug treatment period

食忌 [shí jì]

dietary prohibitions: abbreviation for dietary prohibitions during medication (服药食忌 [fú yào shí jì])

忌口 [jì kǒu]

food taboo: food prohibited from the patient's diet

常用引文 Commonly Used Citations

苦入心。 [kǔ rù xīn]

Drugs bitter in taste act on the heart.

酸入肝。 [suān rù gān]

Drugs sour in taste act on the liver.

甘入脾。 [gān rù pí]

Drugs sweet in taste act on the spleen.

辛入肺。 [xīn rù fèi]

Drugs pungent in taste act on the lung.

咸入肾。 [xián rù shèn]

Drugs salty in taste act on the kidney.

辛散，酸收，甘缓，苦坚，咸软。[xīn sǎn, suān shōu, gān huǎn, kǔ jiān, xián ruǎn]

The pungent causes dispersion, the sour is astringent, the sweet has a moderating effect, the bitter makes firmness, and the salty softens hard masses.

治热以寒，温而行之。[zhì rè yǐ hán, wēn ér xíng zhī]

Treat a heat syndrome with cold-propertied drugs, and the decoction should be taken warm.

治寒以热。凉而行之。[zhì hán yǐ rè, liáng ér xíng zhī]

Treat a cold syndrome with hot-propertied drugs, and the decoction should be taken cool.

用温远温，用热远热，用凉远凉，用寒远寒。[yòng wēn yuǎn wēn, yòng rè yuǎn rè, yòng liáng yuǎn liáng, yòng hán yuǎn hán]

Avoid using warm-propertied medicines in warm weather, hot-propertied medicines in hot weather, cool-propertied medicines in cool weather, and cold-propertied medicines in cold weather.

有毒无毒，所治为主。[yǒu dú wú dú, suǒ zhì wéi zhǔ]

The selection of a drug with toxicity or without toxicity depends upon the case.

大毒治病，十去其六。[dà dú zhì bìng, shí qù qí liù]

The administration of a drug with great toxicity should be ceased

when the disease is 60% removed.

常毒治病，十去其七。[cháng dú zhì bìng, shí qù qí qī]

The administration of a drug with moderate toxicity should be ceased when the disease is 70% removed.

小毒治病，十去其八。[xiǎo dú zhì bìng, shí qù qí bā]

The administration of a drug with minimal toxicity should be ceased when the disease is 80% removed.

无毒治病，十去其九。[wú dú zhì bìng, shí qù qí jiǔ]

The administration of a drug without any toxicity should be ceased when the disease is 90% removed.

有故无殒，亦无殒也。[yǒu gù wú yǔn, yì wú yǔn yě]

If there is enough reason, a toxic drug can also be used without harm.

中药的分类 Classification of Chinese Drugs [Medicinals]

解表药 [jiě biǎo yào]

exterior-releasing drug [medicinal]; superficies-releasing drug [medicinal]: an agent or substance that has the effect of dispelling exogenous pathogenic factors from the superficial, exterior aspect of the body, usually through sweating

发汗解表药 [fā hàn jiě biǎo yào]

diaphoretic exterior-releasing drug [medicinal]: an agent or substance that releases an exterior syndrome through sweating

发表药 [fā biǎo yào]

exterior-effusing drug [medicinal]: synonym for exterior-releasing drug [medicinal] (解表药 [jiě biǎo yào])

发散风寒药 [fā sàn fēng hán yào]

wind-cold dispersing drug [medicinal]: an agent or substance that has the effect of dispersing wind and cold in the treatment of an exterior syndrome

发散风热药 [fā sàn fēng rè yào]

wind-heat dispersing drug [medicinal]: an agent or substance that has the effect of dispersing wind and heat in the treatment of an exterior syndrome

辛温解表药 [xīn wēn jiě biǎo yào]

pungent-warm exterior-releasing drug [medicinal]: an agent or substance pungent in flavor and warm in property, such as *Herba Ephedrae* or *Ramulus Cinnamomi*, which is usually used for treating a wind-cold exterior syndrome

辛凉解表药 [xīn liáng jiě biǎo yào]

pungent-cool exterior-releasing drug [medicinal]: an agent or substance pungent in flavor and cool in property, such as *Herba Menthae* or *Flos Chrysanthemi*, which is usually used for treating a wind-heat exterior syndrome

清热药 [qīng rè yào]

heat-clearing drug [medicinal]: an agent or substance cold or cool in property, which has the effect of clearing up internal heat in cases of externally contracted febrile diseases with high fever and dire thirst, damp-heat dysentery, eruptive epidemic warm diseases, boils, sores and abscess, or fever in cases of yin deficiency

清热泻火药 [qīng rè xiè huǒ yào]

heat-clearing and fire-purging drug [medicinal]: an agent or substance that has the effect of clearing heat from the *qi* system, with high fever, dire thirst, dry yellow tongue coating and rapid surging pulse, or purging fire from the internal organs, such as heart fire, liver fire, etc.

清热凉血药 [qīng rè liáng xuè yào]

heat-clearing and blood-cooling drug [medicinal]: an agent or substance that has the effect of eliminating pathological heat from the nutrient and blood systems in cases of warm diseases marked by fever accompanied by delirium, eruptions and bleeding symptoms, and also in other diseases with bleeding due to heat in the blood

清热燥湿药 [qīng rè zào shī yào]

heat-clearing and dampness-drying drug [medicinal]: an agent or substance bitter in taste and cold in property that is effective for eliminating heat and dampness, usually used in the treatment of diseases caused by damp-heat, such as acute jaundice, acute dysentery, urinary infection, eczema, boils and abscesses

清热解毒药 [qīng rè jiě dú yào]

heat-clearing and toxicity-relieving drug [medicinal]: an agent or substance that counteracts heat toxins or fire toxins, mainly indicated in the treatment of boils, sores, abscess, erysipelas, epidemic infectious diseases, mumps, dysentery, insect or snake bite, and burns

清虚热药 [qīng xū rè yào]

deficiency-heat-clearing drug [medicinal]: an agent or substance that clears heat from deficiency conditions, often indicated in the treatment of heat due to yin deficiency marked by afternoon fever with heat sensation in the palms and soles, night sweats, reddened tongue and scanty coating, but also used in the late stage of a warm disease with residual heat

泻下药 [xiè xià yào]

purgative (drug [medicinal]): an agent or substance that promotes defecation or even causes diarrhea, not only for relieving constipation, but also for driving stagnant matter, excessive heat and retained fluid out of the body

攻下药 [gōng xià yào]

offensive purgative (drug [medicinal]): an agent or substance, usually bitter in taste and cold in property, that has a potent purgative effect for moving the bowels and driving away excessive heat and stagnant matter

温下药 [wēn xià yào]

warm purgative (drug [medicinal]): an agent or substance warm in property, which relieves constipation caused by excessive cold stagnation

润下药 [rùn xià yào]

laxative (drug [medicinal]): an agent or substance that lubricates the intestinal tract to facilitate defecation for relieving constipation in the aged with fluid deficiency, in cases of febrile diseases with fluid impairment and in postpartum blood deficiency

峻下逐水药 [jùn xià zhú shuǐ yào]

drastic hydragogue: a cathartic that causes copious water discharge for reducing accumulated fluid in anasarca, ascites and pleural effusion

祛风湿药 [qù fēng shī yào]

wind-damp-dispelling drug [medicinal]; antirheumatic: an agent or substance that dispels wind and damp, mainly for relieving rheumatism and related conditions

祛风湿散寒药 [qù fēng shī sàn hán yào]

wind-damp-dispelling and cold-dispersing drug [medicinal]: an agent or substance that dispels wind-damp, disperses cold, soothes the tendons and unblocks the collateral meridians, indicated in wind-damp (rheumatic or rheumatoid) arthralgia of cold type

祛风湿清热药 [qù fēng shī qīng rè yào]

wind-damp-dispelling and heat-clearing drug [medicinal]: an agent or substance that dispels wind-damp, unblocks the collateral meridians, clears heat, reduces swelling and alleviates pain, suitable for treating wind-damp (rheumatic or rheumatoid) arthralgia of heat type with redness, swelling, hotness and pain in the joints

祛风湿强筋骨药 [qù fēng shī qiáng jīn gǔ yào]

wind-damp-dispelling and tendon-bone-strengthening drug [medicinal]: an agent or substance that dispels wind-damp, tonifies the liver and kidney and strengthens the tendons and bones, mainly used in the treatment of chronic arthralgia with aching back and weak legs

化湿药 [huà shī yào]

damp-resolving drug [medicinal]: an agent or substance with fragrant odor, warming and drying, that resolves dampness and invigorates the spleen, also called fragrant damp-resolving drug [medicinal] (芳香化湿药 [fāng xiāng huà shī yào])

芳香化湿药 [fāng xiāng huà shī yào]

fragrant damp-resolving drug [medicinal]: a fragrant agent or substance effective for resolving damp, often used in the treatment of damp syndrome marked by anorexia, lassitude, nausea and vomiting, distension in the chest and abdomen, greasy tongue coating and slippery pulse either in cases of febrile diseases or in other miscellaneous diseases

利水渗湿药 [lì shuǐ shèn shī yào]

damp-draining diuretic (drug [medicinal]): an agent or substance that increases urine excretion and water discharge for treating internal retention of dampness

利湿药 [lì shī yào]

damp-draining drug [medicinal]: a synonym for damp-draining diuretic (利水渗湿药 [lì shuǐ shèn shī yào])

利水消肿药 [lì shuǐ xiāo zhǒng yào]

edema-alleviating diuretic (drug [medicinal]): an agent or substance that increases urine excretion for treating edema with oliguria, diarrhea, and retained fluid

利尿通淋药 [lì niào tōng lín yào]

stranguria-relieving diuretic (drug [medicinal]): an agent or substance that increases urine excretion and relieves stranguria, mainly indicated in the treatment of damp-heat in the lower energizer with painful discharge of urine

通淋药 [tōng lín yào]

stranguria-relieving drug [medicinal]: an agent or substance that relieves various kinds of stranguria, including damp-heat stranguria and urolithiasis

利湿退黄药 [lì shī tuì huáng yào]

damp-draining anti-icteric (drug [medicinal]): an agent or substance that drains damp and relieves icterus indicated in the treatment of damp-heat jaundice

利胆退黄药 [lì dăn tuì huáng yào]

bile-draining anti-icteric (drug [medicinal]): an agent or substance that promotes increased flow of bile to relieve jaundice

利尿逐水药 [lì niào zhú shuĭ yào]

diuretic hydragogue (drug [medicinal]): an agent or substance that causes copious discharge of water through catharsis and at the same time increases urine excretion

温里药 [wēn lĭ yào]

interior-warming drug [medicinal]: an agent or substance that warms the interior and expels internal cold, also called cold-expelling drug [medicinal] (祛寒药 [qù hán yào])

祛寒药 [qù hán yào]

cold-expelling drug [medicinal]: a synonym for interior-warming drug [medicinal] (温里药 [wēn lĭ yào])

理气药 [lĭ qì yào]

***qi*-regulating drug [medicinal]:** an agent or substance that regulates the activity of *qi* to treat *qi* stagnation or adverse *qi* flow, also called *qi*-moving drug [medicinal] (行气药 [xíng qì yào])

行气药 [xíng qì yào]

***qi*-moving drug [medicinal]:** an agent or substance that restores the normal movement of *qi*, a synonym for *qi*-regulating drug [medicinal] (理气药 [lĭ qì yào])

消食药 [xiāo shí yào]

digestant (drug [medicinal]): an agent or substance that aids digestion to eliminate accumulated undigested food, also called digestant and evacuant drug [medicinal] (消导药 [xiāo dăo yào])

消导药 [xiāo dăo yào]

digestant and evacuant drug [medicinal]: the full name of digestant (drug [medicinal] (消食药 [xiāo shí yào])

驱虫药 [qū chóng yào]

anthelmintic; worm-expelling drug [medicinal]: an agent or substance that expels or kills parasitic worms

理血药 [lǐ xuè yào]

blood-regulating drug [medicinal]: an agent or substance that has the effects of regulating blood – including arresting bleeding and activating circulation – and tonifying blood

止血药 [zhǐ xuè yào]

hemostatic (drug [medicinal]): an agent or substance that arrests bleeding, either internal or external

凉血止血药 [liáng xuè zhǐ xuè yào]

blood-cooling hemostatic (drug [medicinal]): an agent or substance that arrests bleeding by clearing the blood of heat, indicated in the treatment of blood-heat hemorrhage

化瘀止血药 [huà yū zhǐ xuè yào]

stasis-resolving hemostatic (drug [medicinal]): an agent or substance that arrests bleeding and at the same time removes stagnant blood which may cause further bleeding

收敛止血药 [shōu liǎn zhǐ xuè yào]

astringent hemostatic (drug [medicinal]): an agent or substance that arrests bleeding by its astringent action, indicated in various types of hemorrhage, but not in those associated with excessive pathogens or blood stasis

温经止血药 [wēn jīng zhǐ xuè yào]

meridian-warming hemostatic (drug [medicinal]): an agent or substance, warm or hot in property, that arrests bleeding by warming the internal organs, replenishing spleen yang and strengthening the thoroughfare vessel, effective for treating hemorrhages due to failure of the spleen to control blood or insecurity of the thoroughfare vessel

活血化瘀药 [huó xuè huà yū yào]

blood-activating and stasis-resolving drug [medicinal]: an agent or substance that promotes blood flow and removes stagnant blood, also called blood-activating and stasis-dispelling drug [medicinal] (活血祛瘀药 [huó xuè qù yū yào]), or blood-activating drug [medicinal] (活血药

[huó xuè yào]) and stasis-resolving drug [medicinal] (化瘀药 [huà yū yào]) for short

活血祛瘀药 [huó xuè qù yū yào]

blood-activating and stasis-dispelling drug [medicinal]: a synonym for blood-activating and stasis-resolving drug [medicinal] (活血化瘀药 [huó xuè huà yū yào])

活血药 [huó xuè yào]

blood-activating drug [medicinal]: an agent or substance used in the treatment of retarded or static blood flow

化瘀药 [huà yū yào]

stasis-resolving drug [medicinal]: an agent or substance used in the treatment of blood stasis

活血止痛药 [huó xuè zhǐ tòng yào]

blood-activating analgesic (drug [medicinal]): an agent or substance that activates blood, moves *qi* and alleviates pain, indicated in the treatment of painful conditions caused by stagnation of *qi* and blood

活血行气药 [huó xuè xíng qì yào]

blood-activating and *qi*-moving drug [medicinal]: an agent or substance that activates blood and promotes the flow of *qi*, used primarily in stagnation of *qi* and blood

活血调经药 [huó xuè tiáo jīng yào]

blood-activating and menstruation-regulating drug [medicinal]: an agent or substance that activates blood and regulates menstruation for treating menstrual disorders, dysmenorrhea, amenorrhea and postpartum blood stagnation

活血疗伤药 [huó xuè liáo shāng yào]

blood-activating and trauma-curing drug [medicinal]: an agent or substance that activates blood, reduces swelling, arrests bleeding and promotes the healing of wounds and factures

破血消癥药 [pò xuè xiāo zhēng yào]

blood-breaking and mass-eliminating drug [medicinal]: an agent or substance that, acting drastically, breaks up the stagnant blood and eliminates masses

化痰止咳平喘药 [huà tán zhǐ ké píng chuǎn yào]

phlegm-resolving, cough-stopping [antitussive] and asthma-relieving [antasthmatic] drug [medicinal]: an agent or substance that resolves phlegm, stops coughing and relieves asthma or dyspnea

化痰药 [huà tán yào]

phlegm-resolving drug [medicinal]: an agent or substance that resolves phlegm, either warm in property and drying in action for cold-phlegm, or cold or cool in property for heat-phlegm

温化寒痰药 [wēn huà hán tán yào]

warming phlegm-resolving drug [medicinal]: an agent or substance warm in property, such as *Rhizoma Pinelliae*, used in treating disorders of cold-phlegm or phlegm-dampness

清化热痰药 [qīng huà rè tán yào]

cooling phlegm-resolving drug [medicinal]: an agent or substance cold in property, such as *Bulbus Fritillariae Thunbergii*, used in treating disorders of phlegm-heat

止咳平喘药 [zhǐ ké píng chuǎn yào]

antitussive and antasthmatic (drug [medicinal]): an agent or substance that relieves cough and asthma (or dyspnea), usually by ventilating, clearing or moistening the lung, or directing lung *qi* downward, astringing lung *qi* or resolving phlegm

安神药 [ān shén yào]

tranquilizer; tranquilizing drug [medicinal]: an agent or substance that calms the mind and relieves mental tension

重镇安神药 [zhòng zhèn ān shén yào]

settling tranquilizer; settling tranquilizing drug [medicinal]: an agent or substance, mostly a mineral, fossil bone or shell, that induces tranquilization associated with its settling action

养心安神药 [yǎng xīn ān shén yào]

heart-nourishing tranquilizer; heart-nourishing tranquilizing drug [medicinal]: an agent or substance that nourishes the heart to calm the mind

平肝息风药 [píng gān xī fēng yào]

liver-pacifying and wind-extinguishing drug [medicinal]: an agent or substance that pacifies the liver, suppresses exuberant yang, extinguishes endogenous wind and controls spasms or tremors

平肝抑阳药 [píng gān yì yáng yào]

liver-pacifying and yang-suppressing drug [medicinal]: an agent or substance that pacifies the liver and suppresses exuberant yang for the treatment of headache, dizziness, tinnitus and blurred vision

息风止痉药 [xī fēng zhǐ jīng yào]

wind-extinguishing and spasm-controlling drug [medicinal]: an agent or substance that extinguishes endogenous wind and stops spasms or tremors

芳香开窍药 [fāng xiāng kāi qiào yào]

aromatic stimulant; aromatic orifice-opening drug [medicinal]: an agent or substance, fragrant in flavor, with a resuscitating effect, used for emergency treatment of impairment or loss of consciousness, also called stimulant or orifice-opening drug (开窍药[kāi qiào yào]) for short

开窍药 [kāi qiào yào]

stimulant; orifice-opening drug [medicinal]: a synonym for aromatic stimulants; aromatic orifice-opening drug [medicinal] (芳香开窍药 [fāng xiāng kāi qiào yào])

补益药 [bǔ yì yào]

tonic; tonifying and replenishing drug [medicinal]: an agent or substance that strengthens or supplements what is insufficient or weakened in the body, also called 补养药 [bǔ yǎng yào]

补养药 [bǔ yǎng yào]

tonic; tonifying and nourishing drug [medicinal]: a synonym for tonifying and replenishing drug [medicinal] (补益药 [bǔ yì yào])

补气药 [bǔ qì yào]

***qi* tonic; *qi*-tonifying drug [medicinal]:** an agent or substance that tonifies *qi*, used in treating *qi* deficiency

补阳药 [bǔ yáng yào]

yang tonic; yang-tonifying drug [medicinal]: an agent or substance that tonifies yang-*qi*, used in treating yang deficiency

补肾阳药 [bǔ shèn yang yào]

kidney-yang tonic: an agent or substance that tonifies the kidney yang, used in treating kidney yang deficiency

补血药 [bǔ xuè yào]

blood tonic; blood-tonifying drug [medicinal]: an agent or substance that tonifies the blood in treating blood deficiency of the heart and liver, marked by pallor, dizziness, tinnitus, palpitations, insomnia, oligomenorrhea or amenorrhea, also called blood-nourishing drug [medicinal] (养血药 [yǎng xuè yào])

养血药 [yǎng xuè yào]

blood-nourishing drug [medicinal]: a synonym for blood tonic (补血药 [bǔ xuè yào])

柔肝药 [róu gān yào]

liver-emolliating drug [medicinal]: an agent or substance that replenishes the liver blood or yin in treating deficiency of liver blood or yin with dizziness, tinnitus, insomnia, and blurred vision

补阴药 [bǔ yīn yào]

yin tonic; yin-tonifying drug [medicinal]: an agent or substance that tonifies the yin of the heart, lung, stomach, liver, or kidney

养阴药 [yǎng yīn yào]

yin-nourishing drug [medicinal]: a synonym for yin tonic (补阴药 [bǔ yīn yào])

滋阴药 [zī yīn yào]

yin-replenishing drug [medicinal]: a synonym for yin tonic (补阴药 [bǔ yīn yào])

收涩药 [shōu sè yào]

discharge-arresting drug [medicinal]: an agent or substance that arrests discharges such as sweat, diarrhea, urine, blood, leukorrhea and semen

固涩药 [gù sè yào]

astringent (drug [medicinal]): a synonym for discharge-arresting drug [medicinal] (收涩药 [shōu sè yào])

固表止汗药 [gù biǎo zhǐ hàn yào]

superficies-strengthening anhidrotic: an agent that arrests excessive sweating by strengthening the superficies

敛汗固表药 [liǎn hàn gù biǎo yào]

sweating-arresting and superficies-strengthening drug [medicinal]: an agent that strengthens the superficies by arresting excessive sweating

敛肺涩肠药 [liǎn fèi sè cháng yào]

lung-intestine astringent (drug [medicinal]): an agent that relieves cough and asthma, and arrests chronic diarrhea

涌吐药 [yǒng tù yào]

emetic (drug [medicinal]): an agent that induces vomiting

催吐药 [cuī tù yào]

same as 涌吐药 [yǒng tù yào]

驱虫药 [qū chóng yào]

anthelmintic; worm-expelling drug [medicinal]: an agent or substance that expels or even kills intestinal parasitic worms

解表药 Exterior-releasing Drugs

辛温解表药 Pungent-warm Exterior-releasing Drugs

麻黄 [má huáng]

***Herba Ephedrae,* Ephedra:** the dried herbaceous stem of *Ephedra sinica* Stapf, *Ephedra equisetina* Bunge or *Ephedra intermedia* Schrenk et C.A. Meyer (family Ephedraceae), used (1) to induce sweating for releasing the superficies in cases of wind-cold affliction, (2) to relieve asthma, and (3) to induce diuresis for relieving edema caused by wind

桂枝 [guì zhī]

***Ramulus Cinnamomi,* Cassia Twig:** the dried young stem of *Cinnamomum cassia* Presl. (family Lauraceae), used (1) to induce sweating for releasing the muscles in cases of wind-cold affliction, (2) to warm and unblock the meridians to relieve various pains due to cold and congealing blood, and (3) to stimulate menstrual discharge for treating amenorrhea

生姜 [shēng jiāng]

***Rhizoma Zingiberis Recens,* Fresh Ginger:** the fresh rhizome of *Zingiber officinale* (Willd.) Rosc. (family Zingiberaceae), used as (1) to induce sweating for releasing the superficies in cases of wind-cold affliction, (2) to warm the middle for arresting vomiting

防风 [fáng fēng]

***Radix Saposhnikoviae,* Divaricate Saposhnikovia Root:** the dried root of *Saposhnikovia divaricata* (Turcz.) Schischk. (family Umbelliferae), used (1) to release the superficies for exterior syndromes, (2) to dispel wind in cases of urticaria, (3) to dispel wind-damp and alleviate pain in cases of rheumatalgia, and (4) to relieve spasm in cases of tetanus

白芷 [bái zhǐ]

***Radix Angelicae Dahuricae,* Dahurian Angelica Root:** the dried root of *Angelica dahurica* (Fisch. ex Hoffm.) Benth. et Hook. f. or *Angelica dahurica* var. *formosana* (Boiss.) Shan et Yuan (family Umbelliferae), used (1) to release the superficies, disperse wind and alleviate pain in cases of frontal headache and stuffy nose in colds, rheumatalgia and toothache, (2) to eliminate dampness for checking leukorrhagia, and (3) to discharge pus and reduce swelling for the treatment of boils, sores, abscesses, rhinitis and nasosinusitis

荆芥 [jīng jiè]

***Herba Schizonepetae,* Fineleaf Schizonepeta Herb:** the dried aerial part of *Schizonepeta tenuifolia* Briq. (family Labiatae), used (1) to release the superficies and disperse wind in cases of wind-cold affliction, (2) to promote eruption for treating measles, and (3) to dispel wind for urticaria

荆芥穗 [jīng jiè suì]

***Spica Schizonepetae,* Fineleaf Schizonepeta Spike:** the seed-bearing part of schizonepeta used in a similar way to *Herba Schizonepetae,* fineleaf schizonepeta herb, with stronger actions

荆芥炭 [jīng jiè tàn]

***Herba Schizonepetae Carbonisata*, Carbonized Fineleaf Schizonepeta Herb:** carbonized schizonepeta used as a hemostatic for treating functional uterine bleeding and hematochezia.

紫苏叶 [zǐ sū yè]

***Folium Perillae,* Perilla Leaf:** the dried leaf of *Perilla frutescens* (L.) Britt. (family Labiatae), used (1) to induce sweating for treating wind-cold affliction, (2) to arrest vomiting, and (3) as an antidote for fish and crab poisoning

香薷 [xiāng rú]

***Herba Elshotziae,* Elsholtzia Herb:** the dried aerial part of *Elsholtzia splendens* Nakai ex F. Maekawa (family Labiatae), used (1) to induce sweating and resolve dampness in cases of summer cold, (2) to cause diuresis for relieving edema

细辛 [xì xīn]

***Herba Asari,* Manchurian Wild Ginger:** the entire dried plant of *Asarum heterotropoides* var. *manschuricum* (Maxim.) Kitagawa, *Asarum sieboldii* Miq. var. *seoulense* Nakai (family Aristolochiaceae), used (1) to dispel wind and disperse cold for treating colds, (2) to relieve nasal congestion and alleviate pain for nasosinusitis, headache, toothache or rheumatic pain, and (3) to warm the lung and resolve retained fluid for treating cough with copious, thin expectoration

藁本 [gǎo běn]

***Rhizoma Ligustlci,* Chinese Lovage:** the dried rhizome and root of

Ligustrum sinense Oliver or *Ligustrum jeholense* Nakai et Kitagawa (family Umbelliferae), used to relieve pain in the vertex of the head in cases of wind-cold affliction, and rheumatic arthralgia

辛夷 [xīn yí]

***Flos Magnoliae,* Biond Magnolia Flower:** the dried flower bud of *Magnolia biondii* Pamp., *Magnolia denudata* Desr. or *Magnolia sprengeri* Pamp. (family Magnoliaceae), used for treating stuffy nose and nasal discharge in cases of rhinitis and nasosinusitis

苍耳子 [cāng ěr zǐ]

***Fructus Xanthii,* Siberian Cocklebur Fruit:** the dried ripe fruit of *Xanthium sibiricum* Patrin. (family Compositae), used to disperse wind, eliminate damp, relieve nasal congestion and alleviate pain for the treatment of wind-cold affliction of stuffy nose, rhinitis, nasosinusitis, urticaria with pruritus, and rheumatism

鹅不食草 [é bù shí cǎo]

***Herba Centipedae,* Small Centipeda Herb:** the dried entire plant of *Centipeda minima* (L.) A. Braum et Aschers (family Compositae), used (1) to disperse cold and relieve nasal congestion for the treatment of colds with acute rhinitis, and (2) to arrest cough

辛凉解表药 Pungent-cool Exterior-releasing Drugs

柴胡 [chái hú]

***Radix Bupleuri,* Chinese Thorowax Root:** the dried root of *Bupleurum chinense* DC. or *Bupleurum scorzonerifolium* Willd. (family Umbelliferae), used (1) to reduce fever for relieving alternate spells of chills and fever, (2) to relieve liver *qi* stagnation for alleviating hypochondriac and thoracic pains, and (3) to lift spleen *qi* for correction of visceroptosis

薄荷 [bò he]

***Herba Menthae,* Peppermint:** the dried aerial part of *Mentha haplocalyx* Briq. (family Labiatae), used (1) to disperse wind and heat in the treatment of wind-heat affliction, (2) to clear the head and eyes for relieving headache and conjunctivitis, (3) to promote eruption in the treatment of measles, and (4) to soothe the liver for alleviating hypochondriac and thoracic pain

桑叶 [sāng yè]

***Folium Mori,* Mulberry Leaf:** the dried leaf of White Mulberry, *Morus alba* L. (family Moraceae), used (1) to disperse wind and heat in the treatment of wind-heat affliction, (2) to pacify the liver and brighten the eyes for relieving hyperactivity of the liver with headache and acute conjunctivitis, and (3) to clear and moisten the lung for arresting dry cough

菊花 [jú huā]

***Flos Chrysanthemi,* Chrysanthemum Flower:** the dried flower-head of *Chrysanthemum morifolium* Ramat. (family Compositae), used (1) to disperse wind and heat in the treatment of wind-heat affliction with fever and headache, (2) to pacify the liver and brighten the eyes for treating acute conjunctivitis, and dizziness in hyperactive liver yang, and (3) to clear heat and counteract toxins for treating boils and sores

葛根 [gě gēn]

***Radix Puerariae,* Kudzuvine Root:** the dried root of *Pueraria lobata* (Willd.) Ohwi or *Pueraria thomsonii* Benth. (family Leguminosae), used (1) to reduce heat in cases of exterior syndrome with fever and painful stiffness of the back and nape, (2) to relieve thirst in febrile diseases and diabetes mellitus, (3) to arrest diarrhea in spleen insufficiency, and (4) to promote eruption for measles

牛蒡子 [niú bàng zǐ]

***Fructus Arctii,* Burdock Fruit:** the dried ripe fruit of great burdock, *Arctium lappa* L. (family Compositae), used (1) to disperse wind and heat in the treatment of wind-heat affliction, (2) to promote eruption for measles, and (3) to counteract toxins and reduce swelling for boils, sores, mumps and erysipelas

蔓荆子 [màn jīng zǐ]

***Fructus Viticis,* Shrub Chaste-tree Fruit:** the dried ripe fruit of simple-leaved chaste tree, *Vitex simplicifolia* Cham. or three-leaved chaste tree, *Vitex trifolia* L. (family Verbenaceae), used for treating wind-heat affliction with fever and headache, acute conjunctivitis, blurred vision and dizziness

蝉蜕 [chán tuì]

***Periostracum Cicadae,* Cicada Slough:** slough shed by the nymph of *Cryptotympana pustulata* Fabr. (family Cicadidae), used (1) to disperse wind and heat in the treatment of wind-heat affliction, (2) to promote eruption for measles and relieve itching for urticaria, (3) to remove the nebula and improve eyesight, and (4) to relieve spasm in infantile convulsion and tetanus

蝉衣 [chán yī]

same as 蝉蜕 [chán tuì]

升麻 [shēng má]

***Rhizoma Cimicifugae,* Largetrifoliolious Bugbane Rhizome:** the dried rhizome of *Cimicifuga heracleifolia* Kom., *Cimicifuga dahurica* (Turcz.) Maxim. or *Cimicifuga foetida* L. (family Ranunculaceae), used (1) to promote eruption in the treatment of measles, (2) to clear heat and counteract toxins for treating sore throat and stomatitis, and (3) to restore the normal position of the viscera in cases of splanchnoptosis

淡豆豉 [dàn dòu chǐ]

***Semen Sojae Preparatum,* Fermented Soybean:** the fermented preparation of the ripe seed of *Glycine max* (L.) Merr. (family Leguminosae), used in the early stage of febrile diseases to relieve exterior syndromes and in the late stage to relieve fidgetiness and insomnia

西河柳 [xī hé liǔ]

***Cacumen Tamaricis,* Chinese Tamarisk Twig:** the dried young green twig of *Tamarix chinensis* Lour. (family Tamaricaceae), used for measles to promote eruption, and also for rheumatism to relieve arthralgia

浮萍 [fú píng]

***Herba Spirodelae,* Common Ducksmeat Herb:** the dried entire plant of *Spirodela polyrrhiza* (L.) Schneid. (family Lemnaceae), used to promote eruption for measles, to relieve itching for urticaria, and to induce diuresis for edema

常山 [cháng shān]

***Radix Dichroae,* Antifeverile Dichroa Root:** the dried root of *Dichroa febrifuga* Lour. (family Saxifragaceae), used for treatment of malaria

止咳化痰平喘药 Antitussives, Expectorants and Antiasthmatics

温化寒痰药 Drugs for Resolving Cold-phlegm

半夏 [bàn xià]

***Rhizoma Pinelliae,* Pinellia Tuber:** the dried tuber of *Pinellia ternata*

(Thunb.) Breit. (family Araceae), used as (1) an expectorant for cough with profuse thin phlegm, and (2) an antiemetic for nausea, vomiting and morning sickness

天南星 [tiān nán xīng]

Rhizoma Arisaematis, **Jack-in-the-Pulpit Tuber:** the dried tuber of *Arisaema erubescens* (Wall.) Schott., *Arisaema heterophyllum* Bl. or *Arisaema amurense* Maxim. (family Araceae), used as (1) an expectorant for cough with profuse phlegm, and (2) an anticonvulsive for epilepsy or tetanus

白芥子 [bái jiè zǐ]

Semen Sinapis Albae, **White Mustard Seed:** ripe seed of *Brassica alba* (L.) Boiss. (family Cruciferae), used to warm the lung and resolve phlegm for treating cough with profuse expectoration and stuffy feeling in the chest, and also for treating cold abscess and pleural fluid retention

白附子 [bái fù zǐ]

Rhizoma Typhonii, **Giant Typhonium Tuber:** the dried tuber of *Typhonium giganteum* Engl. (family Araceae), used as (1) an expectorant for cough with profuse phlegm, and (2) an anticonvulsive for epilepsy or tetanus

旋覆花 [xuán fù huā]

Flos Inulae, **Inula Flower:** the dried flower-head of *Inula japonica* Thunb. or *Inula britannica* L. (family Compositae), used as an expectorant for relieving cough and asthma with excessive phlegm, and as an antiemetic for belching and vomiting.

紫菀 [zǐ wǎn]

Radix Asteris, **Tartarian Aster Root:** the dried root and rhizome of *Aster tataricus* L.f. (family Compositae), used as an expectorant and antitussive for cough with profuse phlegm and also for phthisical cough

桔梗 [jié gěng]

Radix Platycodi, **Platycodon Root:** the dried root of *Platycodon grandiflorum* (Jacq.) A. DC. (family Campanulaceae), used to resolve phlegm, soothe the throat and evacuate pus for treating cough with much phlegm, lung abscess with purulent expectoration, painful swelling of the throat and hoarse voice

清化热痰药 Drugs for Resolving Heat-phlegm

瓜蒌 [guā lóu]

***Fructus Trichosanthis,* Snakegourd Fruit:** the dried ripe fruit of *Trichosanthes kirilowii* Maxim. or *Trichosanthes rosthornii* Harms (family Cucurbitaceae), used (1) to clear heat and resolve phlegm for relieving cough and dyspnea caused by heat-phlegm, (2) to soothe the chest for angina pectoris, (3) to reduce swelling in the treatment of lung abscess, appendicitis and mastitis, and (4) to moisten the intestines for opening the bowels

天花粉 [tiān huā fěn]

***Radix Trichosanthis,* Snake-gourd Root:** the dried root of *Trichosanthes kirilowii* Maxim. or *Trichosanthes rosthornii* Harms (family Cucurbitaceae), used to clear heat, promote fluid production, moisten the lung, counteract toxins and reduce swelling for relieving thirst in cases of febrile diseases and diabetes, and treating boils, sores and abscesses

天竺黄 [tiān zhú huáng]

***Concretio Silicea Bambusae,* Tabashir:** the dried masses of secretion in the stem of *Bambusa textilis* McClure or *Schizostachyum chinense* Rendle (family Gramineae), used to clear heat, cleanse the heart of phlegm for the treatment of impaired consciousness in high fever and stroke, and also for infantile convulsion

竹茹 [zhú rú]

***Caulis Bambusae in Taeniam,* Bamboo Shavings:** the dried shavings of the stem of *Bambusa tuldoides* Munro, *Sinocalamus beecheyanus* (Munro) McClure var. *pubescens* P.F. Li or *Phyllostachys nigra* var. *henonis* Stapf (family Gramineae), used to clear heat, resolve phlegm, induce tranquilization and arrest vomiting for relieving cough or insomnia due to phlegm-heat, and vomiting due to stomach heat

南沙参 [nán shā shēn]

***Radix Adenophorae,* Fourleaf Ladybell Root:** the dried root of *Adenophora tetraphylla* (Thunb.) Fisch. or *Adenophora stricta* Miq. (family Campanulaceae), used to nourish yin, clear the lung, resolve phlegm and replenish *qi* for relieving cough in cases of lung yin deficiency, and deficiency of *qi* and fluid in the late stage of a febrile disease

海藻 [hǎi zǎo]

***Sargassum,* Seaweed:** the dried thallus of seaweed, *Sargassum pallidum*

(Turn.) C. Ag. or *Sargassum fusiforme* (Harv.) Setch. (family Sargassaceae), used (1) to eliminate phlegm and soften hard masses for treating goiter, scrofula and swelling of the testis, and (2) to induce diuresis for edema

昆布 [kūn bù]

***Thallus Laminariae seu Eckloniae,* Kelp** or **Tangle:** the dried thallus of Japanese sea tangle, *Laminaria japonica* Aresch. or *Ecklonia kurome* Okam. (family Laminariaceae), used together with seaweed to eliminate phlegm, soften hard masses and induce diuresis

前胡 [qián hú]

***Radix Peucedani,* Hogfennel Root:** the dried root of *Peucedanum praeruptorum* Dunn or *Peucedanum decursivum* Maxim. (family Umbelliferae), used to check the adverse up-flow of *qi*, and resolve phlegm for relieving cough and dyspnea with copious or yellow sticky expectoration

山慈菇 [shān cí gū]

***Pseudobulbus Cremastrae seu Pleiones,* Appendiculate Cremastra Pseudobulb** or **Common Pleiorre Pseudobulb:** the dried ripe pseudobulb of *Cremastra appendiculata* (D. Don) Makino, *Pleione bulbocodioides* (Franch.) Rolfe or *Pleione yunnanensis* Rolfe (family Orchidaceae), used to clear heat for the treatment of boils, sores, scrofula, and snake bite

黄药子 [huáng yào zǐ]

***Rhizoma Dioscoreae Bulbiferae,* Airpotato Yam:** the dried rhizome of *Dioscorea bulbifera* L. (family Dioscoreaceae), used as a blood-cooling hemostatic for arresting various kinds of bleeding, and to counteract toxins for treating boils and sores

金礞石 [jīn méng shí]

***Lapis Micae Aureus,* Mica-schist:** a golden-colored mineral mica-schist, usually made into pills or powders to purge phlegm and arrest convulsions in the treatment of cough and dyspnea with sticky sputum, epilepsy and mania

止咳药 Antitussives

苦杏仁 [kǔ xìng rén]

***Semen Armeniacae Amarum,* Bitter Apricot Seed:** the dried ripe seed or kernel of *Prunus armeniaca* L. var. *ansu* Maxim., *Prunus sibirica* L., *Prunus mandshurica* (Maxim.) Koehne or *Prunus armeniaca* L. (family Rosaceae), used to relieve cough and dyspnea with profuse expectoration, and also to relieve constipation.

白前 [béi qián]

***Rhizoma Cynanchi Stauntonii*, Willowleaf Swallowwort Rhizome:** the dried rhizome and root of *Cynanchum stauntonii* (Decne.) Schltr. ex Lévl. or *Cynanchum glaucescens* (Decne.) Hand.-Mazz. (family Asclepiadaceae), used for the treatment of cough and dyspnea with profuse phlegm

枇杷叶 [pí pa yè]

***Folium Eriobotryae*, Loquat Leaf:** the dried leaf of *Eriobotrya japonica* (Thunb.) Lindl. (family Rosaceae), used (1) to clear the lung and resolve phlegm for arresting coughing in cases of lung heat, and (2) to arrest vomiting due to stomach heat

白果 [bái guǒ]

***Semen Ginkgo*, Ginkgo Seed:** the dried ripe seed of the maiden-hair tree, *Ginkgo biloba* L. (family Ginkgoaceae), used (1) as an antitussive and anti-asthmatic for prolonged cough or asthma with profuse expectoration, (2) to check leukorrhagia, and (3) to reduce urination in cases of enuresis and frequent micturition

沙棘 [shā jí]

***Fructus Hippophae*, Seabuckthorn Fruit:** the dried ripe fruit of *Hippophae rhamnoides* L. (family Elaeagnaceae), used (1) as an antitussive and expectorant for treating cough with profuse phlegm, (2) as a stomachic for dyspepsia and abdominal pain due to undigested food, and (3) to promote blood circulation and remove stasis for treating traumatic wounds and amenorrhea

款冬花 [kuǎn dōng huā]

***Flos Farfarae*, Common Coltsfoot Flower:** the dried flower-bud of *Tussilago farfara* L. (family Compositae), used for treating chronic cough with profuse expectoration and hemoptysis in consumptive diseases.

百部 [bǎi bù]

***Radix Stemonae*, Stemona Root:** the steamed and dried tuberous root of *Stemona sessilifolia* (Miq.) Miq., *Stemona japonica* (Bl.) Miq. or *Stemona tuberosa* Lour. (family Stemonaceae), used to moisten the lung and relieve acute and chronic cough, and externally to kill trichomonads and lice.

浙贝母 [zhè bèi mǔ]

***Bulbus Fritillariae Thunbergii,* Thunbery Fritillary Bulb:** the dried bulb of *Fritillaria thunbergii* Miq. (family Liliaceae), used (1) to clear heat and resolve phlegm in cases of cough with thick expectoration, and (2) to reduce nodulation in cases of mastitis and scrofula

伊贝母 [yī bèi mǔ]

***Bulbus Fritillariae Pallidiflorae,* Sinkiang Fritillary Bulb:** the dried bulb of *Fritillaria walujewii* Regel or *Fritillaria pallidiflora* Schrenk (family Liliaceae), used as thunbery fritillary bulb (浙贝母 [zhebeimu])

川贝母 [chuān bèi mǔ]

***Bulbus Fritillarie Cirrhosae,* Tendrilleaf Fritillary Bulb:** the dried bulb of *Fritillaria cirrhosa* D. Don, *Fritillaria unibracteata* Hsiao et K.C. Hsia, *Fritillaria przewalskii* Maxim. or *Fritillaria delavayi* Franch. (family Liliaceae), used (1) to clear heat, resolve phlegm, moisten the lung for relieving dry cough due to lung heat and chronic cough with bloody sputum in cases of phthisis, and (2) to dissipate nodulation for treating boils, sores, mastitis and lung abscess

平贝母 [píng bèi mǔ]

***Bulbus Fritillarie Ussuriensis,* Ussuri Fritillary Bulb:** the dried bulb of *Fritillaria ussuriensis* Maxim. (family Liliaceae), used to clear the lung of heat, arrest cough and resolve phlegm for the treatment of cough with expectoration of sticky and blood-streaked sputum

罂粟壳 [yīng sù qiào]

***Pericarpium Papaveris,* Poppy Capsule:** the dried pericarp of the ripe fruit of *Papaver somniferum* L. (family Papaveraceae) with the seeds removed, used as an antitussive, antidiarrheal and analgesic for treating chronic cough, chronic diarrhea and abdominal pain

满山红 [mǎn shān hóng]

***Folium Rhododendri Daurici,* Dahurian Rhododendron Leaf:** the dried leaf of *Rhododendron dauricum* L. (Family Ericaceae), used as an antitussive and expectorant for acute and chronic bronchitis

百合 [bǎi hé]

***Bulbus Lilii,* Lily Bulb:** the dried scale leaf of the bulb of *Lilium lancifolium* Thunb., *Lilium brownii* F.E. Brown var. *viridulum* Baker or

Lilium pumilum DC. (family Liliaceae), used (1) to nourish the lung yin and arrest cough in cases of consumptive diseases, and (2) to clear the heart and induce tranquilization for insomnia and fidgetiness in the late stage of febrile diseases with residual heat

桑白皮 [sāng bái pí]

***Cortex Mori,* White Mulberry Root-bark:** the dried root-bark, deprived of the external brown corky part, of *Morus alba* L. (family Moraceae), used (1) to purge the lung and relieve dyspnea for treating lung heat with cough and dyspnea, and (2) to induce diuresis in cases of edema

木蝴蝶 [mù hú dié]

***Semen Oroxyli,* India Trumpetflower Seed:** the dried ripe seed of *Oroxylum indicum* (L.) Vent. (family Bignoniaceae), used to clear the lung of heat, and soothe the throat for the treatment of cough, sore throat, and hoarseness of voice in cases of wind-heat afflictions

暴马子皮 [bào mǎ zǐ pí]

Cortex Syringae, Manchurian Lilac Bark: the dried stem-bark of *Syringa reticulata* (Bl.) Hara var. *mandshurica* (Maxim.) Hara (family Oleaceae), used as an antipyretic, antitussive and diuretic for treating acute or chronic bronchitis, asthma and cardiac edema

胖大海 [pàng dà hǎi]

***Semen Sterculiae Lychnophorae,* Boat-fruited Sterculia Seed:** the dried ripe seed of *Sterculia lychnophora* Hance (family Sterculiaceae), used (1) to clear the lung of heat for relieving sore throat, hoarseness and cough, and (2) to moisten the intestines for relieving constipation.

平喘药 Anti-asthmatics

洋金花 [yáng jīn huā]

***Flos Daturae,* Datura Flower:** the dried flower of *Datura metel* L. (family Solanaceae), used to relieve cough, asthma, gastralgia, rheumatalgia, and epilepsy

葶苈子 [tíng lì zǐ]

***Semen Lepidii seu Descurainiae,* Pepperweed Seed** or **Tansy Mustard Seed:** the dried ripe seed of *Lepidium apetalum* Willd. or Descurainia sophia (L.) Webb ex Prantl. (family Cruciferae), used (1) to purge the lung for relieving cough and dyspnea with excessive phlegm, and (2) to induce diuresis for treating edema

马兜铃 [mǎ dōu líng]

***Fructus Aristolochiae,* Dutchmanspipe Fruit:** the dried ripe fruit of *Aristolochia contorta* Bge. or *Aristolochia debilis* Sieb. et Zucc. (family Aristolochiaceae), used to clear the lung and resolve phlegm for relieving cough and dyspnea due to heat in the lung, and also to remove heat from the large intestine for treating hemorrhoids

紫苏子 [zǐ sū zǐ]

***Fructus Perillae,* Perilla Fruit:** the dried ripe fruit of *Perilla frutescens* (L.) Britt. (family labiatiae), used as an antitussive, antiasthmatic and expectorant for treating chronic bronchitis with thin white phlegm and stuffy feeling in the chest, and also as an aperient for relieving constipation, often simplified as 苏子 [sū zǐ]

苏子 [sū zǐ]

a simplified name for 紫苏子 [zǐ sū zǐ]

天仙子 [tiān xiān zǐ]

***Semen Hyoscyami,* Henbane Seed:** the dried seed of *Hyoscyamus niger* L. (family Solanaceae), used (1) to relieve cough and in cases of asthma for bronchial asthma, (2) to relieve gastralgia, and (3) to induce tranquilization

莨菪子 [làng dàng zǐ]

same as 天仙子 [tiān xiān zǐ]

华山参 [huà shān shēn]

***Radix Physochlainae,* Funneled Physochlaina Root:** the dried root of funnel-shaped physochlaina, *Physochlaina infundibularis* Kuang (family Solanaceae), used to relieve cough and dyspnea, and induce tranquilization

热参 [rè shēn]

same as 华山参 [huà shān shēn]

芸香草 [yún xiāng cǎo]

***Herba Cymbopogonis,* Lemongrass:** the dried aerial part of *Cymbopogon distans* (Nees) A. Camus (family Gramineae), used to relieve cough and dyspnea

清热药 Drugs for Clearing Heat

清热泻火药 Drugs for Clearing Heat and Purging Fire

石膏 [shí gāo]

Gypsum Fibrosum, **Gypsum:** a soft mineral chiefly composed of hydrated calcium sulfate ($CaSO_4 \cdot 2H_2O$), used to clear heat and purge fire for relieving (1) high fever with fidgetiness and thirst in cases of warm diseases, (2) heat in the lung with cough and dyspnea, and (3) heat in the stomach with toothache and painful swelling of the gums, and also externally to promote the healing of wounds and ulcers

知母 [zhī mǔ]

Rhizoma Anemarrhenae, **Common Anemarrhena Rhizome:** the dried rhizome of *Anemarrhena asphodeloides* Bge. (family Liliaceae), used (1) to clear heat and purge fire for relieving high fever with dire thirst in cases of warm diseases, and cough due to heat in the lung, and (2) to nourish yin and moisten the intestines for treating low fever in cases of yin deficiency, diabetes, and constipation

决明子 [jué míng zǐ]

Semen Cassiae, **Cassia Seed:** the dried ripe seed of *Cassia obtusifolia* L. or *Cassia tora* L. (family Leguminosae), used (1) to clear the liver and brighten the eyes for treating acute inflammation of the eye, (2) to moisten the intestines for relieving constipation, and (3) nowadays for reducing high blood pressure and blood cholesterol

青葙子 [qīng xiāng zǐ]

Semen Celosiae, **Feather Cockscomb Seed:** the dried ripe seed of *Celosia argentea* L. (family Amaranthaceae), used to clear the liver of heat, improve vision and remove nebula for the treatment of acute conjunctivitis, blurred eyesight due to nebula, and dizziness due to hyperactivity of the liver

谷精草 [gǔ jīng cǎo]

Flos Eriocauli, **Pipewort Flower:** the dried flower-head with stalk of *Eriocaulon buergerianum* Koern. (family Eriocaulaceae), used to dispel wind and heat for the treatment of acute conjunctivitis, nebula and headache

密蒙花 [mì méng huā]

Flos Buddlejae, **Pale Butterfly-bush Flower:** the dried flower-bud and inflorescence of *Buddleja officinalis* Maxim. (family Loganiaceae), used to clear liver heat and remove nebula for the treatment of acute conjunctivitis with lacrimation and photophobia, and blurred vision due to nebula

木贼 [mù zéi]

***Herba Equiseti Hiemalis,* Common Scouring Rush Herb:** the dried aerial part of *Equisetum hiemale* L. (family Equisetaceae), used in ophthalmology for treating acute infections and removing nebula

淡竹叶 [dàn zhú yè]

***Herba Lophatheri,* Lophatherum Herb:** the dried stem and leaf of *Lophatherum gracile* Brongn. (family Gramineae), used for relieving fidgetiness and thirst in cases of febrile diseases, and dysuria with painful urination, also called 竹叶 [zhú yè]

竹叶 [zhú yè]

another name of *Herba Lophatheri,* Lophatherum Herb (淡竹叶 [dàn zhú yè])

莲子心 [lián zǐ xīn]

***Plumula Nelumbinis,* Lotus Plumule:** the dried plumule and radicle in the ripe seed of *Nelumbo nucifera* Gartn. (family Nymphaeaceae), used (1) to clear the heart and induce tranquilization for treating delirium in cases of acute febrile diseases, insomnia and nocturnal emission, and (2) to arrest seminal discharge and bleeding in cases of seminal emission and hematemesis due to blood heat

芦根 [lú gēn]

***Rhizoma Phragmitis,* Reed Rhizome:** the fresh or dried rhizome of *Phragmites communis* (L.) Trin. (family Gramineae), used (1) to clear heat and promote fluid production in cases of high fever with thirst, (2) to evacuate pus for treating lung abscess, and (3) to arrest vomiting in cases of stomach heat

罗布麻叶 [luó bù má yè]

***Folium Apocyni Veniti,* Dogbane Leaf:** the dried leaf of red dogbane, *Apocynum venetum* L. (family Apocynaceae), used for suppressing hyperactive liver yang, clearing heat and inducing diuresis

夏枯草 [xià kū cǎo]

***Spica Prunellae,* Common Selfheal Fruit-Spike:** the dried fruit-spike of *Prunella vulgaris* L. (family Labiatae), used (1) to clear liver fire for the treatment of acute conjunctivitis, headache and dizziness, and (2) to dissipate nodulation for treating acute mastitis, mumps, scrofula and goiter

清热凉血药 Drugs for Clearing Heat and Cooling the Blood

犀角 [xī jiǎo]

***Cornu Rhinoceri,* Rhinoceros Horn:** the horn of Asiatic rhinoceros, *Rhinoceros unicornis* L., *Rhinoceros sondaicus* Desmarest or *Rhinoceros sumatrensis* Cuvier (family Rhinocerotidae), used in ancient times for treating febrile diseases at the nutrient and blood stages, with delirium, maculation and high fever, and arresting bleeding by clearing heat and cooling blood, but at present replaced by buffalo horn

水牛角 [shuǐ niú jiǎo]

***Cornu Bubali,* Buffalo Horn:** horn of *Bubalus bubalis* L. (family Bovidae), used in a similar way to rhinoceros horn (犀角 [xī jiǎo])

地黄 [dì huáng]

***Radix Rehmanniae,* Rehmannia Root:** the fresh or dried tuberous root of *Rehmannia glutinosa* Libosch (family Scrophulariaceae), used to clear heat, cool blood, nourish yin and promote fluid production for the treatment of febrile diseases at the nutrient and blood stages, bleeding due to blood heat, and thirst in cases of diabetes

生地 [shēng dì]

another name for unprocessed rehmannia root (地黄 [dì huáng])

赤芍 [chì sháo]

***Radix Paeoniae Rubra,* Red Peony Root:** the dried root of *Paeonia lactiflora* Pall. or *Paeonia veitchii* Lynch (family Ranunculaceae), used to remove stagnated blood and dispel heat from the blood for the treatment of epidemic febrile diseases with eruptions, pain due to blood stasis, dysmenorrhea, amenorrhea, traumatic injuries, boils and sores

牡丹皮 [mǔ dān pí]

***Cortex Moutan,* Tree Peony Bark:** the dried root-bark of *Paeonia suffruticosa* Andr. (family Ranunculaceae), used (1) to clear heat and cool the blood for the treatment of febrile diseases with eruptions and bleeding, and (2) to activate blood and eliminate stasis for treating amenorrhea, dysmenorrhea, traumatic injuries, boils, sores and appendicitis

玄参 [xuán shēn]

***Radix Scrophularlae,* Figwort Root:** the dried root of *Scrophularia ningpoensis* Hemsl. (family Scrophulariaceae), used to clear heat, cool the blood, replenish yin and counteract toxins for the treatment of warm diseases at the nutrient level with high fever and delirium or skin eruption, also for treating inflammation of the throat, boils and sores

紫草 [zǐ cǎo]

***Radix Arnebiae seu Lithospermi,* Arnebia Root or Gromwell Root:** the dried root of *Arnebia euchroma* (Royle) Johnst. or *Lithospermum erythrorhizon* Sieb. et Zucc. (family Boraginaceae), used for promoting eruption in cases of measles, and externally for treating burns, frostbite, dermatitis and eczema

地骨皮 [dì gǔ pí]

***Cortex Lycii,* Chinese Wolfberry Bark:** the dried root-bark of *Lycium chinense* Mill. or *Lycium barbarum* L. (family Solanaceae), used for treating chronic fever and hemoptysis in cases of consumptive diseases, and also for diabetes

银柴胡 [yín chái hú]

***Radix Stellariae,* Starwort Root:** the dried root of *Stellaria dichotoma* L. var. *lanceolata* Bge. (family Caryophyllaceae), used for clearing heat of deficiency type and malnutritional fever in children

青蒿 [qīng hāo]

***Herba Artemisiae Annuae,* Sweet Wormwood Herb:** the dried aerial part of *Artemisia annua* L. (family Compositae), used to clear heat of deficiency type for relieving consumptive fever and also for combating malaria

白薇 [bái wēi]

***Radix Cynanchi Atrati,* Blackened Swallowwort Root:** the dried root and rhizome of *Cynanchum atratum* Bge. or *Cynanchum versicolor* Bge. (family Asclepiadaceae), used (1) to clear heat and cool blood for fever in cases of consumptive diseases or cases due to yin deficiency, (2) to induce diuresis in cases of heat stranguria and bloody stranguria, and (3) to counteract toxins in cases of boils and sores

白茅根 [bái máo gēn]

***Rhizoma Imperatae,* Lalang Grass Rhizome:** the dried rhizome of *Imperata cylindrica* Beauv. var. *major* (Nees) C.E. Hubb. (family Graminae), used to cool blood, arrest bleeding, clear heat and induce diuresis for the treatment of epistaxis and hematuria due to blood heat, edema, jaundice, and stranguria associated with heat

清热燥湿药 Drugs for Clearing Heat and Drying Dampness

黄芩 [huáng qín]

***Radix Scutellariae,* Baical Skullcap Root:** the dried root of *Scutellaria baicalensis* Georgi (family Labiatae), used (1) to clear heat and dry dampness for treating damp-warm and damp-heat diseases, (2) to clear the lung of heat for relieving cough in cases of lung heat, (3) to purge fire and counteract toxins for treating boils, sores, painful swelling of the throat, (4) to cool blood for arresting hematemesis, epistaxis, abnormal uterine bleeding, and (5) to prevent miscarriage in cases of threatened abortion

黄连 [huáng lián]

***Rhizoma Coptidis,* Golden Thread:** the dried rhizome of *Coptis chinensis* Franch., *Coptis deltoidea* C.Y. Cheng et Hsiao or *Coptis teeta* Wall. (family Ranunculaceae), used to clear heat, dry dampness, purge fire and counteract toxins for treating dysentery, high fever with restlessness, boils, sores, abscesses, and externally for relieving eczema

黄柏 [huáng bǎi]

***Cortex Phellodendri,* Amur Cork-tree:** the dried bark of Chinese corktree, *Phellodendron chinense* Schneid. or Amur Corktree, *Phellodendron amurense* Rupr. (family Rutaceae), used (1) to clear heat and dry dampness in cases of acute dysentery, jaundice, morbid leukorrhea, and heat stranguria, (2) to purge fire and counteract toxins for treating boils, sores and ulcers, and (3) to relieve fever in cases of yin deficiency with night sweats

三颗针 [sān kē zhēn]

***Radix Berberidis,* Barberry Root:** the dried root of *Berberis soulieana* Schneid, *Berberis wilsonae* Hemsl., *Berberis poiretii* Schneid. or *Berberis vernae* Schneid. (family Berberidaceae), used a similar way to golden thread (黄连 [huáng lián])

龙胆 [lóng dǎn]

***Radix Gentianae,* Chinese Gentian:** the dried root and rhizome of *Gentiana manshurica* Kitag., *Gentiana scabra* Bge., *Gentiana triflora* Pall. or *Gentiana rigescens* Franch. (family Gentianaceae), used to clear heat, dry dampness, and purge the liver and gallbladder fire for the treatment of (1) damp-heat in the liver and gallbladder with morbid leukorrhea, jaundice, or eczema, and (2) liver fire with headache, hypochondriac pain, deafness or convulsions

龙胆草 [lóng dǎn cǎo]

the full name of Chinese gentian (龙胆 [lóng dǎn])

苦参 [kǔ shēn]

Radix Sophorae Flavescentis, **Light-yellow Sophora Root:** the dried root of *Sophora flavescens* Ait. (family Leguminosae), used to clear heat, dry dampness, kill parasitic worms and induce diuresis for treating acute dysentery, jaundice, morbid leucorrhoea, and externally for eczema and scabies

秦皮 [qín pí]

Cortex Fraxini, **Ash Bark:** the dried branch bark or trunk bark of *Fraxinus rhynchophylla* Hance, *Fraxinus chinensis* Roxb., or *Fraxinus stylosa* Lingelsh. (family Oleaceae), used for treating acute dysentery and inflammation of the eye

胡黄连 [hú huáng lián]

Rhizoma Picrorhizae, **Figwortflower Picrorhiza Rhizome:** the dried rhizome of *Picrorhiza scrophulariiflora* Pennell (family Scrophulariaceae), used (1) to remove damp-heat for the treatment of acute dysentery and jaundice, and (2) to relieve consumptive fever in cases of phthisis and infantile malnutrition

鸡骨草 [jī gǔ cǎo]

Herba Abri, **Canton Love-pea Vine:** the dried entire plant of *Abrus cantoniensis* Hance (family Leguminosae), used to clear heat, remove damp, soothe the liver and alleviate pain for treating hepatitis and epigastric pain

白鲜皮 [bái xiān pí]

Cortex Dictamni, **Dittany Root-bark:** the dried root-bark of *Dictamnus dasycarpus* Turcz. (family Rutaceae), used internally or externally for skin diseases with excessive secretion and itching

鸦胆子 [yā dǎn zǐ]

Fructus Bruceae, **Java Brucea Fruit:** the dried ripe fruit of *Brucea javanica* (L.) Merr. (family Simarubaceae), used for treating amebic dysentery and malaria, also used externally for warts, clavus and trichomonas vaginitis

白头翁 [bái tóu wēng]

Radix Pulsatillae, **Chinese Pulsatilla Root:** the dried root of *Pulsatilla*

chinensis (Bge.) Regel (family Ranunculaceae), used for treating bacterial and amebic dysentery, and externally for trichomonas vaginitis

椿皮 [chūn pí]

***Cortex Ailanthi,* Tree-of-heaven Bark:** the dried root bark or stem bark of *Ailanthus altissima* (Mill.) Swingle (family Simarubaceae), used for treating diarrhea, chronic dysentery, abnormal uterine bleeding and leukorrhea

椿根白皮 [chūn gēn bái pí]

same as 椿皮 [chūn pí]

茵陈 [yīn chén]

***Herba Artemisiae Scopariae,* Virgate Wormwood Herb:** the dried young shoot or flowering top of *Artemisia scoparia* Waldst. et Kit. or *Artemisia capillaris* Thunb. (family Compositae), used to eliminate damp-heat in the liver and gallbladder for the treatment of jaundice and also for eczema

茵陈蒿 [yīn chén hāo]

same as virgate wormwood herb (茵陈 [yīn chén])

垂盆草 [chuí pén cǎo]

***Herba Sedi,* Stringy Stonecrop Herb:** the fresh or dried entire plant of *Sedum sarmentosum* Bunge (family Crassulaceae), used to remove damp-heat and counteract toxins for the treatment of acute and chronic hepatitis, jaundice, boils and sores

土茯苓 [tǔ fú líng]

***Rhizoma Smilacis Glabrae,* Glabrous Greenbrier Rhizome:** the dried rhizome of *Smilax glabra* Roxb. (family Libiaceae), used to counteract toxins and eliminate dampness for the treatment of syphilis, morbid leukorrhea and heat stranguria

马齿苋 [mǎ chǐ xiàn]

***Herba Portulacae,* Purslane Herb:** the dried aerial part of *Portulaca oleracea* L. (family Portulacaceae), used for treating dysentery with bloody stools, and externally for boils and sores, eczema, erysipelas, and snake- and insect-bite

黄栌 [huáng lú]

***Folium et Ramulus Cotini,* Smoketree Twig:** the dried leaf and branch of *Cotinus coggygria* Scop. var. *cinera* Engl. (family Anacardiaceae), used for treating hepatitis with jaundice, dysentery, and eczema with pruritus

拳参 [quán shēn]

***Rhizoma Bistortae,* Bistort Rhizome:** the dried rhizome of *Polygonum bistorta* L. (family Polygonaceae), used (1) to clear heat and counteract toxins for treating dysentery, boils and sores, (2) to arrest bleeding for hematemesis, epistaxis, hemorrhoidal bleeding, and (3) externally for trating snake-bite

虎杖 [hǔ zhàng]

***Rhizoma Polygoni Cuspidati,* Giant Knotweed Rhizome:** the dried rhizome of giant or Japanese knotweed, *Polygonum cuspidatum* Sieb. et Zucc. (family Polygonaceae), used (1) to clear heat, counteract toxins, and promote bile flow in cases of hepatitis, jaundice, dysentery, bladder damp-heat, and lung heat with cough, (2) to activate blood and remove stasis for treating amenorrhea and traumatic injuries, and (3) externally for burns and venomous snake-bite

翻白草 [fān bái cǎo]

***Herba Potentillae Discoloris,* Diverse-color Cinquefoil:** the dried entire plant of *Potentilla discolor* Bge. (family Rosaceae), used for treating enteritis, dysentery, pharyngitis, and gastro-intestinal bleeding

栀子 [zhī zǐ]

***Fructus Gardeniae,* Cape-jasmine Fruit:** the dried ripe fruit of *Gardenia jasminoides* Ellis (family Rubiaceae), used (1) to purge fire and calm the mind in cases of fever with fidgetiness and insomnia, and (2) to clear damp-heat from the liver and gallbladder in cases of acute icteric hepatitis, and to cool blood and counteract toxins in cases of bleeding, sores and ulcers

清热解毒药 Drugs for Clearing Heat and Counteracting Toxins

金银花 [jīn yín huā]

***Flos Lonicerae,* Honeysuckle Flower:** the dried flower-bud of *Lonicera japonica* Thunb., *Lonicera hypoglauca* Miq., *Lonicera confusa* DC. or *Lonicera dasystyla* Rehd. (family Caprifoliaceae), used to clear heat, counteract toxins, and disperse wind-heat for treating (1) boils, sores and abscesses, (2) wind-heat afflictions and warm diseases at the early stage, and (3) toxic-heat dysentery

银花 [yín huā]

another name for *Flos Lonicerae,* Honeysuckle Flower (金银花 [jīn yín huā])

忍冬藤 [rěn dōng téng]

***Caulis Lonicerae,* Honeysuckle Stem:** the dried stem and branch of *Lonicera japonica* Thunb. (family Caprifoliaceae), with actions similar to those of honeysuckle flower (金银花 [jīn yín huā]), but more frequently used to clear heat from the meridians and collaterals for treating acute rheumatic arthritis

金银藤 [jīn yín téng]

another name for honeysuckle stem (忍冬藤 [rěn dōng téng])

连翘 [lián qiào]

***Fructus Forsythiae,* Weeping Forsythia Fruit:** the dried fruit of weeping forsythia, *Forsythia suspensa* (Thunb.) Vahl (family Oleaceae), often used together with honeysuckle flower (1) to clear heat, counteract toxins and dissipate nodulation in cases of boils, sores and abscesses, and (2) to disperse wind-heat for wind-heat afflictions and warm diseases at the early stage

板蓝根 [bǎn lán gēn]

***Radix Isatidis,* Isatis Root:** the dried root of *Isatis indigotica* Fort. (family Cruciferae), used to clear heat, counteract toxins and cool the blood in the treatment of warm diseases with fever, headache and sore throat, eruptive epidemic diseases, mumps, boils, sores and erysipelas

大青叶 [dà qīng yè]

***Folium Isatidis*, Dyers Woad Leaf:** the dried leaf of *Isatis indigotica* Fort. (family Cruciferae), used to clear heat, counteract toxins and cool the blood for treating warm diseases at the nutrient and blood stages with eruption, and also for mumps, painful swollen throat and erysipelas

蓼大青叶 [liǎo dà qīng yè]

***Folium Polygoni Tinctorii,* Indigoplant Leaf:** the dried leaf of *Polygonum tinctorium* Ait. (family Polygonaceae), used as dyers woad leaf (大青叶 [dà qīng yè]) with stronger effects

青黛 [qīng dài]

***Indigo Naturalis,* Natural Indigo:** deep blue powder prepared from the leaves of *Baphicacanthus cusia* (Nees) Bremek. (family Acanthaceae), *Polygonum tinctorium* Ait. (family Polygonaceae) or *Isatis indigotica* Fort. (family Cruciferae), used chiefly for the treatment of eruptive epidemic diseases and high fever in children, and used externally for oral ulcers, mumps, and skin infections

蒲公英 [pú gōng yīng]

***Herba Taraxaci,* Dandelion:** the dried entire plant of *Taraxacum mongolicum* Hand.-Mazz., *Taraxacum sinicum* Kitag. or several other *Taraxacum* species (family Compositae), used for boils, sores and other pyogenic infections

野菊花 [yě jú huā]

***Flos Chrysanthemi Indici,* Wild Chrysanthemum Flower:** the dried flower-head of *Chrysanthemum indicum* L. (family Compositae), used to clear heat and counteract toxins for treating boils, sores, carbuncles, erysipelas, acute conjunctivitis, and also externally for eczema and skin itching

紫花地丁 [zǐ huā dì dīng]

***Herba Violae,* Tokyo Violet Herb:** the dried herb of *Viola yedoensis* Makino (family Violaceae), used to clear heat and counteract toxins for the treatment of acute pyogenic infections such as boils, sores and abscesses, and also for venomous snake-bite.

鱼腥草 [yú xīng cǎo]

***Herba Houttuyniae,* Heartleaf Houttuynia Herb:** the dried aerial part of *Houttuynia cordata* Thunb. (family Saururaceae), used to clear heat, counteract toxins, evacuate pus and relieve stranguria for the treatment of lung abscess with purulent expectoration, cough in cases of lung heat, boils and sores, damp-heat stranguria, and acute dysentery

重楼 [chóng lóu]

***Rhizoma Paridis,* Paris Rhizome:** the dried rhizome of *Paris polyphylla* Smith var. *yunnanensis* (Franch.) Hand.-Mazz. or *Paris polyphylla* Smith var. *chinensis* (Franch.) Hara (family Liliaceae), used for treating acute pyogenic inflammations, and also used as an anticonvulsive in the treatment of infantile convulsion

蚤休 [zǎo xīu]

another name for paris rhizome (重楼 [chóng lóu])

败酱草 [bài jiàng cǎo]

***Herba Patriniae,* Patrinia:** the dried entire plant of *Patrinia scabiosaefolia* Fisch. or *Patrinia villosa* Juss. (family Valerianaceae), used for clearing heat, counteracting toxins, evacuating pus, dispelling blood stasis and relieving pain in the treatment of lung abscess, acute appendicitis, boils, sores, ulcers, and postpartum abdominal pain

鸭跖草 [yā zhí cǎo]

***Herba Commelinae,* Common Dayflower Herb:** the dried aerial part of *Commelina communis* L. (family Commelianceae), used (1) to clear heat and counteract toxins for treating warm diseases, boils, sores, and painful swelling of the throat, and (2) to induce diuresis in cases of edema and heat stranguria

穿心莲 [chuān xīn lián]

***Herba Andrographitis,* Common Andrographis Herb:** the dried aerial part of *Andrographis paniculata* (Burm. f.) Nees (family Acanthaceae), used to clear heat, counteract toxins, dry dampness and reduce swelling for the treatment of wind-heat afflictions, warm diseases at the early stage, heat in the lung with cough and dyspnea, lung abscess, damp-heat dysentery, and painful swelling of the throat

白花蛇舌草 [bái huā shé shé cǎo]

***Herba Oldenlandiae,* Oldenlandia:** the dried entire plant of *Oldenlandia diffusa* (Willd.) Roxb., *Oldenlandia corymbosa* L. and other related species (family Rubiaceae), used to clear heat, counteract toxins, remove damp, and relieve stranguria for the treatment of boils, sores, abscesses, venomous snake-bite, and heat stranguria

漏芦 [lòu lú]

***Radix Rhapontici,* Uniflower Swisscentaury Root:** the dried root of *Rhaponticum uniflorum* (L.) DC. (family Compositae), used (1) to clear heat and counteract toxins for mastitis, and (2) to promote lactation in cases of galactostasis

龙葵 [lóng kuí]

***Herba Solani Nigri,* Black Nightshade Herb:** the dried aerial part of *Solanum nigrum* L. (family Solanaceae), used for the treatment of cancer of the stomach and esophagus

半枝莲 [bàn zhī lián]

***Herba Scutellariae Barbatae,* Barbated Skullcap Herb:** the dried entire plant of *Scutellaria barbata* D. Don (family Labiatae), used for the treatment of boils and sore, cirrhosis of the liver with ascites, and snake- and insect-bite

半边莲 [bàn biān lián]

***Herba Lobeliae Chinensis,* Chinese Lobelia Herb:** the dried entire plant of *Lobelia chinensis* Lour. (family Campanulaceae), used to clear heat, counteract toxins and induce dieresis for treating anasarca, ascites, boils and snake- and insect-bite

土牛膝 [tǔ niú xī]

***Radix Achyranthis Asperae,* Native Achyranthes Root:** the dried root of *Achyranthes aspera* L. and other related species (family Amaranthaceae), used for treating sore throat and diphtheria

山豆根 [shān dòu gēn]

***Radix Sophorae Tonkinensis,* Vietnamese Sophora Root:** the dried root and rhizome of *Sophora tonkinensis* Gapnep. (family Leguminosae), used for the treatment of sore throat and gingivitis

广豆根 [guǎng dòu gēn]

same as 山豆根 [shān dòu gēn]

北豆根 [běi dòu gēn]

***Rhizoma Menispermi,* Asiatic Moonseed Rhizome:** the dried rhizome of *Menispermum dauricum* DC. (family Menispermaceae), used in a similar way to Vietnamese sophora root (山豆根 [shān dòu gēn])

射干 [shè gān]

***Rhizoma Belamcandae,* Blackberrylily Rhizome:** the dried rhizome of *Belamcanda chinensis* (L.) DC. (family Iridaceae), used in the relief of painful swelling of the throat, cough and dyspnea with profuse expectoration

马勃 [mǎ bó]

***Lasiosphaera seu Calvatia,* Puff-ball:** the dried sporophore of *Lasiosphaera fenzlii* Reich., *Calvatia gigantea* (Batsch ex Pers.) Lloyd or *Calvatia lilacina* (Mont. et Berk.) LIoyd (family Lycoperdaceae), used to clear heat, counteract toxins, soothe the throat and arrest bleeding for treating painful swelling of the throat and hoarseness of voice in cases of wind-heat afflictions or fire in the lung, and also for epistaxis, hematemesis and traumatic bleeding

青果 [qīng guǒ]

***Fructus Canarii,* Chinese White Olive:** the dried ripe fruit of *Canarium album* Raeusch. (family Burseraceae), used for relieving sore throat and hoarseness in phonation.

锦灯笼 [jǐn dēng lóng]

Calyx seu Fructus Physalis, **Franchet Groundcherry Fruit:** the dried persistent calyx or with the fruit of winter cherry, *Physalis alkekengi* L. var. franchetii (Mast.) Makino (family Solanaceae), used chiefly for treating sore throat

酸浆 [suān jiāng]

another name for 锦灯笼 [jǐn dēng lóng]

葎草 [lǜ cǎo]

Herba Humuli Scandentis, **Climbing Hop Herb:** the dried aerial part of *Humulus scandens* (Lour.) Merr. (family Moraceae),used for the treatment of enteritis, dysentery, acute urinary infection, and also as a tranquilizer in cases of insomnia

祛风湿药 Drugs for Dispelling Wind-Damp

羌活 [qiāng huó]

Rhizoma seu Radix Notopterygii, **Notopterygium Rhizome or Root:** the dried rhizome or root of *Notopterygium incisum* Ting ex H.T. Chang or *Notopterygium forbesii* Boiss. (family Umbelliferae), used to dispel wind, cold and damp for the treatment of wind-cold affliction, and wind-cold-damp (rheumatic or rheumatoid) arthralgia, especially that of the upper part of the body

独活 [dú huó]

Radix Angelicae Pubescentis, **Doubleteeth Pubescent Angelica Root:** the dried root of *Angelica pubescens* Maxim. f. biserrata Shan et Yuan (family Umbelliferae), used to dispel wind-damp, relieve arthralgia and release the superficies for wind-cold-damp (rheumatic or rheumatoid) arthralgia, especially that of the lower part of the body, and affliction of wind-cold with damp

威灵仙 [wēi líng xiān]

Radix Clematidis, **Chinese Clematis Root:** the dried root and rhizome of *Clematis chinensis* Osbeck, *Clematis hexapetala* Pall. or *Clematis manshurica* Rupr. (family Ranunculaceae), used (1) to dispel wind-damp and unblock the collateral meridian for treating wind-damp (rheumatic or rheumatoid) arthralgia, and (2) for the dissolution of fish bone stuck in the throat

秦艽 [qín jiāo]

***Radix Gentianae Macrophyllae,* Large-leaf Gentian Root:** the dried root of *Gentiana macrophylla* Pall., *Gentiana straminea* Maxim., *Gentiana dahurica* Fisch. (family Gentianaceae), used (1) to dispel wind-damp, relieve arthralgia and clear consumptive heat for the treatment of wind-damp (rheumatic or rheumatoid) pain, and also for fever in phthisis, and (2) to remove damp-heat for treating jaundice

木瓜 [mù guā]

***Fructus Chaenomelis,* Common Flowering-quince Fruit:** the dried ripe fruit of *Chaenomeles speciosa* (Sweet) Nakai (family Rosaceae), used (1) to soothe the tendons and unblock collateral meridians for treating wind-damp (rheumatoid) arthralgia with contracture, and (2) to dispel damp and harmonize the stomach for treating vomiting and diarrhea with systremma

豨莶草 [xī xiān cǎo]

***Herba Siegesbeckiae,* Siegesbeckia Herb:** the dried aerial part of *Siegesbeckia orientalis* L., *Siegesbeckia pubescens* Makino or *Siegesbeckia glabrescens* Makino (family Compositae), used (1) to dispel wind-damp and unblock collateral meridians for treating wind-damp (rheumatic or rheumatoid) arthralgia, and (2) to clear heat and counteract toxins for treating boils, sores, abscesses and ulcers

桑枝 [sāng zhī]

***Ramulus Mori,* Mulberry Twig:** the dried young twig of *Morus alba* L. (family Moraceae), used as an antirheumatic for treating arthralgia and shoulder pain

海风藤 [hǎI fēng téng]

***Caulis Piperis Kadsurae*, Kadsura Pepper Stem:** the dried stem of *Piper kadsura* (Choisy) Ohwi. (family Piperaceae), used to dispel wind-damp, unblock the meridian, disperse cold and alleviate pain for treating rheumatalgia of the joints with muscular contracture and traumatic pains

络石藤 [luò shí téng]

***Caulis Trachelospermi*, Chinese Starjasmine Stem:** the dried stem with leaf of *Trachelospermum jasminoides* (Lindl.) Lem. (family Apocynaceae), used to dispel wind-damp, unblock the meridians, cool the blood and reduce swelling in the treatment of rheumatalgia of the joints with muscular contracture, as well as sore throat

千年健 [qiān nián jiàn]

***Rhizoma Homalomenae*, Obscured Homalomena Rhizome:** the dried rhizome of *Homalomena occulta* (Lour.) Schott (family Araceae), used to dispel wind-damp, strengthen tendons and bones, and alleviate rheumatic pain for treating rheumatoid arthritis with cold sensation and pain in the back and knees, and contracture of the lower limbs

蕲蛇 [qí shé]

***Agkistrodon*, Long-noded Pit Viper:** the dried body of *Agkistrodon acutus* (Guenther) (family Viperidae), used to unblock the meridians for relieving chronic and stubborn rheumatalgia, and to relieve spasm for treating hemiplegia, convulsion and tetanus

金钱白花蛇 [jīn qián bái huā shé]

***Bungarus Parvus*, Coin-like White-banded Snake:** the dried body of a young *Bungarus multicinctus* Blyth (family Elapidae), used in a similar way to the long-noded pit viper (蕲蛇 [qí shé])

乌梢蛇 [wū shāo shé]

***Zaocys*, Black-tailed Snake:** the dried body of *Zaocys dhumnades* (Cantor) (family Colubridae), used to dispel wind, unblock the meridian, and relieve convulsion and spasm for treating chronic and stubborn rheumatalgia, hemiplegia in cases of stroke, convulsions and tetanus.

马钱子 [mǎ qián zǐ]

***Semen Strychni*, Nux Vomica:** the dried ripe seed of *Strychnos nux-vomica L. or Strychnos pierriana* A.W. Hill (family Loganiaceae), used to promote the flow of *qi* and blood in collateral meridians, alleviate pain and reduce swelling in cases of rheumatoid arthritis, sequelae of infantile paralysis, and traumatic injuries with pain

五加皮 [wǔ jiā pí]

***Cortex Acanthopanacis*, Slenderstyle Acanthopanax Bark:** the dried root-bark of *Acanthopanax gracilistylus* W.W. Smith (family Araliaceae), used to dispel wind-damp, strengthen the tendons and bones, and induce diuresis in the treatment of rheumatic conditions, and edema

海桐皮 [hǎi tóng pí]

***Cortex Erythrinae*, Coral-bean Bark:** the dried bark of *Erythrina variegata* L. var. *orientalis* (L.) Merr. or *Erythrina arborescens* Roxb. (family Leguminosae), used to dispel wind-damp, unblock the collateral meridians and relieve itching in cases of rheumatalgia, and also externally for treating neurodermatitis and chronic eczema

丝瓜络 [sī guā luò]

***Retinervus Luffae Fructus*, Luffa Vegetable Sponge:** the dried vascular bundles of the ripe fruit of *Luffa cylindrica* (L.) Roem. (family Cucurbitaceae), used to dispel wind, unblock collateral meridians, and relieve toxins for treating rheumatalgia with muscular contracture, and also for treating mastitis

伸筋草 [zhē jīn cǎo]

***Herba Lycopodii*, Common Club-moss Herb:** the dried entire plant of *Lycopodium japonicum* Thunb. (family Lycopodiaceae), used to dispel wind-damp and relieve contracture in cases of arthralgia with stiffness

老鹳草 [lǎo guàn cǎo]

***Herba Erodii seu Geranii*, Heron's Bill** or **Wilford Ganesbill Herb:** the dried aerial part of *Erodium stephanianum* Willd. or *Geranium wilfordii* Maxim. (family Geraniaceae), used to dispel wind-damp, unblock collateral meridians and arrest dysenteric diarrhea in cases of rheumatalgia with muscular contracture, and also for treating enteritis and dysentery

臭梧桐叶 [chòu wú tóng yè]

***Folium Liriodendra Tracheotomy*, Glory bower Leaf:** the dried leaf of *Clerodendrum trichotomum* Thunb. (family Verbenaceae), used to dispel wind-damp and reduce high blood pressure in cases of rheumatism and hypertension

穿山龙 [chuān shān lóng], 穿地龙 [chuān dì lóng]

***Rhizoma Dioscoreae Nipponicae*, Japanese Yam:** the dried rhizome of *Dioscorea nipponica Makino* (family Dioscoreaceae), used to dispel wind-damp, activate blood circulation, unblock collateral meridians and resolve phlegm in the treatment of rheumatalgia, sprain, traumatic pains, and chronic cough with expectoration

徐长卿 [xú cháng qīng]

***Radix Cynanchi Paniculati*, Paniculate Swallowwort Root:** the dried root and rhizome of *Cynanchum paniculatum* (Bge.) Kitag. (family Asclepiadaceae), used to unblock collateral meridians, alleviate pain, relieve toxicity and reduce swelling for treating rheumatalgia, toothache, lumbago, traumatic injuries, dysmenorrhea and eczema

青风藤 [qīng fēng téng]

***Caulis Sinomenii*, Orientvine Stem:** the dried lianoid stem of *Sinomenium acutum* (Thunb.) Rehd. et Wils. or *Sinomenium acutum* var. *cinereum* Rehd. et Wils. (family Menispermaceae), used to dispel wind-damp and alleviate pain in cases of rheumatic arthritis, articular swelling and pain

香加皮 [xiāng jiā pí]

***Cortex Periplocae*, Chinese Silkvine Bark:** the dried root-bark of *Periploca sepium* Bge. (family Asclepiadaceae), used to dispel wind-damp in cases of rheumatic arthritis, and induce diuresis for edema

防己 [fáng jǐ]

***Radix Stephaniae Tetrandrae*, Fourstamen Stephania Root:** the dried root of *Stephania tetrandra* S. Moore (family Menispermaceae), used to dispel wind-damp, induce diuresis in cases of rheumatic arthritis, edema and oliguria

温寒药 Drugs for Dispelling Internal Cold

附子 [fù zǐ]

***Radix Aconiti Lateralis Preparata*, Prepared Daughter Root of Common Monkshood:** the prepared daughter root of *Aconitum carmichaeli* Debx. (family Ranunculaceae), used (1) to restore heart yang for the relief of collapse and shock, (2) to dispel cold for treating deficiency-cold conditions such as gastralgia and abdominal pain with cold sensation, and also for cold rheumatalgia with severe pain, and (3) to reinforce the kidney and spleen for treating edema, chronic diarrhea and impotence.

肉桂 [ròu guì]

***Cortex Cinnamomi*, Cassia Bark:** the dried stem bark of *Cinnamomum cassia* Presl. (family Lauraceae) , used (1) to warm the kidney in the treatment of impotence and chronic diarrhea with coldness of the limbs, (2) to alleviate pain by dispelling cold for epigastric and abdominal pain due to cold attack or deficiency-cold, and (3) to promote menstruation in cases of amenorrhea and dysmenorrhea

干姜 [gān jiāng]

***Rhizoma Zingiberis*, Dried Ginger:** the dried rhizome of *Zingiber officinale* (Willd.) Rosc. (family Zingiberaceae), used (1) to warm the spleen and stomach for the relief of nausea, vomiting, abdominal pain and diarrhea due to deficiency-cold of the spleen and stomach, and (2) to warm the lung for treating chronic cough with thin, white and foamy expectoration

高良姜 [gāo liáng jiāng]

***Rhizoma Alpiniae Officinarum*, Lesser Galangal Rhizome:** the dried rhizome of *Alpinia officinarum* Hance (family Zingiberaceae), used to warm the stomach for relieving gastralgia and vomiting due to cold

花椒 [huā jiāo]

***Pericarpium Zanthoxyli*, Prickly-ash Peel:** the dried ripe pericarp of *Zanthoxylum schinifolium* Sieb. et Zucc. or *Zanthoxylum bungeanum* Maxim. (family Rutaceae), used (1) to warm the stomach for the treatment of gastralgia and dyspepsia due to cold, (2) as an ascaricide, and (3) externally for treating eczema and pruritus.

荜澄茄 [bì chéng qié]

***Fructus Litseae*, Mountain Spicy Fruit:** the dried ripe fruit of *Litsea cubeba* (Lour.) Pers. (family Lauraceae), used to warm the stomach for relieving vomiting, epigastric and abdominal pain due to cold

吴茱萸 [wú zhū yú]

***Fructus Evodiae*, Evodia Fruit:** the dried nearly mature fruit of *Evodia rutaecarpa* (Juss.) Benth., *Evodia rutaecarpa* var. *officinalis* (Dode) Huang or *Evodia rutaecarpa* var. *bodinieri* (Dode) Huang (family Rutaceae), used to warm the stomach and relieve pain in cases of gastralgia, abdominal pain, acid regurgitation and vomiting

丁香 [dīng xiāng]

***Flos Caryophylli*, Cloves:** the dried flower-bud of *Eugenia caryophyllata* Thunb. (family Myrtaceae), used (1) to warm the stomach for the relief of vomiting and hiccups due to cold, and (2) to warm the kidney for treating impotence

小茴香 [xiǎo huí xiāng]

***Fructus Foeniculi*, Fennel Fruit:** the dried fruit of *Foeniculum vulgare* Mill. (family Umbelliferae), used to dispel cold, regulate the *qi* flow and relieve pain for treating cold pain in the lower abdomen, and distending pain in the testis

艾叶 [ài yè]

***Folium Artemisiae Argyi*, Argyi Leaf, Argyi Wormwood Leaf:** the dried leaf of *Artemisia argyi* Levl. et Vant. (family Compositae), used to warm the uterus and stop bleeding in cases of functional uterine bleeding, sterility and dysmenorrhea

川乌 [chuān wū]

***Radix Aconiti*, Mother Root of Common Monkshood:** the dried parent root of *Aconitum carmichaeli* Debx. (family Ranunculaceae), used to dispel cold and wind and to relieve pain in cases of serious rheumatalgia, and cold pain in the abdomen. For internal use, the prepared root is usually employed.

制川乌 [zhì chuān wū]

***Radix Aconiti Preparata*, Prepared Mother Root of Common Monkshood:** cf. *Radix Aconiti*, Mother Root of Common Monkshood (川乌 [chuān wū])

草乌 [cǎo wū]

***Radix Aconiti Kusnezoffii*, Wild Aconite Root, Kusnezoff Monkshood Root:** the dried tuberous root of *Aconitum kusnezoffii* Reichb. (family Ranunculaceae), used in a similar way to mother root of common monkshood (川乌 [chuān wū]), but usually in smaller doses

荜拨 [bì bō]

***Fructus Piperis Longi*, Long Pepper:** the dried nearly ripe or ripe fruit-spike of *Piper longum* L. (family Piperaceae): used to warm the stomach for the treatment of cold and pain in the stomach

芳香化湿药 Drugs with Fragrant Odor for Resolving Dampness

广藿香 [guǎng huò xiāng]

***Herba Pogostemonis*, Cablin Patchouli Herb:** the dried aerial part of *Pogostemon cablin* (Blanco) Benth. (family Labiatae), used to resolve damp for treating nausea, vomiting and diarrhea, especially in cases of summer afflictions

藿香 [huò xiāng]

***Herba Agastachis*, Agastache:** the dried aerial part of *Agastache rugosus* (Fisch. et Mey.) O. Ktze. (family Labiatae), used in a similar way to cablin patchouli (广藿香 [guǎng huò xiāng])

佩兰 [pèi lán]

***Herba Eupatorii*, Fortune Eupatorium Herb:** the aerial part of

Eupatorium fortunei Turcz. (family Compositae), used to resolve damp for relieving nausea, vomiting and abdominal distension, especially in cases of summer afflictions

苍术 [cāng zhú]

***Rhizoma Atractylodis*, Atractylodes Rhizome:** the dried rhizome of *Atractylodes lancea* (Thunb.) DC. or *Atractylodes chinensis* (DC.) Koidz. (family Compositae), used (1) to eliminate dampness and invigorate the spleen for treating damp accumulation in the spleen and stomach, (2) to dispel wind-damp for rheumatic arthritis, and (3) to improve vision in cases of night blindness

豆蔻 [dòu kòu]; 白豆蔻 [bái dòu kòu]

***Fructus Amomi Rotundus*, Round Cardamom Fruit:** the dried ripe fruit of *Amomum kravanh* Pirre ex Gagnep. or *Amomum compactum* Soland ex Maton (family Zingiberaceae), used to resolve damp, move *qi*, and warm the middle for relieving epigastric and abdominal distension, nausea, and vomiting due to accumulation of cold-dampness of stagnation of *qi* in the spleen and stomach

蔻仁 [kòu rén]

***Semen Amomi Rotundus*, Round Cardamom Seed:** the seed of round cardamom freshly removed from the pericarp, which is stronger in activity than the fruit

砂仁 [shā rén]

***Fructus Amomi*, Spiny Amomum Fruit:** the dried ripe fruit of *Amomum villosum* Lour., *Amomum villosum* var. *xanthioides* T.L. Wu et Senjen or *Amomum longiligulare* T.L. Wu (family Zingiberaceae), used (1) to resolve dampness for treating damp accumulation in the spleen and stomach, (2) to warm the middle for treating vomiting and diarrhea due to deficiency-cold of the spleen and stomach, and (3) to prevent miscarriage in cases of threatened abortion

草豆蔻 [cǎo dòu kòu]

***Semen Alpiniae Katsumadai*, Katsumada Galangal Seed:** the dried seed of *Alpinia katsumadai* Hayata (family Zingiberaceae), used to dry dampness, move *qi*, and warm the middle for relieving gastralgia, vomiting and diarrhea due to accumulation of cold-damp or *qi* stagnation in the spleen and stomach

草果 [cǎo guǒ]

***Fructus Tsaoko*, Tsaoko, Caoguo:** the dried ripe fruit of *Amomum tsao-ko* Crevost et Lemaire (family Zigiberaceae), used (1) to remove dampness and warm the stomach in cases of epigastric distension, vomiting and abdominal pain, and (2) for treating malaria

利尿逐水药 Diuretics and Hydragogues

利尿渗湿药 Diuretics

茯苓 [fú líng]

***Poria*, Indian Bread:** the dried sclerotium of the fungus *Poria cocos* (Schw.) Wolf (family Polyporaceae), used (1) as a diuretic in cases of edema and oliguria, (2) to invigorate the spleen for treating anorexia and diarrhea, and (3) to induce tranquilization in cases of palpitation and insomnia

猪苓 [zhū líng]

***Polyporus*, Chuling, Umbellate Polypore:** the dried sclerotium of the fungus *Polyporus umbellatus* (Pers.) Fries (family Polyporaceae), used as a diuretic for edema and oliguria, and also to filter out damp for treating leukorrhagia

泽泻 [zé xiè]

***Rhizoma Alismatis*, Water-plantain Rhizome:** the dried tuber of *Alisma orientalis* (Sam.) Juzep. (family Alismaceae), used (1) to promote urine excretion for oliguria and edema, (2) to filter out damp in cases of diarrhea and leukorrhea, and (3) to purge heat in cases of bladder damp-heat

车前子 [chē qián zǐ]

***Semen Plantaginis*, Plantain Seed:** the dried ripe seed of *Plantago asiatica* L. or *Plantago depressa* Willd. (family Plantaginaceae), used (1) to induce diuresis and filter out damp for treating watery diarrhea, edema, and stranguria, (2) to clear the liver and improve vision in cases of eye diseases, and (3) to clear the lung and resolve phlegm for cases of cough with profuse phlegm

车前草 [chē qián cǎo]

***Herba Plantaginis*, Plantain Herb:** the dried entire plant of *Plantago asiatica* L. or *Plantago depressa* Willd. (family Plantaginaceae), used (1) to induce diuresis in cases of edema, oliguria and stranguria, and (2) to clear heat and counteract toxins in cases of sores, carbuncles, dysentery, and acute pulmonary and urinary infections

滑石 [huá shí]

***Talcum*, Talc:** a very soft mineral composed mainly of hydrous magnesium silicate, used to induce diuresis, clear summer-heat and dispel damp in the treatment of summer afflictions, watery diarrhea, oliguria and urinary infection, and also externally for treating eczema and miliaria

薏苡仁 [yì yǐ rén]

***Semen Coicis*, Coix Seed, Job's-tears Seed:** the dried ripe kernel obtained by removing the hard husk and seed coat of *Coix lacryma-jobi* L. var. *ma-yuen* (Roman.) Stapf (family Graminae), used (1) to invigorate the spleen and dispel dampness for treating diarrhea and edema, (2) to clear heat and discharge pus for treating lung abscess and acute appendicitis, and (3) for treating verruca plana

冬瓜皮 [dōng guā pí]

***Exocarpium Benincasae*, Chinese Wax-gourd Peel:** the dried exocarp of *Benincasa hispida* (Thunb.) Cogn. (family Cucurbitaceae), used to induce diuresis for treating oliguria and edema

青木香 [qīng mù xiāng]

***Radix Aristolochiae*, Dutchmanspipe Root:** the dried root of *Aristolochia debilis* Sieb. et Zucc. (family Aristolochiaceae), used (1) to move *qi* and alleviate pain for treating thoracic, epigastric, hypochondriac and abdominal distension and pain, and (2) to counteract toxins and reduce swelling for treating boils, sores, eczema and venomous snake-bite

大腹皮 [dà fù pí]

***Pericarpium Arecae*, Areca Peel:** the dried pericarp of *Areca catechu* L. (family Palmae), used to induce diuresis and remove stagnant *qi* for relieving abdominal distension and edema

木通 [mù tōng]

***Caulis Aristolochiae Manshuriensis*, Manshurian Dutchmanspipe Stem** (关木通 [guān mù tōng]) or ***Caulis Clematidis Armandii*, Armand Clematis Stem** (川木通 [chuān mù tōng]) (see below)

关木通 [guān mù tōng]

***Caulis Aristolochiae Manshuriensis*, Manchurian Dutchmanspipe Stem:** the dried stem of *Aristolochia manshuriensis* Kom. (family

Aristolochiaceae), used (1) to induce diuresis and relieve stranguria in cases of bladder damp-heat, and (2) as an emmenagogue and galactagogue for amenorrhea and inadequate lactation

川木通 [chuān mù tōng]

***Caulis Clematidis Armandii*, Armand Clematis Stem:** the dried stem of *Clematis armandii* Franch. or *Clematis montana* Buch.-Ham. (family Ranunculaceae), used in a similar way to 关木通 [guān mù tōng]

通草 [tōng cǎo]

***Medulla Tetrapanacis*, Ricepaper-plant Pith:** the stem pith of *Tetrapanax papyriferus* (Hook.) K. Koch (family Araliaceae), used (1) to clear heat and remove damp in cases of stranguria and oliguria, and (2) to promote milk secretion in cases of inadequate lactation

萹蓄 [biǎn xù]

***Herba Polygoni Avicularis*, Common Knotgrass Herb:** the dried aerial part of *Polygonum aviculare* L. (family Polygonaceae), used (1) to promote diuresis and eliminate damp-heat in cases of stranguria with turbid urine and morbid leukorrhea, and (2) to dispel wind-damp in cases of arthralgia

瞿麦 [qú mài]

***Herba Dianthi*, Liliac Pink Herb:** the dried aerial part of *Dianthus superbus* L. or *Dianthus chinensis* L. (family Caryophyllaceae), used to promote diuresis and eliminate damp-heat for the treatment of heat stranguria and blood stranguria, and (2) as an emmenagogue for amenorrhea

苘麻子 [qǐng má zǐ]

***Semen Abutili*, Chingma Abutilon Seed:** the dried ripe seed of *Abutilon theophrastii* Medic. (family Malvaceae), used to remove damp-heat and counteract toxins for the treatment of dysentery, heat stranguria, boils and sores

冬葵果 [dōng kuí guǒ]

***Fructus Malvae*, Cluster Mallow Fruit:** the dried ripe fruit of *Malva verticillata* L. (family Malvaceae), used to clear heat and induce diuresis for treating stranguria, oliguria and edema

萆薢 [bì xiè]

***Rhizoma Dioscoreae Septemlobae*, Seven-lobed Yam Rhizome** (绵萆薢 [mián bì xiè]) or ***Rhizoma Dioscoreae Hypoglaucae*, Hypoglaucous**

Yam Rhizome (粉萆薢 [fěn bì xiè]) (see below)

绵萆薢 [mián bì xiè]

***Rhizoma Dioscoreae Septemlobae*, Seven-lobed Yam Rhizome:** the dried rhizome of *Dioscorea septemloba* Thunb. or *Dioscorea futschauensis* Uline (family Dioscoreaceae), used (1) to eliminate damp-turbidity in cases of chyluria and strangueia with turbid urine, and (2) to dispel wind-damp in cases of rheumatic arthritis

粉萆薢 [fěn bì xiè]

***Rhizoma Dioscoreae Hypoglaucae*, Hypoglaucous Yam Rhizome:** the dried rhizome of *Dioscorea hypoglauca* Palib. (family Dioscoreaceae), used in a similar way to 绵萆薢 [mián bì xiè]

地肤子 [dì fū zǐ]

***Fructus Kochiae*, Belvedere Fruit:** the dried ripe fruit of *Kochia scoparia* (L.) Schrad. (family Chenopodiaceae), used to clear damp-heat in cases of bladder damp-heat with stranguria, and to relieve itch in cases of urticaria, eczema and pruritus

金钱草 [jīn qián cǎo]

***Herba Lysimachiae*, Christina Loosestrife:** the dried entire plant of *Lysimachia christinae* Hance (family Primulaceae), used (1) as a cholagogue, lithagogue and diuretic for the treatment of acute jaundice, biliary and urinary calculi, and (2) to relieve toxicity and reduce swelling in cases of boils and venomous snake-bite

海金沙 [hǎi jīn shā]

***Spora Lygodii*, Japanese Climbing-fern Spores:** spores of *Lygodium japonicum* (Thunb.) Sw. (family Ligodiaceae), used to eliminate damp-heat and as a lithagogue for treating bladder damp-heat and urinary calculi

赤小豆 [chì xiǎo dòu]

***Semen Phaseoli*, Rice Bean:** the dried ripe seed of *Phaseolus calcaratus* Roxb. Or *Phaseolus angularis* Wight (family Leguminosae), used to induce diuresis, counteract toxins and promote the drainage of pus in cases of boils, sores and abscesses

石韦 [shí wěi]

***Folium Pyrrosiae*, Shearer's Pyrrosia Leaf:** the dried leaf of *Pyrrosia sheareri* (Bak.) Ching, *Pyrrosia lingua* (Thunb.) Farwell or *Pyrrosia petiolosa* (Christ) Ching (family Polypodiaceae), used (1) to induce diuresis, relieve dysuria for treating bladder damp-heat, and (2) to clear the lung for relieving cough and dyspnea

葫芦 [hú lú]

***Pericarpium Lagenariae*, Calabash Gourd:** the dried pericarp of *Lagenaria siceraria* (Molina) Standl. var. *depressa* (Ser.) Hara (family Cucurbitaceae), a diuretic for treating severe edema and ascites

抽葫芦 [chōu hú lú]

same as 葫芦 [hú lú]

蝼蛄 [lóu gū]

***Gryllotalpa*, Mole Cricket:** the dried body of *Gyllotalpa africana* Palisot et Beaurois (family Gryllotalpidae), a diuretic for treating severe edema, ascites and retention of urine

路路通 [lù lù tōng]

***Fructus Liquidambaris*, Beautiful Sweetgum Fruit:** the dried strobile (cone) of *Liquidambar formosana* Hance (family Hamamelidaceae), used (1) to induce diuresis for treating edema, (2) to dispel wind-damp in cases of arthralgia, and (3) to promote menstrual discharge in cases of amenorrhea

玉米须 [yù mǐ xū]

***Stigma Maydis*, Corn Stigma:** the dried styles and stigmata of Indian Corn, *Zea mays* L. (family Gramineae), used (1) to induce diuresis for treating edema, (2) to promote bile discharge in cases of jaundice, and (3) to reduce high blood pressure in cases of hypertension

灯心草 [dēng xīn cǎo]

***Medulla Junci*, Common Rush:** the dried pith of *Juncus effusus* L. (family Juncaceae), used (1) to induce diuresis for treating heat stranguria, and (2) to calm the mind for relieving fidgetiness and insomnia

逐水药 Hydragogues or Drastic Purgatives

牵牛子 [qiān niú zǐ]

***Semen Pharbitidis*, Pharbitis Seed:** the dried ripe seed of *Pharbitis nil* (L.) Choisy or *Pharbitis purpurea* (L.) Voigt (family Convolvulaceae), used as a hydragogue for edema and oliguria, and an anthelmintic for ascariasis

黑丑 [hēi chǒu]

Black Pharbitis Seed: pharbitis seed with its surface colored grayish black

白丑 [bái chǒu]

White Pharbitis Seed: pharbitis seed with its surface colored pale yellowish

黑白丑 [hēi bái chǒu]

Black and White Pharbitis Seed: black and white pharbitis seeds mixed in equal quantities.

商陆 [shāng lù]

***Radix Phytolaccae*, Pokeberry Root:** the dried root of *Phytolacca acinosa* Roxb. or *Phytolacca americana* L. (family Phytolaccaceae), used as a diuretic and hydragogue for treating edema and ascites, also used externally for treating boils and sores

巴豆霜 [bā dòu shuāng]

***Semen Crotonis Pulveratum*, Defatted Croton Seed Powder:** partly defatted and powdered seed of *Croton tiglium* L. (family Euphorbiaceae), used as a drastic purgative for treatment of constipation with abdominal distension and pain due to accumulation of cold and stagnation of food

甘遂 [gān suì]

***Radix Euphorbiae Kansui*, Kansui Root:** the dried tuberous root of *Euphorbia kansui* T.N. Liou ex T. P. Wang (family Euphorbiaceae), used as a hydragogue and purgative for hydrothorax and ascites with oliguria and constipation

芫花 [yuán huā]

***Flos Genkwa*, Lilac Daphne Flower Bud:** the dried flower-bud of *Daphne genkwa* Sieb. et Zucc. (family Thymelaeaceae), used as a hydragogue and purgative for treating severe edema, hydrothorax and ascites with oliguria and constipation, and externally for scabies and frostbite

黄芫花 [huáng yuán huā]

***Folium et Flos Wikstroemiae Chamaedaphnis*, Chamaedaphne Leaf and Flower, Yellow Genkwa Leaf and Flower:** leaf and flower-bud of *Wikstroemia chamaedaphne* Meisn. (family Thymeleaceae), used in a similar way to 芫花, and also for treating acute and chronic hepatitis, schizophrenia, and epilepsy

京大戟 [jīng dà jǐ]

***Radix Euphorbiae Peklnensis*, Peking Euphorbia Root:** the dried root of *Euphorbia pekinensis* Rupr. (family Euphorbiaceae), used as a hydragogue and purgative for treating severe edema, hydrothorax and ascites with oliguria and constipation, also used externally for treating scrofula

龙虎草 [lóng hǔ cǎo]

another name of 京大戟 [jīng dà jǐ]

狼毒 [láng dú]

***Radix Euphorbiae Ebractealatae*, Unbracteolated Euphorbia Root:** the dried root of *Euphobia ebracteolata* Hayata or *Euphorbia fischeriana* Steud. (family Euphorbiaceae), used as drastic purgative to remove stagnated food, and as an anthelmintic for the treatment of intestinal parasites, also used for treating scrofula

理气药 Drugs for Regulating the Flow of *Qi*

陈皮 [chén pí]

***Pericarpium Citri Reticulatae*, Dried Tangerine Peel:** the dried ripe pericarp of *Citrus reticulata* Blanco and its cultivated varieties (family Rutaceae), used to regulate *qi*, invigorate the spleen, dry dampness, and resolve phlegm in the treatment of *qi* stagnation in the spleen and stomach, and cough with profuse phlegm

青皮 [qīng pí]

***Pericarpium Citri Reticulatae Viride*, Green Tangerine Peel:** the dried green unripe exocarp of *Citrus reticulata* Blanco and its cultivated varieties (family Rutaceae), used to regulate *qi*, soothe the liver, and remove stagnation for the treatment of liver *qi* stagnation and food retention

橘核 [jú hé]

***Semen Citri Reticulatae*, Tangerine Seed:** the dried ripe seed of *Citrus reticulata* Blanco and its cultivated varieties (family Rutaceae), used to regulate *qi*, dissipate nodulation and alleviate pain for the treatment of hernial pain, nodules in the breast, and swelling and pain of the testis

橘红 [jú hóng]

***Exocarpium Citri Rubrum*, Red Tangerine Peel:** the dried exocarp of *Citrus reticulata* Blanco and its cultivated varieties (family Rutaceae), used in the same way as dried tangerine peel (陈皮 [chén pí]), with stronger action

枳实 [zhǐ shí]

***Fructus Aurantii Immaturus*, Immature Orange Fruit:** the dried small immature fruit of *Citrus aurantium* L. and its cultivated varieties or *Citrus sinensis* Osbeck with a diameter under 2.5 cm (family Rutaceae), used to breakdown the stuffed *qi*, resolve phlegm and remove accumulation for treating dyspepsia, constipation and abdominal distension due to food stagnation, and served in large doses for treating visceroptosis

枳壳 [zhǐ qiào]

***Fructus Aurantii*, Orange Fruit:** the dried immature fruit of *Citrus aurantium* L. and its cultivated varieties with a diameter between 3-5 cm (family Rutaceae), used in the same way as immature orange fruit (枳实 [zhǐ shí]), with a milder effect

厚朴 [hòu pò]

***Cortex Magnoliae Officinalis*, Medicinal Magnolia Bark:** the dried stem bark, root bark or branch bark of *Magnolia officinalis* Rehd. et Wils. or *Magnolia officinalis* var. *biloba* Rehd. et Wils. (family Magnoliaceae), used (1) to promote the flow of *qi* for relieving abdominal distension and pain due to food stagnation, (2) to invigorate the spleen by drying dampness for curing vomiting and diarrhea due to dyspepsia, and (3) to relieve cough and dyspnea with profuse phlegm

紫苏梗 [zǐ sū gěng]

***Caulis Perillae*, Perilla Stem:** the dried stem of *Perilla frutescens* (L.) Britt. (family Labiatae), used to regulate the flow of *qi*, relieve pain and calm the fetus for the treatment of stuffiness in the chest, epigastric pain, eructation, vomiting and threatened abortion

木香 [mù xiāng]

***Radix Aucklandiae*, Common Aucklandia Root:** the dried root of *Aucklandia lappa* Decne. (family Compositae), used to move *qi* and alleviate pain for relieving abdominal distension and pain due to *qi* stagnation, tenesmus in cases of dysentery, and liver *qi* depression with hypochondriac pain and jaundice

香附 [xiāng fù]

***Rhizoma Cyperi*, Nutgrass Galingale Rhizome:** the dried tuber of *Cyperus rotundus* L. (family Cyperaceae), used to soothe liver *qi*, regulate menstruation and alleviate pain for treating chest and abdominal distension with pain, amenorrhea and dysmenorrhea

乌药 [wū yào]

***Radix Linderae*, Combined Spicebush Root:** the dried tuberous root of *Lindera aggregata* (Sims) Kosterm. (family Lauraceae), used to move *qi*, alleviate pain, warm the kidney and dispel cold for relieving distension and pain in the lower abdomen, frequent micturition and enuresis

香橼 [xiāng yuán]

***Fructus Citri*, Citron Fruit:** the dried ripe fruit of *Citrus medica* L. or *Citrus wilsonii* Tanaka (family Rutaceae), used to soothe the liver, regulate *qi*, and resolve phlegm for the treatment of gastric distension with pain and fullness sensation in the chest, as well as cough with profuse phlegm

佛手 [fó shǒu]

***Fructus Citri Sarcodactylis*, Finger Citron:** the dried fruit of *Citrus medica* L. var. *sarcodactylis* Swingle (family Rutaceae), used to soothe the liver, regulate *qi*, harmonize the middle, resolve damp and phlegm for the treatment of *qi* stagnation in the liver or disharmony between the spleen and stomach, as well as chronic cough with profuse expectoration

薤白 [xiè bái]

***Bulbus Allii Macrostemoni*, Longstamen Onion:** the dried bulb of *Allium macrostemon* Bge. (family Liliaceae), used to unblock and regulate yang-*qi* and remove stagnation in the treatment of angina pectoris with stuffiness sensation in the chest, and also for treating tenesmus in cases of dysentery.

甘松 [gān sōng]

***Radix et Rhizoma Nardostachyos*, Nardus Root, Spikenard Root:** the dried rhizome and root of *Nardostachys chinensis* Batal. or *Nardostachys jatamansi* DC. (family Valerianaceae), used to move *qi*, alleviate pain and invigorate the spleen for treating epigastric and abdominal pain and anorexia due to stagnation of *qi*

檀香 [tán xiāng]

***Lignum Santali Albi*, Sandalwood:** heartwood of trunk of *Santalum album* L. (family Santalaceae), used to move *qi*, alleviate pain, disperse cold and regulate the stomach, for treating angina pectoris and gastralgia due to cold

降香 [jiàng xiāng]

***Lignum Dalbergiae Odoriferae*, Rosewood:** heartwood of trunk and root of *Dalbergia odorifera* T. Chen (family Leguminosae), used to regulate *qi*, resolve blood stasis, and alleviate pain for treating angina pectoris, abdominal distension with pain, and various traumatic painful swellings

沉香 [chén xiāng]

***Lignum Aquilariae Resinatum*, Chinese Eagle Wood:** resinous wood of *Aquilaris sinensis* (Lour.) Gilg (family Thymelaeaceae), used to move *qi* for alleviating pain, to warm the middle for arresting vomiting, and to receive *qi* for relieving dyspnea

娑罗子 [suō luó zǐ]

***Semen Aesculi*, Buckeye Seed:** the dried ripe seed of *Aesculus chinensis* Bge., *Aesculus chinensis* var. *chekiangensis* (Hu et Fang) Fang or *Aesculus wilsonii* Rehd. (family Hippocastanaceae), used to regulate *qi*, harmonize the stomach and alleviate pain for relieving distension and stuffiness in the chest and abdomen, and especially gastralgia

荔枝核 [lì zhī hé]

***Semen Litchi*, Lychee Seed:** the dried ripe seed of *Litchi chinensis* Sonn. (family Sapindaceae), used to move *qi*, dissipate nodulation, disperse cold and alleviate pain for treating hernial pain, dysmenorrhea, lower abdominal distension with pain, and swelling and pain of the testis

梅花 [méi huā]

***Flos Mume*, Plum Flower:** the dried flower-bud of *Prunus mume* (Sieb.) Zieb. et Zucc. (family Rosaceae), used to regulate *qi*, ease the mind and resolve phlegm for treating depression, fidgetiness, hypochondriac and epigastric pain, and globus hystericus

绿萼梅 [lǜ è méi]

same as 梅花 [méi huā]

九香虫 [jiǔ xiāng chóng]

***Aspongopus*, Stink-bug:** the dried body of *Aspongopus chinensis* Dallas (family Pentatomidae), used (1) to regulate *qi* and alleviate pain for treating epigastric distension and pain, and (2) to invigorate the kidney for treating impotence and lumbago

柿蒂 [shì dì]

***Calyx Kaki*, Persimmon Calyx:** the dried persistent calyx of *Diospyros kaki* L. f. (family Ebenaceae), used to direct *qi* downward for stopping hiccups

川楝子 [chuān liàn zǐ]

***Fructus Toosendan*, Szechwan Chinaberry:** the dried ripe fruit of *Melia toosendan* Sieb. et Zucc. (family Meliaceae), used to move *qi* for relieving hypochondriac, epigastric and abdominal pain, and (2) to kill parasitic worms in cases of enterobiasis and scabies

理血药 Drugs for Regulating Blood Conditions

止血药 Hemostatics

仙鹤草 [xiān hè cǎo]

***Herba Agrimoniae*, Hairvein Agrimonia Herb:** the dried aerial part of *Agrimonia pilosa* Ledeb. (family Rosaceae), used (1) as an astringent hemostatic for treating various kinds of bleeding including bloody dysentery, and (2) to counteract toxins and reduce swelling for treating boils and sores. It is also used for treating malaria.

三七 [sān qī]

***Radix Notoginseng*, Sanchi:** the dried root of *Panax notoginseng* (Burk.) F.H. Chen (family Araliaceae), used to resolve stasis, stop bleeding, activate the blood and check pain for treating various kinds of external and internal hemorrhage, blood stasis and pain in cases of traumatic injuries, and angina pectoris

白及 [bái jí]

***Rhizoma Bletillae*, Common Bletilla Tuber:** the steamed and dried tuber of *Bletilla striata* (Thunb.) Reichb. f. (family Orchidaceae), used (1) as a hemostatic for treating hemoptysis, hematemesis and traumatic bleeding, and (2) to reduce swelling and promote regeneration for treating boils and burns

大蓟 [dà jì]

***Herba seu Radix Cirsii Japonici*, Japanese Thistle:** the dried aerial part or root of *Cirsium japonicum* DC. (family Compositae), used as a hemostatic for the treatment of hematemesis and hematuria due to blood heat, also used for treating hepatitis and hypertension

小蓟 [xiǎo jì]

***Herba Cirsii*, Field Thistle:** the dried aerial part of *Cirsium setosum* (Willd.) (family Compositae), used (1) to cool blood and stop bleeding, chiefly for the treatment of hematuria, (2) to dissipate stasis and counteract toxin for treating boils, and (3) also used as an antihypertensive

茜草 [qiàn cǎo]

***Radix Rubiae*, Indian Madder Root:** the dried root and rhizome of Indian Madder, *Rubia cordifolia* L. (family Rubiaceae), used to cool the blood, resolve stasis and stop bleeding for treating epistaxis, metrorrhagia and traumatic bleeding

地榆 [dì yú]

***Radix Sanguisorbae*, Garden Burnet Root:** the dried root of *Sanguisorba officinalis* L. or *Sanguisorba officinalis* var. *longifolia* (Bert.) Yu et Li (family Rosaceae), used as a blood-cooling hemostatic for treating various kinds of hemorrhage such as hematemesis, hemoptysis, epistaxis, hematochezia, metrorrhagia, and also used as an important agent for treating burns

槐花 [huái huā]

***Flos Sophorae*, Pagodatree Flower:** the dried flower of *Sophora japonica* L. (family Leguminosae), used (1) to cool blood and stop bleeding in various cases of hemorrhages due to blood heat, particularly hemorrhoidal bleeding, and (2) to clear liver fire for up-flaming of liver fire with headache and also for hypertension

槐米 [huái mǐ]

***Flos Sophorae Immaturus*, Pagodatree Flower-bud:** used in the same way as the flower, with a stronger action

槐角 [huái jiǎo]

***Fructus Sophorae*, Japanese Pagodatree Pod:** the dried ripe fruit of *Sophora japonica* L. (family Leguminosae), used as pagodatree flower (槐花 [huái huā]), chiefly for the treatment of hemorrhoidal bleeding

侧柏叶 [cè bǎi yè]

***Cacumen Platycladi*, Chinese Arborvitae Twig and Leaf:** the dried twig and leaf of *Platycladus orientalis* (L.) Franco (family Cupressaceae), used in the same way as a blood-cooling hemostatic for treating epistaxis, hemoptysis, hematemesis, hematochezia and metrorrhagia, also used for treating premature graying of hair

苎麻根 [zhù má gēn]

***Redix Boehmeriae*, Ramie Root:** the dried root of *Boehmeria nivea* (L.)

Gaud. (family Urticaceae), used to arrest bleeding and prevent miscarriage for the treatment of bleeding in cases of threatened abortion and menorrhagia

血余炭 [xuè yú tàn]

***Crinis Carbonisatus*, Carbonized Hair:** used to arrest bleeding and remove blood stasis for treating various kinds of hemorrhage

棕榈炭 [zōng lǚ tàn]

***Petiolus Trachycarpi Carbonisatus*, Carbonized Windmillpalm Petiole:** carbonized petiole of *Trachycarpus fortunei* H. Wendl. (family Palmae), used as an astringent hemostatic for treating hematemesis, epistaxis, hematochezia, and menorrhagia

花蕊石 [huā ruǐ shí]

***Ophicalcitum*, Ophicalcite:** marble containing green serpentine, used as an astringent hemostatic for treating hemoptysis and hematemesis, and externally for treating incised wounds

荠菜 [jì cài]

***Herba Capsellae*, Shepherd's Purse:** the dried entire plant of *Capsella bursa-pastoris* (L.) Medic. (family Cruciferae), used (1) as a blood-cooling hemostatic for treating menorrhagia, postpartum hemorrhage and hematuria, and (2) as a diuretic for treating nephritic edema and hypertension

瓦松 [wǎ sōng]

***Herba Orostachyos*, Roof Stonecrop:** the dried aerial part of *Orostachys fimbriatus* (Turcz.) Berg. (family Crassalaceae), used as a hemostatic mainly for treating hematochezia and hematemesis, and externally for treating skin ulcers

藕节 [ǒu jié]

***Nodus Nelumbinis Rhizomatis*, Lotus Rhizome Node:** the dried node of the rhizome of *Nelumbo nucifera* Gaertn. (family Nymphaeaceae), used to cool blood, arrest bleeding and remove blood stasis for the treatment of nasal bleeding, hemoptysis, hematuria and abnormal uterine bleeding

墨旱莲 [mò hàn lián]

***Herba Ecliptae, Eclipta*, Yerbadetajo Herb:** the aerial part of *Eclipta prostrata* L. (family Compositae), used (1) as a blood-cooling hemostatic for various hemorrhages due to excessive heat in the blood, and (2) as a tonic to nourish the liver and kidney for the treatment of dizziness, tinnitus, premature graying of hair, and aching and weakness in the back and legs

牛西西 [niú xī xī]

***Radix Rumecis Patientiae*, Patient Dock Root:** the dried root of *Rumex patientia* L. (family Polygonaceae), used as a blood-cooling hemostatic for various types of hemorrhage due to excessive heat in the blood

活血化瘀药 Drugs for Activating Blood and Resolving Stasis

川芎 [chuān xiōng]

***Rhizome Chuanxiong*, Szechwan Lovage Rhizome:** the dried rhizome of *Ligusticum chuanxiong* Hort. (family Umbelliferae), used (1) to activate blood circulation and promote the flow of *qi* for the treatment of irregular menstruation, dysmenorrhea, amenorrhea and coronary heart disease, and (2) to dispel wind and alleviate pain for relieving headache and rheumatalgia

红花 [hóng huā]

***Flos Carthami*, Safflower:** the dried flower of *Carthamus tinctorius* L. (family Compositae), used to activate blood flow, eliminate stasis and alleviate pain for the treatment of amenorrhea, chest pain, abdominal mass, and traumatic injuries

西红花 [xī hóng huā]

***Stigma Croci, Crocus*, Saffron:** the dried stigma of *Crocus sativus* L. (family Iridaceae), used in the same way as 红花 [hóng huā], with a stronger effect

番红花 [fān hóng huā]

another name for *Stigma Croci, Crocus*, Saffron 西红花 [xī hóng huā]

藏红花 [zàng hōng huā]

another name for *Stigma Croci, Crocus*, Saffron 西红花 [xī hóng huā]

桃仁 [táo rén]

***Semen Persicae*, Peach Seed:** the dried ripe seed of *Prunus persica* (L.) Batsch or *Prunus davidiana* (Carr.) Franch. (family Rosaceae), used (1) to promote blood flow and remove stasis for the treatment of amenorrhea, dysmenorrhea, abdominal masses, and traumatic injuries, and (2) as an aperient for constipation in the aged and debilitated

川牛膝 [chuān niú xī]

***Radix Cyathulae*, Medicianl Cyathula Root:** the dried root of *Cyathula*

officinalis Kuan (family Amaranthaceae), used (1) to promote blood flow for the treatment of amenorrhea, dysmenorrhea, and traumatic injuries, (2) to tonify the liver and kidney and strengthen the tendons and bones for lumbago and aching joints, and (3) to direct fire and blood downward for treating headache, epistaxis and hematemesis

丹参 [dā shēn]

***Radix Salviae Miltiorrhizae*, Danshen Root:** the dried root and rhizome of *Salvia miltiorrhiza* Bge. (family Labiatae), used (1) to promote blood circulation and to remove blood stasis for the treatment of dysmenorrhea, amenorrhea, abdominal masses due to stagnation of blood, as well as ischemic apoplexy and coronary heart disease, (2) to remove heat from the blood for treating boils and sores, and (3) to induce tranquilization for treating palpitation and insomnia

郁金 [yù jīn]

***Radix Curcumae*, Turmeric Root Tuber:** steamed and dried tuberous root of *Curcuma wenyujin* Y. H. Chen et C. Ling, *Curuma longa* L., *Curcuma kwangsiensis* S. G. Lee et C. F. Liang, or *Curcuma phaeocaulis* Val. (family Zingiberaceae), used (1) to activate blood and move *qi* for relieving pain in the chest, abdomen or costal regions due to *qi* stagnation and blood stasis, (2) to cool the blood for treating various types of hemorrhage due to upward perversion of *qi* and fire, (3) to calm the mind in the treatment of delirium, mania and epilepsy, and (4) as a cholagogue for the treatment of jaundice

姜黄 [jiāng huáng]

***Rhizoma Curcumae Longae*, Turmeric:** the steamed and dried rhizome of *Curcuma longa* L. (family Zingiberaceae), used to activate blood, move *qi*, unblock meridians and relieve pain in cases of rheumatalgia, dysmenorrhea, epigastric, abdominal and costal pains, and traumatic injuries

片姜黄 [piàn jiāng huáng]

***Rhizoma Wenyujin Concisa*, Wenyujin Concise Rhizome:** the dried rhizome of *Curcuma wenyujin* Y.H. Chen et C. Ling (family Zingiberaceae), used to resolve blood stasis and relieve pain in cases of dysmenorrhea, rheumatalgia, shoulder pain and traumatic injuries

莪术 [é zhú]

***Rhizoma Curcumae*, Zedoary Rhizome:** the steamed and dried rhizome of *Curcuma zedoaria* Rosc., *Curcuma phaeocaulis* Valeton, or *Curcuma kwangsiensis* S. G. Lee et C.F. Liang or *Curcuma wenyujin* Y.H. Chen et C. Ling (family Zingiberaceae), used to relieve pain caused by retention of food and activate blood circulation and remove blood stasis for the treatment of abdominal mass and amenorrhea, also used as an anticancer agent, especially for cervical cancer of the uterus.

温莪术 [wēn é zhú]

a specific name for the rhizome of *Curcuma wenyujin* Y.H. Chen et C. Ling (family Zingiberaceae)

水红花子 [shuǐ hōng huā zǐ]

***Fructus Polygoni Orientalis*, Prince's-feather Fruit:** the dried ripe fruit of *Polygonum orientalis* L. (family Polygonaceae), used to eliminate blood stasis in the treatment of abdominal pain, and relieve epigastric pain due to food stagnation

鸡血藤 [jī xuè téng]

***Caulis Spatholobi*, Suberect Spatholobus Stem:** the dried lianoid stem of *Spatholobus suberectus* Dunn (family Leguminosae), used to move and tonify the blood, regulate menstruation and unblock collateral meridians for the treatment of menstrual disorders due to blood deficiency together with blood stasis, inflammation of peripheral vessels or thrombosis, numbness of the body and limbs, and also effective for leucopenia

延胡索 [yán hú suǒ]

***Rhizoma Corydalis*, Yanhusuo:** the steamed and dried tuber of *Corydalis turtschaninovii* Bess (family Papaveraceae), used to activate blood and move *qi* for relieving pain in the chest and abdomen, dysmenorrhea and traumatic pain

元胡 [yuán hú]

another name of *Rhizoma Corydalis*, Yanhusuo 延胡索 [yán hú suǒ]

五灵脂 [wǔ líng zhī]

***Faeces Trogopterorum*, Trogopterus Dung:** the dried faeces of *Trogopterus xanthipes* Milne-Edwards (family Petauristidae), used to relieve pain by eliminating blood stasis mainly for the treatment of gastric and abdominal pain, and dysmenorrhea

蒲黄 [pú huáng]

***Pollen Typhae*, Cat-tail Pollen:** the dried pollen of *Typha angustifolia* L.,

Typha orientalis Presl. or related species (family Typhaceae), used to promote the circulation of the blood and relieve pain by eliminating blood stasis for the treatment of dysmenorrhea, postpartum abdominal pain and gastralgia

蒲黄炭 [pú huáng tàn]

***Pollen Typhae Carbonisatum*, Carbonized Cat-tail Pollen:** used as a stasis-removing hemostatic

穿山甲 [chuān shān jiǎ]

***Squama Manitis*, Pangolin Scale:** the scale of anteater *Manis pentadactyla* L. (family Manidae), used (1) as an emmenagogue and galactagogue for amenorrhea and deficiency of lactation, and (2) to reduce swelling and dispel pus for treating acute suppurative inflammation

皂角刺 [zào jiǎo cì]

***Spina Gleditsiae*, Chinese Honeylocust Spine:** the dried spine of *Gleditsia sinensis* Lam. (family Leguminosae), used (1) to reduce swelling and dispel pus for treating acute suppurative inflammation with the effect of promoting local rupture, and (2) as an antipruritic in the treatment of skin diseases

王不留行 [wáng bù liú xíng]

***Semen Vaccariae*, Cow-Herb Seed:** the dried ripe seed of *Vaccaria segetalis* (Neck.) Garcke (family Caryophyllaceae), used as an emmenagogue and galactagogue for treating amenorrhea and lack of lactation, and also used for treating urinary calculus.

水蛭 [shuǐ zhì]

***Hirudo*, Leech:** the dried body of *Whitmania pigra* Whitman, *Whitmania acranulata* Whitman or *Hirudo nipponica* Whitman (family Hirudinidae), used to break stasis and reduce swellings for the treatment of severe cases of blood stasis, such as hematoma, amenorrhea, gynecological masses, and contusions

虻虫 [méng chóng]

***Tabanus*, Gadfly:** the dried female insect of *Tabanus bivittatus* Matsum. (family Tabanidae), used to break stasis and reduce swellings for the treatment of severe cases of blood stasis, such as amenorrhea and gynecological mass

䗪虫 [zhè chóng]

***Eupolyphaga seu Steleophaga*, Ground Beetle:** the dried female insect of *Eupolyphaga sinensis* Walk. or *Steleophaga plancyi* (Bol.) (family Corydiidae), used (1) to break stasis for the treatment of amenorrhea and gynecological mass, and (2) to promote the healing of bone fracture

土鳖虫 [tǔ biē chóng]

another name of *Eupolyphaga seu Steleophaga,* Ground Beetle (土鳖虫 [tǔ biē chóng])

苏木 [sū mù]

***Lignum Sappan*, Sappan Wood:** the dried heart wood of *Caesalpinia sappan* L. (family Leguminosae), used to activate blood and remove stasis, mainly for the treatment of contused wounds, dysmenorrhea and amenorrhea

益母草 [yì mǔ cǎo]

***Herba Leonuri*, Motherwort Herb:** the dried aerial part of *Leonurus heterophyllus* Sweet (family Labiatae), used (1) to activate blood flow and regulate the menstrual discharge in cases of menstrual disorders, and (2) as a diuretic in cases of nephritic edema

坤草 [kūn cǎo]

another name of *Herba Leonuri*, Motherwort Herb 益母草 [yì mǔ cǎo]

马鞭草 [mǎ biān cǎo]

***Herba Verbenae*, European Verbena Herb:** the dried aerial part of *Verbena officinalis* L. (family Verbenaceae), used (1) to activate the blood and promote menstrual flow for the treatment of amenorrhea and dysmenorrhea, (3) to counteract toxins for treating boils and other types of suppurative inflammation, and also (2) as an antimalarial agent for treating malarial splenomegaly

三棱 [sān léng]

***Rhizoma Sparganii*, Common Burreed Tuber:** peeled and dried tuber of *Sparganium stoloniferum* Buch.-Ham. (family Sparganiaceae), used to break blood stasis and eliminate masses for the treatment of dysmenorrhea, amenorrhea and abdominal masses

泽兰 [zé lán]

***Herba Lycopi*, Bugleweed Herb:** the dried aerial part of *Lycopus lucidus* Turcz. var. *hirtus* Regel (family Labiatae), used (1) to activate the blood, remove stasis and regulate menstruation for the treatment of irregular menstruation and postpartum abdominal pain, (2) to reduce swelling for treating traumatic injuries, boils and sores, and (3) to induce diuresis for treating edema and ascites

毛冬青 [máo dōng qīng]

***Radix llicis Pubescentis*, Pubescent Holly Root:** the dried root of *Ilex pubescens* Hook. et Arn. (family Aquifoliaceae), used (1) to invigorate blood circulation and unblock the meridians and collaterals for the treatment of thromboangitis obliterans and angina pectoris, (2) to clear heat and counteract toxins for treating inflammations such as acute tonsillitis, and (3) as antitussive and expectorant for treating acute bronchitis

乳香 [rǔ xiāng]

***Olibanum,* Frankincense:** gum-resin obtained from *Boswellia carterii* Birdwood and possibly other species of *Boswellia* (family Burseraceae), used to relieve pain and swelling in cases of traumatic injury by activating the local blood circulation

没药 [mò yào]

***Myrrha,* Myrrh:** gum-resin obtained from the stem of *Commphora molmol* Engler and probably other species (family Burseraceae), used in the relief of pain and swelling in cases of traumatic injury

自然铜 [zì rán tóng]

***Pyritum*, Pyrite:** a brassy yellow mineral, iron disulphide, cube-like crystals, used for promoting the healing of fractures and relieving traumatic pain

芳香开窍药 Aromatic Stimulants

冰片 [bīng piàn]

***Borneolum*, Borneol:** a crystalline organic compound obtained synthetically or from *Dryobalanops aromatica* Gaertn. f., used (1) as an aromatic stimulant for treating loss of consciousness and convulsion due to high fever, and (2) topically to clear heat and alleviate pain for treating pharyngitis, tonsillitis, laryngitis and stomatitis

牛黄 [niú huáng]

***Calculus Bovis*, Cow-Bezoar:** the dried gallstone of domestic cattle, *Bos taurus domesticus* Gmelin (family Bovidae), used to arrest convulsions, resolve phlegm, restore consciousness, clear heat and counteract toxins for treating delirium and convulsion in cases of acute febrile diseases, infantile convulsion, inflammation of the pharynx, larynx and mouth, boils and sores

石菖蒲 [shí chāng pú]

***Rhizoma Acori Tatarinowii*, Grass-leaved Sweetflag Rhizome:** the dried rhizomes of *Acorus tatarinowii* Schott. (family Araceae), used (1) as an aromatic stimulant for treating impaired consciousness, insanity and epilepsy, and (2) to resolve dampness and harmonize the stomach for treating accumulation of dampness in the middle with anorexia, epigastric stuffiness and abdominal distension

苏合香 [sū hé xiāng]

***Styrax*, Storax:** purified, semi-fluid, viscid balsam obtained from the trunk of *Liquidamber orientalis* Miller (family Hamamelidaceae), used as an aromatic stimulant for treating loss of consciousness due to apoplexy, and also for relieving angina pectoris

麝香 [shè xiāng]

***Moschus*, Musk:** the dried secretion obtained from the musk sac of adult male musk deer, *Muschus berezovskii* Flerov, *Moschus sifanicus* Przewalski or *Moschus moschiferus* L. (family Cervidae), used as an aromatic stimulant for treating loss of consciousness in cases of high fever and apoplexy, (2) to activate blood and alleviate pain for the treatment of painful swellings of boils, carbuncles and thromboangitis obliterans, and (3) to expedite child delivery in cases of difficult labor and detention of the afterbirth

安息香 [ān xī xiāng]

***Benzoinum*, Benzoin:** the dried resin obtained from Tokin Snowbell, *Styrax tonkenensis* (Pierre) Craib ex Hart. (family Styracaceae), used (1) as an aromatic stimulant for restoring consciousness in cases of apoplexy, and (2) to relieve pain of the chest and abdomen by activating the flow of *qi* and blood

安神药 Tranquilizers

朱砂 [zhū shā]

***Cinnabaris*, Cinnabar:** a mineral composed of red mercuric sulphide, used (1) as a settling tranquilizer for the treatment of palpitation, insomnia, infantile convulsion and epilepsy, and (2) as a detoxicant for boils and carbuncles

琥珀 [hǔ pò]

***Succinum*, Amber:** a yellowish or brownish fossil resin, used as (1) a sedative for the treatment of insomnia, dream-disturbed sleep, palpitation and convulsion, and (2) as a diuretic and hemostatic for urodynia and hematuria due to acute urinary infection and urinary calculus

磁石 [cí shí]

***Magnetitum*, Magnetite:** magnetic iron ore composed mainly of ferriferrous oxide (Fe_3O_4), used as a settling tranquilizer and antiasthmatic for the treatment of tinnitus, palpitation, insomnia, epilepsy and mania, and also used for relieving asthma.

酸枣仁 [suān zǎo rén]

***Semen Ziziphi Spinosae*, Spine Date Seed:** the dried ripe seed of *Ziziphus jujuba* Mill. var. *spinosa* (Bunge) Hu ex H. F. Chou (family Rhamnaceae), used (1) as a tranquilizer for the treatment of fidgetiness, insomnia and palpitation, and (2) to arrest excessive sweating in cases of spontaneous perspiration and night sweats

远志 [yuǎn zhì]

***Radix Polygalae*, Thin-leaf Milkwort Root:** the dried root of *Polygala tenuifolia* Willd. or *Polygala sibirica* L. (family Polygalaceae), used (1) as a tranquilizer in cases of palpitation and insomnia due to disharmony of the heart and kidney, (2) as an expectorant in cases of acute or chronic cough with profuse sputum, (3) to expel phlegm for treating epilepsy and mania due to obstruction of the heart orifice by phlegm, and (4) to reduce swelling in cases of boils and sores

合欢皮 [hé huān pí]

***Cortex Albiziae*, Silktree Albizia Bark:** the dried bark of *Albizia julibrissin* Durazz. (family Leguminosae), used (1) as a tranquilizer for palpitations and insomnia due to anxiety, and (2) to relieve pain by activating blood circulation for treating painful traumatic swellings or boils and sores

合欢花 [hé huān huā]

***Flos Albiziae*, Albizia Flower:** the dried flower-head of *Albizia julibrissin* Durazz. (family Leguminosae), used as a tranquilizer for treating fidgetiness and insomnia

首乌藤 [shǒu yū téng]

Caulis Polygoni Multiflori, Fleece-flower Stem: the dried lianoid stem of *Polygonum multiflorum* Thunb. (family Polygonaceae), used (1) as a heart-nourishing tranquilizer for treating insomnia and dream-disturbed sleep, (2) to activate blood circulation in collaterals for the treatment of aching limbs

夜交藤 [yè jiāo téng]

another name of *Caulis Polygoni Multiflori*, Fleece-flower Stem 首乌藤 [shǒu yū téng]

灵芝 [líng zhī]

Ganoderma Lucidum, Lucid Ganoderma: the dried fructifications of the fungus, *Ganoderma lucidum* (Leyss. ex Fr.) Karst. (family Polyporaceae), used (1) as a tranquilizer for treating dizziness and insomnia, and (2) as a tonic for treating weakness or debility

缬草 [xié cǎo]

Rhizoma Valerianae, Valerian Rhizome: the dried rhizome of *Valeriana officinalis* L.(family Valerianaceae), used (1) as a tranquilizer for treating insomnia, and (2) to regulate the flow of *qi* for relieving abdominal distension and pain

珍珠 [zhēn zhū]

Margarita, Pearl: lustrous concretion found in certain bivalve shell-fish, e.g., *Pteria martensii* (Dunker) (family Pteriidae), *Hyriopsis cumingii* (Lea), *Cristaria plicata* (Leach) (family Unionidae), used (1) as a settling tranquilizer and anticonvulsive agent for the treatment of convulsion due to high fever or infantile convulsion, (2) externally to hasten the healing of wounds.

珍珠母 [zhēn zhū mǔ]

Concha Margaritifera Usta, Nacre: the calcined shell of certain pearl-yielding shell-fish, *Hyriopsis cumingii* (Lea), *Cristaria plicata* (Leach) (family Unionidae) or *Pteria martensii* (Dunker) (family Pteriidae), used (1) as a settling tranquilizer for the treatment of palpitation, insomnia, mania, and (2) to pacify the liver and subdue exuberant yang for relieving headache and dizziness

柏子仁 [bǎi zǐ rén]

Semen Platycladi, Chinese Arborvitae Seed: the kernel of dried ripe seed of *Platycladus orientalis* (L.) Franco (family Cupressaceae), used (1)

to nourish the heart and relieve mental strain for the treatment of palpitations and insomnia in deficiency of heart blood, and (2) as an aperient for constipation in debilitated patients.

茯神 [fú shén]

***Poria cum Radice Pino*, Fu-shen:** The drug consists of *poria* with a piece of pine root embedded in it, used as a tranquilizer for treating palpitations and insomnia.

紫贝齿 [zǐ bèi chǐ]

***Concha Mauritiae*, Purple Cowry Shell:** the dried shell of *Mauritia (Arabica) arabica* (L.) (family Cypaeidae), used as a settling tranquilizer for treating palpitations and infantile convulsion

龙骨 [lóng gǔ]

***Os Draconis*, Dragon's Bone:** fossil bone of an ancient large mammal, such as *Stegodon orientalis* or *Rhinocerus sinensis*, used (1) as a settling tranquilizer for the treatment of palpitation, insomnia, and dream-disturbed sleep, (2) to pacify the liver and subdue exuberant yang for relieving dizziness or vertigo, and (3) to arrest discharge for treating enuresis, seminal emission, spermatorrhea and leukorrhagia, and (4) externally for absorbing exudate in cases of skin diseases

龙齿 [lóng chǐ]

***Dens Draconis*, Dragon's Teeth:** the fossil teeth from an ancient large mammal, such as *Stegodon orientalis* or *Rhinocerus sinensis*, used in a similar way to *Os Draconis*, Dragon's Bone 龙骨 [lóng gǔ], with a stronger action

牡蛎 [mǔ lì]

***Concha Ostreae*, Oyster Shell:** the shell of *Ostrea gigas* Thunb., *Ostrea talienwhanensis* Crosse or *Ostrea rivularis* Gould (family Ostreidae), used (1) as a settling tranquilizer for the treatment of headache, dizziness, palpitation and insomnia, and (2) to soften and disperse hard lumps in cases of scrofula

平肝熄风药

Drugs for Pacifying the Liver and Extinguishing Wind

天麻 [tiān má]

***Rhizoma Gastrodiae*, Gastrodia Tuber:** the dried tuber of *Gastrodia elata* Bl. (family Orchidaceae), used (1) to extinguish wind and relieve spasm for treating convulsion and hemiplegia in cases of apoplexy, (2) to pacify the liver and subdue exuberant yang for relieving headache, dizziness and vertigo, and (3) to relieve rheumatalgia

钩藤 [gōu téng]

***Ramulus Uncariae cum Uncis*, Gambir Plant:** the dried hook-bearing stem branch of *Uncaria rhynchophylla* (Miq.) Jack., *Uncaria macrophylla* Wall., *Uncaria hirsuta* Havil., *Uncaria sinensis* (Oliv.) Havil. or *Uncaria sessilifructus* Roxb. (family Rubiaceae), used to extinguish wind, relieve spasm, clear heat and pacify the liver for treating convulsions due to high fever, and for headache, dizziness and vertigo due to liver heat

全蝎 [quán xiē]

***Scorpio*, Scorpion:** the boiled and dried body of *Buthus martensii* Karsch (family Buthidae), used to subdue endogenous wind for the treatment of various kinds of tics, convulsion, tetanus and sequelae of cerebrovascular accidents.

全虫 [quán chóng]

same as **全蝎** [quán xiē]

蜈蚣 [wú gōng]

***Scolopendra*, Centipede:** the dried body of *Scolopendra subspinipes mutilans* L. Koch (family Scolopendridae), used (1) to extinguish wind and relieve spasms for the treatment of tics, convulsion, tetanus and facial paralysis, (2) to unblock collateral meridians and alleviate pain in cases of stubborn arthralgia and intractable migraine, and (3) as a detoxicant for treating scrofula and venomous snake-bite

僵蚕 [jiāng cán]

***Bombyx Batryticatus*, Stiff Silkworm:** the dried body of the 4-5th stage larva of *Bombyx mori* L., dead and stiffened due to *Beauveria bassiana* fungus infection, used (1) to extinguish endogenous wind for relieving convulsions, (2) to resolve phlegm and dissipate nodulation for the treatment of scrofula, and (3) to dispel exogenous wind in the case of wind-heat afflictions such as sore throat, hoarseness of voice and urticaria

白僵蚕 [bái jiāng cán]

same as **僵蚕** [jiāng cán]

羚羊角 [líng yáng jiǎo]

***Cornu Saigae Tataricae*, Antelope Horn:** the horn of *Saiga tatarica* L. (family Bovidae), used to pacify the liver, extinguish wind, clear heat and counteract toxins for the treatment of (1) liver wind with impaired consciousness and convulsions, (2) liver fire with headache, dizziness and acute conjunctivitis, and (3) high fever with delirium

地龙 [dì lóng]

***Lumbricus*, Earthworm:** the dried body of *Pheretima aspergillum* (Perrier) or *Allolobophora caliginosa* (Savigny) *trapezoides* (Ant. Duges) (family Megascolecidae), used to clear heat, extinguish wind, unblock collateral meridians, relieve asthma and induce diuresis, for the treatment of convulsions due to high fever, rheumatalgia, hemiplegia, bronchial asthma and accumulated heat in the bladder with dysuria

赭石 [zhě shí]

***Haematitum*, Hematite:** a dark-brown colored iron ore mainly composed of ferric oxide (Fe_2O_3), used (1) to pacify the liver and subdue exuberant yang for treating up-rising of liver yang with headache, vertigo and tinnitus, (2) to check the upward adverse flow of *qi* for relieving belching, nausea, vomiting and asthma, and (3) as a blood-cooling hemostatic in cases of hematemesis and epistaxis

代赭石 [dài zhě shí]

a synonym for 赭石 [zhě shí]

石决明 [shí jué míng]

***Concha Haliotidis*, Sea-ear Shell:** the shell of *Haliotis diversicolor* Reeve, *Haliotis discus hanai* Ino or *Haliotis ovina* Gmelin, *Haliotis ruber* (Leach), *Haliotis asinina* L. or *Haliotis Laevigata* (Donovan) (family Haliotidae), used (1) to pacify the liver and subdue exuberant yang for the treatment of up-rising of liver yang with headache and vertigo, and (2) to clear liver heat and improve vision for the treatment of glaucoma and cataracts.

蒺藜 [jí lí]

***Fructus Tribuli*, Puncture-vine Caltrop Fruit:** the dried fruit of *Tribulus terrestris* L. (family Zygophylaceae), used (1) to pacify and soothe the liver for treating headache, vertigo, thoracic and hypochondriac pain, and mastitis due to depressed liver *qi*, (2) to improve vision in cases of conjunctivitis and nebula, and (3) to dispel wind in cases of urticaria and pruritus

刺蒺藜 [cì jí lí]

same as *Fructus Tribuli,* Puncture-vine Caltrop Fruit (蒺藜 [jí lí])

玳瑁 [dài mào]

***Carapax Eretmochelydis*, Hawksbill Shell:** the carapace of a hawksbill turtle, *Eretmochelys imbricata* (L.) (family Chelonidae), used to extinguish wind, clear heat and counteract toxins for the treatment of convulsion and delirium in cases of febrile diseases

熊胆 [xióng dǎn]

***Fel Ursi*, Bear Gall:** the dried gall-bladder of a bear, *Selenarctos thibetanus* Cuvier or *Ursus arctos* L. (family Ursidae), used (1) to extinguish wind, clear heat, and counteract toxins for treating febrile convulsions, epilepsy, and externally for boils, sores and hemorrhoidal swelling, and (2) to clear the liver and improve vision in cases of conjunctivitis and nebula

补养药 Tonics

补气药 Drugs for Replenishing *Qi* (Qi Tonics)

人参 [rén shēn]

***Radix Ginseng*, Ginseng:** the dried root of *Panax ginseng* C. A. Mey. (family Araliaceae), used (1) to powerfully replenish *qi* and to promote fluid production for the treatment of prostration, general weakness, diabetes mellitus, impotence or frigidity, heart failure and cardiogenic shock, (2) to tonify the spleen and lung for the treatment of anorexia, cough and shortness of breath, and (3) as a tranquillizer for treating cardiac palpitation and insomnia

党参 [dǎng shēn]

***Radix Codonopsis*, Tangshen:** the dried root of *Codonopsis pilosula* (Franch.) Nannf., *Codonopsis pilosula* var. *modesta* (Nannf.) L.T. Shen or *Codonopsis tangshen* Oliv. (family Campanulaceae), used to replenish *qi*, promote fluid production and nourish blood for treating (1) deficiency of the middle *qi* with general debility, anorexia, lassitude and loose stools, and (2) deficiency of both *qi* and yin, with shortness of breath, pallor, dizziness and palpitations

太子参 [tài zǐ shēn]

***Radix Pseudostellariae*, Heterophylly Falsestarwort Root:** the dried tuberous root of *seudostellaria heterophylla* (Miq.) Pax ex Pax et Hoffm. (family Caryophyllaceae), used in a similar way to *Radix Codonopsis*, Tangshen (党参 [dǎng shēn]), less active as a tonic, but more active in promoting the production of body fluids

孩儿参 [hái ér shēn]

another name of *Radix Pseudostellariae,* Heterophylly Falsestarwort Root (太子参 [tài zǐ shēn])

黄芪 [huáng qí]

***Radix Astragali*, Milkvetch Root:** the dried root of *Astragalus membranaceus* (Fisch.) Bge. or *Astragalus membranaceus* var. *mongholicus* (Bge.) Hsiao (family Leguminosae), used (1) to replenish *qi* for the treatment of general weakness, anorexia and loose stools, prolapse of the uterus or anus, spontaneous sweating, and chronic nephritis with edema and proteinuria, and (2) to dispel pus and accelerate the healing of chronic ulcers

红芪 [hóng qí]

***Radix Hedysari*, Sweetvetch Root:** the dried root of *Hedysarum polybotrys* Hand.-Mazz. (family Leguminosae), used as a substitute for *Radix Astragali*, Milkvetch Root (黄芪 [huáng qí])

甘草 [gān cǎo]

***Radix Glycyrrhizae*, Licorice Root:** the dried root and rhizome of *Glycyrrhiza uralensis* Fisch., *Glycyrrhiza inflata* Bat. or *Glycyrrhiza glabra* L. (family Leguminosae), used (1) to replenish *qi* and tonify the heart for treating arrythmia in cases of heart *qi* deficiency, (2) to tonify the spleen for treating lassitude, anorexia and loose bowels in cases of spleen insufficiency, (3) to relieve epigastric colic and spastic pain of the limbs, (4) to dispel phlegm and arrest cough, (5) to clear heat and counteract toxins for treating sore throat, boils, sores and drug overdose, and (6) most frequently for modulating the ingredients in a prescription

炙甘草 [zhì gān cǎo]

***Radix Glycyrrhizae Preparata*, Prepared Licorice Root:** the processed *Radix Glycyrrhizae*, Licorice Root by stir-baking with honey, used to tonify the spleen and heart, and particularly used for treating arrhythmia

刺五加 [cì wǔ jiā]

***Radix Acanthopanacis Senticosi*, Thorny Acathopanax Root:** the dried root and rhizome of *Acanthopanax senticosus* (Rupr. et Maxim.) Harms (family Aralicaceae), used to replenish *qi*, strengthen the spleen, tonify the kidney, and induce tranquilization for the treatment of general weakness, anorexia, aching back and knees, and insomnia and dream-disturbed sleep

白术 [bái zhú]

***Rhizoma Atractylodis Macrocephalae*, Largehead Atractylodes Rhizome:** the dried rhizome of *Atractylodes macrocephala* Koidz. (family Compositae), used (1) to replenish *qi*, invigorate the spleen for the treatment of general weakness, anorexia, dyspepsia and chronic diarrhea, (2) to arrest excessive sweating, and (3) to calm the fetus when treating threatened abortion

山药 [shān yào]

***Rhizoma Dioscoreae*, Common Yam Rhizome:** the dried rhizome of *Dioscorea opposita* Thunb. (family Dioscoreaceae), used (1) to replenish *qi* and yin, tonify the spleen, lung and kidney for the treatment of (1) weakness of the spleen and stomach with poor appetite and chronic diarrhea, (2) lung insufficiency with chronic cough, (3) insecurity of the kidney with nocturnal emission, polyuria and leukorrhagia, and (4) yin deficiency in cases of diabetes

白扁豆 [bái biǎn dòu]

***Semen Lablab Album*, White Hyacinth Bean:** the dried ripe seed of *Dolichos lablab* L. (family Leguminosae), used to strengthen the spleen and resolve dampness for the treatment of (1) weakness of the spleen and stomach with anorexia, loose stools and leukorrhagia, and (2) vomiting and diarrhea due to summer dampness

大枣 [dà zǎo]

***Fructus Jujubae*, Jujube, Chinese Date:** the dried ripe fruit of *Ziziphus jujuba* Mill. (family Rhamnaceae), used to replenish the middle *qi*, nourish the blood and induce tranquilization, and also used to moderate drug actions

黄精 [huáng jīng]

***Rhizoma Polygonati*, Solomonseal Rhizome:** the steamed and dried rhizome of *Polygonatum sibiricum* Red., *Polygonatum kingianum* Coll. et Hemsl. or *Polygonatum cyrtonema* Hua (family Liliaceae), used (1) to replenish spleen *qi* for the treatment of general debility and poor appetite, and (2) to nourish lung yin for the treatment of chronic dry cough in cases of phthisis

饴糖 [yí táng]

***Extractum Malti*, Malt Extract:** amber or yellowish brown, viscous liquid, with an agreeable odor and a sweet taste, prepared from malted grains of barley, *Hordeum vulgare* L. or malted grains of wheat, *Triticum aestivum* L., used as a tonic to replenish the middle *qi* for treating general debility, also used as an antitussive for treating chronic cough

补血药 Drugs for Nourishing the Blood (Blood Tonics)

当归 [dāng guī]

***Radix Angelicae Sinensis*, Chinese Angelica:** the dried root of *Angelica sinensis* (Oliv.) Diels (family Umbelliferae), used (1) to nourish the blood for treating blood deficiency of the heart and liver, (2) activate the blood flow and regulate menstruation for treating menstrual disorders, and (2) as an emollient and laxative for treating chronic constipation in the aged and debilitated

白芍 [bái sháo]

***Radix Paeoniae Alba*, White Peony Root:** the peeled and dried root of *Paeonia lactiflora* Pall. (family Ranunculaceae), used (1) to nourish the blood and regulate menstruation for treating menstrual disorders, (2) to pacify the liver and alleviate pain for relieving headache, hypochondriac pain, and spastic pain of the limbs, and (3) to arrest excessive sweating

阿胶 [ē jiāo]]

***Colla Corii Asini*, Ass-hide Glue:** solid glue prepared from the skin of ass, *Equus asinus* L. (family Equidae), used (1) to nourish the blood for blood deficiency, (2) to arrest bleeding for treating all kinds of hemorrhages, and (3) to nourish yin for the treatment of insomnia and dry cough

紫河车 [zǐ hé chē]

***Placenta Hominis*, Human Placenta:** the dried human placenta, used to replenish *qi*, nourish blood and supplement essence for treating deficiency of *qi* and blood, general weakness, sterility, impotence, chronic cough and asthma

龙眼肉 [lóng yǎn ròu]

***Arillus Longan*, Longan Aril:** the dried aril of *Dimocarpus longan* Lour.

(family Sapindaceae), used to nourish the blood and induce tranquilization for the treatment of palpitation, dizziness and insomnia

熟地黄 [shú dì huáng]

***Radix Rehmanniae Praeparata*, Prepared Rehmannia Root:** the steamed and dried tuberous root of *Rehmannia glutinosa* Libosch. (family Scrophulariaceae), used as (1) the main blood tonic for treating blood deficiency with pallor, dizziness, palpitation, menstrual disorders, and (2) an important kidney-yin tonic for the treatment of chronic tidal fever, night sweats, lumbago, nocturnal emission and diabetes

补阴药 Drugs for Replenishing Yin (Yin Tonics)

西洋参 [xī yáng shēn]

***Radix Panacis Quinquefolii*, American Ginseng:** the dried root of *Panax quinquefolium* L. (family Araliaceae), used to replenish *qi*, nourish yin, reduce the internal heat and promote fluid production, for treating (1) yin deficiency with exuberant fire with cough and blood-streaked sputum, and (2) impairment of both *qi* and yin in cases of febrile diseases with fidgetiness and thirst

石斛 [shí hú]

***Herba Dendrobii*, Dendrobium:** the fresh or dried stem of *Dendrobium loddigesii* Rolfe., *Dendrobium chrysanthum* Wall., *Dendrobium fimbriatum* var. *oculatum* Hook., *Dendrobium candidum* Wall. ex Lindl. or *Dendrobium nobile* Lindl. (family Orchidaceae), used to replenish stomach yin, clear heat, and promote fluid production for treating chronic febrile diseases with thirst and dry mouth, deficiency of stomach yin with epigastric distress and pain, and also for improving vision in cases of cataracts

玉竹 [yù zhú]

***Rhizoma Polygonati Odorati*, Fragrant Solomonseal Rhizome:** the steamed and dried rhizome of *Polygonatum odoratum* (Will.) Druce (family Liliaceae), used to nourish yin and promote fluid production for the treatment of dipsosis, dry throat and dry cough in cases of febrile diseases and diabetes

麦冬 [mài dōng]

***Radix Ophiopogonis*, Dwarf Lilyturf Root:** the dried tuberous root of *Ophiopogon japonicus* (Thunb.) Ker-Gawl. (family Liliaceae), used (1) to replenish and promote fluid production for the treatment of dipsosis, dry throat, dry cough and bloody sputum in cases of acute febrile diseases and yin deficiency of the lung and stomach, and (2) to calm the mind for the treatment of fidgetiness and insomnia

麦门冬 [mài mén dōng]

a synonym for 麦冬 [mài dōng]

天冬 [tiān dōng]

***Radix Asparagi*, Asparagus Root:** the steamed peeled and dried tuberous root of *Asparagus cochinchinensis* (Lour.) Merr. (family Liliaceae), used to replenish yin and promote fluid production for the treatment of dipsosis, dry throat, cough with sticky phlegm, bloody sputum and constipation

天门冬 [tiān mén dōng]

synonym for 天冬 [tiān dōng]

北沙参 [běi shā shēn]

***Radix Glehniae*, Coastal Glehia Root:** the dried root of *Glehnia littoralis* Fr. Schmidt ex Miq. (family Umbelliferae), used to replenish yin of the lung and stomach and promote fluid production for the treatment of dipsosis, dry throat and dry cough

枸杞子 [gǒu qǐ zǐ]

***Fructus Lycii*, Barbary Wolfberry Fruit:** the dried ripe fruit of *Lycium barbarum* L. (family Solanaceae), used to replenish liver and kidney yin for the treatment of aching back and legs, impotence and nocturnal emission, vertigo and decreased eyesight

山茱萸 [shān zhū yú]

***Fructus Corni*, Asiatic Cornelian Cherry Fruit:** the dried ripe sarcocarp of *Cornus officinalis* Sieb. et Zucc. (family Cornaceae), used (1) to replenish liver and kidney yin for the treatment of aching back, weakened knees, vertigo and impotence, and (2) to arrest discharge for nocturnal emission, enuresis, abnormal uterine bleeding, and excessive perspiration

何首乌 [hé shǒu wū]

***Radix Polygoni Multiflori*, Fleeceflower Root:** the dried tuberous root of *Polygonum multiflorum* Thunb. (family Polygonaceae), used as a laxative for constipation and also as an antimalarial agent

首乌 [shǒu wū]

a synonym for 何首乌 [hé shǒu wū]

制何首乌 [zhì hé shǒu wū]

***Radix Polygoni Multiflori Preparata*, Prepared Fleeceflower Root:** fleeceflower root processed with black bean juice, used to replenish liver and kidney yin and nourish blood for the treatment of blood deficiency of the liver and essence deficiency of the kidney with dizziness, tinnitus, aching black and knees, and early graying of the hair

牛膝 [niú xī]

***Radix Achyranthis Bidentatae*, Twoteethed Achyranthes Root:** the dried root of *Achyranthes bidentata* Bl. (family Amaranthaceae), used (1) to nourish the liver and kidney and to strengthen the sinews and bones for the treatment of aching back and knees, and asthenia of the lower limbs, (2) to activate blood flow for treating amenorrhea, dysmenorrhea and irregular menstruation, as well as traumatic injuries, and (3) to direct fire or blood downward in the treatment of headache and dizziness due to up-rising of liver yang, epistaxis and hemoptysis due to up-flaming of fire

怀牛膝 [huái niú xī]

synonym for 牛膝 [niú xī]

沙苑子 [shā yuàn zǐ]

***Semen Astragali Complanati*, Flatstem Milkvetch Seed:** the dried ripe seed of *Astragalus complanatus* R. Br. (family Leguminosae), used to replenish liver and kidney yin for the treatment of dizziness, blurred vision, seminal emission, premature ejaculation, impotence, frequent micturition and leukorrhagia

潼蒺藜 [tóng jí lí]

synonym for 沙苑子 [shā yuàn zǐ]

女贞子 [nǚ zhēn zǐ]

***Fructus Ligustri Lucidi*, Glossy Privet Fruit:** the dried ripe fruit of *Ligustrum lucidum* Ait. (family Oleaceae), used to replenish liver and kidney yin, darken the hair and improve the eyesight for the treatment of early graying of the hair, dim eyesight, lumbago and low fever in cases of yin deficiency

桑寄生 [sāng jì shēng]

***Ramulus Taxilli*, Mulberry Mistletoe:** the dried leaf-bearing stem and branch of *Taxillus chinensis* (DC.) Danser (family Loranthaceae), used (1) to replenish liver and kidney yin, strengthen the sinews and bones and dispel wind-damp for the treatment of arthralgia with aching back and limbs, and (2) to nourish the blood and prevent miscarriage for the treatment of menorrhagia and threatened abortion

鹿衔草 [lù xián cǎo]

***Herba Pyrolae*, Pyrola Herb:** the dried entire plant of *Pyrola calliantha* H. Andres or *Pyrola decorata* H. Andres (family Pyrolaceae), used to replenish kidney yin, strengthen the sinews and bones, dispel wind-damp and arrest bleeding for the treatment of lumbago, rheumatism, menorrhagia, bloody sputum and epistaxis

龟甲 [guī jiǎ]

***Carapax et Plastrum Testudinis*, Tortoise Shell:** the carapace and plastron of a fresh-water tortoise, *Chinemys reevesii* (Gray) (family Testudinidae), used to replenish liver and kidney yin and check hyperactive liver yang, for the treatment of vertigo, chronic tidal fever, night sweats, dry mouth and throat, aching back and knees with asthenia, osteomalacia and rickets

龟板 [guī bǎn]

***Plastrum Testudinis*, Tortoise Plastron:** the ventral shell of a fresh-water tortoise with the same uses as *carapax et plastrum testudinis*, tortoise shell (龟甲 [guī jiǎ])

鳖甲 [biē jiǎ]

***Carapax Trionycis*, Turtle Shell:** the dorsal shell of a soft-shelled turtle, *Trionyx sinensis* Wiegmann (family Trionychidae), used to replenish yin, check exuberant yang, and soften and resolve hard lumps for the treatment of (1) chronic tidal fever and night sweats in cases of yin deficiency, and (2) splenomegaly in cases of chronic malaria

桑椹 [sāng shèn]

***Fructus Mori*, Mulberry Fruit:** the dried fruit-spike of *Morus alba* L. (family Moraceae), used (1) to replenish yin and nourish the blood for the treatment of dizziness, tinnitus, blurred vision in cases of deficiency of yin and blood, and (2) to promote fluid production for relieving dipsosis in cases of diabetes

补阳药 Drugs for Reinforcing Yang (Yang Tonics)

鹿茸 [lù róng]

***Cornu Cervi Pantotrichum*, Hairy Deer-horn:** the hairy, unossified young horn of male sika deer, *Cervus nippon* Temminck or red deer, *Cervus elaphus* L. (family Cervidae), used to reinforce the kidney yang and strengthen the bones and muscles for the treatment of intolerance of cold, loss of strength, impotence, spontaneous seminal emission, leukorrhagia and other symptoms of yang deficiency in cases of chronic diseases

鹿角 [lù jiǎo]

***Cornu Cervi*, Antler, Deer-horn:** the ossified horn of the male red deer, *Cervus elaphus* L. or sika deer *Cervas nippon* Temminck (family Cervidae), used in a similar way to hairy deer-horn (鹿茸 [lù róng]), but less active, also used to remove blood stasis for the treatment of traumatic wounds

鹿角胶 [lù jiǎo jiāo]

***Colla Cornus Cervi*, Deer-horn Gelatin:** gelatin prepared from a decoction of deer-horn, with a kidney-nourishing action superior to that of deer-horn (鹿角 [lù jiǎo]), and additional effects of nourishing the blood and stopping bleeding

鹿角霜 [lù jiǎo shuāng]

***Cornu Cervi Degelatinatum*, Degelatinated Deer-horn:** by-product of making deer-horn glue, the residual deer-horn left after the decoction is taken out and dried, with an action similar but inferior to that of deer-horn (鹿角 [lù jiǎo])

肉苁蓉 [ròu cōng róng]

***Herba Cistanchis*, Desert-living Cistanche:** the dried fleshy stem with scales of *Cistanche deserticola* Y.C. Ma (family Orobanchaceae), used (1) to reinforce kidney yang for the treatment of impotence and premature ejaculation, and (2) as a mild laxative for treating chronic constipation in the aged

大芸 [dà yún]

a synonym for 肉苁蓉 [ròu cōng róng]

益智仁 [yì zhì rén]

***Semen Alpiniae Oxyphyllae*, Sharpleaf Galangal Seed:** the dried ripe seed of *Alpinia oxyphylla* Miq. (family Zingiberaceae), used to warm the spleen and kidney for the treatment of (1) chronic diarrhea with cold and pain in the abdomen, and (2) enuresis, frequent micturition and seminal emission

仙茅 [xiān máo]

***Rhizoma Curculiginis*,Common Curculigo Rhizome:** the dried rhizome of *Curculigo orchioides* Gaertn. (family Amaryllidaceae), used to warm the kidney, reinforce yang, strengthen the tendons and bones, and dispel cold-damp for the treatment of aching back and knees with intolerance of cold, impotence, enuresis, stubborn arthralgia, chronic diarrhea

淫羊藿 [yín yáng huò]

***Herba Epimedii*, Epimedium Herb:** the dried aerial part of *Epimedium brevicornum* Maxim., *Epimedium sagittatum* (Sieb.et Zucc.) Maxim., *Epimedium koreanum* Nakai, *Epimedium pubescens* Maxim. or *Epimedium wushanense* T. S. Ying (family Berberidaceae), used (1) to replenish kidney yang for the treatment of impotence, sterility and frequent micturition, and (2) to strengthen the tendons and bones and dispel wind-damp for rheumatalgia, contracture and numbness

仙灵脾 [xiān líng pí]

a synonym for 淫羊藿 [yín yáng huò]

核桃仁 [hé táo rén]

***Semen Juglandis*, English Walnut Seed:** the dried ripe seed of *Juglans regia* L.(family Juglandeceae), used to tonify the kidney and lung for treating aching back and knees, cough and dyspnea of deficiency-cold type, seminal emission and impotence

锁阳 [suǒ yáng]

***Herba Cynomorii*, Songaria Cynomorium Herb:** the dried fleshy stem of *Cynomorium songaricum* Rupr. (family Cynomoriaceae), used (1) to reinforce kidney yang for the treatment of impotence, seminal emission, and (2) as a mild laxative for chronic constipation in the aged

巴戟天 [bā jǐ tiān]

***Radix Morindae Officinalis*, Morinda Root:** the dried root of *Morinda officinalis* How (family Rubiaceae), used to reinforce kidney yang for the treatment of impotence and premature ejaculation in men, and frigidity in women

葫芦巴 [hú lú bā]

***Semen Trigonellae*, Common Fenugreek Seed:** the dried ripe seed of *Trigonella foenum-graecum* L. (family Leguminosae), used to warm the kidney, dispel cold and relieve pain for the treatment of cold pain in the testis, hernial pain, weakness and edema of the legs due to cold-damp

补骨脂 [bǔ gǔ zhī]

***Fructus Psoraleae*, Malaytea Scurfpea Fruit:** the dried ripe fruit of *Psoralea corylifolia* L. (family Leguminosae), used to warm the kidney and spleen, and reinforce yang for the treatment of impotence, nocturnal emission, frequent micturition, chronic asthma due to kidney insufficiency, and diarrhea occurring daily just before dawn due to deficiency of spleen and kidney yang

菟丝子 [tù sī zǐ]

***Semen Cuscutae*, Dodder Seed:** the dried ripe seed of *Cuscuta chinensis* Lam. (family Convolvulaceae), used to tonify the liver and kidney, to improve eyesight and prevent miscarriage, for the treatment of nocturnal emission, impotence, enuresis, diabetes, decreased eyesight and threatened abortion

杜仲 [dù zhòng]

***Cortex Eucommiae*, Eucommia Bark:** the dried stem-bark of *Eucommia ulmoides* Oliv. (family Eucommiaceae), used to tonify the liver and kidney, strengthen the tendons and bones, and prevent miscarriages for the treatment of aching back and knees, impotence, frequent micturition, threatened abortion and nowadays for hypertension

狗脊 [gǒu jǐ]

***Rhizoma Cibotii*, Cibot Rhizome:** the dried rhizome of *Cibotum barometz* (L.) J. Sm. (family Dicksoniaceae), used to tonify the liver and kidney, strengthen the back and knees and dispel wind-damp, for the treatment of insecurity of the kidney with enuresis and leukorrhagia, aching back and knees, rheumatic pain in the back, and strained lumbar muscles

续断 [xù duàn]

***Radix Dipsaci*, Himalayan Teasel Root:** the dried root of *Dipsacus asperoides* C.Y. Cheng et T.M. Ai (family Dipsacaceae), used (1) to tonify the liver and kidney and strengthen the tendons and bones for the treatment of aching back and joints, rheumatic pain in the lumbar region, (2) to improve the healing of fractures, and (3) to stop bleeding and prevent miscarriage, for treating functional uterine bleeding and threatened abortion

骨碎补 [gǔ suì bǔ]

***Rhizoma Drynariae*, Fortunes's Drynaria Rhizome:** the dried rhizome of *Drynaria fortunei* (Kunze) J. Sm. or *Drynaria baronii* (Christ) Diels (family Polypodiaceae), used (1) to tonify the kidney for the treatment of lumbago, impaired hearing and tinnitus, (2) to promote the healing of traumatic injuries and bone fracture, and (3) externally for alopecia areata and vitiligo

冬虫夏草 [dōng cóng xià cǎo]

***Cordyceps*, Chinese Caterpillar Fungus:** the dried body of stroma of the fungus, *Cordyceps sinensis* (Berk.) Sacc. (family Hypocreaceae) growing on the larvae of certain insect (family Hepialidae) and the dead caterpillars, used to reinforce kidney yang and tonify the lung for the treatment of impotence, nocturnal emission, night sweats, chronic cough with hemoptysis in cases of phthisis

蛤蚧 [gé jiè]

***Gecko*, Tokay Gecko:** the dried body, with the viscera removed, of a lizard, *Gekko gecko* L. (family Geckonidae), used to reinforce kidney yang and replenish lung *qi* for the treatment of chronic asthma

海马 [hǎi mǎ]

***Hippocampus*, Sea-Horse:** the dried body of *Hippocampus kelloggi* Jordan et Snyder, *H. histrix* Kaup, *H.* kuda Bleeker, *H. trimaculatus* Leach or *H. japonicus* Kaup. (family Syngnathidae), used (1) to tonify kidney yang for the treatment of impotence and frigidity, (2) to reduce swelling of abdominal masses and traumatic wounds, and (3) also used externally for treating boils and sores

固涩药 Astringents and Hemostatics

浮小麦 [fú xiǎo mài]

***Fructus Tritici Levis*, Light Wheat:** the dried light grains of *Triticum aestivum* L. (family Graminae), used as an antihidrotic agent for spontaneous sweating or night sweats

麻黄根 [má huáng gēn]

***Radix Ephedrae*, Ephedra Root:** the dried root and rhizome of *Ephedra sinica* Stapf. or *Ephedra intermedia* Schrenk et C.A. Mey (family Ephedraceae), used as an anhidrotic agent for the treatment of spontaneous perspiration and night sweats

五倍子 [wǔ bèi zǐ]

***Galla Chinensis*, Chinese Gall:** the gall produced mainly by aphides of *Melaphis chinensis* (Bell) Baker on the leaf of various Sumac, *Rhus chinensis* Mill., *Rhus potaninii* Maxim., *Rhus punjabensis* Stew. var. *sinica* (Diels) Rehd. et Wils. (family Anacardiaceae), used as an astringent agent for the treatment of persistent cough, night sweats, chronic diarrhea, bloody stool and enuresis, and used externally for treating burns, traumatic bleeding, hemorrhoids and oral ulcers

诃子 [hē zǐ]

***Fructus Chebulae*, Terminalia Fruit:** the dried ripe fruit of *Terminalia chebula* Retz. or *Terminalia chebula* var. *tomentella* Kurt. (family Combretaceae), used as an antidiarrhetic and antitussive agent for the treatment of chronic diarrhea or dysentery, persistent cough and hoarse voice.

石榴皮 [shí liú pí]

***Pericarpium Granati*, Pomegranate Rind:** the dried pericarp of *Punica granatum* L. (family Punicaceae), used as an antidiarrhetic for the treatment of chronic diarrhea or dysentery, also used as an anthelmintic for intestinal taeniasis and ascariasis

赤石脂 [chì shí zhī]

***Halloysitum Rubrum*, Red Halloysite:** a mineral, hydrated aluminum silicate, in red color due to the presence of iron oxides, used as an antidiarrhetic and hemostatic agent for the treatment of chronic diarrhea, menorrhagia and leukorrhagia

莲子 [lián zǐ]

***Semen Nelumbinis*, Lotus Seed:** the dried ripe seed of *Nelumbo nucifera* Gaertn. (family Nymphaeaceae), used as an astringent for the treatment of chronic diarrhea, spontaneous emission and leukorrhagia

莲须 [lián xū]

***Stamen Nelumbinis*, Lotus Stamen:** the dried stamen of Lotus, *Nelumbo nucifera* Gaertn. (family Nymphaeaceae), used as an astringent to consolidate kidney *qi* for the treatment of seminal emission and leukorrhagia

芡实 [qiàn shí]

***Semen Euryales*, Gordon Euryale Seed:** the dried kernel of ripe seed of *Euryale ferox* Salisb. (family Nymphaeaceae), used as an astringent for the treatment of chronic diarrhea, spontaneous emission, enuresis and leukorrhagia

禹余粮 [yǔ yú liáng]

***Limonitum*, Limonite:** brownish iron ore, mainly composed of basic iron oxide [FeO(OH)], used as an astringent for the treatment of chronic diarrhea or dysentery, menorrhagia and leukorrhagia.

禹粮石 [yǔ liáng shí]

a synonym for 禹余粮 [yǔ yú liáng]

伏龙肝 [fú lóng gān]

***Terra Flava Usta*, Calcined Yellow Earth:** clean calcined yellow earth in small lumps, used as (1) an anti-emetic for the treatment of nausea and vomiting due to chronic stomach diseases or pregnancy, (2) an antidiarrhetic for chronic diarrhea, and (3) a hemostatic for bleeding due to failure of the spleen to control the blood

乌梅 [wū méi]

***Fructus Mume*, Smoked Plum:** the dried nearly ripe fruit of Japanese Apricot, *Prunus Mume* (Sieb.) Sieb. et Zucc. (family Rosaceae) , used as an antidiarrhetic, antitussive, antidiptic and anthelmintic agent for treating chronic diarrhea, persistent cough, morbid thirst and ascariasis

肉豆蔻 [ròu dòu kòu]

***Semen Myristicae*, Nutmeg:** the dried kernel of *Myristica fragrans* Houtt. (family Myristicaceae), used as an antidiarrhetic agent by warming the spleen and stomach for the treatment of chronic diarrhea

肉果 [ròu guǒ]

a synonym for 肉豆蔻 [ròu dòu kòu]

罂粟壳 [yīng sù qiào]

***Pericarpium Papaveris*, Poppy Capsule:** the dried ripe capsule of Opium Poppy, *Papaver somniferum* L. (family Papaveraceae), used as an antidiarrhetic, antitussive and analgesic agent for the treatment of chronic diarrhea, persistent cough and abdominal pain

米壳 [mǐ qiào]

a synonym for 罂粟壳 [yīng sù qiào]

五味子 [wǔ wèi zǐ]

***Fructus Schisandrae*, Chinese Magnoliavine Fruit:** the dried ripe fruit of *Schisandra chinensis* (Turcz.) Baill. or *Schisandra sphenanthera* Rehd. et Wils. (family Magnoliaceae), used as an astringent for the treatment of dry cough, asthma, night sweats, seminal emission and chronic diarrhea, also used as a tranquilizer for palpitation and insomnia.

桑螵蛸 [sāng piāo xiāo]

***Oötheca Mantidis*, Egg Capsule of Mantid:** the dried egg capsule of a praying mantis, *Tenodera sinensis* Saussure, *Statilja maculata* (Thunb.) or *Hierodula patellifera* (Serville) (family Mantidae), used as an astringent for the treatment of frequent micturition, enuresis, seminal emission and leukorrhagia

海螵蛸 [hǎi piāo xiāo]

***Os Sepiae*, Cuttlebone:** the dried internal shell of *Sepiella maindroni* de Rochebrune or *Sepia esculenta* Hoyle (family Sepiadae), used as a hemostatic and antacid agent for the treatment of hematemesis, bloody stool, menorrhagia, acid regurgitation and leukorrhagia

乌贼骨 [wū zéi gǔ]

a synonym for 海螵蛸 [hǎi piāo xiāo]

瓦楞子 [wǎ léng zǐ]

***Concha Arcae*, Arc Shell:** the shell of *Arca subcrenata* Lischke, *Arca granosa* L. or *Arca inflata* Reeve (family Arcidae), used to eliminate phlegm and soften hard lumps for treating scrofula and goiter

煅瓦楞 [duàn wǎ léng]

***Concha Arcae Usta*, Calcined Arc Shell:** the calcined shell of *Arca subcrenata* Lischke, *Arca granosa* L. or *Arca inflata* Reeve (family Arcidae), used as an antacid agent for the treatment of acid regurgitation

煅龙骨 [duàn lóng gǔ]

***Os Draconis Ustum*, Calcined Dragon's Bone:** the calcined fossil bone of large ancient mammals, such as *Stegodon orientalis* and *Rhinocerus sinensis*, used as an astringent for the treatment of seminal emission, night sweats, leukorrhagia and uterine bleeding

煅牡蛎 [duàn mǔ lì]

***Concha Ostreae Usta*, Calcined Oyster Shell:** the calcined shell of oyster, *Ostrea gigas* Thunb., *Ostrea talienwhanensis* Crosse or *Ostrea rivularis* Gould (family Ostreidae), used as an astringent and antacid for the treatment of excessive sweating, seminal emission, leukorrhagia and acid regurgitation

金樱子 [jīn yīng zǐ]

***Fructus Rosae Laevigatae*, Cherokee Rose Fruit:** the dried ripe fruit of Cherokee Rose, *Rosa laevigata* Mickx. (family Rosaceae), used as an astringent for the treatment of seminal emission, enuresis, frequent micturition and chronic diarrhea

覆盆子 [fù pén zǐ]

***Fructus Rubi*, Palmleaf Raspberry Fruit:** the steamed and dried fruit of *Rubus chingii* Hu (family Rosaceae), used as an astringent for the treatment of frequent micturition, enuresis and seminal emission

消导药 Digestives and Evacuants

山楂 [shān zhā]

***Fructus Crataegi*, Hawthorn Fruit:** the dried ripe fruit of Large Chinese Hawthorn, *Crataegus pinnatifida* Bge. var. *major* N.E. Br. or Chinese Hawthorn, *Crataegus pinnatifida* Bge. (family Rosaceae), used to improve digestion and relieve food stagnation for the treatment of dyspepsia and stagnation of fatty food, also to activate blood flow for treating amenorrhea and postpartum abdominal pain due to blood stasis

焦山楂 [jiāo shān zhā]

***Fructus Crataegi Preparatus*, Charred Hawthorn Fruit:** hawthorn fruit stir-baked to a brown color, used to improve digestion and relieve food stagnation for the treatment of dyspepsia and stagnation of fatty food

麦芽 [mài yá]

***Fructus Hordei Germinatus*, Germinated Barley:** the dried germinated grain of barley, *Hordeum vulgare* L. (family Graminae), used (1) to improve digestion for treating dyspepsia, and (2) to inhibit milk secretion for stopping lactation

焦麦芽 [jiāo mài yá]

***Fructus Hordei Germinatus Preparatus*, Charred Germinated Barley:** germinated grain of barley stir-baked to a brown color, used to improve digestion for treating dyspepsia induced by cereal food and infantile lactodyspepsia

稻芽 [dào yá]

***Fructus Oryzae Germinatus*, Rice-grain Sprout:** the dried germinated grains of rice, *Oryza sativa* L. (family Graminae), used to improve digestion for the treatment of poor appetite and dyspepsia

谷芽 [gǔ yá]

***Fructus Setariae Germinatus*, Millet Sprout:** the dried germinated grains of millet, *Setaria italica* (L.) Beauv. (family Graminae), used in the same way same as rice-grain sprout (稻芽 [dào yá]) to improve digestion for the treatment of poor appetite and dyspepsia

粟芽 [sù yá]

a synonym for 谷芽 [gǔ yá]

神曲 [shén qū]

***Massa Fermentata Medicinalis*, Medicated Leaven:** the dried mass of a fermented mixture of wheat flour, fresh aerial parts of *Artemisia annua*, *Xanthium sibiricum*, and *Polygonum hydropiper*, used to improve digestion for the treatment of dyspepsia and abdominal distension due to food stagnation.

焦三仙 [jiāo sān xiān]

Charred Triplet: a mixture that consists of equal parts of charred medicated leaven, charred hawthorn fruit and charred germinated barley, and has a stronger effect for improving digestion than each of them alone

鸡内金 [jī nèi jīn]

***Endothelium Corneum Gigeriae Galli*, Chicken's Gizzard-skin:** the dried lining membrane of the gizzard of common fowl, *Gallus gallus domesticus* Briss. (family Phasianidae), used to improve the appetite and digestion for the treatment of poor appetite and dyspepsia

莱菔子 [lá fú zǐ]

***Semen Raphani*, Radish Seed:** the dried ripe seed of garden radish, *Raphanus sativus* L. (family Cruciferae), used (1) to improve the digestion and direct *qi* downward for the treatment of food stagnation with abdominal distension and pain, and (2) to resolve phlegm for cough and dyspnea with profuse expectoration

泻下药 Purgatives

蜂蜜 [fēng mì]

***Mel*, Honey:** a saccharine fluid made by the hive-bee, *Apis cerana* Fabr. or *Apis mellifera* L. (family Apidae), used as an antitussive for dry cough, and as an aperient for constipation in the aged

郁李仁 [yù lǐ rén]

***Semen Pruni*, Chinese Dwarf Cherry Seed:** the dried ripe seed of *Prunus humilis* Bge., *Prunus japonica* Thunb. or *Prunus pedunculata*

Maxim. (family Rosaceae), used as an aperient for the treatment of constipation, and a diuretic for relieving edema

火麻仁 [huǒ má rén]

***Fructus Cannabis*, Hemp Seed:** the dried ripe fruit of *Cannabis sativa* L.(family Moraceae), used as an aperient for the treatment of constipation in the debilitated or aged

大黄 [dà huáng]

***Radix et Rhizoma Rhei*, Rhubarb:** the dried root and rhizome of *Rheum palmatum* L., *Rheum tanguticum* Maxim. ex Balf. or *Rheum officinale* Baill. (family Polygonaceae), used to induce catharsis, clear heat, purge fire, arrest bleeding, counteract toxins and remove blood stasis, for treating (1) constipation with gastrointestinal accumulation, (2) warm diseases with high fever, delirium and constipation, (3) postpartum abdominal pain, amenorrhea due to blood stasis, (4) hemoptysis, hematemesis and epistaxis associated with excessive heat in the blood, and, externally, (5) for burns, boils and sores

番泻叶 [fān xiè yè]

***Folium Sennae*, Senna Leaf:** the dried leaflet of *Cassia angustifolia* Vahl or *Cassia acutifolia* Delile (family Leguminosae), used as a purgative for the treatment of constipation, especially habitual constipation

芒硝 [máng xiāo]

***Natrii Sulfas*, Sodium Sulfate, Glauber's Salt:** crystalline hydrated sodium sulfate, usually made from natural sources, used (1) as a purgative for the treatment of constipation, and, externally, (2) to soften hard masses for treating acute mastitis

玄明粉 [xuán míng fěn]

***Natrii Sulfas Exsiccatus*, Exsiccated Sodium Sulfate:** a white powder composed of sodium sulfate, used as a purgative for the treatment of constipation

芦荟 [lú huì]

***Aloe*, Aloes:** the dried leaf juice of *Aloe barbadensis* Mill., *Aloe ferox* Mill. or related species (family Liliaceae), used (1) as a purgative for constipation, (2) to clear the liver for treating liver fire with dizziness, headache and irritability, and (3) to kill intestinal parasitic worms

驱虫药 Anthelmintics

苦楝皮 [kǔ liàn pí]

***Cortex Meliae*, Szechwan Chinaberry Bark:** the dried stem- or root-bark of *Melia toosendan* Sieb. et Zucc. or *Melia azedarach* L. (family Meliaceae), used as an antiparasitic for the treatment of helminths, and externally for scabies

使君子 [shǐ jūn zǐ]

***Fructus Quisqualis*, Rangoon-creeper Fruit:** the dried ripe fruit of *Rangoon* Creeper, *Quisqualis indica* L. (family Combretaceae), used as an anthelmintic for the treatment of ascariasis, enterobiasis and infantile malnutrition associated with intestinal parasitosis

槟榔 [bīng láng]

***Semen Arecae*, Areca Seed:** the dried ripe seed of Betel Palm, *Areca catechu* L. (family Palmae), used (1) to expel helminths for the treatment of ascariasis, fasciolopsiasis, ancylostomiasis, oxyuriasis and particularly taeniasis, (2) to remove undigested food for relieving abdominal distension and diarrhea with tenesmus in cases of food stagnation, (3) to induce diuresis for treating edema, and (4) to arrest malarial episodes

南瓜子 [nán guā zǐ]

***Semen Cucurbitae*, Pumpkin Seed:** the dried seed of *Cucurbita moschata* Duch. (family Cucurbitaceae), used as an anthelmintic for the treatment of taeniasis, schistosomiasis and clonorchiasis

榧子 [fěi zǐ]

***Semen Torreyae*, Grand Torreya Seed:** the dried ripe seed of Chinese Torreya, *Torreya grandis* Fort. (family Taxaceae), used as an anthelmintic and laxative for the treatment of taeniasis, enterobiasis, ancylostomiasis, ascariasis and fasciolopsiasis

雷丸 [léi wán]

***Omphalia*, Thunder Ball:** the dried sclerotium of *Omphalia lapidescens* Schroet. (family Polyporaceae), used as an anthelmintic for the treatment of taeniasis, ancylostomiasis, and ascariasis

鹤虱 [hè shī]

***Fructus Carpesii*, Common Carpesium Fruit:** the dried ripe fruit of *Carpesium abrotanoides* L. (family Compositae), used as an anthelmintic for the treatment of ascariasis, enterobiasis and taeniasis

北鹤虱 [běi hè shī]

same as 鹤虱 [hè shī]

南鹤虱 [nán hè shī]

***Fructus Carotae*, Carrot Fruit:** the dried ripe fruit of *Daucus carota* L. (family Umbelliferae), used (1) to kill parasitic worms in cases of ascariasis, oxyuriasis and taeniasis, and (2) to remove undigested food for treating food stagnation

鹤草芽 [hè cǎo yá]

***Gemma Agrimoniae*, Agrimonia Bud:** the dried bud, with a short piece of rhizome attached, of *Agrimonia pilosa* Ledeb. (family Rosaceae), used as an anthelmintic for the treatment of taeniasis

外用药 Drugs for External Use

硫黄 [liú huáng]

***Sulfur*, Sulfur:** obtained from natural sources after purification, used (1) externally as an antiparasitic for treating scabies, and (2) internally to reinforce yang for the treatment of impotence and chronic asthma.

雄黄 [xióng huáng]

***Realgar*, Realgar:** a mineral, orange to reddish in color, mainly composed of arsenic disulfide (As_2S_2), used externally as a detoxicant and antiparasitic agent for snake and insect bites, boils and scabies

信石 [xìn shí]

***Arsenicum Trioxidum*, Arsenic Trioxide:** used (1) externally as a caustic to remove dead tissue for the treatment of boils, ulcers, scrofula and hemorrhoids, and (2) internally in minute quantities as an expectorant and antiasthmatic agent for trreating asthma with thin and frothy phlegm

白砒 [bái pī]

a synonym for 信石 [xìn shí]

轻粉 [qīng fěn]

***Calomelas*, calomel:** crystalline mercurous chloride (Hg_2Cl_2), used (1) externally as an antiparasitic for treating scabies, tinea, neurodermatitis and eczematous lesions, and (2) internally in small quantities to remove phlegm and cause purgation

甘汞 [gān gǒng]

a synonym for 轻粉 [qīng fěn]

白矾 [bái fán]

***Alumen*, Alum:** a crystalline mineral salt, hydrated potassium aluminum sulfate, used (1) externally to kill parasites, arrest discharges and relieve itching in cases of scabies, tinea, neurodermatitis and eczematous lesions, and (2) internally to dispel wind-phlegm for treating epilepsy and mania

明矾 [míng fán]

a synonym for 白矾 [bái fán]

枯矾 [kū fán]

***Alumen Ustum,* Calcined Alumen:** calcined potassium aluminum sulfate, used to arrest discharges, promote the healing of ulcers, stop bleeding, and cause cauterization, externally for the treatment of eczema, excessive leukorrhea with pudendal itching, and nasal polyp, and internally as an astringent for chronic diarrhea and bloody stool

炉甘石 [lú gān shí]

***Calamina*, Calamine:** calcined and elutriated powder of smithsonite, mainly composed of zinc carbonate ($ZnCO_3$) with a pink tint due to the presence of a small amount of ferric oxide, used externally as an astringent for chronic ulcers, eczema, conjunctivitis and keratitis.

血竭 [xuè jié]

***Sanguis Draconis*, Dragon's Blood:** red resin secreted from the fruit of *Daemonorops draco* Bl. (family Palmae), used to eliminate blood stasis, relieve pain and promote the healing of wounds for the treatment of traumatic injuries

硇砂 [náo shā]

***Sal Purpureum*, Purple Rocksalt** and ***Sal Ammoniacum*, Sal Ammoniac:** mineral salts containing ammonium chloride, used externally for treating nebula and pterygium, and internally for treating cancer of the esophagus

紫硇砂 [zǐ náo shā]

***Sal Purpureum*, Purple Rocksalt:** a purple-colored rocksalt

白硇砂 [bái náo shā]

***Sal Ammoniacum*, Sal Ammoniac:** a colorless crystalline mineral salt mainly containing ammonium chloride

硼砂 [péng shā]

***Borax*, Borax:** a colorless crystalline mineral salt, hydrated sodium tetraborate, used externally as gargle for treating oral ulcers and acute tonsillitis, and internally as an expectorant

蛇床子 [shé chuáng zǐ]

***Fructus Cnidii*, Common Cnidium Fruit:** the dried ripe fruit of *Cnidium monnieri* (L.) Cuss. (family Umbelliferae), used (1) externally as an astringent and antiparasitic for treating eczema, pruritus vulvae and trichomonas vaginitis, and (2) internally to warm the kidney and promote virility for the treatment of impotence

巴豆 [bā dòu]

***Semen Crotonis*, Croton Seed:** the dried ripe seed of *Croton tiglium* L. (family Euphorbiaceae), used externally for treating scabies, tinea, and warts (cf.. 巴豆霜 [bā dòu shuāng])

斑蝥 [bān máo]

***Mylabris*, Mylabris, Blister Beetle:** the dried body of *Mylabris phalerata* Pall. or *Mylabris cichorii* L. (family Meloidae), used (1) externally as a rubefacient, irritant and caustic to promote local blood circulation, remove dead tissue and accelerate the healing of wounds for the treatment of psoriasis, neurodermatitis, chronic ulcers and scrofula, and (2) internally in small quantities for the treatment of swelling of the lymph glands, and rabies

蟾酥 [chán sū]

***Venenum Bufonis*, Toad Venom:** the dried secretion of the skin glands of a toad, *Bufo bufo gargarizans* Cantor or *Bufo melanostictus* Schneider (family Bufonidae), used as a detoxicant, discutient and anodyne, applied externally and taken internally for the treatment of boils, sores, ulcers, tumors, chronic osteomyelitis and sore throat

蜂房 [fēng fáng]

***Nidus Vespae*, Wasp's Nest:** the nest of wasps or hornets, *Polistes olivaceus* (DeGeer), *Polistes japonicus* Sauss. or *Parapolybia varia* Fabr. (family Vespidae), used (1) externally for treating tinea, (2) as gargles for trreating painful swelling of the gums, and (3) internally for treating convulsions, urticaria and chronic cough

儿茶 [ér chá]

***Catechu*, Cutch, Black Catechu:** a dry extract prepared from the peeled stem and branches of *Acacia catechu* (L.) Willd. (family Leguminosae), used externally as an astringent for chronic ulcer, eczema and traumatic bleeding

方剂 Formulas

方剂 [fāng jì]

formula; prescription; recipe: direction of the preparation (including the ingredients and doses) and administration of a remedy, also called 方 [fāng] for short

方 [fāng]

an abbreviation for 方剂 [fāng jì]

单方 [dān fāng]

simple formula: a formula consisting of one or two medicinal substances for treating a particular illness in uncomplicated condition

奇方 [jī fāng]

odd-numbered formula [prescription]: (1) a formula or prescription with ingredients odd in number; (2) a formula or prescription with one single ingredient

偶方 [ǒu fāng]

even-numbered formula [prescription]: (1) a formula or prescription with ingredients even in number; (2) a formula or prescription with two ingredients

复方 [fù fāng]

compound formula [prescription]: a formula or prescription that is formed by (1) two or more set formulas; (2) one formula with additional ingredients

成方 [chéng fāng]

set formula: a formula that has already been set and recorded

验方 [yàn fāng]

proved formula: a formula that has been proved effective in the treatment of a certain morbid condition

良方 [liáng fāng]

well-tried formula: a formula that often shows good results in treating a certain illness

秘方 [mì fāng]

secret formula: a formula that is kept unknown to others, also called forbidden formula (禁方 [jìn fāng])

禁方 [jìn fāng]

forbidden formula: a formula that is kept unknown to others

祖传秘方 [zǔ chuán mì fāng]

secret formula handed down from the ancestors

偏方 [piān fāng]

special but irregular recipe: a simple recipe with special effect in treating a certain illness

土方 [tǔ fāng]

folk recipe: a simple recipe used by the people living in a certain area

土法 [tǔ fǎ]

folk treatment: a simple treatment used by the people living in a certain area

经方 [jīng fāng]

classical formula: (1) formula recorded in the *Canon of Medicine*" or Zhang Zhong-jing's works; (2) formula recorded in Zhang Zhong-jing's works only

时方 [shí fāng]

contemporary formula: formula introduced by physicians after the time of the great physician Zhang Zhongjing

大方 [dà fāng]

major [heavy] formula: (1) a formula or prescription which consists of many ingredients with strong actions; (2) large dosage of medicine given at one time for a strong action; and (3) a formula or prescription for the treatment of a serious disease or a disease of the lower energizer

小方 [xiǎo fāng]

minor [mild] formula: (1) a mild formula or prescription which consists of only a few ingredients for treating a mild illness; (2) small dosage of medicine for the treatment of an uncomplicated disease or a disease of the upper energizer

缓方 [huǎn fāng]

slow-acting formula: a formula or prescription which is composed of ingredients that act slowly or counteract each other to moderate the effect, and is indicated in the treatment of cases of chronic debilitation

急方 [jí fāng]

quick-acting formula: a formula or prescription which is employed for immediate effect in the treatment of emergency or critical cases

配方 [pèi fāng]

dispense a prescription: prepare a medicine according to the prescription

汤头 [tāng tóu]

decoction formula: a formula that indicates the preparation of a decoction

汤头歌 [tāng tóu gē]

formulas in rhyme: formulas put into rhyme to make them easier to memorize

方剂配伍 [fāng jì pèi wǔ]

ingredient combination in a formula [prescription]: combination of various ingredients in a formula or prescription for producing the desired therapeutic effect in unison, and reducing toxic or side effects

君臣佐使 [jūn chén zuǒ shǐ]

sovereign [chief], minister [associate], adjuvant [assistant] and courier [guide]: the ingredients in a formula or prescription that play different roles

君药 [jūn yào]

sovereign [chief] ingredient: the ingredient that provides the principal curative action

臣药 [chén yào]

minister [associate] ingredient: the ingredient that helps strengthen the principal action

佐药 [zuǒ yào]

adjuvant [assistant] ingredient: the ingredient that relieves secondary symptoms or tempers the action of the principal ingredient when the latter is too potent

使药 [shǐ yào]

courier [guide] ingredient: the ingredient that directs action to the affected meridian or site

主辅佐引 [zhǔ fǔ zuǒ yǐn]

principal, adjuvant, auxiliary and conductant ingredients: alternative names for sovereign, minister, adjuvant and courier ingredients (君臣佐使 [jūn chén zuǒ shǐ])

引经报使 [yǐn jīng bào shǐ]

directing to the affected meridian or site: the action of a conductant ingredient in directing other ingredients to work on the affected meridian or site, e.g., *Radix Bupleuri* directing to the *shaoyang* meridian, *Radix Platycodi* to the throat, *Radix Cyathulae* to the lower extremities

药引子 [yào yǐn zi]

extra conductant ingredient: an extra ingredient in a formula or prescription, used to strengthen the efficacy of the whole recipe

反佐 [fǎn zuǒ]

using a corrigent: adding a conductant ingredient with a property opposite to the other ingredients, e.g., adding an ingredient cold in property to a recipe hot in nature, or an ingredient hot in property to a recipe cold in nature

相须 [xiāng xū]

mutual reinforcement: two ingredients with similar properties used in combination to reinforce each other's action

相使 [xiāng shǐ]

mutual assistance: two or more ingredients in a prescription used in combination, one being the principal substance while the others play a subsidiary role to reinforce the action of the former

相畏 [xiāng wèi]

mutual restraint: the mutual restraining effect of different ingredients to weaken or neutralize each other's action

相恶 [xiāng wù]

mutual inhibition; counteraction: property of one ingredient to weaken the action of another ingredient

相杀 [xiāng shā]

mutual suppression; neutralization: property of one ingredient to neutralize the toxicity of another ingredient

相反 [xiāng fǎn]

mutual antagonism; incompatibility: property of one ingredient being unsuitable for combination with another ingredient, which may result in severe side effects if these ingredients are used together

十八反 [shí bā fǎn]

eighteen antagonisms: incompatible medicinals which, if given in combination, are believed to have serious side effects: *Radix Glycyrrhizae* being antagonistic to *Radix Euphorbiae Pekinensis, Flos*

Genkwa, Radix Euphorbiae Kansui, and *Sargassum; Radix Aconiti* being antagonistic to *Bulbus Fritillariae, Fructus Trichosanthis, Rhizoma Pinelliae*, *Radix Ampelopsis* and *Rhizoma Bletillae*; and *Radix Veratri Nigri* being antagonistic to *Radix Ginseng, Radix Salviae Miltiorrhizae, Radix Adenophorae, Radix Sophorae Flavescentis, Radix Scrophulariae, Herba Asari* and *Radix Paeoniae*

十九畏 [shí jiǔ wèi]

nineteen incompatibilities: medicinals of mutual restraint which, if used in combination, may restrain or neutralize each other's action: sulfur restraining crude sodium sulfate; mercury restraining arsenic trioxide; *Radix Euphorbiae Ebracteolatae* restraining litharge; *Semen Crotonis* restraining *Semen Pharbitidis; Flos Caryophylli* restraining *Radix Curcumae*; crystalline sodium sulfate restraining *Rhizoma Sparganii; Radix Aconiti* and *Radix Aconiti Kuznezoffi* restraining *Cornu Rhinoceri; Radix Ginseng* restraining *Faeces Trogopterorum;* and *Cortex Cinnamomi* restraining *Halloysitum Rubrum*

十剂 [shí jì]

ten categories of formulas

通剂 [tōng jì]

obstruction-removing formula: a formula used in treating stasis or obstruction, e.g., amenorrhea, galactostasis and arthralgia, due to obstruction of *qi* and blood in the collateral meridians

宣剂 [xuān jì]

dispelling formula: a formula indicated for removal of stasis, reducing phlegm, and inducing emesis

补剂 [bǔ jì]

tonifying formula: a formula used in treating various deficiency conditions and building up health

泄剂 [xiè jì]

purgative formula: formula used not only for relieving constipation, but also for removing excessive heat, eliminating accumulated cold and purging retained fluid

轻剂 [qīng jì]

light (diaphoretic) formula: a formula composed of light dispersing ingredients to release the superficies from exogenous pathogens

重剂 [zhòng jì]

heavy formula: a formula that contains weighty drugs with tranquillizing action

滑剂 [huá jì]

lubrication formula: a formula that relieves dysuria and aids discharge of calculi

涩剂 [sè jì]

astringent formula: a formula that arrests discharge, often used for treating excessive sweating, seminal emission and protracted diarrhea

燥剂 [zào jì]

desiccating formula: a formula that has the effect of removing pathogenic dampness, often used for treating edema and retention of excessive fluid and phlegm

湿剂 [shī jì]

moistening formula: a formula that has the action of replenishing body fluid

十二剂 [shí èr jì]

twelve categoris of formulas: the ten categories of formulas plus cooling and warming formulas

寒剂 [hán jì]

cooling formula: a formula with drugs cool or cold in property, used in treating heat syndromes

热剂 [rè jì]

warming formula: a formula with drugs warm or hot in property, used in treating cold syndromes

十四剂 [shí sì jì]

fourteen categories of formulas: the twelve categories of formulas plus elevating formula and depressant formula

升剂 [shēng jì]

elevating formula: a formula with elevating effect for the treatment of prolapse of the rectum, prolapse of the uterus, and other kinds of visceroptosis

降剂 [jiàn jì]

depressant formula: a formula with the effect of checking the upward adverse flow of *qi,* air or gas, for the treatment of cough, hiccups, belching and vomiting

解表剂 [jiě biǎo jì]

exterior-releasing formula: formula to dispel pathogenic factors from the superficies of the body for the treatment of an exterior syndrome

辛温解表剂 [xīn wēn jiě biǎo jì]

pungent-warm exterior-releasing formula: formula mainly consisting of ingredients pungent in flavor and warm in property to dispel pathogenic factors from the superficies of the body for the treatment of exterior syndrome of wind-cold afflictions

麻黄汤 [má huáng tāng]

***Mahuang* Decoction; Ephedra Decoction:** decoction composed of 麻黄 *Herba Ephedrae,* 桂枝 *Ramulus Cinnamomi*, 苦杏仁 *Semen Armeniacae Amarum* and 甘草 *Radix Glycyrrhizae*, used as a diaphoretic and antasthmatic for the treatment of exterior excess syndrome of wind-cold afflictions

桂枝汤 [guì zhī tāng]

***Guizhi* Decoction; Cassia-twig Decoction:** decoction composed of 桂枝 *Ramulus Cinnamomi*, 白芍 *Radix Paeoniae Alba*, 生姜 *Rhizoma Zingiberis Recens*, 甘草 *Radix Glycyrrhizae* and 大枣 *Fructus Ziziphi Jujubae*, used to expel exogenous pathogenic factors from the superficial muscles and rectify derangement of the constructive and defensive systems for the treatment of exterior deficiency syndrome of wind-cold afflictions

九味羌活汤 [jiǔ wèi qiāng huó tāng]

***Jiuwei Qianghuo* Decoction; Nine-ingredient Decoction with Notopterygium:** a formula composed of 羌活 *Rhizoma seu Radix Notopterygii*, 防风 *Radix Saposhnikoviae*, 苍术 *Rhizoma Atractylodis,* 川芎 *Rhizoma Chuanxiong*， 细辛 *Herba Asari*, 白芷 *Radix Angelicae Dahuricae*,生地黄 *Radix Rehmanniae* and 甘草 *Radix Glycyrrhizae*, used to induce sweating, dispel dampness and clear internal heat for external contraction of wind-cold-damp complicated by internal heat

香薷散 [xiāng rú sǎn]

***Xiangru* Powder; Elshotzia Powder:** a formula composed of 香薷 *Herba Elshotziae,* 白扁豆 *Semen Lablab Album* and 厚朴 *Cortex Magnoliae Officinalis*, used to dispel summer-heat, release the exterior, resolve dampness and harmonize the middle for colds in summer

小青龙汤 [xiǎo qīng lóng tāng]

***Xiao Qinglong* Decoction; Blue Dragon Minor Decoction:** decoction composed of 麻黄 *Herba Ephedrae*, 桂枝 *Ramulus Cinnamomi*, 细辛 *Herba Asari*, 干姜 *Rhizoma Zingiberis*, 制半夏 *Rhizoma Pinelliae Praeparata*, 五味子 *Fructus Schisandrae*, 白芍 *Radix Paeoniae Alba* and 甘草 *Radix Glycyrrhizae*, used to release the exterior, disperse cold, warm the lung and resolve the retained fluid in treating cold in the exterior and retained fluid in the interior

止嗽散 [zhǐ sòu sǎn]

***Zhisou* Powder; Antitussive Powder:** a formula composed of 桔梗 *Radix Platycodi*, 荆芥 *Herba Schizonepetae*, 紫菀 *Radix Asteris*, 百部 *Radix Stemonae,* 白前 *Rhizoma Cynanchi Stauntonii*，甘草 *Radix Glycyrrhizae* and 陈皮 *Pericarpium Citri Reticulatae*, used to disperse wind and stop coughing in treating wind attack of the lung

辛凉解表剂 [xīn liáng jiě biǎo jì]

pungent-cool exterior-releasing formula: a formula mainly consisting of ingredients pungent in flavor and cool in property to disperse wind-heat in the treatment of exterior syndrome of wind-heat afflictions or warm diseases at the early stage

辛凉平剂 [xīn liáng píng jì]

moderate pungent-cool formula: formula composed of pungent and cool ingredients to release wind-heat exterior syndrome with a moderate action, e.g., lonicera-forsythia powder

辛凉轻剂 [xīn liáng qīng jì]

mild pungent-cool formula: formula composed of pungent and cool ingredients to release wind-heat exterior syndrome with a mild action, e.g., morus-chrysanthemum decoction

辛凉重剂 [xīn liáng zhòng jì]

drastic pungent-cool formula: formula composed of pungent and cool ingredients to release wind-heat exterior syndrome with a drastic action

银翘散 [yín qiào sǎn]

***Yin Qiao* Powder; Lonicera-Forsythia Powder:** a formula composed of 金银花 *Flos Lonicerae*, 连翘 *Fructus Forsythiae*, 牛蒡子 *Fructus Arctii*, 薄荷 *Herba Menthae*, 荆芥 *Herba Schizonepetae*, 豆豉 *Semen Sojae Praeparatum*, 桔梗 *Radix Platycodi*, 甘草 *Radix Glycyrrhizae*, 淡竹叶 *Herba Lophatheri* and 芦根 *Rhizoma Phragmitis*, used as an exterior-releasing, heat-clearing and toxin-counteracting remedy for warm diseases at the early stage

桑菊饮 [sāng jú yǐn]

***Sang Ju Yin*; Morus-Chrysanthemum Decoction:** decoction composed of 桑叶 *Folimu Mori*, 菊花 *Flos Chrysanthemi*, 薄荷 *Herba Menthae*, 苦杏仁 *Semen Armeniacae Amarum*, 桔梗 *Radix Platycodi*, 甘草 *Radix Glycyrrhizae*, 淡竹叶 *Herba Lophatheri* and 芦根 *Rhizoma Phragmitis*, used to disperse wind, clear heat and stop coughing in the treatment of wind-warm at the early stage

麻杏石甘汤 [má xìng shí gān tāng]

***Ma Xing Shi Gan* Decoction; Decoction of Ephedra, Apricot Kernel, Gypsum and Liquorice:** a formula composed of 麻黄 *Herba Ephedrae*, 苦杏仁 *Semen Armeniacae Amarum*, 石膏 *Gypsum Fibrosum*, 甘草 *Radix Glycyrrhizae*, used to ventilate the lung with pungent-coolness and clear the lung of heat for treating lung heat with cough and dyspnea combined with un-released exterior syndrome

柴葛解肌汤 [chái gě jiě jī tāng]

***Chai Ge Jieji* Decoction; Bupleurum-Pueraria Muscle-releasing Decoction:** a formula composed of 柴胡 *Radix Bupleuri*, 葛根 *Radix Puerariae*, 甘草 *Radix Glycyrrhizae*, 黄芩 *Radix Scutellariae*, 羌活 *Rhizoma seu Radix Notopterygii*, 白芷 *Radix Angelicae Dahuricae* and 桔梗 *Radix Platycodi*, used to release the muscles and clear heat for treating wind-cold affliction with heat transformation

升麻葛根汤 [shēng má gě gēn tāng]

***Shenma Gegen* Decoction; Cimicifuga-Pueraria Decoction:** a formula composed of 升麻 *Rhizoma Cimicifugae*, 葛根 *Radix Puerariae*，芍药 *Radix Paeoniae* and 甘草 *Radix Glycyrrhizae*, used to release the muscles and promote eruption for measles at the early stage

扶正解表剂 [fú zhèng jiě biǎo jì]

normal-*qi*-supportive exterior-releasing formula: formula to relieve exterior syndrome in patients with weak constitution

败毒散 [bài dú sǎn]

Baidu Powder; Antiphlogistic Powder: a formula composed of 柴胡 *Radix Bupleuri*, 前胡 *Radix Peucedani,* 川芎 *Radix Chuanxiong,* 枳壳 *Fructus Aurantii,* 羌活 *Rhizoma seu Radix Notopterygii*, 独活 *Radix Angelicae Pubescentis,* 桔梗 *Radix Platycodi*, 茯苓 *Poria*, 人参 *Radix Ginseng* and 甘草 *Radix Glycyrrhizae*, used to dispel cold, remove dampness, replenish *qi* and release the exterior for the treatment of external contraction in cases of *qi* deficiency

荆防败毒散 [jīng fáng bài dú sǎn]

***Jingfang Baidu* Powder; Schizonepeta-Saposhnikovia Antiphlogistic Powder:** a formula composed of 荆芥 *Herba Schizonepetae*, 防风 *Radix Saposhnikoviae*, 羌活 *Rhizoma seu Radix Notopterygii*, 独活 *Radix Angelicae Pubescentis,* 川芎 *Radix Chuanxiong,* 桔梗 *Radix Platycodi*, 枳壳 *Fructus Aurantii,* 茯苓 *Poria*, 甘草 *Radix Glycyrrhizae* and 薄荷 *Herba Menthae*, used to induce sweating, release the exterior, disperse wind and dispel damp in treating external contraction of wind, cold and dampness

参苏饮 [shēn sū jǐn]

***Shen Su Yin*; Ginseng-Perilla Decoction:** a formula composed of 人参 *Radix Ginseng,* 紫苏叶 *Folium Perillae,* 葛根 *Radix Puerariae,* 桔梗 *Radix Platycodi,* 半夏 *Rhizoma Pinelliae,* 前胡 *Radix Peucedani,* 茯苓 *Poria*, 木香 *Radix Aucklandiae,* 枳壳 *Fructus Aurantii,* 陈皮 *Pericarpium Citri Reticulatae* and 炙甘草 *Radix Glycyrrhizae Preparata*, used to replenish *qi,* release the exterior, regulate *qi* and resolve phlegm for wind-cold affliction in a weak patient with phlegm-fluid in the interior

加减葳蕤汤 [jiā jiǎn wēi ruí tāng]

***Jiajian Weirui* Decoction; modified Solomon's Seal Decoction:** a formula composed of 葳蕤 *Rhizoma Polygoni odorati*, 桔梗 *Radix Platycodi,* 白薇 *Radix Cynanchi Atrati,* 淡豆豉 *Semen Sojae Preparatum,* 薄荷 *Herba Menthae* and 炙甘草 *Radix Glycyrrhizae Preparata*, used to nourish yin and release the exterior in the treatment of wind-heat affliction in cases of yin deficiency

泻下剂 [xiè xià jì]

purgative formula: formula used for relieving constipation and purging various kinds of pathogenic factors from the interior of the body

寒下剂 [hán xià jì]

cold purgative formula: formula indicated in the treatment of interior accumulation and stagnation of heat

大承气汤 [dà chéng qì tāng]

***Da Chengqi* Decoction; Drastic Purgative Decoction:** a classical formula composed of 大黄 *Radix et Rhizoma Rhei*, 芒硝 *Natrii Sulfas*, 枳实 *Fructus Aurantii Immaturus* and 厚朴 *Cortex Magnoliae Officinalis*, used to purge the bowels drastically of accumulated heat in treating excess syndrome of *yangming fu*-syndrome, fecal impaction with watery discharge, excessive internal heat with heat syncope, convulsions or mania

小承气汤 [xiǎo chéng qì tāng]

***Xiao Chengqi* Decoction; Mild Purgative Decoction: a** classical formula composed of 大黄 *Radix et Rhizoma Rhei*, 枳实 *Fructus Aurantii Immaturus* and 厚朴 *Cortex Magnoliae Officinalis*, used to purge the bowels gently of accumulated heat

大黄牡丹汤 [dà huáng mǔ dān tāng]

***Dahuang Mudan* Decoction; Rhubarb-Peony Decoction:** a classical formula composed of 大黄 *Radix et Rhizoma Rhei*, 牡丹皮 *Cortex Moutan*, 桃仁 *Semen Persicae*, 冬瓜子 *Semen Benincasae Hispidae* and 芒硝 *Natrii Sulfas*, used to purge heat, break stasis and dissipate swelling for treating appendicitis at the early stage

温下剂 [wēn xià jì]

warm purgative formula: formula used for treating interior accumulation and stagnation of excessive cold

大黄附子汤 [dà huáng fù zǐ tāng]

***Dahuang Fuzi* Decoction; Rhubarb-Aconite Decoction:** a classical formula composed of 大黄 *Radix et Rhizoma Rhei*, 附子 *Radix Aconiti Lateralis Preparata* and 细辛 *Herba Asari*, used to warm the interior, dispel cold, move the bowels and alleviate pain for treating abdominal pain caused by accumulated cold

温脾汤 [wēn pí tāng]

***Wenpi* Decoction; Spleen-warming Decoction:** a formula composed of 大黄 *Radix et Rhizoma Rhei*, 当归 *Radix Angelicae Sinensis*, 干姜 *Rhizoma Zingiberis*, 附子 *Radix Aconiti Lateralis Preparata*, 人参 *Radix Ginseng*, 芒硝 *Natrii Sulfas* and 甘草 *Radix Glycyrrhizae*, used to drive away accumulated cold and warm-tonify the spleen for relieving abdominal pain caused by cold accumulation

润下剂 [rùn xià jì]

lubricant laxative formula: formula indicated in the relief of constipation caused by insufficiency of intestinal fluid

五仁丸 [wǔ rén wán]

Wuren Pill; Five-Seed Pill: a formula composed of 桃仁 *Semen*

Persicae, 杏仁 *Semen Armenicae,* 柏子仁 *Semen Platycladi*, 松子仁 *Semen Pini Tabulaeformis,* 郁李仁 *Semen Pruni* and 陈皮 *Pericarpium Citri Reticulatae*, used to moisten the intestines and move the bowels for relieving constipation caused by consumption of fluid

麻子仁丸 [má zǐ rén wán]

***Maziren* Pill; Hemp-seed Pill:** a formula composed of 麻子仁 *Fructus Cannabis*, 芍药 *Radix Paeoniae,* 枳实 *Fructus Aurantii Immaturus*, 大黄 *Radix et Rhizoma Rhei,* and 杏仁 *Semen Armenicae,* used to moisten the intestines, purge heat, promote *qi* flow and move the bowels for treating splenic constipation

脾约丸 [pí yuē wán]

another name of hemp-seed pill (麻子仁丸 [má zǐ rén wán])

逐水剂 [zhú shuǐ jì]

hydragogue formula: formula to expel retained fluid drastically, indicated in excess case of accumulation and retention of water in the interior

十枣汤 [shí zǎo tāng]

***Shizao* Decoction; Ten-Dates Decoction:** a formula composed of 甘遂 *Radix Euphorbiae Kansui*, 芫花 *Flos Genkwa* and 大戟 *Radix Euphorbiae* together with ten pieces of date, used to drive away retained fluid in cases of anasarca or pleural fluid retention

和解剂 [hé jiě jì]

harmonizing formula: formula that regulates the correlation of viscera, meridians, *qi* and blood, so as to remove pathogenic factors and restore normal functions

和解少阳剂 [hé jiě shào yáng jì]

***shaoyang*-harmonizing formula:** formula useful for treating cold pathogens in the *shaoyang* meridian, marked by alternate chills and fever, discomfort in the chest and hypochondriac region, loss of appetite, fidgetiness, nausea, dryness of the throat and bitterness in the mouth, dizziness and stringy pulse

小柴胡汤 [xiǎo chái hú tāng]

***Xiao Chaihu* Decoction; Minor [Mild] Bupleurum Decoction:** a classical formula composed of 柴胡 *Radix Bupleuri*, 黄芩 *Radix Scutellariae*, 大枣 *Fructus Ziziphi Jujubae*, 生姜 *Rhizoma Zingiberis Recens*, 制半夏 *Rhizoma Pinelliae Praeparata*, 甘草 *Radix Glycyrrhizae*

and 党参 *Radix Codonopsis Pilosulae*, used to harmonize *shaoyang* in the treatment of *shaoyang* syndrome in cases of cold-induced diseases and heat in a woman's blood chamber

蒿芩清胆汤 [hāo qín qīng dǎn tāng]

***Hao Qin Qingdan* Decoction; Arteminsia-Scutellaria Gallbladder-clearing Decoction:** a formula composed of 青蒿 *Herba Artemisiae Annuae*，竹茹 *Caulis Bambusae in Taeniam*，制半夏 *Rhizoma Pinelliae Praeparata*, 黄芩 *Radix Scutellariae*, 枳壳 *Fructus Aurantii,* 陈皮 *Pericarpium Citri Reticulatae* and 碧玉散 jasper powder, used for clearing the gallbladder, removing dampness, harmonizing the stomach and resolving phlegm in cases of *shaoyang* damp-heat syndrome

调和肝脾剂 [tiáo hé gān pí jì]

liver-spleen harmonizing formula: formula indicated in treating disharmony between the liver and spleen

四逆散 [sì nì sǎn]

***Sini* Powder; Counterflow-relieving Powder:** a formula composed of 柴胡 *Radix Bupleuri*, 白芍 *Radix Paeoniae Alba*, 枳实 *Fructus Aurantii Immaturus* and 甘草 *Radix Glycyrrhizae*, the principal formula for restoring the normal function of a depressed liver in which there is stagnancy of *qi* in the interior with coldness in the extremities, accompanied by costal or abdominal pain and menstrual complaints

逍遥散 [xiāo yáo sǎn]

***Xiaoyao* Powder; Carefree Powder:** a formula composed of 柴胡 *Radix Bupleuri*, 当归 *Radix Angelicae Sinensis*, 白芍 *Radix Paeoniae Alba*, 白术 *Rhizoma Atractylodis Macrocephalae*, 茯苓 *Poria*, 甘草 *Radix Glycyrrhizae*, 煨生姜 *Rhizoma Zingiberis Praeparata* and 薄荷 *Herba Menthae*, used to soothe the liver, relieve depression, nourish the blood and strengthen the spleen in treating a syndrome with depressed liver, deficient blood and weakened spleen

痛泻要方 [tòng xiè yào fāng]

***Tongxie Yaofang*; Important Formula for Painful Diarrhea:** a formula composed of 白术 *Rhizoma Atractylodis Macrocephalae*, 白芍 *Radix Paeoniae Alba*, 陈皮 *Pericarpium Citri Reticulatae* 防风 *Radix Saposhnikoviae*, used to tonify the spleen, mollify the liver and dispel dampness for stopping diarrhea associated with abdominal pain

调和寒热剂 [tiáo hé hán rè jì]

cold-heat harmonizing formula: formula indicated in the relief of binding of cold and heat in the middle energizer, marked by epigastric stuffiness, nausea, vomiting, borborygmus and diarrhea

半夏泻心汤 [bàn xià xiè xīn tāng]

Banxia Xiexin Decoction; Pinellia Heart-purging Decoction: a classical formula composed of 制半夏 *Rhizoma Pinelliae Praeparata,* 黄芩 *Radix Scutellariae*, 黄连 *Rhizoma Coptidis*, 干姜 *Rhizoma Zingiberis*, 人参 *Radix Ginseng,* 大枣 *Fructus Ziziphi Jujubae* and 甘草 *Radix Glycyrrhizae*, used to regulate cold and heat, and eliminate stuffiness

表里双解剂 [biǎo lǐ shuāng jiě jì]

exterior-interior releasing formula: formula that releases the exterior and interior simultaneously

大柴胡汤 [dà chái hú tāng]

***Da Chaihu* Decoction; Major Bupleurum Decoction:** a classical formula composed of 柴胡 *Radix Bupleuri*, 黄芩 *Radix Scutellariae*, 白芍 *Radix Paeoniae Alba*, 制半夏 *Rhizoma Pinelliae Praeparata,* 大黄 *Radix et Rhizoma Rhei*, 枳实 *Fructus Aurantii Immaturus*, 大枣 *Fructus Ziziphi Jujubae* and 生姜 *Rhizoma Zingiberis Recens*, used to treat combined syndrome of *shaoyang* and *yangming* meridians

防风通圣散 [fáng fēng tōng shèng sǎn]

***Fangfeng Tongsheng* Powder, Miraculous Powder of Saposhnikovia:** a formula composed of 防风 *Radix Saposhnikoviae*, 连翘 *Fructus Forsythiae*, 麻黄 *Herba Ephedrae*, 栀子 *Fructus Gardeniae*, 大黄 *Radix et Rhizoma Rhei*, 石膏 *Gypsum Fibrosum*, 黄芩 *Radix Scutellariae*, 白芍 *Radix Paeoniae Alba*, 川芎 *Rhizoma Chuanxiong*, etc., used to disperse wind and release the exterior, clear heat and move the bowels for the treatment of wind-heat affliction with excessiveness in both the exterior and interior

葛根黄芩黄连汤 [gě gēn huáng qín huáng lián tāng]

***Gegen Huangqi Huanglian* Decoction; Pueraria-Scutellaria-Coptis Decoction:** a formula composed of 葛根 *Radix Puerariae*, 黄芩 *Radix Scutellariae*, 黄连 *Rhizoma Coptidis* and 甘草 *Radix Glycyrrhizae*, used to release the exterior and clear the interior for treating dysentery with fever

清热剂 [qīng rè jì]

heat-clearing formula: any formula that is mainly composed of heat-clearing ingredients and used for clearing heat, purging fire, cooling the blood, or counteracting toxins

清气分热剂 [qīng qì fēn rè jì]

***qi*-phase heat-clearing formula:** formula used for treating febrile diseases at the *qi* stage marked by high fever, profuse sweating, dire thirst and gigantic surging pulse

白虎汤 [bái hǔ tāng]

***Baihu* Decoction; White Tiger Decoction:** a classical formula composed of 石膏 *Gypsum Fibrosum*, 知母 *Rhizoma Anemarrhenae*, 甘草 *Radix Glycyrrhizae*, and 粳米 *Semen Oryzae Nonglutinosae*, used to clear heat at the *qi* stage with high fever, dire thirst, sweating and gigantic full pulse

竹叶石膏汤 [chú yè shí gāo tāng]

***Zhuye Shigao* Decoction; Laphatherum-Gypsum Decoction:** a classical formula composed of 淡竹叶 *Herba Laphatheri*, 石膏 *Gypsum Fibrosum*, 麦冬 *Radix Ophiopogonis*, 半夏 *Rhizoma Pinelliae*, 人参 *Radix Ginseng* or 党参 *Radix Codonopsis Pilosulae*, 粳米 *Semen Oryzae Nonglutinosae* and 甘草 *Radix Glycyrrhizae*, used to clear heat, promote the production of fluid, replenish *qi*, and harmonize the stomach for the treatment of febrile diseases at the stage of restoration with lingering heat and impaired *qi* and body fluid

清营凉血剂 [qīng yíng liáng xuè jì]

nutrient-blood-phase heat-clearing formula: formula used in the treatment of febrile diseases at the nutrient or blood stage

清营汤 [qīng yíng tāng]

***Qingying* Decoction; Nutrient-clearing Decoction:** a formula composed of 水牛角 *Cornu Bubali,* 生地黄 *Radix Rehmanniae,* 元参 *Radix Scrophularlae,* **麦冬** *Radix Ophiopogonis,* 竹叶 *Herba Lophatheri,* 丹参 *Radix Salviae Miltiorrhizae,* 黄连 *Rhizoma Coptidis,* 银花 *Flos Lonicerae* and 连翘 *Fructus Forsythiae,* used for treating febrile diseases at the nutrient stage

犀角地黄汤 [xī jiǎo dì huáng tāng]

Xijiao Dihuang Decoction; Decoction of Rhinoceros Horn and Rehmannia: a formula composed of 水牛角 *Cornu Bubali,* 生地黄 *Radix Rehmanniae*, 赤芍 *Radix Paeoniae Rubra* and 牡丹皮 *Cortex Moutan*, used for treating febrile diseases at the blood stage

清热解毒剂 [qīng rè jiě dú jì]

heat-clearing toxin-counteracting formula: formula indicated in treating epidemic pestilence, toxic warm diseases, boils, sores, and abscesses

黄连解毒汤 [huáng lián jiě dú tāng]

***Huanglian Jiedu* Decoction; Detoxicant Coptis Decoction:** a formula composed of 黄连 *Rhizoma Coptidis*, 黄芩 *Radix Scutellariae*, 黄柏 *Cortex Phellodendri* and 栀子 *Fructus Gardeniae*, used to purge fire and counteract toxins for curing various pyogenic infections

普济消毒饮 [pǔ jì xiāo dú yǐn]

***Puji Xiaodu Yin*; Universal Antitoxic Decoction:** a formula composed of 黄芩 *Radix Scutellariae,* 黄连 *Rhizoma Coptidis,* 元参 *Radix Scrophularlae,* 柴胡 *Radix Bupleuri,* 连翘 *Fructus Forsythiae,* 桔梗 *Radix Platycodi,* 板蓝根 *Radix Isatidis,* 马勃 *Lasiosphaera seu Calvatia*， 升麻 *Rhizoma Cimicifugae,* 薄荷 *Herba Menthae,* etc., mainly used for the treatment of facial erysipelas

清脏腑热剂 [qīng zàng fǔ rè jì]

***zang-fu* heat-clearing formula:** formula that clears heat from a certain *zang-fu* organ

导赤散 [dǎo chì sǎn]

***Daochi* Powder; Redness-removing Powder:** a formula composed of 生地黄 *Radix Rehmanniae*, 竹叶 *Herba Lophatheri*, 木通 *Caulis Aristolochiae* and 甘草 *Radix Glycyrrhizae*, used to clear the heart, induce diuresis and nourish yin for treating fire syndrome of the heart meridian marked by oral ulceration or passage of reddened urine with pain

清胃散 [qīng wèi sǎn]

***Qingwei* Powder; Stomach-clearing Powder:** a formula composed of 黄连 *Rhizoma Coptidis*, 当归 *Radix Angelicae Sinensis*, 生地黄 *Radix Rehmanniae*, 升麻 *Rhizoma Cimicifugae* and 丹皮 *Cortex Moutan*, used to clear the stomach and cool the blood for relieving toothache caused by stomach fire

龙胆泻肝汤 [lóng dǎn xiè gān tāng]

***Longdan Xiegan* Decoction; Gentian Liver-purging Decoction:** a formula composed of 龙胆 *Radix Gentianae*, 黄芩 *Radix Scutellariae*, 栀子 *Fructus Gardeniae*, 泽泻 *Rhizoma Alismatis*, 关木通 *Caulis*

Aritolochiae Manshuriensis, 车前子 *Semen Plantaginis*, 当归 *Radix Angelicae Sinensis*, 生地黄 *Radix Rehmanniae*, 柴胡 *Radix Bupleuri* and 甘草 *Radix Glycyrrhizae*, used for clearing the liver and gallbladder fire and purging damp-heat from the lower energizer

泻白散 [xiè bái sǎn]

***Xiebai* Powder; Lung-purging Powder:** a formula composed of 地骨皮 *Cortex Lycii,* 桑白皮 *Cortex Mori,* and 甘草 *Radix Glycyrrhizae*, used to clear and purge the lung of heat for treating lung heat with cough and dyspnea, also called 泻肺散 [xiè fèi sǎn]

泻肺散 [xiè fèi sǎn]

a synonym for 泻白散 [xiè béi sǎn]

白头翁汤 [bái tóu wēng tāng]

***Baitouweng* Decoction; Pulsatilla Decoction:** a formula composed of 白头翁 *Radix Pulsatillae,* 黄连 *Rhizoma Coptidis,* 黄柏 *Cortex Phellodendri* and 秦皮 *Cortex Fraxini*, used to clear heat, counteract toxins and cool the blood for treating heat-toxic dysentery

清热祛暑剂 [qīng rè qù shǔ jì]

summerheat-clearing formula: formula that clears summer heat for treating heat syndromes occurring in summer

六一散 [liù yī sǎn]

Liu Yi Powder; Six-to-one Powder: a formula composed of 滑石 *Talcum* and 甘草 *Radix Glycyrrhizae* at a ratio of six to one in weight, used to relieve summer heat with damp

清虚热剂 [qīng xū rè jì]

deficiency-heat-clearing formula: formula indicated in the treatment of febrile diseases at the late stage with lingering pathogens and impaired yin fluid

青蒿鳖甲汤 [qīng hāo biē jiǎ tāng]

***Qinghao Biejia* Decoction; *Chinghao* and Turtle Shell Decoction:** a formula composed of 青蒿 *Herba Artemisiae Chinghao*, 鳖甲 *Carapax Trionycis*, 生地黄 *Radix Rehmanniae*, 知母 *Rhizoma Anemarrhenae*, 牡丹皮 *Cortex Moutan*, used to nourish yin and expel heat in the treatment of warm diseases at the late stage when the pathogens are hiding in the yin system

清骨散 [qīng gǔ sǎn]

***Qinggu* Powder; Bone-clearing Powder:** a formula composed of 银柴

胡 *Radix Stellariae,* 秦艽 *Radix Gentianae Macrophyllae,* 胡黄连 *Rhizoma Picrorhizae,* 青蒿 *Herba Artemisiae Chinghao,* 鳖甲 *Carapax Trionycis,* 地骨皮 *Cortex Lycii,* 青蒿 *Herba Artemisiae Chinghao,* 知母 *Rhizoma Anemarrhenae* and 甘草 *Radix Glycyrrhizae*, used to clear deficiency-heat in treating consumptive fever

温里剂 [wēn lǐ jì]

interior-warming formula: warming formula used for the treatment of interior cold

温中祛寒剂 [wēn zhōng qù hán jì]

center-warming cold-expelling formula: formula that warms the middle energizer and expels pathogenic cold for the treatment of deficiency-cold of the spleen and stomach

理中汤 [lǐ zhōng tāng]

***Lizhong* Decoction; Center-regulating Decoction:** a classical formula composed of 党参 *Radix Codonopsis Pilosulae*, 干姜 *Rhizoma Zingiberis*, 白术 *Rhizoma Atractylodis Macrocephalae* and 炙甘草 *Radix Glycyrrhizae Praeparata,* used to warm the middle energizer, dispel cold, replenish *qi* and strengthen the spleen in treating deficiency-cold of the spleen and stomach

小建中汤 [xiǎo jiàn zhōng tāng]

***Xian Jianzhong* Decoction; Minor Center-constructing Decoction:** a classical formula composed of 白芍 *Radix Paeoniae Alba*, 桂枝 *Ramulus Cinnamomi*, 炙甘草 *Radix Glycyrrhizae Praeparata*, 生姜 *Rhizoma Zingiberis Recens*, 大枣 *Fructus Ziziphi Jujubae* and 饴糖 malt extract, used for warming and tonifying the middle energizer and relieving spasmodic pains for the treatment of abdominal pain in deficiency conditions

吴茱萸汤 [wú zhū yú tāng]

***Wuzhuyu* Decoction; Evodia Decoction:** a classical formula composed of 吴茱萸 *Fructus Evodiae*, 人参 *Radix Ginseng* 大枣 *Fructus Ziziphi Jujubae* and 生姜 *Rhizoma Zingiberis Recens*, used to arrest deficiency-cold vomiting

回阳救逆剂 [huí yáng jiù nì jì]

yang-restoring emergency formula: formula for emergency treatment of failure of yang-*qi* with exuberant yin cold or even repelling of yang

祛寒剂 [qù hán jì]

cold-dispelling formula: formula composed chiefly of drugs warm or hot in property and indicated in the treatment of cold syndrome

四逆汤 [sì nì tāng]

***Sini* Decoction; Cold-extremities Decoction:** a formula composed of 制附子 *Radix Aconiti Lateralis Praeparata*, 干姜 *Rhizoma Zingiberis* and 炙甘草 *Radix Glycyrrhizae Praeparata*, used to restore yang from collapse or shock with cold limbs

温经散寒剂 [wēn jīng sàn hán jì]

meridian-warming cold-dispersing formula: formula that warms the meridians and disperses pathogenic cold for the treatment of blood blockage in the meridians

当归四逆汤 [dāng guī sì nì tāng]

***Danggui Sini* Decoction; Angelica Cold-extremities Decoction:** a classical formula composed of 当归 *Radix Angelicae Sinensis,* 桂枝 *Ramulus Cinnamomi,* 芍药 *Radix Paeoniae,* 细辛 *Herba Asari,* 炙甘草 *Radix Glycyrrhizae Praeparata,* 通草 *Medulla Tetrapanacis* and 大枣 *Fructus Ziziphi Jujubae*, used to warm the meridians, dispel cold, nourish the blood and unblock the vessels for treating blood deficiency with syncope

黄芪桂枝五物汤 [huáng qí guì zhī wǔ wù tāng]

***Huangqi Guizhi Wuwu* Decoction; Five-ingredient Decoction with Milkvetch and Cassia Twig:** a classical formula composed of 黄芪 *Radix Astragali*, 芍药 *Radix Paeoniae,* 桂枝 *Ramulus Cinnamomi*, 生姜 *Rhizoma Zingiberis Recens* and 大枣 *Fructus Ziziphi Jujubae*, used to replenish *qi*, warm the meridians, harmonize the blood and remove blockage for the treatment of numbness

阳和汤 [yáng hé tāng]

***Yanghe* Decoction; Yang-harmonizing Decoction:** a formula composed of 熟地黄 *Rhizoma Rehmanniae Praeparata,* 肉桂 *Cortex Cinnamomi,* 麻黄 *Herba Ephedrae,* 白芥子 *Semen Sinapis Albae,* 姜炭 *Rhizoma Zingiberis Carbonisatum* and 甘草 *Radix Glycyrrhizae,* used to warm yang, tonify the blood, dispel cold and remove stagnation for the treatment of yin cellulitis

补益剂 [bǔ yì jì]

tonifying formula: any formula that reinforces yang, replenishes *qi*, nourishes the blood or supplements yin in deficiency conditions

补气剂 [bǔ qì jì]

***qi*-tonifying formula:** formula that replenishes *qi*, mainly indicated in cases of deficiency of the lung *qi* or spleen *qi*

四君子汤 [sì jūn zǐ tāng]

***Sijunzi* Decoction; Decoction of Four Noble Ingredients:** a formula composed of 人参 *Radix Ginseng* or 党参 *Radix Codonopsis Pilosulae*, 茯苓 *Poria*, 白术 *Rhizoma Atractylodis Macrocephalae* and 炙甘草 *Radix Glycyrrhizae Praeparata*, the basic formula for replenishing *qi* and strengthening the spleen, used for treating *qi* deficiency of the spleen and stomach

参苓白术散 [shēn líng bǎi zhú sǎn]

***Shenling Baizhu* Powder; Ginseng-Poria-Atractylodes Powder:** a formula composed of 人参 *Radix Ginseng*, 茯苓 *Poria*, 白术 *Rhizoma Atractylodis Macrocephalae*, 山药 *Rhizoma Dioscoreae*, 莲子 *Semen Nelumbinis*, 砂仁 *Fructus Amomi*, etc., used for replenishing *qi*, strengthening the spleen, draining damp and arresting diarrhea, for the treatment of spleen insufficiency complicated by dampness

补中益气汤 [bǔ zhōng yì qì tāng]

***Buzhong Yiqi* Decoction; Center-tonifying *Qi*-replenishing Decoction:** a formula composed of 黄芪 *Radix Astragali*, 人参 *Radix Ginseng* or 党参 *Radix Codonopsis Pilosulae*, 当归 *Radix Angelicae Sinensis*, 陈皮 *Pericarpium Citri Reticulatae*, 甘草 *Radix Glycyrrhizae*, 白术 *Rhizoma Atractylodis Macrocephalae*, 升麻 *Rhizoma Cimicifugae* and 柴胡 *Radix Bupleuri*, used to tonify the middle energizer, replenish *qi* and elevate yang for treating deficiency of spleen and stomach *qi*, sinking of *qi*, and fever in *qi* deficiency

玉屏风散 [yù píng fēng sǎn]

***Yupingfeng* Powder; Jade-Screen Powder:** formula composed of 黄芪 *Radix Astragali*, 白术 *Rhizoma Atractylodis Macrocephalae*, and 防风 *Radix Saposhnikoviae*, used to replenish *qi,* consolidate the superficies and check perspiration for treating superficial deficiency with spontaneous sweating

补血剂 [bǔ xuè jì]

blood-tonifying formula: formula suitable for treating blood deficiency

四物汤 [sì wù tāng]

***Siwu* Decoction; Four-Drug Decoction:** a formula composed of 熟地黄

Radix Rehmanniae Praeparata, 白芍 *Radix Paeoniae Alba*, 当归 *Radix Angelicae Sinensis* and 川芎 *Rhizoma Chuanxiong*, used to tonify and harmonize the blood for the treatment of deficiency and stagnation of nutrient-blood

当归补血汤 [dāng guī bǔ xuè tāng]

Danggui Buxue **Decoction; Angelica Blood-tonifying Decoction:** a formula composed of 当归 *Radix Angelicae Sinensis*, and 黄芪 *Radix Astragali*, used to replenish *qi* and promote blood production for the treatment of blood deficiency with fever

归脾汤 [guī pí tāng]

Guipi **Decoction; Spleen-restoring Decoction:** a formula composed of 党参 *Radix Codonopsis Pilosulae*, 白术 *Rhizoma Atractylodis Macrocephalae*, 黄芪 *Radix Astragali*, 茯神 *Poria cum Radice Pino*, 炙甘草 *Radix Glycyrrhizae Praeparata*, 当归 *Radix Angelicae Sinensis*, 酸枣仁 *Semen Ziziphi Spinosae*, 龙眼肉 *Arillus Longan*, 远志 *Radix Polygalae*, 木香 *Radix Aucklandiae*, 生姜 *Rhizoma Zingiberis Recens* and 大枣 *Fructus Ziziphi Jujubae*, used to replenish *qi*, tonify the blood, strengthen the spleen and nourish the heart, for treating deficiency of spleen *qi* and heart blood, and also for treating failure of the spleen to control the blood

气血双补剂 [qì xuè shuāng bǔ jì]

***qi*-blood tonifying formula:** formula that tonifies both *qi* and blood for the treatment of dual *qi*-blood deficiency

八珍汤 [bā zhēn tāng]

Bazhen **Decoction, Eight-Treasure Decoction:** a formula composed of 人参 *Radix Ginseng* or 党参 *Radix Codonopsis Pilosulae*, 白术 *Rhizoma Atractylodis Macrocephalae*, 茯苓 *Poria*, 甘草 *Radix Glycyrrhizae*, 当归 *Radix Angelicae Sinensis*, 白芍 *Radix Paeoniae Alba*, 川芎 *Rhizoma Chuanxiong* and 熟地黄 *Rhizoma Rehmanniae Praeparata*, used for replenishing *qi* and tonifying blood in the treatment of dual *qi*-blood deficiency

十全大补汤 [shí quán dà bǔ tāng]

Shiquan Dabu **Decoction; All-inclusive Grand Tonic Decoction:** a formula composed of 人参 *Radix Ginseng* or 党参 *Radix Codonopsis Pilosulae*, 白术 *Rhizoma Atractylodis Macrocephalae*, 茯苓 *Poria*, 甘草 *Radix Glycyrrhizae*, 当归 *Radix Angelicae Sinensis*, 白芍 *Radix*

Paeoniae Alba, 川芎 *Rhizoma Chuanxiong*, 熟地黄 *Rhizoma Rehmanniae Praeparata*, 肉桂 *Cortex Cinnamomi* and 黄芪 *Radix Astragali*, used for warming and tonifying *qi* and blood in cases of general debility with dual *qi*-blood deficiency

补阴剂 [bǔ yīn jì]

yin-replenishing formula: formula indicated in the treatment of yin deficiency

六味地黄丸 [liù wèi dì huáng wán]

Liuwei Dihuang Pill; Six-Ingredient Rehmannia Pill: a formula composed of 熟地黄 *Radix Rehmanniae Praeparata*, 山茱萸 *Fructus Corni*, 山药 *Rhizoma Dioscoreae*, 泽泻 *Rhizoma Alismatis*, 茯苓 *Poria* and 牡丹皮 *Cortex Moutan*, used to nourish and tonify the liver and kidney in the treatment of kidney yin deficiency, originally called *Dihuang* Pill, Rehmannia Pill (地黄丸 [dì háung wán])

地黄丸 [dì háung wán]

Dihuang Pill; Rehmannia Pill: another name for *Liuwei Dihuang* Pill; Six-ingredient Rehmannia Pill (六味地黄丸 [liù wèi dì huáng wán])

左归丸 [zuǒ guī wán]

***Zuo Gui* Pill; Yin-restoring Pill:** a formula composed of 熟地黄 *Radix Rehmanniae Praeparata*, 山药 *Rhizoma Dioscoreae*, 山茱萸 *Fructus Corni*, 枸杞子 *Fructus Lycii*, 菟丝子 *Semen Cuscuta*, 川牛膝 *Radix Cyathulae*, 鹿角胶 *Colla Cornus Cervi* and 龟板胶 *Colla Plastri Testudinis*, used to nourish yin and tonify the kidney for the treatment of kidney yin deficiency

一贯煎 [yī guàn jiān]

Yiguan Jian; Ever-Effective Decoction: a formula composed of 沙参 *Radix Glehniae*, 麦冬 *Radix Ophiopogonis*, 生地黄 *Radix Rehmanniae*, 当归 *Radix Angelicae Sinensis*, 枸杞子 *Fructus Lycii*, and 川楝子 *Fructus Toosendan*, used to nourish yin and soothe the liver for the treatment of yin deficiency of the liver and kidney with restraint of liver *qi*

补阳剂 [bǔ yáng jì]

yang-tonifying formula: formula used for treating deficiency of yang-qi

肾气丸 [shèn qì wán]

***Shenqi* Pill; Kidney *Qi* Pill:** a classical formula composed of 附子 *Radix Aconiti Lateralis Praeparata*, 肉桂 *Cortex Cinnamomi*, 熟地黄

Radix Rehmanniae Praeparata, 山茱萸 *Fructus Corni*, 山药 *Rhizoma Dioscoreae*, 泽泻 *Rhizoma Alismatis*, 茯苓 *Poria* and 牡丹皮 *Cortex Moutan*, used to tonify the kidney and support yang for the treatment of kidney yang deficiency

右归丸 [yòu guī wán]

***You Gui* Pill; Yang-restoring Pill:** formula composed of 熟地黄 *Radix Rehmanniae Praeparata*, 山茱萸 *Fructus Corni*, 山药 *Rhizoma Dioscoreae*, 枸杞子 *Fructus Lycii*, 菟丝子 *Semen Cuscuta*, 鹿角胶 *Colla Cornus Cervi*, 杜仲 *Cortex Eucommiae*, 肉桂 *Cortex Cinnamomi*, 当归 *Radix Angelicae Sinensis* and 附子 *Radix Aconiti Lateralis Preparata*, used to warm and tonify kidney yang for the treatment of kidney yang deficiency with decline of the life fire

阴阳并补剂 [yīn yáng bìng bǔ jì]

simultaneous yin-yang tonifying formula: formula that tonifies yin and yang simultaneously, suitable for treating deficiency of both yin and yang

龟鹿二仙胶 [guī lù èr xiān jiāo]

***Gui Lu Erxian* Glue; Two-elixir Glue of Tortoise Plastron and Deer Horn:** a formula composed of 鹿角, *Cornu Cervi*, 龟板 *Plastron Testudinis*, 人参 *Radix Ginseng* and 枸杞子 *Fructus Lycii*, used to nourish yin, supplement essence, replenish *qi* and invigorate yang

二仙汤 [èr xiān tāng]

***Erxian* Decoction; Two-elixir Decoction:** a formula composed of 仙茅 *Rhizoma Curculiginis*, 仙灵脾 *Herba Epimedii*, 巴戟天 *Radix Morindae Officinalis*, 当归 *Radix Angelicae Sinensis*, 黄柏 *Cortex Phellodendri* and 知母 *Rhizoma Anemarrhenae*, used to tonify both yin and yang of the kidney for the treatment of menopausal syndrome and hypertension

固涩剂 [gù sè jì]

astringent formula: formula that arrests discharges, including excessive perspiration, persistent diarrhea, seminal emission, incontinence of urine, profuse uterine bleeding and leukorrhea

固表止汗剂 [gù biǎo zhǐ hàn jì]

superficies-consolidating sweating-arresting formula: formula that consolidates the superficies and arrests excessive sweating, for strengthening the superficial body resistance

牡蛎散 [mǔ lì sǎn]

***Muli* Powder; Ostrea Powder:** a formula composed of 黄芪 *Radix*

Astragali, 麻黄根 *Radix Ephedrae*, and 牡蛎 *Concha Ostreae,* used to replenish *qi* and consolidate the superficies, and astringe yin for arresting spontaneous sweating and night sweats

敛肺止咳剂 [liǎn fèi zhǐ ké jì]

lung-astringing antitussive formula: formula to stop coughing by astringing the lung

涩肠固脱剂 [sè cháng gù tuō jì]

intestine-astringing antidiarrheal formula: formula to check protracted diarrhea by astringing the intestines

四神丸 [sì shén wán]

***Sishen* Pill; Four-miracle Pill:** a formula composed of 补骨脂 *Fructus Psoraleae*, 五味子 *Fructus Schisandrae*, 肉豆蔻 *Semen Myristicae* and 吴茱萸 *Fructus Evodiae*, used to warm the kidney and spleen, and astringe the intestines for relieving diarrhea daily before dawn

涩精止遗剂 [sè jīng zhǐ yí jì]

semen-astringing enuresis-checking formula: astringent formula to check seminal emission or involuntary discharge of urine

固精丸 [gù jīng wán]

Gujing Pill; Semen-securing Pill: a formula composed of 潼蒺藜 *Semen Astragali Complanati*, 芡实 *Semen Euryales*, 莲须 *Stamen Nelumbinis*, 煅龙骨 *Os Draconis Usta* and 煅牡蛎 *Concha Ostreae Usta*, used for treating nocturnal and spontaneous emission due to kidney insufficiency, also called 金锁固精丸 [jīn suǒ gù jīng wán]

金锁固精丸 [jīn suǒ gù jīng wán]

***Jinsuo Gujing* Pill; Golden-lock Semen-securing Pill:** another name for Gujing Pill, Semen-securing Pill (固精丸 [gù jīng wán])

缩泉丸 [suō niào wán]

***Suoquan* Pill; Stream-reducing Pill:** a formula composed of 乌药 *Radix Linderae* and 益智仁 *Semen Alpiniae Oxyphyllae*, used to warm the kidney, dispel cold, reduce urination and check involuntary discharge of urine in cases of deficiency-cold of the bladder

理气剂 [lǐ qì jì]

***qi*-regulating formula:** formula that regulates and normalizes the flow of *qi*

行气剂 [xíng qì jì]

***qi*-moving formula:** formula that facilitates the smooth movement of *qi*, indicated in relieving stagnation or retardation of *qi* flow

瓜蒌薤白半夏汤 [guā lóu xiè bái bàn xià tāng]

***Gualou Xiebai Banxia* Decoction; Trichosanthes-Allium-Pinellia Decoction:** a classical formula composed of 瓜蒌 *Fructus Trichosanthis*, 薤白 *Bulbus Allii Macrostemi*, 白酒 *Spiritus* and 制半夏 *Rhizoma Pinelliae Praeparata*, used for relieving chest pain due to *qi* obstruction with phlegm, such as angina pectoris

半夏厚朴汤 [bàn xià hòu pò tāng]

Banxia Houpo* Decoction; Pinellia-Magnolia Decoction:** a classical formula composed of 制半夏 *Rhizoma Pinelliae Praeparata,* 厚朴 *Cortex Magnoliae Officinalis,* 茯苓 *Poria,* 生姜 *Rhizoma Zingiberis Recens* and 紫苏叶 *Folium Perillae,** used for moving *qi,* dissipating nodulation and resolving phlegm in the treatment of globus hystericus

良附丸 [liáng fù wán]

***Liang Fu* Pill; Alpinia-Cyperus Pill:** a formula composed of 高良姜 *Rhizoma Alpiniae Officinarum* and 香附 *Rhizoma Cyperi*, used to move *qi,* soothe the liver and dispel cold, for relieving epigastric, hypochondriac and abdominal pain due to *qi* congealed by cold

金铃子散 [jīn líng zǐ sǎn]

***Jinlingzi* Powder; Toosendan Powder:** a formula composed of 金铃子 *Fructus Toosendan* and 玄胡索 *Rhizoma Corydalis*, used to soothe the liver, purge heat, activate the blood and alleviate pain, for treating fire transformation of the depressed liver

暖肝煎 [nuǎn gān jiān]

***Nuangan* Decoction; Liver-warming Decoction:** a formula composed of 当归 *Radix Angelicae Sinensis*, 枸杞子 *Fructus Lycii*, 小茴香 *Fructus Foeniculi*, 肉桂 *Cortex Cinnamomi*, 乌药 *Radix Linderae*, 沉香 *Lignum Aquilariae Resinatum* and 茯苓 *Poria*, used to warm and tonify the liver and kidney, move *qi* and alleviate pain for the treatment of deficiency-cold of the liver and kidney with testicular or lower abdominal pain

加味乌药汤 [jiā wèi wū yào tāng]

Jiawei Wuyao Decoction; Supplemented Lindera Decoction: a formula composed of 乌药 *Radix Linderae*, 砂仁 *Fructus Amomi*, 延胡索 *Rhizoma Corydalis*, 香附 *Rhizoma Cyperi*, 香附 *Rhizoma Cyperi*, 木香 *Radix Aucklandiae*, and 甘草 *Radix Glycyrrhizae*, used to move *qi,* activate the blood, regulate menstruation and alleviate pain for treating dysmenorrhea

降气剂 [jiàng qì jì]

***qi*-descending formula:** formula that brings down the upward adverse flow of *qi,* usually for relieving asthma or vomiting

定喘汤 [dìng chuǎn tāng]

***Dingchuan* Decoction; Asthma-arresting Decoction:** a formula composed of 白果 *Semen Ginkgo,* 麻黄 *Herba Ephedrae,* 桑白皮 *Cortex Mori Radicis,* 苏子 *Fructus Perillae,* 苦杏仁 *Semen Armenizacae Amarum,* 黄芩 *Radix Scutellariae,* 款冬花 *Flos Farfarae,* 制半夏 *Phizoma Pinelliae Preparata* and 甘草 *Radix Glycyrrhizae*, used for relieving asthma with heat and phlegm

旋复代赭汤 [xuán fù dài zhě tāng]

***Xuanfu* Daizhe Decoction; Inula-Haematite Decoction:** a classical formula composed of 旋复花 *Flos Inulae*, 赭石 *Haematitum*, 生姜 *Rhizoma Zingiberis Recens*, 制半夏 *Rhizoma Pinelliae Praeparata*, 炙甘草 *Radix Glycyrrhizae Praeparata*, 大枣 *Fructus Ziziphi Jujubae* and 党参 *Radix Codonopsis Pilosulae*, used to relieve nausea and arrest vomiting due to dysfunction of the stomach with retention of phlegm

丁香柿蒂汤 [dīng xiāng shì dì tāng]

***Dingxiang Shidi* Decoction; Decoction of Cloves and Persimon Calyx:** a formula composed of 丁香 *Flos Caryophylli*, 柿蒂 *Calyx Kaki*, 人参 *Radix Ginseng* and 生姜 *Rhizoma Zingiberis Recens*, used to warm the middle, replenish *qi,* and bring down the upward reverse flow of *qi* for stopping deficiency-cold hiccups

橘皮竹茹汤 [jú pí zhú rú tāng]

***Jupi Zhuru* Decoction; Decoction of Tangerine Peel and Bamboo Shavings:** a formula composed of 橘皮 *Pericarpium Citri Reticulatae,* 竹茹 *Caulis Bambusae in Taeniam*, 生姜 *Rhizoma Zingiberis Recens,* 甘草 *Radix Glycyrrhizae*, 人参 *Radix Ginseng*, and 大枣 *Fructus Ziziphi Jujubae*, used to bring down the upward reversed flow of *qi* for stopping stomach-heat hiccups

理血剂 [lǐ xuè jì]

blood-regulating formula: any formula that regulates the blood, including blood-tonifying formula, blood-activating and stasis-removing formula, and hemostatic formula

活血祛瘀剂 [huó xuè qù yū jì]

blood-activating and stasis-removing formula: formula that activates the blood flow and removes blood stasis, indicated in various conditions of blood aggregation and stagnation

血府逐瘀汤 [xuè fǔ zhú yū tāng]

***Xuefu Zhuyu* Decoction; Thoracic Stasis-expelling Decoction:** a formula composed of 当归 *Radix Angelicae Sinensis*, 赤芍 *Radix Paeoniae Rubra*, 生地黄 *Radix Rehmanniae*, 川芎 *Rhizoma Ligustici Chuanxiong*, 桃仁 *SemenPersicae*, 红花 *Flos Carthami*, 柴胡 *Radix Bupleuri*, 枳壳 *Fructus Aurantii*, 桔梗 *Radix Platycodi*, 甘草 *Radix Glycyrrhizae* and 牛膝 *Radix Achyranthis Bidentatae*, used to activate the blood, remove stasis, move *qi* and alleviate pain for the treatment of blood stasis in the chest

补阳还五汤 [bǔ yáng huán wǔ tāng]

***Buyang Huanwu* Decoction; Yang-tonifying Five-tenths-restoring Decoction:** a formula composed of 黄芪 *Radix Astragali*, 当归 *Radix Angelicae Sinensis*, 赤芍 *Radix Paeoniae Rubra*, 川芎 *Rhizoma Chuanxiong*, 桃仁 *Semen Persicae*, 红花 *Flos Carthami* and 地龙 *Lumbricus*, used to supplement *qi*, activate the blood and unblock collateral meridians for treating post-apoplectic hemiplegia

生化汤 [shēng huà tāng]

***Shenghua* Decoction; Generation and Resolution Decoction:** a formula composed of 当归 *Radix Angelicae Sinensis*, 川芎 *Rhizoma Chuanxiong*, 桃仁 *Semen Persicae*, 炮姜 *Rhizoma Zingiberis Praeparata* and 炙甘草 *Radix Glycyrrhizae Praeparata*, used to resolve blood stasis, generate new blood, warm meridians and alleviate pain for the treatment of retention of lochia and lower abdominal pain after childbirth

止血剂 [zhǐ xuè jì]

styptic formula: formula that checks bleeding

小蓟饮子 [xiǎo jì yǐn zi]

***Xiaoji Yinzi*; Cirsium Decoction:** a formula composed of 生地黄 *Radix Rehmanniae*, 小蓟 *Herba Cirsii*, 滑石 *Pulvis Talci*, 木通 *Caulis Aristolochiae Manshuriensis*, 炒蒲黄 *Pollen Typhae Carbonizatum*, 藕节 *Nodus Nelumbinis Rhizomatis*, 淡竹叶 *Herba Lophatheri*, 当归 *Radix Angelicae Sinensis*, 栀子 *Fructus Gardeniae* and 甘草 *Radix*

Glycyrrhizae, used to cool the blood, check bleeding, induce diuresis and relieve stranguria in treating hematuria and bloody stranguria

黄土汤 [huáng tǔ tāng]

***Huangtu* Decoction; Oven-earth Decoction:** a formula composed of 甘草 *Radix Glycyrrhizae*， 地黄 *Radix Rehmanniae,* 白术 *Rhizoma Atractylodis Macrocephalae*, 附子 *Radix Aconiti Lateralis Praeparata*, 黄芩 *Radix Scutellariae* and 灶心土 *Terra Flava Usta,* used to check hematochezia in cases of yang deficiency

治风剂 [zhì fēng jì]

wind-treating formula: formula that dispels or extinguishes pathogenic wind, either exogenous or endogenous

疏散外风剂 [shū sàn wài fēng jì]

exogenous-wind-dispersing formula: formula that disperses exogenous wind, used for treating various external wind afflictions

独活寄生汤 [dú huó jì shēng tāng]

***Duhuo Jisheng* Decoction; Pubescent Angelica and Loranthus Decoction:** a formula composed of 独活 *Radix Angelicae Pubescentis*, 桑寄生 *Ramulus Taxilli*, 川芎 *Rhizoma Chuanxiong*, 细辛 *Herba Asari*, 秦艽 *Radix Gentianae Macrophyllae*, 防风 *Radix Saposhnikoviae*, 牛膝 *Radix Achyranthis Bidentatae*, 杜仲 *Cortex Eucommiae*, 当归 *Radix Angelicae sinensis*, 白芍 *Radix Paeoniae Alba*, 熟地黄 *Radix Rehmanniae Praeparata*, 茯苓 *Poria*, 党参 *Radix Codonopsis Pilosulae*, 桂枝 *Ramulus Cinnamomi* and 甘草 *Radix Glycyrrhizae,* used to dispel wind-damp, tonify the liver and the kidney, replenish *qi* and blood, and relieve arthralgia for treating chronic rheumatic or rheumatoid troubles

牵正散 [qiān zhèng sǎn]

***Qianzheng* Powder; Pulling-aright Powder:** a formula composed of 白附子 Rhizoma Typhonii, 白僵蚕 *Bombyx Batryticatus* and 全蝎 *Scorpio*, used for treating facial paralysis

平熄内风剂 [píng xī nèi fēng jì]

endogenous-wind-extinguishing formula: formula used for treating endogenous wind, also called wind-extinguishing formula for short

熄风剂 [xī fēng jì]

wind-extinguishing formula: abbreviation of endogenous-wind-extinguishing formula (平熄内风剂 [píng xī nèi fēng jì])

天麻钩藤饮 [tiān má gōu téng yǐn]

***Tianma Gouteng Yin*; Gastrodia-Uncaria Decoction:** a formula composed of 天麻 *Rhizoma Gastrodiae*, 钩藤 *Ramulus Uncariae cum Uncis*, 生石决明 *Concha Hallotidis*, 桑寄生 *Ramulus Taxilli*, 杜仲 *Cortex Eucommiae*, 栀子 *Fructus Gardeniae*, 黄芪 *Radix Astragali*, 牛膝 *Radix Achyranthis Bidentatae*, 益母草 *Herba Leonuri*, 茯神 *Poria cum Radice Pino* and 首乌藤 *Caulis Polygoni Multiflori*, used to pacify the liver, extinguish wind, clear heat, activate the blood and tonify the liver and kidney for treating exuberant liver yang with embarrassing wind

治燥剂 [zhì zào jì]

dryness-treating formula: formula that relieves dryness syndromes, either exogenous or endogenous

轻宣外燥剂 [qīng xuān wài zào jì]

exogenous-dryness-dispersing formula: formula used for the treatment of externally contracted cool dryness or warm dryness

杏苏散 [xìng sū sǎn]

***Xing Su* Powder; Apricot-Seed and Perilla-Leaf Powder:** a formula composed of 苦杏仁 *Semen Armeniacae Amarum,* 紫苏叶 *Folium Perillae* 半夏 *Rhizoma Pinelliae,* 前胡 *Radix Peucedani,* 桔梗 *Radix Platycodi,* 茯苓 *Poria,* 枳壳 *Fructus Aurantii,* 陈皮 *Pericarpium Citri Reticulatae,* 甘草 *Radix Glycyrrhizae,* 生姜 *Rhizoma Zingiberis Recens* and 大枣 *Fructus Ziziphi Jujubae,* used to treat externally contracted cool-dryness

清燥救肺汤 [qīng zào jiù fèi tāng]

***Qingzao Jiufei* Decoction; Dryness-clearing Lung-saving Decoction:** a formula composed of 桑叶 *Folium Mori*，石膏 *Gypsum Fibrosum,* 甘草 *Radix Glycyrrhizae,* 人参 *Radix Ginseng*，阿胶 *Colla Corii Asini,* 麦冬 *Radix Ophiopogonis,* 杏仁 *Semen Armeniacae Amarum* and 枇杷叶 *Folium Eriobotryae,* used to clear dryness and moisten the lung for the treatment of warm-dryness damage to the lung

滋阴润燥剂 [zī yīn rùn zào jì]

yin-nourishing moistening formula: formula used for treating internal dryness due to fluid consumption in the *zang-fu* organs

麦门冬汤 [mài mén dōng tāng]

***Maimendong Decoction;* Ophiopogon Decoction:** a formula composed of 麦冬 *Radix Ophiopogonis*, 半夏 *Rhizoma Pinelliae,* 人参、*Radix Ginseng*，甘草 *Radix Glycyrrhizae*, 大枣 *Fructus Ziziphi Jujubae* and non-glutinous rice, used to moisten the lung for treating lung atrophy

养阴清肺汤 [yǎng yīn qīng fèi tāng]

***Yangyin Qingfei* Decoction; Yin-nourishing and Lung-clearing Decoction:** a formula composed of 生地黄 *Radix Rehmanniae*, 麦冬 *Radix Ophiopogonis*, 玄参 *Radix Scrophulariae*, 牡丹皮 *Cortex Moutan*, 川贝母 *Bulbus Fritillariae Cirrhosae*, 甘草 *Radix Glycyrrhizae*, 薄荷 *Herba Menthae* and 白芍 *Radix Paeoniae Alba*, used for nourishing yin, clearing the lung, counteracting toxins and soothing the throat, and particularly for treating diphtheria

祛湿剂 [qù shī jì]

damp-dispelling formula: formula that has the effect of resolving damp, removing water and relieving stranguria, for the treatment of water-damp ailments

化湿和胃剂 [huà shī hé wèi jì]

damp-resolving stomach-pacifying formula: formula for relieving internal accumulation of damp-turbidity with disharmony of the spleen and stomach

平胃散 [píng wèi sǎn]

***Pingwei* Powder; Stomach-pacifying Powder:** a formula composed of 苍术 *Rhizoma Atractylodis,* 厚朴 *Cortex Magnoliae Officinalis,* 陈皮 *Pericarpium Citri Reticulatae* and 甘草 *Radix Glycyrrhizae,* used to dry dampness, invigorate the spleen and harmonize the stomach for treating damp stagnation in the spleen and stomach

藿香正气散 [huò xiāng zhèng qì sǎn]

***Huoxiang Zhenqi* Powder; Health-restoring Agastache Powder:** a formula composed of 藿香 *Herba Agastachis*, 紫苏叶 *Folium Perillae*, 白芷 *Radix Angelicae Dahuricae*, 大腹皮 *Pericarpium Arecae*, 茯苓 **Poria**, 白术 *Rhizoma Atractylodis Macrocephalae* or 苍术 *Rhizoma Atractylodis*, 陈皮 *Pericarpium Citri Reticulatae*, 半夏曲 *Massa Pinelliae Fermentata*, 厚朴 *Cortex Magnoliae Officinalis*, 桔梗 *Radix Platycodi* and 甘草 *Radix Glycyrrhizae*, used for treating wind-cold affliction with internal stagnation of dampness

清热祛湿剂 [qīng rè qù shī jì]

heat-clearing damp-dispelling formula: formula used to treat damp-heat, externally contracted, internally exuberant or downward pouring

茵陈蒿汤 [yīn chén hāo tāng]

***Yinchenhao* Decoction; Oriental Wormwood Decoction:** a classical formula composed of 茵陈 *Herba Artemisiae Scopariae*, 栀子 *Fructus Gardeniae* and 大黄 *Radix et Rhizoma Rhei*, used to clear heat, remove damp and relieve icterus for the treatment of damp-heat jaundice

五苓散 [wǔ líng sǎn]

***Wuling* Powder; Powder of Five Drugs with Poria:** a formula composed of 茯苓 *Poria*, 猪苓 *Polypolus umbellatus*, 白术 *Rhizoma Atractylodis Macrocephalae*, 泽泻 *Rhizoma Alismatis* and 桂枝 *Ramulus Cinna-momi*, commonly used to induce diuresis for treating various kinds of edema and oliguria

消食剂 [xiāo shí jì]

digestant formula: formula to promote digestion and remove stagnated food

保和丸 [bǎo hé wán]

***Baohe* Pill; Lenitive Pill:** a formula composed of 山楂 *Fructus Crataegi*, 神曲 *Massa Fermentata Medicinalis*, 莱服子 *Semen Raphani*, 茯苓 *Poria*, 陈皮 *Pericarpium Citri Reticulatae*, 半夏 *Rhizoma Pinelliae* and 连翘 *Fructus Forsythiae*, used to remove stagnated food and harmonize the stomach for the treatment of dyspepsia

祛痰剂 [qù tán jì]

phlegm-expelling formula: formula used for expelling or dissipating phlegm

二陈汤 [èr chén tāng]

***Erchen* Decoction; Decoction of Two Old Drugs:** a formula composed of 陈皮 *Pericarpium Citri Reticulatae*, 制半夏 *Rhizoma Pinelliae Praeparata*, 茯苓 *Poria* and 炙甘草 *Radix Glycyrrhizae Praeparata*, used to resolve phlegm by drying internal dampness and regulating the function of the spleen and the stomach for the treatment of damp-phlegm syndromes

真武汤 [zhēn wǔ tāng]

***Zhenwu* Decoction:** a formula composed of 茯苓 *Poria*,白术 *Rhizoma Atractylodis Macrocephalae*, 白芍 *Radix Paeoniae Alba*, 生姜 *Rhizoma Zingiberis Recens* and 制附子 *Radix Aconiti Lateralis Praeparata*, used to relieve water retention by invigorating the kidney and the spleen, indicated in the treatment of edema and prolonged diarrhea (Zhenwu supposedly being the god who controls water)

八正散 [bā zhèng sǎn]

***Bazheng* Powder; Eight-ingredient Rectification Powder:** a formula composed of 车前子 *Semen Plantaginis*, 关木通 *Caulis Aristolochiae Manshuriensis*, 瞿麦 *Herba Dianthi*, 萹蓄 *Herba Polygoni Avicularis*, 滑石 *Pulvis Talci*, 甘草 *Radix Glycyrrhizae*, 栀子 *Fructus Gardeniae*, 熟大黄 *Radix et Rhizoma Rhei Praeparata* and 灯芯草 *Medulla Junci*, used to clear evil heat and dispel dampness by promoting urination for the treatment of damp-heat stranguria

安神剂 [ān shén jì]

sedative or tranquilizing formula: formula that causes sedation or tranquilization

重镇安神剂 [zhòng zhèn ān shén jì]

settling tranquilizing formula: formula that causes sedation by using ingredients heavy in weight, and is indicated for treating exuberant heart yang or fire, manifested by insomnia, fidgetiness, palpitation or even epilepsy

朱砂安神丸 [zhū shā ān shén wán]

***Zhusha Anshen* Pill; Cinnabar Tranquilizing Pill:** a formula composed of 朱砂 *Cinnabaris*, 黄连 *Rhizoma Coptidis*, 炙甘草 *Radix Glycyrrhizae Preparata*, 当归 *Radix Angelicae Sinensis* and 生地黄 *Radix Rehmanniae*, used in the treatment of exuberant heart fire with deficiency of yin-blood marked by insomnia, fidgetiness and palpitation

磁朱丸 [cí zhū wán]

***Ci Zhu* Pill; Cinnabar-Magnetite Pill:** a formula composed of 朱砂 *Cinnabaris*, and 磁石 *Magnetitum*, used for treating disharmony between the heart and kidney with insomnia and palpitation, and also for epilepsy

补养安神剂 [bǔ yǎng ān shén jì]

tonifying tranquilizing formula: tranquilizing formula used in treating blood deficiency of the heart and liver marked by insomnia, palpitation, fidgetiness and forgetfulness

酸枣仁汤 [suān zǎo rén tāng]

***Suanzaoren* Decoction; Spiny Jujube Seed Decoction:** aformula composed of 酸枣仁 *Semen Ziziphi Spinosae*, 知母 *Rhizoma Anemarrhenae*, 茯苓 *Poria*, 川芎 *Rhizoma Chuanxiong*, and 炙甘草 *Radix Glycyrrhizae Praeparata*, used to nourish the blood, clear heat and cause tranquilization for treating insomnia with fidgetiness

甘麦大枣汤 [gān mài dà zǎo tāng]

Gan Mai Dazao **Decoction; Decoction of Liquorice, Wheat and Jujube:** a formula composed of 炙甘草 *Radix Glycyrrhizae Praeparata*, 大枣 *Fructus Ziziphi Jujubae* and 浮小麦 *Fructus Tritici Levis*), used as a tranquilizer especially for treating hysteria

成药 Patent Medicines

感冒清热冲剂 [gǎn mào qīng rè chōng jì]

Ganmao Qingre **Granules; Antipyretic Granules for Colds:** granules for infusion prepared from 荆芥穗 *Spica Schizonepetae*, 薄荷 *Herba Menthae*, 防风 *Radix Saposhnikoviae*, 柴胡 *Radix Bupleuri*, 紫苏叶 *Folium Perillae*, 葛根 *Radix Puerariae*, 桔梗 *Radix Platycodi*, 苦杏仁 *Semen Armeniacae Amarum*, 白芷 *Radix Angelicae Dahuricae*, 苦地丁 *Herba Corydalis Bungeanae* and 芦根 *Rhizoma Phragmitis*, used for treating colds with headache, fever, chills, general aching, stuffed running nose and cough

感冒退热冲剂 [gǎn mào tuì rè chōng jì]

Ganmao Tuire **Granules; Antiphlogistic Granules for Flu:** granules for infusion prepared from 大青叶 *Folium Isatidis*, 板蓝根 *Radix Isatidis*, 连翘 *Fructus Forsythiae* and 拳参 *Rhizoma Bistortae*, used for treating upper respiratory infection, acute tonsillitis and pharyngitis

小儿感冒冲剂 [xiǎo ér gǎn mào chōng jì]

Xiao'er Ganmao **Granules; Children's Colds Granules:** granules for infusion prepared from 广藿香 *Herba Pogostemonis*, 菊花 *Flos Chrysanthemi*, 连翘 *Fructus Forsythiae*, 大青叶 *Folium Isatidis*, 板蓝根 *Radix Isatidis*, 生地黄 *Radix Rehmanniae*, 地骨皮 *Cortex Lycii*, 白薇 *Radix Cynanchi Atrati*, 薄荷 *Herba Menthae* and 生石膏 *Gypsum Fibrosum*, used to remove heat and induce diaphoresis for treating colds and influenza with fever in children

板蓝根冲剂 [bǎn lán gēn chōng jì]

Banlangen **Granules; Isatis-root Granules:** granules for infusion prepared from 板蓝根 *Radix Isatidis*, used for the treatment of tonsillitis, mumps, sore throat, and for the prevention and treatment of infectious hepatitis and measles

银翘解毒丸[片] [yín qiào jiě dú wán/piàn]

***Yinqiao Jiedu* Pills [Tablets]; Detoxicant Pills [Tablets] of Lonicera and Forshythia:** pills [tablets] prepared from 金银花 *Flos Lonicerae*, 连翘 *Fructus Forsythiae*, 薄荷 *Herba Menthae*, 桔梗 *Radix Platycodi*, 牛蒡子 *Fructus Arctii*, 荆芥 *Herba Schizonepetae* etc., used to expel toxic heat from the exterior of the body, for the treatment of wind-heat affliction with chills and fever, headache, and sore throat

防风通圣丸 [fáng fēng tōng shèng wán]

***Fangfeng Tongsheng* Pills; Miraculous Saposhnikovia Pills:** pills prepared from 防风 *Radix Saposhnikoviae*, 连翘 *Fructus Forsythiae*,麻黄 *Herba Ephedrae*, 栀子 *Fructus Gardeniae*, 大黄 *Radix et Rhizoma Rhei*, 石膏 *Gypsum Fibrosum*, 黄芩 *Radix Scutellariae*, 白芍 *Radix Paeoniae Alba*, 川芎 *Rhizoma Chuanxiong* etc., used for the treatment of wind-heat affliction marked by headache, sore throat, fullness in the chest, constipation, skin eruption or ulcers

通宣理肺丸[片] [tōng xuān lǐ fèi wán/piàn]

***Tongxuan Lifei* Pills [Tablets]; Lung-Ventilating Pills [Tablets]:** pills [tablets] prepared from 紫苏叶 *Folium Perillae*, 麻黄 *Herba Ephedrae*, 苦杏仁 *Semen Armeniacae Amarum*, 前胡 *Radix Peucedani*, 桔梗 *Radix Platycodi*, 黄芩 *Radix Scutellariae*, 陈皮 *Pericarpium Citri Reticulatae*, 半夏 *Rhizoma Pinelliae* etc., used to cure cough, stuffed nose and headache in cases of wind-cold affliction

二母宁嗽丸[片] [èr mǔ níng sòu wán/piàn]

***Ermu Ningsou* Pills [Tablets]; Cough Pills [Tablets] with Anemarrhena and Fritillary:** pills [tablets] prepared from 知母 *Rhizoma Anemarrhenae*, 川贝母 *Bulbus Fritillariae Cirrhosae*, 桑白皮 *Cortex Mori*, 瓜蒌仁 *Semen Trichosanthis*, 石膏 *Gypsum Fibrosum*, 栀子 *Fructus Gardeniae*, 陈皮 *Pericarpium Citri Reticulatae*, 茯苓 *Poria*, etc., used to clear the lung of heat for relieving cough with yellow sputum

复方川贝精片 [fù fāng chuān bèi jīng piàn]

***Fufang Chuanbeijing* Tablets; Compound Tablets of Fritillary Extract:** tablets prepared from 川贝母 *Bulbus Fritillariae Cirrhosae*, 麻黄 *Herba Ephedrae*, 甘草 *Radix Glycyrrhizae*, 五味子 *Fructus Schisandrae*, 陈皮 *Pericarpium Citri Reticulatae* etc., used for relieving cough and asthma due to wind-cold affliction

川贝枇杷糖浆 [chuān bèi pí bā táng jiāng]

***Chuanbei Pipa* Syrup; Fritillary-Loquat Syrup:** syrup prepared from 川贝母流浸膏 *Extractum Bulbus Fritillariae Cirrhosae Liquidum*, 枇杷叶 *Folium Eriobotryae*, 桔梗 *Radix Platycodi* and 薄荷脑 *Mentholum*, used to clear the lung of heat and resolve phlegm for treating cough in cases of colds and bronchitis

蛇胆川贝散 [shé dǎn chuān bèi sǎn]

***Shedan Chuanbei* Powder; Snake-bile and Tendrilled-Fritillary Powder:** powder prepared from 蛇胆汁 *Fel Serpentis Liquidum* and 川贝 *Bulbus Fritilleriae Cirrhosae*, used to remove heat from the lung, arrest cough and eliminate phlegm for treating bronchitis

蛇胆陈皮散 [shé dǎn chén pí sǎn]

Shedan Chenpi Powder; Snake-bile and Tangerine-peel Powder: powder prepared from 蛇胆汁 *Fel Serpentis Liquidum* and 陈皮 *Pericarpium Citri Reticulatae*, used to relieve cough, resolve phlegm and promote digestion for treating cough and expectoration with nausea and vomiting in cases of colds

橘红丸[片] [jú hóng wán/piàn]

***Juhong* Pills [Tablets]; Red Tangerine Pills [Tablets]:** pills [tablets] prepared from 橘红 *Exocarpium Citri Rubrum*, 款冬花 *Flos Farfarae*, 茯苓 *Poria*, 紫菀 *Radix Asteris*, 瓜蒌仁 *Semen Trichosanthis*, 生石膏 *Gypsum Fibrosum* etc, used to remove pathogenic heat from the lung and resolve phlegm for relieving cough and dyspnea with sticky or yellow sputum in cases of acute or chronic bronchitis

定喘丸 [dìng chuǎn wán]

***Dingchuan* Pills; Antasthmatic Pills:** pills prepared from 紫苏子 *Fructus Perillae*, 苦杏仁 *Semen Armeniacae Amarum*, 川贝母 *Bulbus Fritillariae Cirrhosae*, 黄芪 *Radix Astragali*, 阿胶 *Colla Corii Asini*, 款冬花 *Flos Farfarae* etc., used to relieve cough and asthma in chronic cases by replenishing and regulating lung *qi*

气管炎丸 [qì guǎn yán wán]

Bronchitis Pills: pills prepared from 麻黄 *Herba Ephedrae*, 款冬花 *Flos Farfarae*, 苦杏仁 *Semen Armeniacae Amarum*, 川贝母 *Bulbus Fritillariae Cirrhosae* etc., used to expel phlegm and relieve cough and dyspnea for the treatment of chronic bronchitis

养阴清肺膏 [yǎng yīn qīng fèi gāo]

***Yangyin Qingfei* Extract; Yin-nourishing Lung-clearing Extract:** extract prepared from 生地 *Radix Rehmanniae*, 麦冬 *Radix Ophiopogonis*, 玄参 *Radix Scrophulariae*, 川贝母 *Bulbus Fritillariae Cirrhosae*, 白芍 *Radix Paeoniae Alba*, 牡丹皮 *Cortex Moutan*, 薄荷 *Herba Menthe* and 甘草 *Radix Glycyrrhizae*, used for treating lung-yin deficiency marked by dryness and pain in the throat, and dry cough with scanty expectoration or bloody sputum

玉屏风口服液 [yù píng fēng kǒu fú yè]

***Yupingfeng* Oral Liquid; Jade-screen Liquid:** an oral liquid prepared from 黄芪 *Radix Astragali*, 防风 *Radix Saposhnikoviae* and 白术 *Rhizoma Atractylodis Macrocephalae*, used to replenish *qi*, strengthen the superficial resistance and arrest excessive sweating, for treating spontaneous sweating and liability to colds

牛黄上清丸 [niú huáng shàng qīng wán]

***Niuhuang Shangqing* Pills, Bezoar Pills for Clearing the Upper:** pills prepared from 牛黄 *Calculus Bovis*, 黄连 *Rhizoma Coptidis*, 大黄 *Radix et Rhizoma Rhei*, 黄芩 *Radix Scutellariae*, 连翘 *Fructus Forsythiae*, 栀子 *Fructus Gardeniae*, 生石膏 *Gypsum Fibrosum* 菊花 *Flos Chrysanthemi* etc., used to clear toxic heat particularly in the upper part of the body marked by headache, dizziness, redness of eyes, tinnitus, ulceration of the mouth and tongue, swelling and pain of the gums, and constipation

牛黄解毒丸[片] [niú huáng jiě dú wán/piàn]

***Niuhuang Jiedu* Pills [Tablets]; Bezoar Detoxicant Pills [Tablets]:** pills [tablets] prepared from 黄芩 *Radix Scutellariae*, 黄连 *Rhizoma Coptidis*, 黄柏 *Cortex Phellodendri*, 大黄 *Radix et Rhizoma Rhei*, 连翘 *Fructus Forsythiae*, 金银花 *Flos Lonicerae*, 牛黄 *Calculus Bovis* etc., used to clear toxic heat for the treatment of intense heat or fire in the liver and stomach, marked by headache and dizziness, red eyes, tinnitus, oral ulcers, periodontitis and constipation

牛黄清心丸[片] [niú huáng qīng xīn wán/piàn]

***Niuhuang Qingxin* Pills (Tablets); Bezoar Sedative Pills (Tablets):** pills (tablets) prepared from 牛黄 *Calculus Bovis*, 麝香 *Moschus*, 犀角 *Corni Rhinoceri*, 羚羊角 *Cornu Saigae Tataricae*, 朱砂 *Cinnabaris* etc., used to clear evil heat from the heart and induce sedation, and for the treatment of excessive heat in the heart meridian marked by vertigo, irritability, delirium, and even convulsion

牛黄降压丸 [niú huáng jiàng yā wán]

***Niuhuang Jiangya* Pills; Bezoar Antihypertensive Pills:** pills prepared from 牛黄 *Calculus Bovis*, 羚羊角 *Cornu Saigae Tataricae*, 珍珠 *Magarita*, 冰片 *Borneolum Syntheticum*, 黄芪 *Radix Astragali*, 郁金 *Radix Curcumae*, 白芍 *Radix Paeoniae Alba* etc., used to induce sedation and reduce high blood pressure for treating hypertension

血脂宁丸 [xuè zhī níng wán]

***Xuezhining* Pills; Blood-lipid Lowering Pills:** pills prepared from 山楂 *Fructus Crataegi*, 何首乌 *Radix Polygoni Multiflori*, 荷叶 *Folium Nelumbinis* etc., used to lower the blood lipids, soften the blood vessels and increase the coronary blood circulation for treating hyperlipemia and arrhythmia

脑立清 [nǎo lì qīng]

***Nao Li Qing*; Head-clearing Pills:** pills prepared from 赭石 *Haematitum*, 半夏 *Rhizoma Pinelliae*, 牛膝 *Radix Achyranthis Bidentatae*, 珍珠母 *Concha Margaritifera Usta*, etc., used to quench fire in the liver for treating hypertension due to deficiency of liver yin with exuberance of yang marked by dizziness, tinnitus and insomnia

补心丹 [pǔ xīn dān]

***Buxin* Pills, Mind-Tonic Pills:** pills prepared from 茯苓 *Poria*,人参 *Radix Ginseng*, 麦冬 *Radix Ophiopogonis*, 酸枣仁 *Semen Zizyphi Spinosae*, 柏子仁 *Semen Boitae*, 远志 *Radix Polygalae*, 当归 *Radix Angelica Sinensis*, etc., used to calm the mind by nourishing heart blood, for the treatment of heart blood deficiency with restlessness, insomnia and forgetfulness

朱砂安神丸 [zhū shā ān shén wán]

***Zhusha Anshen* Pills; Cinnabar Sedative Pills:** pills prepared from 朱砂 *Cinnabaris*, 龙齿 *Dens Draconis*, 当归 *Radix Angelicae Sinensis*, 黄连 *Rhizoma Coptidis*, 酸枣仁 *Semen Zizyphi Spinosae*, 熟地黄 *Radix Rehmanniae Preparata* etc., used to calm the mind for the treatment of fidgetiness and insomnia, forgetfulness, palpitation and shortness of breath due to deficiency of *qi* and blood of the heart

柏子养心丸 [bǎi zǐ yǎng xīn wán]

***Baizi Yangxin* Pills; Mind-tonic Pills of Arborvitae Seed:** pills prepared from 柏子仁 *Semen Biotae*, 人参 *Radix Ginseng*, 黄芪 *Radix Astragali*, 酸枣仁 *Semen Zizyphi Spinosae*, 当归 *Radix Angelicae Sinensis*, 五味子 *Fructus Schizandrae*, 远志 *Radix Polygalae* etc., used to relieve anxiety and mental strain, also for treating palpitation, insomnia and amnesia

败酱片 [bài jiàng piàn]

***Baijiang* Tablets; Dahurican Patrinia Tablets:** tablets prepared from extract of 黄花败酱 *Rhizoma et Radix Patriniae Scabiosaefoliae*, used as a sedative for treating insomnia in cases of neurasthenia and psychoses

麻仁丸 [má rén wán]

***Maren* Pills; Cannabis-Seed Pills:** pills prepared from 火麻仁 *Semen Cannabis*, 大黄 *Radix et Rhizoma Rhei*, 苦杏仁 *Semen Armeniacae Amarum*, 厚朴 *Cortex Magnoliae Officinalis*, 枳实 *Fructus Aruantii Immaturus* and 白芍 *Radix Paeoniae Alba*, used to relieve constipation due to deficiency of fluids and constipation in the aged and debilitated

香连丸 [xiāng lián wán]

***Xianglian* Pills; Aucklandia-Coptis Pills:** pills prepared from 黄连 *Rhizoma Coptidis* and 木香 *Radix Aucklandiae*, used to eliminate damp-heat, promote the flow of *qi* and relieve pain, for treating dysentery with tenesmus, abdominal pain and diarrhea

舒肝丸 [shū gān wán]

***Shugan* Pills; Liver-soothing Pills:** pills prepared from 厚朴 *Cortex Magnoliae Officinalis*, 姜黄 *Rhizoma Curcumae Longae*, 沉香 *Lignum Aquilariae Resinatum*, 红豆蔻 *Fructus Galangae*, 柴胡 *Radix Bupleuri*, 元胡 *Rhizoma Corydalis* etc., used for removing stagnancy of liver *qi* manifested by depression, pain and fullness over the hypochondriac and epigastric regions, eructation and acid regurgitation

逍遥丸 [xiāo yáo wán]

***Xiaoyao* Pills; Carefree Pills:** formula composed of 柴胡 *Radix Bupleuri*, 当归 *Radix Angelicae Sinensis*, 白芍 *Radix Paeoniae Alba*, 白术 *Rhizoma Atractylodis Macrocephalae*, 茯苓 *Poria*, 甘草 *Radix Glycyrrhizae*, 煨生姜 *Rhizoma Zingiberis Preparata*, 薄荷 *Herba Menthae*, used to soothe the liver, invigorate the spleen, nourish the blood and regulate menstruation for the treatment of depressed liver *qi* marked by hypochondriac distension and pain, dizziness, impaired appetite and menstrual disorders

加味逍遥丸 [jiā wèi xiāo yáo wán]

***Jiawei Xiaoyao* Pills: Modified Carefree Pills:** pills prepared from 柴胡 *Radix Bupleuri*, 当归 *Radix Angelicae Sinensis*, 白芍 *Radix Paeoniae Alba*, 白术 *Rhizoma Atractylodis Macrocephalae*, 茯苓 *Poria*, 甘草 *Radix Glycyrrhizae*, 煨生姜 *Rhizoma Zingiberis Preparata*, 牡丹皮 *Cortex Moutan*,栀子 *Fructus Gardeniae* and 薄荷 *Herba Menthae*, used to remove stagnant liver *qi,* clear heat and invigorate the spleen and stomach, for the treatment of stagnation of the liver and disharmony between the liver and stomach marked by distension and pain of the hypochondriac region, dizziness, anorexia, menoxenia, and abdominal distension and pain

木香顺气丸 [mù xiāng shùn qì wán]

***Muxiang Shunqi* Pills; Aucklandia Carminative Pills:** pills prepared from 木香 *Radix Aucklandiae*, 青皮 *Pericarpium Citri Reticulatae Viride*, 厚朴 *Cortex Magnoliae Officinalis*, 乌药 *Radix Linderae*, 大黄 *Radix et Rhizoma Rhei*, 牵牛子 *Semen Pharbitidis*, etc., used to relieve stagnancy of food and gas, for the treatment of indigestion with flatulence and constipation

大山楂丸 [dà shān zhā wán]

***Danshanzha* Pills; Large Haw Pills:** pills prepared from 山楂 *Fructus Crataegi*, 六神曲 *Massa Fermentata Medicinalis* and 麦芽 *Fructus Hordei Germinatus*, used to promote the appetite and digestion, for the treatment of indigestion with anorexia and epigastric distension

启脾丸 [qǐ pí wán]

***Qipi* Pills; Spleen-activating Pills:** pills prepared from 人参 *Radix Genseng*, 白术 *Rhizoma Atractylodis Macrocephalae*, 茯苓 *poria*, 甘草 *Radix Glycyrrhizae*, 陈皮 *Pericarpium Citri Reticulatae*, 山药 *Rhizoma Dioscoreae*, 莲子 *Semen Nelumbinis*, 山楂 *Fructus Crataegi*, 六神曲 *Massa Medicata Fermentata*, 麦芽 *Fructus Hordei Germinatus* and 泽泻 *Rhizoma Alismatis*, used for the treatment of spleen insufficiency marked by dyspepsia, abdominal distension and loose bowels

附子理中丸 [fù zǐ lǐ zhōng wán]

***Fuzi Lizhong* Pills; Aconite Middle-regulating Pills:** pills prepared from 附子 *Radix Aconiti Lateralis Preparata*，党参 *Radix Codonopsis Pilosulae*, 白术 *Rhizoma Atractylodis Macrocephalae*, 干姜 *Rhizoma Zingiberis* and 甘草 *Radix Glycyrrhizae*, used to warm and invigorate the spleen and stomach for the treatment of deficiency-cold of the spleen and stomach with epigastric pain with cold sensation, vomiting, diarrhea and cold limbs

香砂养胃丸 [xiāng shā yǎng wèi wán]

***Xiangsha Yangwei* Pills; Cyperus-Amomum Stomach-nourishing Pills:** pills prepared from 香附 *Rhizoma Cypri*, 砂仁 *Fructus Amomi*, 木香 Radix *Aucklandiae*, 白术 *Rhizoma Atractylodis Macrocephalae*, 陈皮 *Pericarpium Citri Reticulatae*, 厚朴 *Cortex Magnoliae Officinalis* etc., used for treating dyspepsia due to weakness of the stomach marked by epigastric distension, vomiting, belching and acid regurgitation

香砂六君丸 [xiāng shā liù jūn wán]

***Xiangsha Liujun* Pills; Cyperus-Amomum Six-Noble Pills:** pills prepared from 党参 *Radix Codonopsis Pilosulae*, 茯苓 *Poria*, 白术 *Rhizoma Atractylodis Macrocephalae*, 甘草 *Radix Glycyrrhizae*, 陈皮 *Pericarpium Citri Reticulatae*, 半夏 *Rhizoma Pinelliae*, 木香 *Radix Aucklandiae* and 砂仁 *Fructus Amomi*, used to invigorate the spleen and regulate the stomach for the treatment of dyspepsia, belching, anorexia, epigastric and abdominal distension, and loose bowels

参苓白术丸 [shēn líng bái zhú wán]

***Shenling Baizhu* Pills; Ginseng-Poria-Atractylodes Pills:** pills prepared from 人参 *Radix Ginseng*, 茯苓 *Poria*, 白术 *Rhizoma Atractylodis Macrocephalae*, 山药 *Rhizoma Dioscoreae*, 莲子 *Semen Nelumbinis*, 砂仁 *Fructus Amomi* etc., used for the treatment of diminished function of the spleen and the stomach marked by loss of appetite, abdominal distension, diarrhea and lassitude

人参健脾丸 [rén shēn jiàn pí wán]

***Renshen Jianpi* Pills; Ginseng Spleen-strengthening Pills:** pills prepared from 人参 *Radix Ginseng*, 茯苓 *Poria*, 山药 *Rhizoma Dioscoreae*, 黄芪 *Radix Astragali*, 白术 *Rhizoma Atractylodis Macrocephalae*, 陈皮 *Pericarpium Citri Reticulatae* etc., used for the treatment of diminished function of the spleen and stomach marked by emaciation, general weakness, loss of appetite, and alternate diarrhea and constipation

八珍丸 [bā zhēn wán]

***Bazhen* Pills; Eight-Treasure Pills:** pills prepared from 人参 *Radix Ginseng* or 党参 *Radix Codonopsis Pilosulae*, 白术 *Rhizoma Atractylodis Macrocephalae*, 茯苓 *Poria*, 甘草 *Radix Glycyrrhizae*, 当归 *Radix*

Angelicae Sinensis, 白芍 *Radix Paeoniae Alba*, 川芎 *Rhizoma Chuanxiong* and 熟地黄 *Rhizoma Rehmanniae Preparata*, used to improve the function of the spleen and stomach, reinforce *qi* and nourish the blood for treating general debility, loss of appetite, lassitude, etc.

十全大补丸 [shí quán dà bǔ wán]

***Shiquan Dabu* Pills; All-inclusive Grand Tonic Pills:** pills prepared from 人参 *Radix Ginseng* or 党参 *Radix Codonopsis Pilosulae*, 白术 *Rhizoma Atractylodis Macrocephalae*, 茯苓 *Poria*, 甘草 *Radix Glycyrrhizae*, 当归 *Radix Angelicae Sinensis*, 白芍 *Radix Paeoniae Alba*, 川芎 *Rhizoma Chuanxiong*, 熟地黄 *Rhizoma Rehmanniae Preparata*, 肉桂 *Cortex Cinnamomi* and 黄芪 *Radix Astragali*, used to replenish both *qi* and blood for general debility after illness

补中益气丸 [bǔ zhōng yì qì wán]

***Buzhong Yiqi* Pills; Middle-reinforcing *Qi*-replenishing Pills:** prepared from 黄芪 *Radix Astragali*, 人参 *Radix Ginseng* or 党参 *Radix Codonopsis Pilosulae*, 黄芪 *Radix Astragali*, 白术 *Rhizoma Atractylodis Macrocephalae*, 当归 *Radix Angelicae Sinensis*, 陈皮 *Pericarpium Citri Reticulatae*, 甘草 *Radix Glycyrrhizae*, 白术 *Rhizoma Atractylodis Macrocephalae*,升麻 *Rhizoma Cimicifugae* and 柴胡 *Radix Bupleuri*, used to reinforce spleen *qi* for the treatment of general debility, lassitude and somnolence, prolonged diarrhea, uterine bleeding, or accompanied by prolapse of the rectum or the uterus

生脉饮 [shēng mài yǐn]

***Shengmai Yin*; Pulse-activating Drink:** solution prepared from 人参 *Radix Ginseng*, 麦冬 *Radix Ophiopogonis* and 五味子 *Fructus Schisandrae*, used to replenish *qi* and yin, for the treatment of cardiac palpitation, shortness of breath, faint pulse and spontaneous sweating

大补阴丸 [dà bǔ yīn wán]

***Dabuyin* Pills; Large Yin-nourishing Pills:** pills prepared from 熟地黄 *Radix Rehmanniae Preparata*, 知母 *Rhizoma Anemarrheanae*, 黄柏 *Cortex Phellodendri*, 龟板 *Carapax et Plastrum Testudinis* and 猪脊髓 *Medulla Spinalis Suis*, used to nourish yin and reduce fire, for the treatment of yin deficiency manifested by afternoon fever, night sweats, cough, hemoptysis, tinnitus, and seminal emission

河车大造丸 [hé chē dà zào wán]

***Heche Dazao* Pills; Restorative Placenta Pills:** pills prepared from 紫河

车 *Placenta Hominis*, 麦冬 *Radix Ophiopogonis*, 天冬 *Radix Asparagi*, 杜仲 *Cortex Eucommiae*, 龟板 *Plastrum Testudinis*, 熟地黄 *Rhizoma Rehmanniae Preparata* etc., used to nourish kidney essence for the treatment of general debility, night sweats, nocturnal emission, lassitude, tidal fever and maldevelopment.

五子衍宗丸 [wǔ zǐ yǎn zōng wán]

***Wuzi Yanzong* Pills; Pills of Five Kinds of Seeds for Offspring:** pills prepared from 枸杞子 *Fructus Lycii*, 菟丝子 *Semen Cuscutae*, 复盆子 *Fructus Rubi*, 五味子 *Fructus Schisandrae* and 车前子 *Semen Plantaginis*, used to replenish kidney essence for the treatment of dribbling of urine after micturition, seminal emission, premature ejaculation, impotence and sterility

六味地黄丸 [liù wèi dì huáng wán]

***Liuwei Dihuang* Pills; Six-ingredient Rehmannia Pills:** pills prepared from 熟地黄 *Radix Rehmanniae Preparata*, 山茱萸 *Fructus Corni*, 山药 *Rhizoma Dioscoreae*, 泽泻 *Rhizoma Alismatis*, 茯苓 *Poria* and 牡丹皮 *Cortex Moutan*, used to replenish kidney yin for the treatment of yin deficiency marked by dizziness, tinnitus, aching and limpness of loins and knees, night sweats, and also used for the treatment of diabetes

杞菊地黄丸 [qǐ jú dì huáng wán]

***Qiju Dihuang* Pills; Wolfberry-Chrysanthemum Rehmannia Pills:** pills prepared from 枸杞子 *Fructus Lycii*, 菊花 *Flos Chrysanthemi*, 熟地黄 *Radix Rehmanniae Preparata*, 山茱萸 *Fructus Corni*, 山药 *Rhizoma Dioscoreae*, 泽泻 *Rhizoma Alismatis*, 茯苓 *Poria* and 牡丹皮 *Cortex Moutan*, used to nourish liver and kidney yin for treating yin deficiency of the liver and kidney with dizziness, tinnitus and blurred vision

知柏地黄丸 [zhī bǎi dì huáng wán]

***Zhibai Dihuang* Pills; Amenarrhena-Phellodendron Rehmannia Pills:** pills prepared from 知母 *Rhizoma Anemarrheanae*, 黄柏 *Cortex Phellodendri*, 熟地黄 *Radix Rehmanniae Preparata*, 山茱萸 *Fructus Corni*, 山药 *Rhizoma Dioscoreae*, 泽泻 *Rhizoma Alismatis*, 茯苓 *Poria* and 牡丹皮 *Cortex Moutan*, used to nourish yin and reduce fire, for the treatment of yin deficiency with up-flaming of fire marked by daily recurring fever, night sweats, dryness of the mouth, sore throat and tinnitus

麦味地黄丸 [mài wèi dì huáng wán]

***Maiwei Dihuang* Pills; Lilyturf-Magnoliavine Rehmannia Pills:** pills prepared from 麦冬 *Radix Ophiopogonis*, 五味子 *Fructus Schisandrae*, 熟地黄 *Radix Rehmanniae Preparata*, 山茱萸 *Fructus Corni*, 山药 *Rhizoma Dioscoreae*, 泽泻 *Rhizoma Alismatis*, 茯苓 *Poria* and 牡丹皮 *Cortex Moutan*, used to nourish kidney and lung yin for the treatment of yin deficiency of the lung and kidney marked by recurring fever, night sweats, dryness of the throat, hemoptysis, dizziness, tinnitus, and also used for the treatment of diabetes

桂附地黄丸 [guì fù dì huáng wán]

***Guifu Dihuang* Pills; Cassia-Aconite Rehmannia Pills:** Pills prepared from 肉桂 *Cortex Cinnamomi*, 附子 *Radix Aconiti Lateralis Preparata* 熟地黄 *Radix Rehmanniae Preparata*, 山茱萸 *Fructus Corni*, 山药 *Rhizoma Dioscoreae*, 泽泻 *Rhizoma Alismatis*, 茯苓 *Poria* and 牡丹皮 *Cortex Moutan*, used to reinforce kidney yang for the treatment of kidney yang deficiency marked by cold sensation in the loins and knees, edema of the legs, oliguria, or for the treatment of diabetes

龟龄集 [guī líng jí]

***Guilingji* Capsules; Longevity Capsules:** granules in capsules prepared from 人参 *Radix Ginseng*, 鹿茸 *Cornu Cervi Pantotrichum*, 海马 *Hippocampus*, 淫羊藿 *Herba Epimedii*, 雀脑 sparrow's brain etc., used to invigorate kidney yang for treating impotence, sterility, amnesia and mental debility

全鹿丸 [quán lù wán]

***Quanlu* Pills; Deer Tonic Pills:** pills prepared from 人参 *Radix Ginseng*, 鹿茸 *Cornu Cervi Pantotrichum*, 锁阳 *Herba Cynomorii*, 巴戟天 *Radix Morindae Officinalis*, 当归 *Radix Angelicae Sinensis*, 沉香 *Lignum Aquilariae Resinatum*, 熟地黄 *Rhizoma Rehmanniae Preparata* etc., used as a tonic for kidney insufficiency marked by asthenia, lassitude, amnesia, insomnia, night sweats and spontaneous emission, or metrorrhagia, leukorrhagia and miscarriage

参茸卫生丸 [shēn róng wèi shēng wán]

***Shenrong Weisheng* Pills; Ginseng-Antler Life-preserving Pills:** pills prepared from 人参 *Radix Ginseng*, 鹿茸 *Cornu Cervi Pantotrichum*, 莲子 *Semen Nelumbinis*, 酸枣仁 *Semen Zizyphi Spinosae*, 锁阳 *Herba Cynomorii*, 巴戟天 *Radix Morindae Officinalis*, 枸杞子 *Fructus Lycii*

etc., used to replenish *qi* and blood, nourish essence of both the liver and the kidney, and invigorate the functions of the spleen and stomach, for the treatment of deficiency of *qi* and blood and kidney insufficiency with lassitude, fatigue, poor appetite, spermatorrhea, anemia, early graying of the hair, etc.

人参养荣丸 [rén shēn yǎng róng wán]

***Renshen Yangrong* Pills; Ginseng Nutritive Pills:** pills prepared from 人参 *Radix Ginseng*, 白术 *Rhizoma Atractylodis Macrocephalae*, 茯苓 *Poria*, 甘草 *Radix Glycyrrhizae*, 当归 *Radix Angelicae Sinensis*, 熟地 *Radix Rehmanniae Preparata*, 白芍 *Radix Paeoniae Alba*, 黄芪 *Radix Astragali*, 陈皮 *Pericarpium Citri Reticulatae*, 远志 *Radix Polygalae*, 肉桂 *Cortex Cinnamomi* and 五味子 *Fructus Schisandrae*, used to warm and tonify *qi* and blood for treating deficiency syndrome of both the heart and the spleen with insufficiency of *qi* and blood marked by emaciation, lassitude, anorexia, and loose stools, and also for weakness during convalescence

参茸固本片 [shēn róng gù běn piàn]

***Shenrong Guben* Tablets; Ginseng-Antler Restorative Tablets:** tablets prepared from 当归 *Radix Angelicae Sinensis*, 山药 *Rhizoma Dioscoreae*, 茯苓 *Poria*, 山茱萸 *Fructus Corni*, 杜仲 *Cortex Eucommiae*, 枸杞子 *Fructus Lycii*, 熟地黄 *Radix Rehmanniae Preparata*, 菟丝子 *Fructus Cuscutae*, 人参 *Radix Ginseng*, 鹿茸 *Cornu Cervi Pantotrichum* etc., used to tonify *qi* and blood for treating various kinds of deficiency syndromes with tinnitus, dizziness and lassitude

再造丸 [zài zào wán]

***Zaizao* Pills; Restorative Pills:** pills prepared from 蕲蛇 *Agkistrodon deprived of head, scales and bones*, 全蝎 *Scorpio*, 水牛角浓缩粉 *Pulvis Cornus Bubali Concentratus*, 牛黄 *Calculus Bovis*, 天麻 *Rhizoma Gastrodiae*, 人参 *Radix Ginseng*, 麝香 *Moschus* etc., used for treating apoplectic coma and hemiplegia by dispelling wind-phlegm and promoting blood circulation.

人参再造丸 [rén shēn zài zào wán]

***Renshen Zaizao* Pills; Ginseng Restorative Pills:** synonym for 再造丸 [zài zào wán]

紫雪 [zǐ xuě]

***Zixue* Powder; Purple Snowy Powder:** powder prepared from 水牛角浓

缩粉 *Pulvis Cornus Bubali Concentratus*, 羚羊角 *Cornu Saigae Tataricae*, 麝香 *Moschus*, 沉香 *Lignum Aquilariae Resinatum*, 石膏 *Gypsum Fibrosum*, etc., used to clear up evil heat, relieve convulsions and promote the restoration of consciousness, for treating high fever with restlessness, delirium and convulsion

安宫牛黄丸 [ān gōng niú huáng wán]

***Angong Niuhuang* Pills; Bezoar Resurrection Pills:** pills prepared from 牛黄 *Calculus Bovis*, 水牛角浓缩粉 *Pulvis Cornus Bubali Concentratus*, 珍珠 *Margarita*, 麝香 *Moschus*, 栀子 *Fructus Gardeniae* etc., used to eliminate toxic heat and bring the patient back to consciousness from coma, and relieve convulsions due to high fever or cerebral hemorrhage

苏合香丸 [sū hé xiāng wán]

***Suhexiang* Pills; Storax Pills:** pills prepared from 苏合香 *Styrax*, 安息香 *Benzoinum*, 冰片 *Borneolum Syntheticum*, 水牛角 *Cornu Bubali*, 麝香 *Moschus*, 檀香 *Lignum Santali Albi*, 沉香 *Lignum Aquilariae Resinatum*, 丁香 *Flos Caryophylli*, 香附 *Rhizoma Cyperi*, 木香 *Radix Aucklandiae*, 乳香 *Olibanum* etc., used to promote the restoration of consciousness as an aromatic stimulant, to promote the flow of *qi* and relieve pain for emergency treatment of apoplexy and heatstroke with loss of consciousness, and also for precordial and epigastric pain due to *qi* stagnation

小活络丸[丹] [xiǎo huó luò wán/dān]

***Xiaohuoluo* Pills; Collateral-activating Pills (mild recipe):** pills prepared from 制川乌 *Radix Aconiti Preparata*, 制草乌 *Radix Aconiti Kusnezoffii Preparata*, 胆南星 *Arisaema cum Bile*, 乳香 *Olibanum*, 没药 *Myrrha* and 地龙 *Lumbricus*, used to relieve rheumatic pain, numbness and difficulty in movement of joints by dispelling wind and dampness, and invigorating blood flow in collaterals

大活络丸[丹] [dà huó luò wán/dān]

***Dahuoluo* Pills; Collateral-activating Pills (heavy recipe):** pills prepared from 蕲蛇 *Agkistrodon*, 乌梢蛇 *Zaocys*, 天麻 *Rhizoma Gastrodiae*, 人参 *Radix Ginseng*, 牛黄 *Calculus Bovis*, 麝香 *Moschus*, 水牛角浓缩粉 *Pulvis Cornus Bubali Concentratus*, 地龙 *Lumbricus*, 血竭 *Sanguis Draconis* etc., used to dispel wind and dampness, activate blood flow in collateral meridians, relax the contracture of limbs, and treat apoplectic hemiplegia

木瓜丸 [mù guā wán]

***Mugua* Pills; Chaenomeles Pills:** pills prepared from 木瓜 *Fructus Chaenomelis*, 当归 *Radix Angelicae*, 川芎 *Rhizoma Chuanxiong*, 白芷 *Radix Angelicae Dahuricae*, 威灵仙 *Radix Clematis*, 狗脊 *Rhizoma Ciboti*, 牛膝 *Radix Achyranthis Bidentatae*, 鸡血藤 *Caulis Statholobi*, 海风藤 *Caulis Piperis Kadsurae*, 人参 *Radix Ginseng*, 制川乌 *Radix Aconiti Preparata* and 制草乌 *Radix Aconiti Kusnezoffii Preparata*, used to dispel wind-cold, remove obstructions from collateral meridians and relieve pain for the treatment of rheumatic and rheumatoid arthritis

豨莶丸 [xī xiān wán]

***Xixian* Pills; Siegesbeckia Pills:** pills prepared from 豨莶草 *Herba Siegesbeckiae,* used to relieve rheumatic conditions and to improve the motility of joints, for treating rheumatic arthralgia with aching and weakness of the loins and knees, and numbness of the limbs

国公酒 [guó gōng jiǔ]

***Guogong* Wine:** medicinal wine prepared from 当归 *Radix Angelicae Sinensis*, 川芎 *Rhizoma Chuanxiong*, 独活 *Radix Angelicae Pubescentis*, 牛膝 *Radix Achyranthis Bidentatae*, 佛手 *Fructus Citri Sarcodactylis*, 玉竹 *Rhizoma Polygonati Odorati*, 陈皮 *Pericarpium Citri Reticulatae*, etc., used to relieve muscular contracture in cases of rheumatoid arthritis

冠心苏合丸 [guàn xīn sū hé wán]

***Guanxin Suhe* Pills; Coronary Storax Pills:** pills prepared from 苏合香 *Styrax*, 冰片 *Borneolum*, 乳香 *Olibanum*, 檀香 *Lignum Santali Albi* and 青木香 *Radix Aristolochiae*, used to regulate the flow of *qi* in the chest and relieve pain for the treatment of angina pectoris with stuffy sensation in the chest

复方丹参片 [fù fāng dān shēn piàn]

***Fufang Danshen* Tablets; Compound Salvia Tablets:** tablets prepared from 丹参 *Salviae Miltiorrhzae*, 三七 *Radix Notoginseng* and 冰片 *Borneolum*, used to activate blood circulation and eliminate blood stasis for the treatment of angina pectoris

当归丸 [dāng guī wán]

***Danggui* Pills; Chinese Angelica Pills:** pills prepared from 当归 *Radix Angelicae Sinensis*, used to cure menstrual disturbance such as infrequent menstruation, menorrhalgia and morbid leukorrhea, by activating and tonifying blood

乌鸡白凤丸 [wū jī bái fèng wán]

***Wuji Baifeng* Pills; White Phoenix Pills:** pills prepared from 乌鸡 white-feathered chicken with dark skin, 人参 *Radix Ginseng*, 当归 *Radix Angelicae Sinensis*, 香附 *Rhizoma Cyperi*, 地黄 *Radix Rehmanniae*, 黄芪 *Radix Astragali*, 鹿角胶 *Colla Cornus Cervi* etc., used for treating menstrual disturbances and morbid leukorrhea due to deficiency of *qi* and blood

艾附暖宫丸 [ài fù nuǎn gōng wán]

***Aifu Nuangong* Pills; Argyi-Cyperus Uterus-warming Pills:** pills prepared from 艾叶 *Folium Artemisiae Argyi*, 香附 *Rhizoma Cyperi*, 吴茱萸 *Fructus Evodiae*, 肉桂 *Cortex Cinnamomi*, 当归 *Radix Angelicae Sinensis*, 川芎 *Rhizoma Chuanxiong*, 黄芪 *Radix Astragali* etc., used to replenish *qi,* warm the uterus and regulate menstruation, for the treatment of menstrual disorders of deficiency-cold type

痛经丸 [tòng jīng wán]

***Tongjing* Pills; Dysmenorrhea Pills:** pills prepared from 当归 *Radix Angelicae Sinensis*, 白芍 *Radix Paeoniae Alba*, 川芎 *Rhizoma Chuanxiong*, 熟地黄 *Radix Rehmanniae Preparatae*, 香附 *Rhizoma Cyperi*, 木香 *Radix Aucklandiae*, 元胡 *Rhizoma Corydalis*, 炮姜 *Rizoma Zingiberis*, 肉桂 *Cortex Cinnamomi*, 丹参 *Radix Salviae Miltiorrhizae*, 红花 *Flosn Carthami*, 益母草 *Herba Leonuri* etc., used to promote blood flow, dispel cold, regulate menstruation and relieve pain in cases of dysmenorrhea

八珍益母丸 [bā zhēn yì mǔ wán]

***Bazhen Yimu* Pills; Eight-Precious Motherwort Pills:** pills prepared from 益母草 *Herba Leonuri*, 党参 *Radix Codonopsis Pilosulae*, 白术 *Rhizoma Atractylodis Macrocephalae*, 茯苓 *Poria*, 甘草 *Radix Glycyrrhizae*, 当归 *Radix Angelicae Sinensis*, 白芍 *Radix Paeoniae Alba*, 川芎 *Rhizoma Chuanxiong* and 熟地黄 *Rhizoma Rehmanniae Preparata*, used to replenish *qi* and blood and to regulate menstruation, for the treatment of deficiency of *qi* and blood in women with general weakness and menstrual disorders

妇科十味片 [fù kē shí wèi piàn]

***Fuke Shiwei* Tablets: Ten-Ingredient Gynecological Tables:** tablets prepared from 党参 *Radix Codonopsis Pilosulae*, 白术 *Rhizoma Atractylodis Macrocephalae*, 当归 *Radix Angelicae Sinensis*, 地黄 *Radix*

Rehmanniae, 大枣 *Fructus Zizyphi Jujubae*, 香附 *Rhizoma Cyperi*, 茯苓 *Poria*, 川芎 *Rhizoma Chuanxiong*, 白芍 *Radix Paeoniae Alba* and 甘草 *Radix Glycyrrhizae*, used to regulate menstrual disturbances by replenishing *qi* and blood

更年安 [gēng nián ān]

Gengnian'an **Tablets; Climacteric Peace Tablets:** pills prepared from 熟地黄 *Radix Rehmanniae Preparata*, 何首乌 *Radix Polygoni Multiflori*, 泽泻 *Rhizoma Alismatis*, 茯苓 *Poria*, 五味子 *Fructus Schisandrae*, 珍珠母 *Concha Margaritifera Usta*, 玄参 *Radix Scrophulariae*, 浮小麦 *Fructus Tritici Levis* etc., used to nourish yin, remove heat, ease the mind and induce tranquilization, for treating menopausal syndrome marked by afternoon fever, excessive sweating, dizziness, tinnitus, insomnia and unsteady blood pressure

小金丸[丹] [xiǎo jīn wán/dān]

Xiaojin **Pills; Minor Panacea:** pills prepared from 麝香 *Moschus*, 乳香 *Olibanum*, 当归 *Radix Angelicae Sinensis*, 制草乌 *Radix Aconiti Kusnezoffii Preparata* etc., used to cure traumatic wounds by promoting blood circulation, removing blood stasis and reducing swelling, also for the treatment of scrofula, carbuncles, cutaneous abscesses and ulcers

六神丸 [liù shén wán]

Liushen **Pills; Miraculous Pills of Six Ingredients:** pills prepared from 牛黄 *Calculus Bovis*, 麝香 *Moschus*, 珍珠 *Margarita*, 冰片 *Borneol*, 樟脑 *Camphora*, 蟾酥 *Venenum Bufonis* and 雄黄 *Realgar*, used as an antiphlogistic for treating acute tonsillitis, sore throat and boils

金不换膏 [jīn bù huàn gāo]

Jinbuhuan **Plaster, Priceless Plaster:** plaster prepared from 大黄 *Radix et Rhizoma Rhei*, 没药 *Myrrha*, 血竭 *Sanguis Draconis*, 蜈蚣 *Scolopendra*, 麻黄 *Herba Ephedrae*, 草乌 *Radix Aconiti Kusnezoffii* etc., used externally to expel wind and cold, promote blood circulation and relieve pain, for the treatment of muscle and joint pains due to cold, also for sprains and other injuries

伤湿止痛膏 [shāng shī zhǐ tòng gāo]

Shangshi Zhitong Gao; **Rheumatic-Pain-Relieving Plaster:** plaster prepared from 川乌 *Radix Aconiti*, 乳香 *Olibanum*, 没药 *Myrrha*, 肉桂 *Cortex Cinnamomi*, 丁香 *Flos Caryophylli*, 薄荷脑 *Mentholum*, 马钱子 *Semen Strychni* etc., used externally for treating rheumatic pains, sprains and other injuries

七厘散 [qī lí sǎn]

***Qili* Powder; Anti-Bruise Powder:** powder prepared from 血竭 *Sanguis Draconis*, 红花 *Flos Carthami*, 乳香 *Olibanum*, 没药 *Myrrha*, 儿茶 *Catechu*, 冰片 *Borneolum*, 麝香 *Moschus*, etc., used to promote blood circulation and relieve pain in cases of traumatic wounds with local ecchymosis

冰硼散 [bīng péng sǎn]

***Bingpeng* Powder; Borneolum-Borax Powder:** powder prepared from 冰片 *Borneolum*, 硼砂 *Borax*, 朱砂 *Cinnabaris* and 玄明粉 *Natrii Sulfas Exsiccatus*, used externally for treating sore throat, painful swelling of the gums, and ulcers in the mouth or on the tongue

如意金黄散 [rú yì jīn huáng sǎn]

***Ruyi Jinhuang* Powder; Golden Powder for Alleviation:** powder prepared from 姜黄 *Rhizoma Curcumae Longae*, 大黄 *Radix et Rhizoma Rhei*, 黄柏 *Cortex Phellodendri*, 苍术 *Rhizoma Atractylodis*, 厚朴 *Cortex Magnoliae Officinalis*, 天南星 *Rhizoma Arisaematis*, 白芷 *Radix Angelicae Dahuricae* etc., used externally to promote the subsidence of swelling and alleviate pain for the treatment of abscesses, erysipelas and traumatic wounds

养血生发胶囊 [yǎng xuè shēng fà jiāo náng]

***Yangxue Shengfa* Capsules; Blood-nourishing Hair-growing Capsules:** capsules prepared from 何首乌 *Radix Polygoni Multiflori*, 当归 *Radix Angelicae Sinensis*, 熟地黄 *Radix Rehmanniae Preparata*, 天麻 *Rhizoma Gastrodiae*, 川芎 *Rhizoma Chuanxiong*, 木瓜 *Fructux Chaenomelis* etc., used to promote the growth of hair in cases of alopecia areata, seborrheic alopecia, and alopecia occurring after childbirth or after a serious disease

石斛夜光丸 [shí hú yè guāng wán]

***Shihu Yeguang* Pills; Dendrobium Eyesight-improving Pills:** pills prepared from 石斛 *Herba Dendrobi*, 人参 *Radix Ginseng*, 肉苁蓉 *Herba Cistanches*, 枸杞子 *Fructus Lycii*, 菟丝子 *Semen Cuscutae*, 地黄 *Radix Rehmanniae*, 五味子 *Fructus Schisandrae*, 天冬 *Radix Asparagi*, 麦冬 *Radix Ophiopogonis*, 川芎 *Rhizoma Chuanxiong*, 黄连 *Rhizoma Coptidis*, 牛膝 *Radix Achyanthis Bidentatae*, 菊花 *Flos Chrysanthemi*, 蒺藜 *Fructus Tribuli*, 青葙子 *Semen Celosiae*, 决明子 *Semen Cassiae*,

水牛角 *Cornu Bubali*, 羚羊角 *Cornu Saigae Tataricae* etc., used to replenish kidney yin, quench liver fire and improve eyesight for the treatment of cataracts

耳聋左慈丸 [ěr lóng zuǒ cí wán]

***Erlong Zuoci* Pills; *Zuoci's* Deafness Pills:** pills prepared from 磁石 *Magnetitum*, 熟地黄 *Radix Rehmanniae Preparata*, 山茱萸 *Fructus Corni*, 牡丹皮 *Cortex Moutan*, 山药 *Rhizoma Discoreae*, 茯苓 *Poria*, 泽泻 *Rhizoma Alismatis* and 竹叶柴胡 *Radix Bupleuri Marginati*, used to replenish the kidney and subdue hyperactivity of the liver for the treatment of tinnitus and impairment of hearing

针灸学 Acupuncture and Moxibustion

针法 Acupuncture

针灸学 [zhēn jiǔ xué]

(science of) acupuncture and moxibustion: a branch of traditional Chinese medicine which mainly involves the theory of meridians, location, usage, indications and combinations of acupoints, needling manipulations and application of ignited moxa in disease treatment through regulation of *qi*, blood and *zang-fu* functions

针灸医生 [zhēn jiǔ yī shēng]

acupuncturist: one who practices acupuncture and moxibustion

针法 [zhēn fǎ]

needling; acupuncture: a traditional Chinese therapy in which the functions of the body are regulated for curing diseases by stimulating certain sites on the body with special needles

刺法 [cì fǎ]

puncturing: a synonym for needling (针法 [zhēn fǎ])

刺灸法 [cì jiǔ fǎ]

puncturing and moxibustion: a collective term for the techniques of acupuncture and moxibustion

针灸 [zhēn jiǔ]

acupuncture-moxibustion: a collective term for acupuncture and moxibustion

同身寸 [tóng shēn cùn]

***cun*; proportional body *cun*:** unit of length for measurement in locating acupoints. A certain part of the patient's body is divided into certain divisions of equal length, each of which is taken as one proportional unit for measurement.

中指同身寸 [zhōng zhǐ tóng shēn cùn]

middle finger *cun*: the length between the two medial ends of the twisted folds of the patient's middle finger when bent, which is taken as one *cun*, a unit of measurement (Fig. 1)

拇指同身寸 [mǔ zhǐ tóng shēn cùn]

thumb *cun*: the width of the phalangeal joint of the patient's thumb, which is taken as one *cun*, a unit of measurement. (Fig. 2)

目横同身寸 [mù héng tóng shēn cùn]

eye *cun*: the length between the medial canthus and lateral canthus of the patient's eye, which is taken as one *cun*, a unit of measurement

一夫法 [yī fū fǎ]

palm measurement: The maximal width of the four fingers (namely, the first finger, middle finger, ring finger and little finger) held together with the hand open is taken as a unit of measurement of 3 *cun*. (Fig. 3)

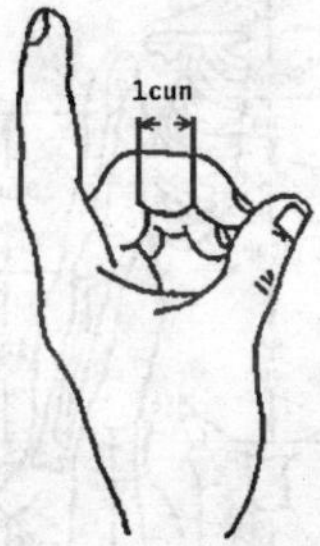

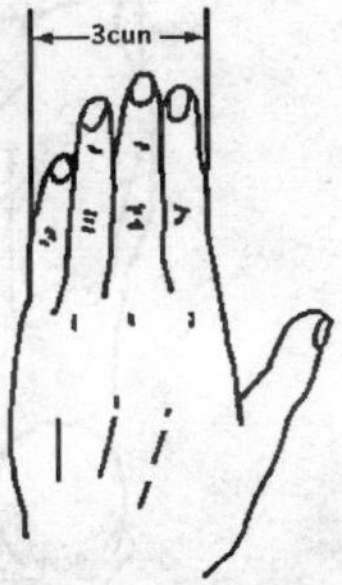

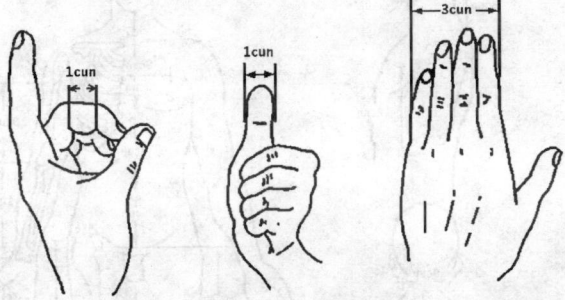

Fig.1 Middle finger cun Fig.2 Thumb cun Fig.3 Palm measurement

骨度法 [gǔ dù fǎ]

bone-length measurement: The length of equally divided portions of a certain long bone or of the distance between two anatomical landmarks is taken as one *cun*, a unit of measurement. (Fig. 4)

针尖 [zhēn jiān]

needle tip: the pointed end of the needle (Fig. 5)

针体 [zhēn tǐ]

needle body: the part of the needle between the tip and the handle (Fig. 5)

针根 [zhēn gēn]

needle root: junction between the handle and the body of the needle (Fig. 5)

针柄 [zhēn bǐng]

needle handle: that part of the needle held with the fingers in use (Fig. 5)

毫针 [háo zhēn]

filiform needle: a most commonly used acupuncture needle, with length ranging from 15 to 125mm, and caliber ranging from gauge 26 to gauge 32 (Fig. 5)

三棱针 [sān léng zhēn]

three-edged needle: a special kind of acupuncture needle with a triangular head and sharp point used for quick puncture and bloodletting

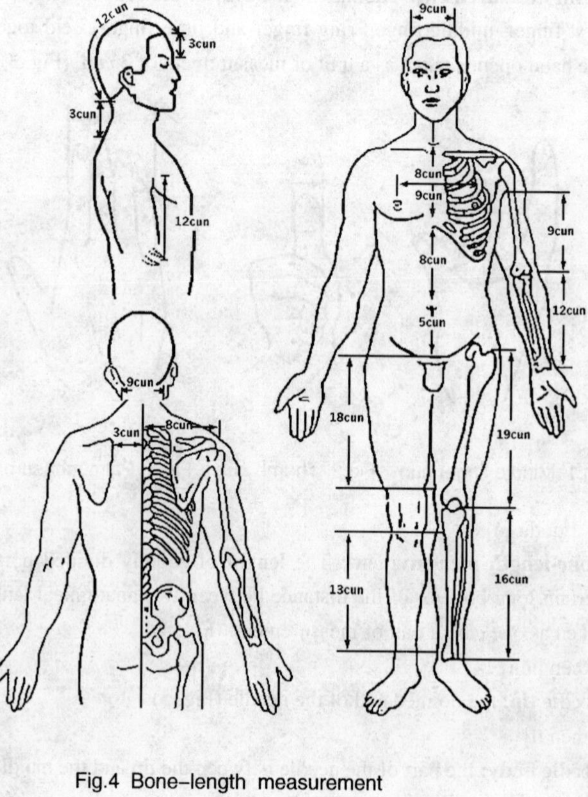

Fig.4 Bone-length measurement

三棱针法 [sān léng zhēn fǎ]

three-edged needling: a variety of therapeutic method to relieve or cure illness by using a three-edged needle, including pricking, open picking, scattered needling, and collateral puncture

点刺 [diǎn cì]

pricking: a fast piercing method in acupuncture, usually with a three-edged needle

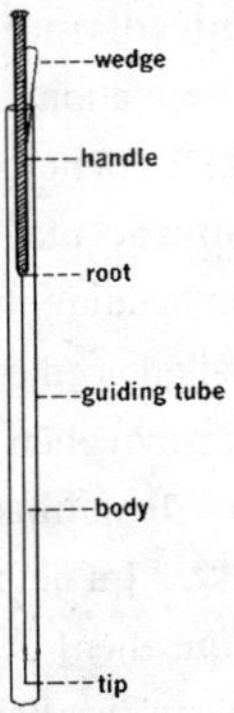

Fig.5 A filiform acupuncture needle

散刺 [sǎn cì]

scattered puncturing: a method of treatment by pricking with a three-edged needle around the local lesion, also known as leopard-spot puncturing (豹文刺 [bào wén cì])

豹文刺 [bào wén cì]

leopard-spot puncturing: another name for scattered puncturing (散刺 [sǎn cì])

刺络 [cì luò]

collateral puncturing: a therapeutic method using a three-edged needle, in which a vein at the cubital or popliteal fossa is pierced after sterilization of the local skin for letting out a small amount of blood

挑刺 [tiǎo cì]

open picking: a therapeutic method using a three-edged needle, in which the skin is fixed by pressing with one hand, and pierced 1-2 mm and picked open with the other hand

皮肤针 [pí fū zhēn]

dermal needle: a variety of needling instrument, including plumb-blossom needle and seven-star needle, composed of several short needles used for tapping and pricking certain points or areas of the body

皮肤针法 [pí fū zhēn fǎ]

dermal needling: a treatment for relieving or curing illness by using cutaneous needles

梅花针 [méi huā zhēn]

plum-blossom needle: a type of cutaneous needle with a bundle of five short fine needles fixed vertically at the end of a handle, the tips of which are clustered in the pattern of the plum blossom petals

七星针 [qī xīng zhēn]

seven-star needle: a type of cutaneous needle with seven short needles attached vertically to the end of a handle

皮内针 [pí nèi zhēn]

intradermal needle: a small needle embedded in the skin for continuous stimulation

皮内针法 [pī nèi zhēn fǎ]

intradermal needling: a treatment for relieving or curing illness by embedding in the skin a small needle or needles at a certain point(s), also called needle-embedding method (埋针法 [mái zhēn fǎ])

埋针法 [mái zhēn fǎ]

needle-embedding method: another name for intradermal needling (皮内针法 [pí nèi zhēn fǎ])

揿针 [qìn zhēn]

press needle: a small needle which is usually embedded in the auricle, also called thumbtack-type needle (图钉型针 [tú dīng xíng zhēn])

图钉型针 [tú dīng xíng zhēn]

thumbtack-type needle: a small needle for subcutaneous embedding with a head like a thumbtack, also known as press needle (揿针 [qìn zhēn])

麦粒型针 [mài lì xíng zhēn]

wheatgrain-like needle: a small needle with the head resembling a grain of wheat, which may be embedded subcutaneously at any part of the body

火针 [huǒ zhēn]

fire needle: heated needle, also known as burnt needle (燔针 [fán zhēn], 烧针 [shāo zhēn])

火针法 [huǒ zhēn fǎ]

fire needling: an acupuncture procedure which involves heating the needles, inserting them into the diseased part immediately and withdrawing them at once, often used for treating scrofula and rheumatism

燔针；烧针 [fán zhēn; shāo zhēn]

burnt needle: another name for fire needle (火针 [huǒ zhēn])

砭石 [biān shí]

stone needle: needle made of stone, used in acupuncture and surgical operation in ancient times

九针 [jiǔ zhēn]

nine needles: a collective term for the various kinds of needles used in ancient times, namely, 镵针 [chán zhēn] shear needle, 圆针 [yuán zhēn] round needle, 鍉针 [chí zhēn] spoon needle, 锋针 [fēng zhēn] lance needle, 铍针 or 铍针 [pī zhēn] stilletto needle, 圆利针 [yuán lì zhen] round-sharp needle, 毫针 [háo zhēn] filiform needle, 长针 [cháng zhēn], long needle and 大针 [dà zhēn] big needle

鑱针 [chán zhēn]

shear needle: one of the nine needles used in ancient times, marked by a big head and sharp tip, used for reducing yang-*qi*

圆针 [yuán zhēn]

round needle: one of the nine needles used in ancient times, marked by a round end, used for massage as in the treatment of rheumatic conditions

鍉针 [chí zhēn]

spoon needle: one of the nine needles used in ancient times, marked by a round and slightly pointed tip, used to press the meridian vessels for directing *qi* and blood

锋针 [fēng zhēn]

lance needle: one of the nine needles used in ancient times, also called three-edged needle (三棱针 [sān léng zhēn])

铍针；铧针 [pī zhēn]

stiletto needle: one of the nine needles used in ancient times, used for draining pus

圆利针 [yuán lìzhēn]

round-sharp needle: one of the nine needles used in ancient times, a small needle 1.6 *cun* long with a somewhat large and round-sharp end, used for treating abscesses and rheumatic conditions

长针 [cháng zhēn]

long needle: one of the nine needles used in ancient times, a needle with a length of 7 *cun*, used for deep puncturing

大针 [dà zhēn]

big needle: one of the nine needles used in ancient times, a large-gauge needle with a length of 4 *cun*, primarily used to treat edema

针灸铜人 [zhēn jiǔ tóng rén]

bronze figure with acupoints: human figure made of bronze marked with acupuncture points, used for teaching purposes, originated in the 11th century

进针 [jìn zhēn]

needle insertion: penetration of the skin with the tip of the needle to a certain depth

进针法 [jìn zhēn fǎ]

method of needle insertion: technique of inserting the needle through the skin (Fig. 6)

直刺 [zhí cì]

perpendicular insertion: insertion in which the needle enters the skin at a 90° angle (Fig. 6)

斜刺 [xié cì]

oblique insertion: needle insertion at a 40°–60° angle to the skin surface (Fig. 6)

平刺 [píng cì]

horizontal insertion: needle insertion at a 10°–25° angle to the skin surface (Fig. 6)

透刺 [tòu cì]

joined puncture: puncture of two or more adjoining points in one insertion of the needle

指切进针法 [zhǐ qiē jìn zhēn fǎ]

fingernail-pressing method of insertion: insertion of the needle with the help of finger-tip pressure — a method of insertion for short filiform needles

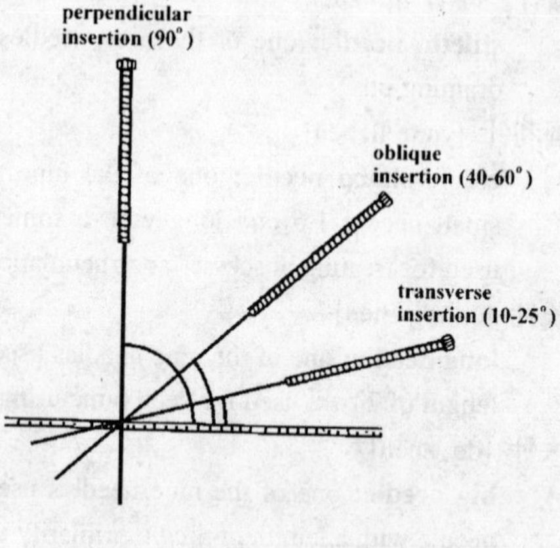

Fig.6 Methods of needle insertion

行针 [xíng zhēn]

needle manipulation: manipulating the needle after insertion to produce the desired effect

留针 [liú zhēn]

retaining of needle: retaining the needle in the point for a time to maintain and prolong the effect

出针 [chū zhēn]

needle withdrawal: taking the needle away from the point in which it has been inserted

出针法 [chū zhēn fǎ]

needle-withdrawal method: method of taking the needle out of the point in which it has been inserted

引针 [yǐn zhēn]

withdrawal of needle, synonymous with needle withdrawal (出针 [chū zhēn])

得气 [dé qì]

getting the *qi*: getting the acupuncture feeling, with soreness, heaviness, numbness and distension felt by the patient and tightness of the needle by the practitioner, which are normal sensations of successful acupuncture

补泻法 [bǔ xiè fǎ]

method of reinforcement and reduction: Reinforcement means to activate and restore a decreased function to normal, while reduction means to expel pathogenic factors and thus to restore hyperactivity to normal.

提插补泻 [tí chā bǔ xiè]

lifting-thrusting reinforcement-reduction: a form of needle manipulation in which reinforcement or reduction is attained by lifting and thrusting with different degrees of force

提插补泻法 [tí chā bǔ xiè fǎ]

lifting-thrusting reinforcement-reduction method: For reinforcement the needle is thrust in heavily and lifted gently, and for reduction, thrust in gently and lifted with force.

捻转补泻 [niǎn zhuǎn bǔ xiè]

twirling reinforcement-reduction: a form of needle manipulation in which the differentiation of reinforcing and reducing is based on the degree of twirling and the strength with which the needle is twirled.

捻转补泻法 [niǎn zhuǎn bǔ xiè fǎ]

twirling reinforcing-reducing method: For reduction, the degree of twirling should exceed 360°, with heavy manipulation. For reinforcement, the degree of twirling should be less than 180°, with gentle manipulation.

呼吸补泻 [hū xī bǔ xiè]

breathing reinforcement-reduction: a form of needle manipulation in which reinforcement or reduction is achieved by timing the insertion and withdrawal of the needle according to the phases of the patient's respiration.

呼吸补泻法 [hū xī bǔ xiè fǎ]

breathing reinforcing-reducing method: For reinforcement, the needle is inserted when the patient exhales and withdrawn when the patient has inhaled to the fullest capacity. For reduction, insertion is made during the patient's inspiration, and withdrawal at the end of expiration.

迎随补泻 [yíng suí bǔ xiè]

directional reinforcement-reduction: a form of needle manipulation in which reinforcement or reduction is achieved by the direction of needle insertion

迎随补泻法 [yíng suí bǔ xiè fǎ]

directional reinforcing-reducing method: During insertion, the needle is pointed obliquely along the run of the meridian for reinforcement, and against the run of the meridian for reduction.

开阖补泻 [kāi hé bǔ xiè]

open-close reinforcement-reduction: a form of needle manipulation in which reinforcement or reduction is achieved by closing or opening the acupuncture hole after withdrawing the needle

开阖补泻法 [kāi hé bǔ xiè fǎ]]

open-close reinforcement-reduction method: Reinforcement is achieved if the acupuncture hole after withdrawing the needle is closed with light finger pressure to prevent the *qi* from escaping, and reduction by leaving the hole open to let pathogenic factors out.

疾徐补泻 [jī xú bǔ xiè]

rapid-slow reinforcement-reduction: a form of needle manipulation in which reinforcement or reduction is achieved by insertion and withdrawal of the needle at different speeds

疾徐补泻法 [jī xú bǔ xiè fǎ]

rapid-slow reinforcing-reducing method: For reinforcement, the insertion is slow, while the withdrawal is rapid, and for reduction, the insertion is swift, while the withdrawal is slow.

平补平泻 [píng bǔ píng xiè]

uniform reinforcement-reduction: a form of needle manipulation indicated in a case with combined excess and deficiency or no distinct excess or deficiency

平补平泻法 [píng bǔ píng xiè fǎ]

uniform reinforcing-reducing method: The needle is lifted, thrust and twirled evenly with a proper amplitude and favorable angle.

白虎摇头 [bái hǔ yáo tóu fǎ]

"white tiger shaking its head": a form of needle manipulation, in which the practitioner whirls the needle to the left while inserting, and whirls it to the right while lifting, and then shakes it gently to promote blood circulation

青龙摆尾 [qīng lóng bǎi wěi fǎ]

"green dragon wagging the tail": a form of needle manipulation, in which the practitioner directs the inserted needle toward the diseased site and gently moves its handle from side to side in order to guide the flow of *qi*

烧山火 [shāo shān huǒ]

"burning the mountain": a form of needle manipulation to achieve reinforcement with a local or generalized feeling of intense heat

透天凉 [tòu tiān liáng]

"cooling the sky": a form of needle manipulation to achieve reduction with a local or generalized feeling of cooling

行气法 [xíng qì fǎ]

***qi*-conducting method:** a method of conducting the *qi* or acupuncture feeling to a certain site, usually the diseased site.

指压行气法 [zhǐ yā xíng qì fǎ]

finger-pressure conduction of *qi*: a method of inducing the acupuncture feeling to travel proximally or distally along the meridian by applying pressure with the finger to the meridian distal or proximal to the acupoint, respectively.

针向行气法 [zhēn xiàng xíng qì fǎ]

needle-direction conduction of *qi*: a method of inducing the transmission of the acupuncture feeling by varying the direction of insertion, i.e., inserting the needle in the same direction as that of the desired *qi* transmission

晕针 [yūn zhēn]

fainting during acupuncture: one of the acupuncture complications, manifested by dizziness, dim eyesight, pale complexion, nausea, palpitations, cold sweats and drop of blood pressure

滞针 [zhì zhēn]

sticking of the needle: one of the abnormal conditions occurring in acupuncture, when the needle is impossible to be whirled, lifted, thrust, or even withdrawn after it is inserted

弯针 [wān zhēn]

bending of the needle: one of the abnormal conditions occurring during acupuncture after insertion of the needle, often due to change of the patient's posture

折针 [zhé zhēn]

breaking of the needle: acupuncture accident mostly due to using needles of poor quality, too forceful manipulation that causes powerful muscle contraction, or sudden change of the patient's posture

经络 Meridian System

经络学说 [jīng luò xué shuō]

theory of meridians: an important component part of traditional Chinese medical theory, according to which there exists within the human body a system of conduits through which *qi* and blood circulate, and by which the internal organs are connected with the superficial organs and tissues, and the body is made an organic whole

经络 [jīng luò]

meridian system; channels and collaterals: conduits through which *qi* and blood circulate and by which the internal organs are related to superficial organs and tissues, making the body an organic whole

经脉 [jīng mài]

meridians; channels: cardinal conduits of *qi* and blood coursing vertically, composed of the twelve regular meridians and the eight extra meridians

络脉 [luò mài]

collaterals: the branches of the meridians, serving as the network linking the various aspects of the body, and consisting of the fifteen collaterals (十五络脉 [shí wǔ luò mài]), superficial collaterals (浮络 [fú luò]), and lesser collaterals (孙络 [sūn luò])

十二经 [shí èr jīng]

twelve meridians, also known as the regular meridians (正经 [zhèng jīng]). They are the lung meridian of hand *taiyin* (LU), the large intestine meridian of hand *yangming* (LI), the stomach meridian of foot *yangming* (ST), the spleen meridian of foot *taiyin* (SP), the heart meridian of hand *shaoyin* (HT), the small intestine meridian of hand *taiyang* (SI), the bladder meridian of foot *taiyang* (BL), the kidney meridian of foot *shaoyin* (KI), the pericardium meridian of hand *jueyin* (PC), the triple energizer meridian of hand *shaoyang* (TE), the gallbladder meridian of foot *shaoyang* (GB), and the liver meridian of foot *jueyin* (LR). They are the main passages of *qi* and blood.

十二经脉 [shí èr jīng mài]

twelve meridians, same as 十二经 [shí èr jīng]

正经 [zhèng jīng]

regular meridians: another name of the twelve meridians (十二经 [shí èr jīng])

手三阴经 [shǒu sān yīn jīng]

three yin meridians of the hand: the meridians running through the anterior side of the upper limbs from the chest to the hands, namely, the lung meridian, the heart meridian, and the pericardium meridian

手三阳经 [shǒu sān yáng jīng]

three yang meridians of the hand: the meridians running through the posterior side of the upper limbs from the hands to the head, namely, the large intestine meridian, the small intestine meridian, and the triple energizer meridian

足三阳经 [zú sān yáng jīng]

three yang meridians of the foot: the meridians running from the head through the trunk downward to the feet, namely, the stomach meridian, the bladder meridian, and the gallbladder meridian

足三阴经 [zú sān yīn jīng]

three yin meridians of the foot: the meridians running through the inner side of the lower limbs from the feet to the abdomen and chest, namely, the spleen meridian, the kidney meridian, and the liver meridian

六经 [liù jīng]

six meridians: a collective term for *taiyang* meridian, *yangming* meridian, *shaoyang* meridian, *taiyin* meridian, *shaoyin* meridian, and *jueyin* meridian, which, in conformity with the twelve meridians, may be subdivided into the six meridians of the hand and the six meridians of the foot

阳经 [yáng jīng]

yang meridians: a collective term for the three yang meridians of the hand and the foot, governor vessel, yang link vessel, and yang heel vessel

阴经 [yīn jīng]

yin meridians: a collective term for the three yin meridians of the hand and the foot, conception vessel, thoroughfare vessel, yin link vessel, and yin heel vessel

三阴 [sān yīn]

(1) the three yin: a collective name for the three yin meridians of both the hand and the foot, six in all; **(2) the third yin:** *taiyin* meridian

二阴 [èr yīn]

the second yin: *shaoyin* meridian

一阴 [yī yīn]

the first yin: *jueyin* meridian

三阳 [sān yáng]

(1) the three yang: a collective name for the three yang meridians of both the hands and the feet, six in all; **(2) the third yang:** *taiyang* meridian

二阳 [èr yáng]

the second yang: *yangming* meridian

一阳 [yī yáng]

the first yang: *shaoyang* meridian

十四经 [shí sì jīng]

fourteen meridians: the twelve meridians plus the governor and conception vessels

手太阴肺经 [shǒu tài yīn fèi jīng]

lung meridian of hand *taiyin*; lung meridian (LU): one of the twelve meridians, which begins internally in the middle energizer, descends to connect with the large intestine, then ascends to the lung and throat, courses laterally and exits superficially at *zhongfu* (LU1), and then descends along the lateral side of the arm and forearm, terminates at *shaoshang* (LU11), with 11 points on either side (Fig. 7)

手阳明大肠经 [shǒu yáng míng dà cháng jīng]

large intestine meridian of hand *yangming*; large intestine meridian (LI): one of the twelve meridians, which originates at *shangyang* (LI1) and ascends the dorsal surface of the hand and forearm, the lateral side of the arm, the dorsal side of the shoulder to *jugu* (LI16), where the meridian enters internally and travels posteriorly to *dazhui* (GV14), and then courses anteriorly to the supraclavicular fossa, where it descends past the diaphragm to connect with the large intestine. The superficial supraclavicular branch ascends the anterior lateral neck and the mandible, connects internally with the lower teeth, encircles the lips and terminates at the opposite *yingxiang* (LI20). There are 20 points on either side of the body. (Fig. 8)

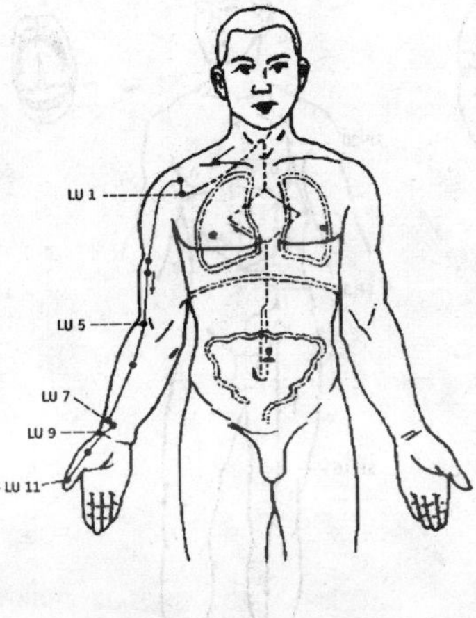

Fig.7 Lung Meridian

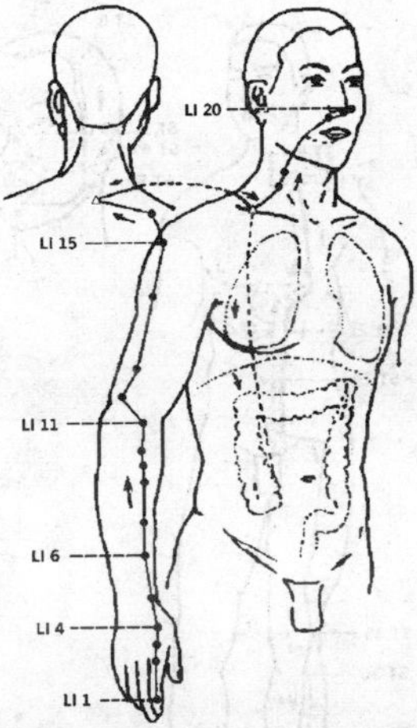

Fig.8 Large Intestine Meridian

足阳明胃经 [zú yáng míng wèi jīng]

stomach meridian of foot *yangming*; stomach meridian (ST): one of the twelve meridians which originates internally at the lateral edge of the nose, ascends to the medial canthus of the eye, then continues to the first superficial point *chenqi* (ST1) at the inferior border of the orbit, descends to the upper gum, courses around the mouth, and travels up to *touwei* (ST8) at the hairline of the temple. From here it continues internally to terminate at *shenting* (GV24). The facial branch descends from *daying* (ST5), where it turns internally and descends past the diaphragm to connect with the stomach and spleen. The supraclavicular fossa branch descends along the midclavicular line to *qichong* (ST30) in the inguinal region, then anteriorly along the lateral margin of the femur to the patella, terminating at *lidui* (ST45) on the lateral side of the tip of the second toe. The gastric branch descends internally past the umbilicus and terminates at *qichong* (ST30). The tibial branch leaves *zusanli* (ST36) and descends along the fibula, terminating at the lateral side of the tip of the middle toe. The dorsal foot branch leaves *chongyang* (ST42) and descends to the medial side of the great toe at *yinbai* (SP1). There are 45 points on either side of the body. (Fig.9)

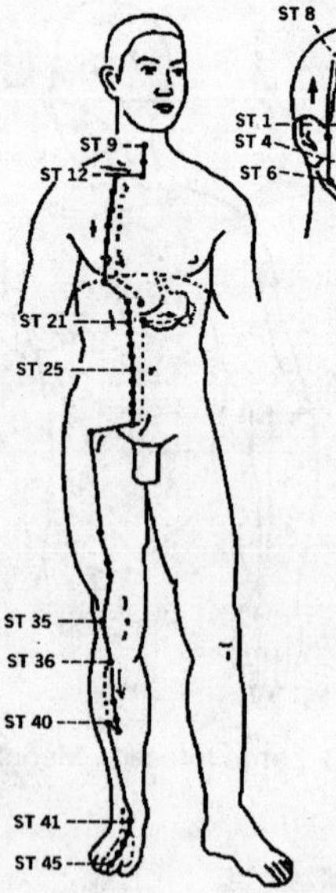

Fig.9 Stomach Meridian

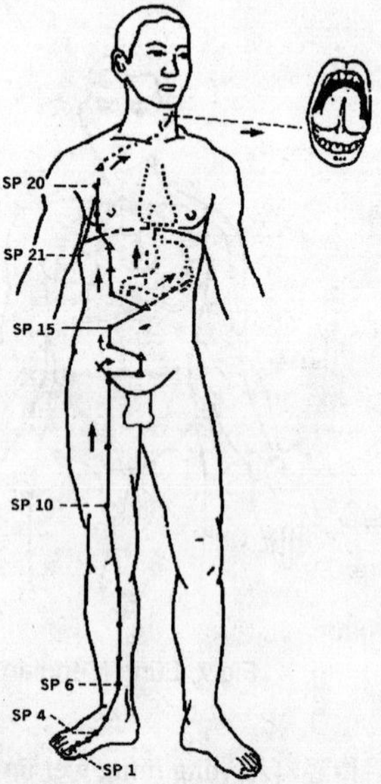

Fig.10 Spleen Meridian

足太阴脾经 [zú tài yīn pí jīng]

spleen meridian of foot *taiyin*; spleen meridian (SP): one of the twelve meridians, which runs from *yinbai* (SP 1) at the medial side of the great toe, ascends along the medial side of the foot and tibia and anteromedial side of the thigh to the lower abdomen. It then enters the abdomen, and connects with the spleen and stomach. The meridian ascends the abdomen at a distance of 4.0 *cun* lateral to the conception vessel, and terminates superficially at *dabao* (SP21) in the sixth intercostal space on the midaxillary line. The meridian continues internally past the supraclavicular fossa and terminates at the base of the tongue. The gastric branch leaves the stomach and ascends ınternally past the diaphragm, and connects with the heart. There are 21 points on either side of the body. (Fig. 10)

手少阴心经 [shǒu shào yīn xīn jīng]

heart meridian of hand *shaoyin*; heart meridian (HT): one of the twelve meridians, which originates in the heart, descends internally past the diaphragm, and connects with the small intestine. The cardiac branch ascends internally paralateral to the esophagus, and terminates at the eye. The main branch leaves the heart, traverses the lung and emerges superficially in the midaxilla at *jiquan* (HT1) and descends along the ulnar side of the forearm medially, terminating at *shaochong* (HT9) on the radial side of the tip of the small finger, with 9 points on either side. (Fig. 11)

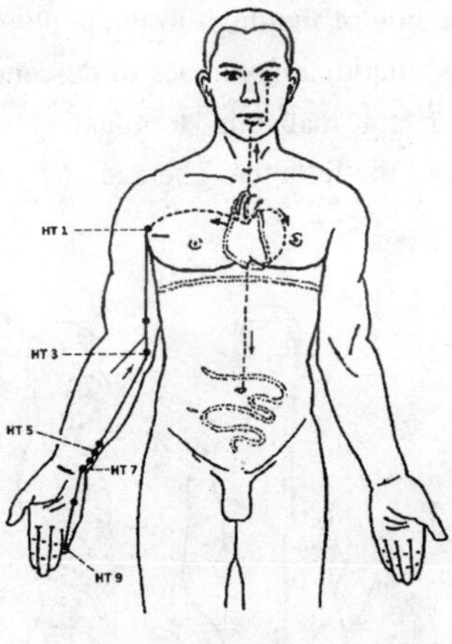

Fig.11 Heart Meridian

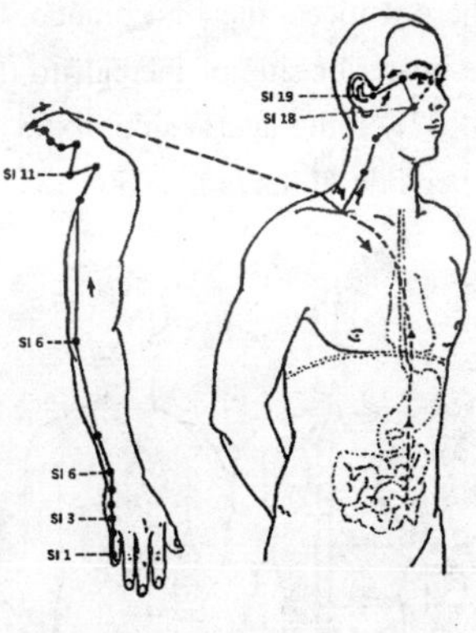

Fig.12 Small Intestine Meridian

手太阳小肠经 [shǒu tài yáng xiǎo cháng jīng]

small intestine meridian of hand *taiyang*; small intestine meridian (SI): one of the twelve meridians which originates at *shaoze* (SI1) at the ulnar side of the little finger, ascends the ulnar side of the forearm, the arm, over the scapula to *dazhui* (GV14) between the spinous processes of the 7th cervical and 1st thoracic vertebrae. The meridian then descends internally to the heart, and follows the esophagus past the diaphragm, to connect with the small intestine. The supraclavicular fossa branch ascends superficially along the lateral side of the neck, past the cheek to the lateral corner of the eye, and terminates at *tinggong* (SI19). The buccal branch leaves the main meridian at the cheek, and ascends to the medial canthus of the eye. There are 19 points on either side. (Fig. 12)

足太阳膀胱经 [zú tài yáng páng guāng jīng]

bladder meridian of foot *taiyang*; bladder meridian (BL): one of the twelve meridians which runs from *jingming* (BL1) at the medial canthus of the eye, ascends the forehead to the vertex and then enters the brain, and exits at the nape of the neck, where it divides into two parallel branches: The first branch descends the back at a distance of 1.5 *cun* from the spine, and during its course it connects with the kidney and the urinary bladder, and continues along the posterior side of the thigh to the popliteal fold; the second branch descends the back at a distance of 3 *cun* from the spine, continues along the latero-posterior side of the thigh to the popliteal fold, where it meets the first branch. The meridian continues to descend along the posterior side of the calf to the lateral malleolus, terminating at *zhiyin* (BL67) on the lateral side of the tip of the little toe. There are 67 points on either side of the body. (Fig. 13)

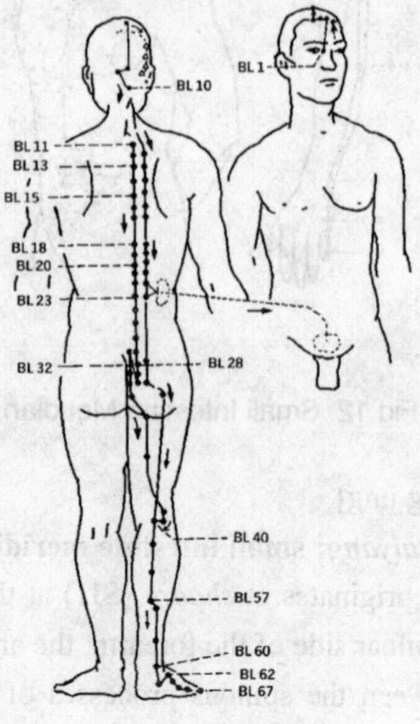

Fig.13 Bladder Meridian

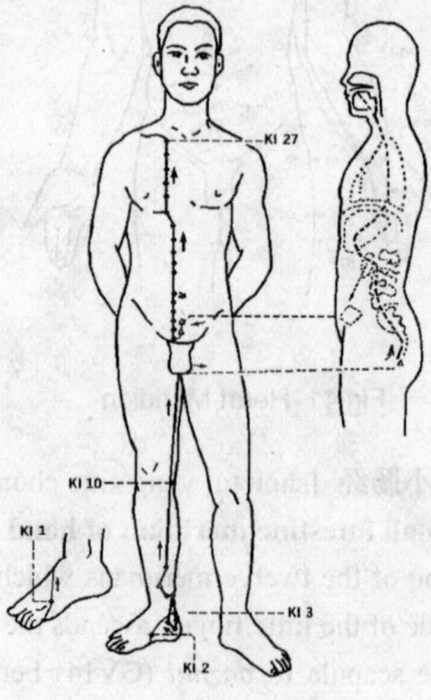

Fig.14 Kidney Meridian

足少阴肾经 [zú shào yīn shèn jīng]

kidney meridian of foot *shaoyin*; kidney meridian (KI): one of the twelve meridians which begins on the plantar tip of the little toe and travels to *yongquan* (KI1) in the center of the sole, continues along the inner side of the lower limb to the symphysis pubis, turns internally to the kidney and urinary bladder, and back to the symphysis pubis, descending along the abdomen and chest up to *shufu* (KI27) in the depression between the first rib and the lower border of the clavicle, with 27 points on either side (Fig. 14)

手厥阴心包经 [shǒu jué yīn xīn bāo jīng]

pericardium meridian of hand *jueyin*; pericardium meridian (PC): one of the twelve meridians which originates in the center of the thorax, connects with the pericardium, and descends to the lower abdomen, linking all the three energizers. The thoracic branch exits superficially at *tianchi* (PC1) near the nipple, and descends along the midline of the anterior side of the arm to *zhongchong* (PC9) at the midpoint of the tip of the middle finger, with 9 points on either side. (Fig. 15)

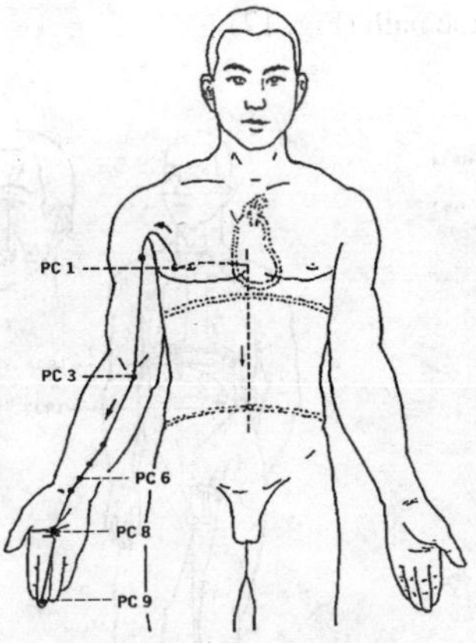

Fig.15 Pericardium Meridian

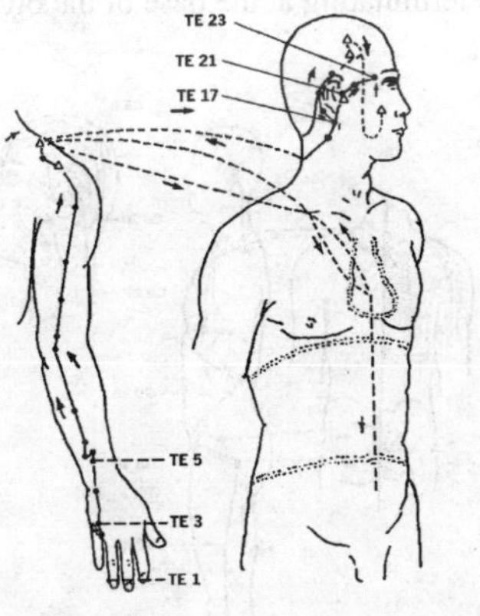

Fig.16 Triple Energizer Meridian

手少阳三焦经 [shǒu shào yáng sān jiāo jīng]

triple energizer meridian of hand *shaoyang*; triple energizer meridian (TE): one of the twelve meridians, which runs from *guanchong* (TE1) at the ulnar side of the ring finger, travels along the midline of the posterior side of the arm and through the regions of the shoulder, neck, ear and eye, and terminates at *sizhukong* (TE23) at the lateral canthus, with 23 points on either side. A branch extends from the supraclavicular fossa to the pericardium and down through the thorax and abdomen, linking the upper, middle and lower energizers. (Fig. 16)

足少阳胆经 [zú shào yáng dǎn jīng]

gallbladder meridian of foot *shaoyang*; gallbladder meridian (GB): one of the twelve meridians, which runs from *tongziliao* (GB1) at the lateral canthus of the eye, through the regions of the temple, ear, neck, shoulder, flank, and the outer side of the lower limb, terminating at *zuqiaoyin* (GB44) on the lateral side of the tip of the 4th toe, with 44 points on either side. The post-auricular branch travels into the ear and down to the supraclavicular fossa where it joins the original branch. It continues down into the chest, past the diaphragm, connecting with the gallbladder and liver, and travels down to the lower abdomen into the inguinal canal. The dorsal foot branch leaves the main meridian at *zulinqi* (GB41) and descends between the first and second metatarsals, terminating at the base of the big toe nail. (Fig. 17)

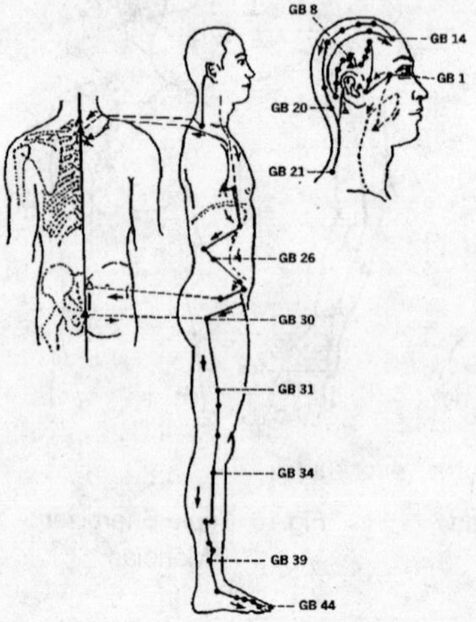

Fig.17 Gallbladder Meridian

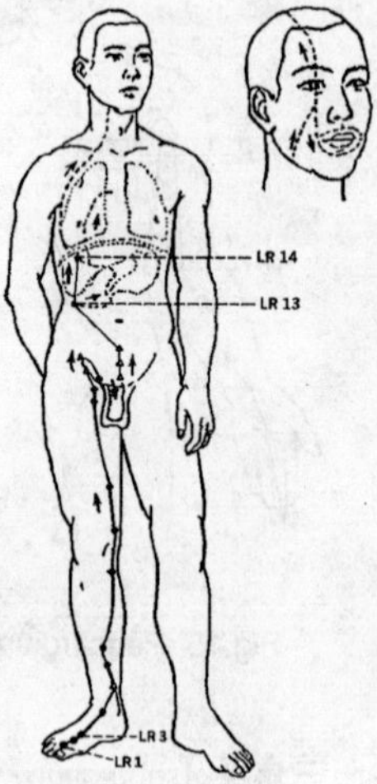

Fig.18 Liver Meridian

足厥阴肝经 [zú jué yīn gān jīng]

liver meridian of foot *jueyin*; liver meridian (LR): one of the twelve meridians, which runs from dadun (LR1) on the big toe just behind the nail, through the inner side of the lower limb, external genitalia and abdomen, to *qimen* (LR14), a point about 2 *cun* below the nipple, with 14 points on either side. From *qimen* (LR14) the meridian enters the abdomen, travels the stomach para-laterally, to connect with the liver and gallbladder. From the liver, the meridian ascends past the diaphragm along the trachea, larynx, and sinus cavity, connecting with the eye, and then ascends to the vertex, where it meets the governor vessel. (Fig. 18)

奇经八脉 [jì jīng bā mài]

eight extra meridians: governor vessel, conception vessel, thoroughfare vessel, belt vessel, yin heel vessel, yang heel vessel, yin link vessel, and yang link vessel

督脉 [dū mài]

governor vessel (GV): one of the eight extra meridians which begins at *changqiang* (GV1), a point at the back of the anus, sending one branch forward to *huiyin* (CV1). The main portion of the meridian ascends along the midline of the back to the top of the head, and then descends the midline of the face down to *yinjiao* (GV28), a point between the upper lip and the upper gum in the labia frenum, with 28 points. (Fig. 19)

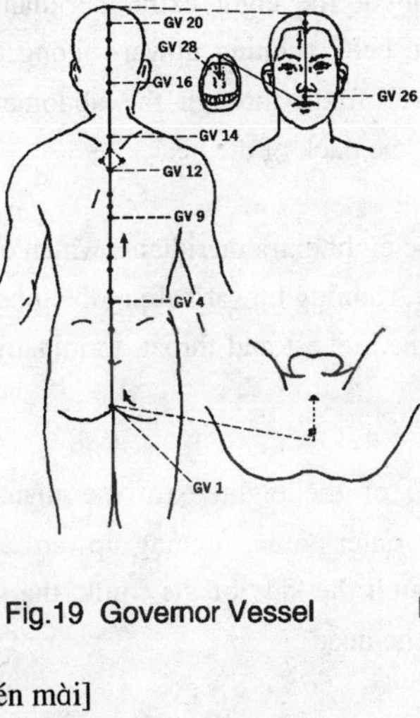

Fig.19 Governor Vessel

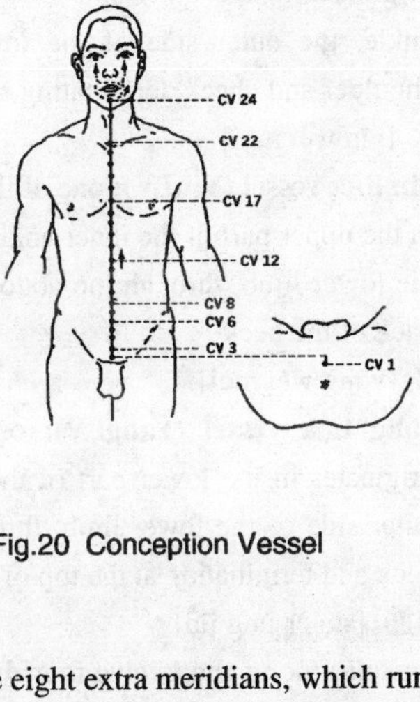

Fig.20 Conception Vessel

任脉 [rén mài]

conception vessel (CV): one of the eight extra meridians, which runs from *huiyin* (CV1), a point in the center of perineum, ascends the midline of the abdominal wall and chest to *chengjiang* (CV24), the midpoint of the mentolabial sulcus, with 24 points. The internal portion of this meridian ascends from *chengjiang* (CV24), encircling the mouth and traveling to the eyes. Another branch travels internally from the pelvic cavity, and ascends the spine to the throat. (Fig. 20)

冲脉 [chōng mài]

thoroughfare vessel (TV): one of the eight extra meridians, which originates in the uterus or *guanyuan* (CV4), comes into confluence with the kidney meridian, and then runs upward along the two sides of the abdomen to the chest

带脉 [dài mài]

belt vessel (BV): one of the eight extra meridians which originates from the lower part of the hypochondria and goes round the waist

阴跷脉 [yīn qiāo mài]

yin heel vessel (YinHV): one of the eight extra meridians, which originates in the inner side of the heel, running upward along the inner side of the lower limb, through the front private parts, the abdomen, chest, neck and either side of the nose, and terminating in the eye

阳跷脉 [yáng qiāo mài]

yang heel vessel (YangHV): one of the eight extra meridians, which originates in the outer side of the heel, running upward along the outer ankle, the outer side of the lower limb, through the abdomen, chest, shoulder and cheek, terminating at the back of the neck

阴维脉 [yīn wéi mài]

yin link vessel (YinLV): one of the eight extra meridians, which originates in the upper part of the inner ankle, running upward along the inner side of the lower limb, through the abdomen, chest and throat, terminating at the back of the neck

阳维脉 [yáng wéi mài]

yang link vessel (YangLV): one of the eight extra meridians, which originates in the lower part of the outer ankle, running upward along the outer side of the lower limb, through the side of the trunk, the shoulder, neck and terminating at the top of the head

十二经筋 [shí èr jīng jīn]

muscles along the twelve meridians: the muscle systems distributed and nourished by the *qi* of the twelve meridians, also called muscles along meridians (经筋 [jīng jīn]) for short

经筋 [jīng jīn]

muscles along meridians: abbreviation for muscles along the twelve meridians (十二经筋 [shí èr jīng jīn])

十二经别 [shí èr jīng bié]

twelve divergent meridians: the divergent passages of the regular meridians going deep into the body to strengthen the communication between the interior and exterior, and to serve as supplementary passages for the flow of *qi* of the regular meridians, also called divergent meridians (经别 [jīng bié]) for short

经别 [jīng bié]

divergent meridians: abbreviation for the divergent passages of the regular meridians (十二经别 [shí èr jīng bié])

十二皮部 [shí èr pí bù]

twelve cutaneous regions: the regions of the skin reflecting the functioning of the twelve regular meridians respectively

十五络脉 [shí wǔ luò mài]

fifteen main collaterals: Each of the fourteen meridians has a main collateral – together with the great collateral of the spleen, there are fifteen in all – which communicate with the exterior and interior of the body.

脾之大络 [pí zhī dà luò]

great collateral of the spleen: the collateral that issues from *dabao* (SP21) and spreads over the thoracic and hypochondriac regions

孙络 [sūn luò]

tertiary collateral: (1) subdivided small branch of the meridian; (2) capillary

浮络 [fú luò]

superficial collateral: collateral lying just beneath the skin

鱼络 [yú luò]

thenar collateral: collateral on the thenar eminence, the congestion of which shows disorder of the large intestinal meridian.

胞络 [bāo luò]

uterine collateral: vessels distributed on the uterus

胞脉 [bāo mài]

uterine vessels: vessels that connect with the uterus, chiefly the conception vessel and thoroughfare vessel, governing menstruation, conception and pregnancy

阴络 [yīn luò]

yin collateral: (1) collateral or branch of the yin meridian of the hand or foot; (2) collateral going downward or deep

阳络 [yáng luò]

yang collateral: (1) collateral or branch of yang meridian of hand or foot; (2) collateral or branch running upward or superficially

俞穴 Acupoints

经穴 Meridian Points

经穴 [jīng xué]

meridian point: acupuncture point of a regular meridian

手太阴肺经穴 [shǒu tài yīn fèi jīng xué]

points of lung meridian: acupuncture-moxibustion points distributed on the lung meridian (LI)

中府 [zhōng fǔ]

***zhongfu* (LU1):** point in the superior lateral part of the anterior thoracic wall, on the level of the 1st intercostal space, 6 *cun* lateral to the anterior midline (Fig. 24)

云门 [yún mén]

***yunmen* (LU2):** point in the depression of the infraclavicular fossa, 6 *cun* lateral to the anterior midline (Fig. 24)

天府 [tiān fǔ]

***tianfu* (LU3):** point on the medial side of the upper arm, 3 *cun* below the anterior end of the axillary fold (Fig. 21)

侠白 [xiá bái]

***xiabai* (LU4):** point on the medial side of the upper arm, 4 *cun* below the anterior end of the axillary fold (Fig. 21)

尺泽 [chǐ zé]

***chize* (LU5):** point in the cubital crease, in the depression of the radial side of the tendon of the biceps muscle of the arm (Fig. 21)

孔最 [kǒng zuì]

***kongzui* (LU6):** point on the radial side of the palmar surface of the forearm, 7 *cun* above the cubital crease (Fig. 21)

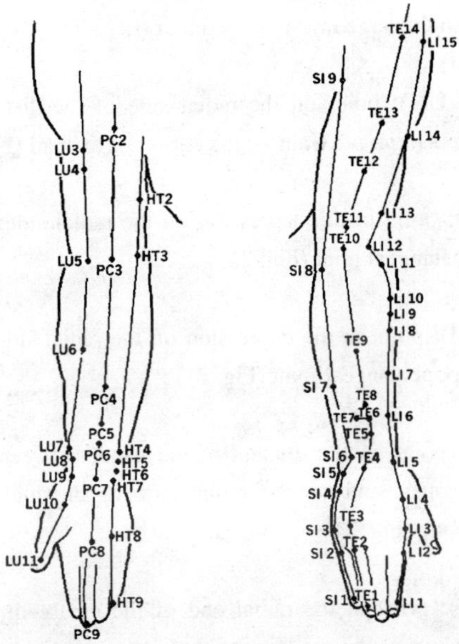

Fig.21 Regular points on the upper limb

列缺 [liè quē]

***lieque* (LU7):** point on the radial side of the forearm, proximal to the styloid process of the radius, 1.5 *cun* above the crease of the wrist (Fig. 21)

经渠 [jīng qú]

***jingqu* (LU8):** point on the radial side of the palmar surface of the forearm, 1 *cun* above the crease of the wrist (Fig. 21)

太渊 [tài yuān]

***taiyuan* (LU9):** point at the radial end of the crease of the wrist, where the pulsation of the radial artery is palpable (Fig. 21)

鱼际 [yú jì]

***yuji* (LU10):** point on the radial side of the midpoint of the 1st metacarpal bone, and on the junction of the red and white skin (Fig. 21)

少商 [shào shāng]

***shaoshang* (LU11):** point on the radial side of the distal segment of the thumb, 0.1 *cun* from the corner of the fingernail (Fig. 21)

手阳明大肠经穴 [shǒu yáng míng dà cháng jīng xué]

points of large intestine meridian: acupuncture-moxibustion points distributed on the large intestine meridian (LI)

商阳 [shāng yáng]

***shangyang* (LI1):** point on the radial side of the distal segment of the index finger, 0.1 *cun* proximal to the corner of the nail (Fig. 21)

二间 [èr jiān]

***erjian* (LI2):** point in the depression on the radial side, distal to the 2nd metacarpophalangeal joint (Fig. 21)

三间 [sān jiān]

***sanjian* (LI3):** point in the depression on the radial side, proximal to the 2nd metacarpophalangeal joint (Fig. 21)

合谷 [hé gǔ]

***hegu* (LI4):** point on the dorsum of the hand, between the 1st and 2nd metacarpal bones, and on the radial side of the midpoint of the 2nd metacarpal bone (Fig. 21)

阳溪 [yáng xī]

***yangxi* (LI5):** point at the radial end of the crease of the wrist, in the depression between the tendons of the short extensor and long extensor muscles of the thumb when the thumb is tilted upward (Fig. 21)

偏历 [piān lì]

***pianli* (LI6):** point on the radial side of the dorsal surface of the forearm, 3 *cun* above the crease of the wrist (Fig. 21)

温溜 [wēn liù]

***wenliu* (LI7):** point on the radial side of the dorsal surface of the forearm, 5 *cun* above the crease of the wrist (Fig. 21)

下廉 [xià lián]

***xialian* (LI8):** point on the radial side of the dorsal surface of the forearm, 4 *cun* below the cubital crease (Fig. 21)

上廉 [shàng lián]

***shanglian* (LI9):** point on the radial side of the dorsal surface of the forearm, 3 *cun* below the cubital crease (Fig. 21)

手三里 [shǒu sān lǐ]

***shousanli* (LI10):** point on the radial side of the dorsal surface of the forearm, 2 *cun* below the cubital crease (Fig. 21)

曲池 [qū chí]

***quchi* (LI11):** point at the lateral end of the cubital crease with the elbow flexed (Fig. 21)

肘髎 [zhǒu liáo]

***zhouliao* (LI12):** point on the lateral side of the upper arm, 1 *cun* above *quchi* (LI11) with the elbow flexed, on the border of the humerus (Fig. 21)

手五里 [shǒu wǔ lǐ]

***shouwuli* (LI13):** point on the lateral side of the upper arm, 3 *cun* above *quchi* (LI11) (Fig. 21)

臂臑 [bì nào]

***binao* (LI14):** point on the lateral side of the arm, 7 *cun* above *quchi* (LI11) (Fig. 21)

肩髃 [jiān yú]

***jianyu* (LI15):** point on the shoulder, in the depression anterior and inferior to the acromion when the arm is abducted (Fig. 21)

巨骨 [jù gǔ]

***jugu* (LI16):** point on the shoulder, in the depression between the acromial extremity of the clavicle and scapular spine (Fig. 24)

天鼎 [tiān dǐng]

***tianding* (LI17):** point on the lateral side of the neck, at the posterior border of the sternocleidomastoid muscle beside the laryngeal protuberance (fig. 23a,b)

扶突 [fú tū]

***futu* (LI18):** point on the lateral side of the neck, beside the laryngeal protuberance, between the anterior and posterior borders of the sternocleidomastoid muscle (fig. 23a,b)

口禾髎 [kǒu hé liáo]

***kouheliao* (LI19):** point on the upper lip, directly below the lateral border of the nostril, on the level of *shuigou* (GV26) (fig. 23a,b)

禾髎 [hé liáo]

***heliao* (LI19),** same as 口禾髎 [kǒu hé liáo]

迎香 [yíng xiāng]

***yingxiang* (LI20):** point in the nasolabial groove, beside the midpoint of the lateral border of the nasal ala (fig. 23a,b)

足阳明胃经穴 [zú yáng míng wèi jīng xué]

points of stomach meridian: acupuncture-moxibustion points distributed on the stomach meridian (ST)

承泣 [chéng qì]

***chengqi* (ST1):** point on the face, directly below the pupil, between the eyeball and the infraorbital ridge (Fig. 23a,b)

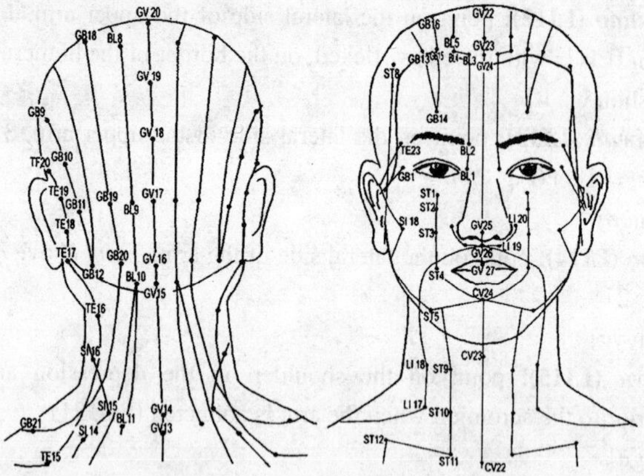

Fig.23a Regular points on the head

四白 [sì bái]

***sibai* (ST2):** point on the face, directly below the pupil, in the depression of the infraorbital foramen (Fig. 23a,b)

巨髎 [jù liáo]

***juliao* (ST3):** point on the face, directly below the pupil, on the level of the lower border of the nasal ala (Fig. 23a,b)

地仓 [dì cāng]

***dicang* (ST4):** point on the face, directly below the pupil, beside the mouth angle (Fig. 23a,b)

大迎 [dà yíng]

***daying* (ST5):** point anterior to the mandibular angle, on the anterior border of the masseter muscle, where the pulsation of the facial artery is palpable (Fig. 23a,b)

颊车 [jiá chē]

***jiache* (ST6):** point on the cheek, one finger breadth anterior and superior to the mandibular angle (Fig. 23a,b)

下关 [xià guān]

***xiaguan* (ST7):** point on the face, anterior to the ear, in the depression between the zygomatic arch and mandibular notch (Fig. 23a,b)

头维 [tóu wéi]

***touwei* (ST8):** point on the lateral side of the head, 0. 5 *cun* above the anterior hairline at the corner of the forehead (Fig. 23a,b)

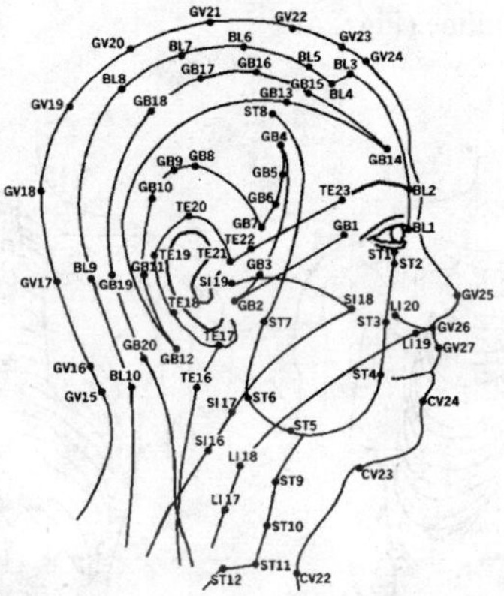

Fig.23b Regular points on the head

人迎 [rén yíng]

***renying* (ST9):** point on the neck, beside the laryngeal protuberance, and on the anterior border of the sternocleidomastoid muscle where the pulsation of the common carotid artery is palpable (Fig. 23a,b)

水突 [shuǐ tū]

***shuitu* (ST10):** point on the neck and on the anterior border of the sternocleidomastoid muscle, at the midpoint of the line connecting *renying* (ST9) and *qishe* (ST11) (Fig. 23a,b)

气舍 [qì shè]

***qishe* (ST11):** point on the neck and on the upper border of the medial end of the clavicle, between the sternal and clavicular heads of the sternocleidomastoid muscle (Fig. 23a,b)

缺盆 [quē pén]

***quepen* (ST12):** point at the center of the supraclavicular fossa, 4 *cun* lateral to the anterior midline (Fig. 23a,b)

气户 [qì hù]

***qihu* (ST13):** point on the chest, below the midpoint of the lower border of the clavicle, 4 *cun* lateral to the anterior midline (Fig. 24)

库房 [kù fáng]

kufang **(ST14):** point on the chest, in the 1st intercostal space, 4 *cun* lateral to the anterior midline (Fig. 24)

屋翳 [wū yì]

wuyi **(ST15):** point on the chest, in the 2nd intercostal space, 4 *cun* lateral to the anterior midline (Fig. 24)

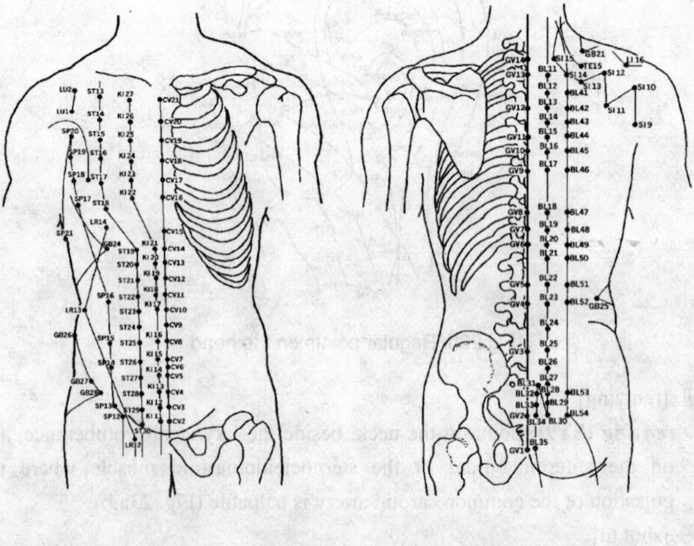

Fig.24 Regular points on the trunk

膺窗 [yīng chuāng]

yingchuang **(ST16):** point on the chest, in the 3rd intercostal space, 4 *cun* lateral to the anterior midline (Fig. 24)

乳中 [rǔ zhōng]

ruzhong **(ST17):** point at the center of the nipple (Fig. 24)

乳根 [rǔ gēn]

rugen **(ST18):** point on the chest, in the 5th intercostal space, 4 *cun* lateral to the anterior midline (Fig. 24)

不容 [bù róng]

burong **(ST19):** point on the upper abdomen, 6 *cun* above the center of the umbilicus and 2 *cun* lateral to the anterior midline (Fig. 24)

承满 [chéng mǎn]

***chengman* (ST20):** point on the upper abdomen, 5 *cun* above the center of the umbilicus and 2 *cun* lateral to the anterior midline (Fig. 24)

梁门 [liáng mén]

***liangmen* (ST21):** point on the upper abdomen, 4 *cun* above the center of the umbilicus and 2 *cun* lateral to the anterior midline (Fig. 24)

关门 [guān mén]

***guanmen* (ST22):** point on the upper abdomen, 3 *cun* above the center of the umbilicus and 2 *cun* lateral to the anterior midline (Fig. 24)

太乙 [tài yǐ]

***taiyi* (ST23):** point on the upper abdomen, 2 *cun* above the center of the umbilicus and 2 *cun* lateral to the anterior midline (Fig. 24)

滑肉门 [huá ròu mén]

***huaroumen* (ST24):** point on the upper abdomen, 1 *cun* above the center of the umbilicus and 2 *cun* lateral to the anterior midline (Fig. 24)

天枢 [tiān shū]

***tianshu* (ST25):** point on the middle abdomen, 2 *cun* lateral to the center of the umbilicus (Fig. 24)

外陵 [wài líng]

***wailing* (ST26):** point on the lower abdomen, 1 *cun* below the center of the umbilicus and 2 *cun* lateral to the anterior midline (Fig. 24)

大巨 [dà jù]

***daju* (ST27):** point on the lower abdomen, 2 *cun* below the center of the umbilicus and 2 *cun* lateral to the anterior midline (Fig. 24)

水道 [shuǐ dào]

***shuidao* (ST28):** point on the lower abdomen, 3 *cun* below the center of the umbilicus and 2 *cun* lateral to the anterior midline (Fig. 24)

归来 [guī lái]

***guilai* (ST29):** point on the lower abdomen, 4 *cun* below the center of the umbilicus and 2 *cun* lateral to the anterior midline (Fig. 24)

气冲 [qì chōng]

***qichong* (ST30):** point slightly above the inguinal groove, 5 *cun* below the center of the umbilicus and 2 *cun* lateral to the anterior midline (Fig. 24)

髀关 [bì guān]

***biguan* (ST31):** point on the anterior side of the thigh and on the line connecting the anteriosuperior iliac spine and the superiolateral corner of the patella, in the depression lateral to the sartorius muscle (Fig. 22)

伏兔 [fú tù]

***futu* (ST32):** point on the anterior side of the thigh, 6 *cun* above the superiolateral corner of the patella (Fig. 22)

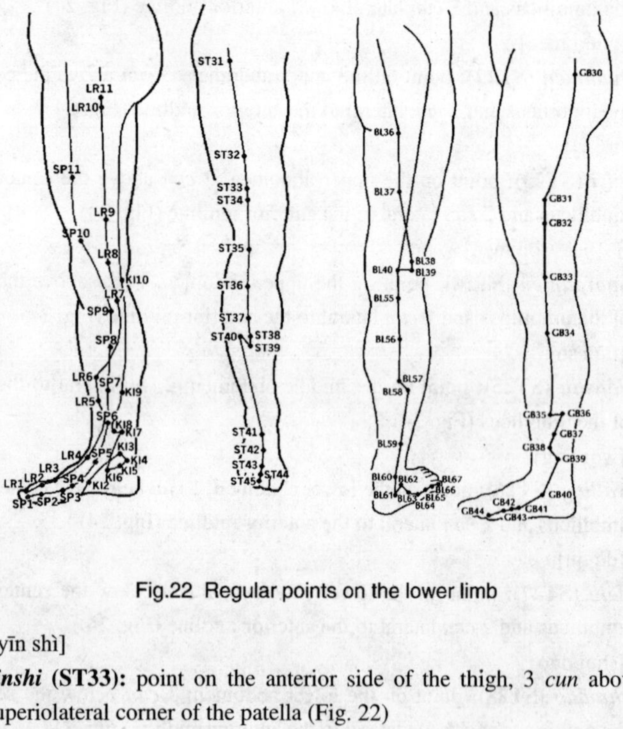

Fig.22 Regular points on the lower limb

阴市 [yīn shì]

***yinshi* (ST33):** point on the anterior side of the thigh, 3 *cun* above the superiolateral corner of the patella (Fig. 22)

梁丘 [liáng qīu]

***liangqiu* (ST34):** point on the anterior side of the thigh, 2 *cun* above the superiolateral corner of the patella (Fig. 22)

犊鼻 [dú bí]

***dubi* (ST35):** point on the knee, in the depression lateral to the patella and its ligament when the knee is flexed (Fig. 22)

足三里 [zú sān lǐ]

***zusanli* (ST36):** point on the anteriolateral side of the leg, 3 *cun* below dubi (ST35), one finger breadth from the anterior crest of the tibia (Fig. 22)

上巨虚 [shàng jù xū]

***shangjuxu* (ST37):** point on the anteriolateral side of the leg, 6 *cun* below *dubi* (ST35), one finger breadth from the anterior crest of the tibia (Fig. 22)

条口 [tiáo kǒu]

***tiaokou* (ST38):** point on the anteriolateral side of the leg, 8 *cun* below dubi (ST35), one finger breadth from the anterior crest of the tibia (Fig. 22)

下巨虚 [xià jù xū]

***xiajuxu* (ST39):** point on the anteriolateral side of the leg, 9 *cun* below *dubi* (ST35), one finger breadth from the anterior crest of the tibia (Fig. 22)

丰隆 [fēng lóng]

***fenglong* (ST40):** point on the anteriolateral side of the leg, 8 *cun* above the tip of the external malleolus, lateral to *tiaokou* (ST38), and two finger breadths from the anterior crest of the tibia (Fig. 22)

解溪 [jiě xī]

***jiexi* (ST41):** point in the central depression of the crease between the instep of the foot and the leg (Fig. 22)

冲阳 [chōng yáng]

***chongyang* (ST42):** point on the dome of the instep of the foot, where the pulsation of the dorsal artery of the foot is palpable (Fig. 22)

陷谷 [xiàn gǔ]

***xiangu* (ST43):** point on the instep of the foot, in the depression distal to the commissure of the 2nd and 3rd metatarsal bone (Fig. 22)

内庭 [nèi tíng]

***neiting* (ST44):** point on the instep of the foot, at the junction of the red and white skin proximal to the margin of the web between the 2nd and 3rd toes (Fig. 22)

厉兑 [lì duì]

***lidui* (ST45):** point on the lateral side of the distal segment of the 2nd toe, 0.1 *cun* proximal to the corner of the nail (Fig. 22)

足太阴脾经穴 [zú tài yīn pí jīng xué]

points of spleen meridian: acupuncture-moxibustion points distributed on the spleen meridian (SP)

隐白 [yǐn bái]

***yinbai* (SP1):** point on the medial side of the distal segment of the big toe, 0.1 *cun* proximal to the corner of the nail (Fig. 22)

大都 [dà dū]

***dadu* (SP2):** point on the medial border of the foot, in the depression just distal to the metatarsophalangeal joint (Fig. 22)

太白 [tài bái]

***taibai* (SP3):** point on the medial border of the foot, in the depression proximal and inferior to the metatarsophalangeal joint (Fig. 22)

公孙 [gōng sūn]

***gongsun* (SP4):** point on the medial border of the foot, anterior and inferior to the proximal end of the 1st metatarsal bone (Fig. 22)

商丘 [shāng qīu]

***shangqiu* (SP5):** point on the medial side of the ankle in the depression anterior and inferior to the medial malleolus (Fig. 22)

三阴交 [sān yīn jiāo]

***sanyinjiao* (SP6):** point on the medial side of the leg, 3 *cun* above the tip of the medial malleolus, just posterior to the tibia (Fig. 22)

漏谷 [lòu gǔ]

***lougu* (SP7):** point on the medial side of the leg, 6 *cun* above the tip of the medial malleolus, just posterior to the tibia (Fig. 22)

地机 [dì jī]

***diji* (SP8):** point on the medial side of the leg, 3 *cun* below *yinlingquan* (SP9) (Fig. 22)

阴陵泉 [yīn líng quán]

***yinlingquan* (SP9):** point on the medial side of the leg, in the depression posterior and inferior to the medial condyle of the tibia (Fig. 22)

血海 [xuè hǎi]

***xuehai* (SP10):** point with the flexed knee, on the medial side of the thigh, 2 *cun* above the superior medial corner of the patella, on the prominence of the medial head of the quadriceps muscle (Fig. 22)

箕门 [jī mén]

***jimen* (SP11):** point on the medial side of the thigh, on the line connecting *xuehai* (SP10) and *chongmen* (SP12), and 6 *cun* above *xuehai* (SP10) (Fig. 22)

冲门 [chōng mén]

chongmen **(SP12):** point at the lateral end of the inguinal groove, 3.5 *cun* lateral to the midpoint of the upper border of the symphysis pubis, lateral to the pulsating external iliac artery (Fig. 24)

府舍 [fǔ shè]

fushe **(SP13):** point on the lower abdomen, 4 *cun* below the center of the umbilicus, 0.7 *cun* above *chongmen* (SP12) , and 4 *cun* lateral to the anterior midline (Fig. 24)

腹结 [fù jié]

fujie **(SP14):** point on the lower abdomen, 1.3 *cun* below *daheng* (SP15), and 4 *cun* lateral to the anterior midline (Fig. 24)

大横 [dà héng]

daheng **(SP15):** point on the middle abdomen, 4 *cun* lateral to the center of the umbilicus (Fig. 24)

腹哀 [fù āi]

fu'ai **(SP16):** point on the upper abdomen, 3 *cun* above the center of the umbilicus, and 4 *cun* lateral to the anterior midline (Fig. 24)

食窦 [shí dòu]

shidou **(SP17):** point on the lateral side of the chest and in the 5th intercostal space, 6 *cun* lateral to the anterior midline (Fig. 24)

天溪 [tiān xī]

tianxi **(SP18):** point on the lateral side of the chest and in the 4th intercostal space, 6 *cun* lateral to the anterior midline (Fig. 24)

胸乡 [xiōng xiāng]

xiongxiang **(SP19):** point on the lateral side of the chest and in the 3rd intercostal space, 6 *cun* lateral to the anterior midline (Fig. 24)

周荣 [zhōu róng]

zhourong **(SP20):** point on the lateral side of the chest and in the 2nd intercostal space, 6 *cun* lateral to the anterior midline (Fig. 24)

大包 [dà bāo]

dabao **(SP21):** point on the lateral side of the chest and on the middle axillary line, in the 6th intercostal space (Fig. 24)

手少阴心经穴 [shǒu shào yīn xīn jīng xué]

points of heart meridian: acupuncture-moxibustion points distributed on the heart meridian (HT)

极泉 [jí quán]

***jiquan* (HT1):** point at the apex of the axillary fossa, where the pulsation of the axillary artery is palpable (Fig. 11)

青灵 [qīng líng]

***qingling* (HT2):** point on the medial side of the arm, 3 *cun* above the cubital crease, in the groove medial to the biceps muscle (Fig. 21)

少海 [shào hǎi]

***shaohai* (HT3):** point at the midpoint of the line connecting the medial end of the cubital crease and the medial epicondyle of the humerus when the elbow is flexed (Fig. 21)

灵道 [líng dào]

***lingdao* (HT4):** point on the palmar side of the forearm and on the radial side of the tendon of the ulnar flexor muscle of the wrist, 1.5 *cun* proximal to the crease of the wrist (Fig. 21)

通里 [tōng lǐ]

***tongli* (HT5):** point on the palmar side of the forearm and on the radial side of the tendon of the ulnar flexor muscle of the wrist, 1 *cun* proximal to the crease of the wrist (Fig. 21)

阴郄 [yīn xì]

***yinxi* (HT6):** point on the palmar side of the forearm and on the radial side of the tendon of the ulnar flexor muscle of the wrist, 0.5 *cun* proximal to the crease of the wrist (Fig. 21)

神门 [shén mén]

***shenmen* (HT7):** point on the wrist, at the ulnar end of the crease of the wrist, in the depression of the radial side of the tendon of the ulnar flexor muscle of the wrist (Fig. 21)

少府 [shào fǔ]

***shaofu* (HT8):** point in the palm, between the 4th and 5th metacarpal bones, at the part of the palm touching the tip of the little finger when a fist is made (Fig. 21)

少冲 [shào chōng]

***shaochong* (HT9):** point on the radial side of the distal segment of the little finger, 0.1 *cun* proximal to the corner of the nail (Fig. 21)

手太阳小肠经穴 [shǒu tài yáng xiǎo cháng jīng xué]

points of small intestine meridian: acupuncture-moxibustion points distributed on the small intestine meridian (SI)

少泽 [shào zé]

***shaoze* (SI1):** point on the ulnar side of the distal segment of the little finger, 0.1 *cun* proximal to the corner of the nail (Fig. 21)

前谷 [qián gǔ]

***qiangu* (SI2):** a point at the junction of the red and white skin along the ulnar border of the hand, at the ulnar end of the crease of the 5th metacarpophalangeal joint when a loose fist is made (Fig. 21)

后溪 [hòu xī]

***houxi* (SI3):** a point at the junction of the red and white skin along the ulnar border of the hand, at the ulnar end of the distal palmar crease, proximal to the 5th metacarpophalangeal joint when a loose fist is made (Fig. 21)

腕骨 [wàn gǔ]

***wangu* (SI4):** a point on the ulnar border of the hand, in the depression between the proximal end of the 5th metacarpal bone and hamate bone, and at the junction of the red and white skin (Fig. 21)

阳谷 [yáng gǔ]

***yanggu* (SI5):** a point on the ulnar border of the wrist, in the depression between the styloid process of the ulna and triangular bone (Fig. 21)

养老 [yǎng lǎo]

***yanglao* (SI6):** a point on the ulnar side of the posterior surface of the forearm, in the depression proximal to and on the radial side of the head of the ulna (Fig. 21)

支正 [zhī zhèng]

***zhizheng* (SI7):** a point on the ulnar side of the posterior surface of the forearm, 5 *cun* proximal to the dorsal crease of the wrist (Fig. 21)

小海 [xiǎo hǎi]

***xiaohai* (SI8):** a point on the medial side of the elbow, in the depression between the olecranon of the ulna and the medial epicondyle of the humerus (Fig. 21)

肩贞 [jiān zhēn]

***jianzhen* (SI9):** a point posterior and inferior to the shoulder joint, 1 *cun* above the posterior end of the axillary fold with the arm adducted (Fig. 21 and 24)

臑俞 [nào shù]

***naoshu* (SI10):** a point on the shoulder, above the posterior end of the axillary fold, in the depression below the lower border of the scapular spine (Fig. 24)

天宗 [tiān zōng]

***tianzong* (SI11):** a point on the scapula, in the depression of the center of the subscapular fossa, and on the level of the 4th thoracic vertebra (Fig. 24)

秉风 [bǐng fēng]

***bingfeng* (SI12):** a point on the scapula, at the center of the suprascapular fossa, in the depression found when the arm is raised (Fig. 24)

曲垣 [qū yuán]

***quyuan* (SI13):** a point on the scapula, at the medial end of the suprascapular fossa, at the midpoint of the line connecting *naoshu* (SI10) and the spinous process of the 2nd thoracic vertebra (Fig. 24)

肩外俞 [jiān wài shù]

***jianwaishu* (SI14):** a point on the back, below the spinous process of the 1st thoracic vertebra, 3 *cun* lateral to the posterior midline (Fig. 24)

肩中俞 [jiān zhōng shù]

***jianzhongshu* (SI15):** a point on the back, below the spinous process of the 7th cervical vertebra, 2 *cun* lateral to the posterior midline (Fig. 24)

天窗 [tiān chuāng]

***tianchuang* (SI16):** a point on the lateral side of the neck, posterior to the sternocleidomastoid muscle and *futu* (LI18), on the level of the laryngeal protuberance (Fig. 23b)

天容 [tiān róng]

***tianrong* (SI17):** a point on the lateral side of the neck, posterior to the mandibular angle, in the depression of the anterior border of the sternocleidomastoid muscle (Fig. 23b)

颧髎 [quán liáo]

***quanliao* (SI18):** a point on the face, directly below the outer canthus, in the depression below the zygomatic bone (Fig. 23a,b)

听宫 [tīng gōng]

***tinggong* (SI19):** a point on the face, anterior to the tragus and posterior to the mandibular condyloid process, in the depression found when the mouth is open (Fig. 23b)

足太阳膀胱经穴 [zú tài yáng páng guāng jīng xué]

points of bladder meridian: acupuncture-moxibustion points distributed on the bladder meridian (BL)

睛明 [jīng míng]

***jingming* (BL1):** a point on the face, in the depression slightly above the inner canthus (Fig. 23a,b)

攒竹 [cuán zhú]

***cuanzhu* (BL2):** a point on the face, in the depression of the medial end of the eyebrow, at the supraorbital notch (Fig. 23a,b)

眉冲 [méi chōng]

meichong (BL3): a point on the head, directly above *cuanzhu* (BL2), 0.5 *cun* above the anterior hairline (Fig. 23a,b)

曲差 [qū chā][qū chāi]

***qucha* (*quchai*) (BL4):** a point on the head, 0.5 *cun* above the anterior hairline and 1.5 *cun* lateral to *shenting* (GV24) (Fig. 23a,b)

五处 [wǔ chù]

***wuchu* (BL5):** a point on the head, 1 *cun* directly above the midpoint of the anterior hairline and 1.5 *cun* lateral to the midline (Fig. 23a,b)

承光 [chéng guāng]

***chengguang* (BL6):** a point on the head, 2.5 *cun* directly above the midpoint of the anterior hairline and 1.5 *cun* lateral to the midline (Fig. 23a)

通天 [tōng tiān]

***tongtian* (BL7):** a point on the head, 4 *cun* directly above the midpoint of the anterior hairline and 1.5 *cun* lateral to the midline (Fig. 23b)

络却 [luò què]

***luoque* (BL8):** a point on the head, 5.5 *cun* directly above the midpoint of the anterior hairline and 1.5 *cun* lateral to the midline (Fig. 23a,b)

玉枕 [yù zhěn]

***yuzhen* (BL9):** a point on the occiput, 2.5 *cun* directly above the midpoint of the posterior hairline and 1.3 *cun* lateral to the midline, in the depression on the level of the upper border of the external occipital protuberance (Fig. 23a,b)

天柱 [tiān zhù]

***tianzhu* (BL10):** a point on the nape, in the depression of the lateral border of the trapezius muscle and 1. 3 *cun* lateral to the midpoint of the posterior hairline (Fig. 23a,b)

大杼 [dà zhù]

***dazhu* (BL11):** a point on the back, below the spinous process of the 1st thoracic vertebra, 1.5 *cun* lateral to the posterior midline (Fig. 23a and 24)

风门 [fēng mén]

***fengmen* (BL12):** a point on the back, below the spinous process of the 2nd thoracic vertebra, 1.5 *cun* lateral to the posterior midline (Fig. 24)

肺俞 [fèi shù]

***feishu* (BL13):** a point on the back, below the spinous process of the 3rd thoracic vertebra, 1.5 *cun* lateral to the posterior midline (Fig. 24)

厥阴俞 [jué yīn shù]

***jueyinshu* (BL14):** a point on the back, below the spinous process of the 4th thoracic vertebra, 1.5 *cun* lateral to the posterior midline (Fig. 24)

心俞 [xīn shù]

***xinshu* (BL15):** a point on the back, below the spinous process of the 5th thoracic vertebra, 1.5 *cun* lateral to the posterior midline (Fig. 24)

督俞 [dū shù]

***dushu* (BL16):** a point on the back, below the spinous process of the 6th thoracic vertebra, 1.5 *cun* lateral to the posterior midline (Fig. 24)

膈俞 [gé shù]

***geshu* (BL17):** a point on the back, below the spinous process of the 7th thoracic vertebra, 1.5 *cun* lateral to the posterior midline (Fig. 24)

肝俞 [gān shù]

***ganshu* (BL18):** a point on the back, below the spinous process of the 9th thoracic vertebra, 1.5 *cun* lateral to the posterior midline (Fig. 24)

胆俞 [dǎn shù]

***danshu* (BL19):** a point on the back, below the spinous process of the 10th thoracic vertebra, 1.5 *cun* lateral to the posterior midline (Fig. 24)

脾俞 [pí shù]

***pishu* (BL20):** a point on the back, below the spinous process of the 11th thoracic vertebra, 1.5 *cun* lateral to the posterior midline (Fig. 24)

胃俞 [wèi shù]

***weishu* (BL21):** a point on the back, below the spinous process of the 12th thoracic vertebra, 1.5 *cun* lateral to the posterior midline (Fig. 24)

三焦俞 [sān jiāo shù]

***sanjiaoshu* (BL22):** a point on the lower back, below the spinous process of the 1st lumbar vertebra, 1.5 *cun* lateral to the posterior midline (Fig. 24)

肾俞 [shèn shù]

***shenshu* (BL23):** a point on the lower back, below the spinous process of the 2nd lumbar vertebra, 1.5 *cun* lateral to the posterior midline (Fig. 24)

气海俞 [qì hǎi shù]

***qihaishu* (BL24):** a point on the lower back, below the spinous process of the 3rd lumbar vertebra, 1.5 *cun* lateral to the posterior midline (Fig. 24)

大肠俞 [dà cháng shù]

***dachangshu* (BL25):** a point on the lower back, below the spinous process of the 4th lumbar vertebra, 1.5 *cun* lateral to the posterior midline (Fig. 24)

关元俞 [guān yuán shù]

***guanyuanshu* (BL26):** a point on the lower back, below the spinous process of the 5th lumbar vertebra, 1.5 *cun* lateral to the posterior midline (Fig. 24)

小肠俞 [xiǎo cháng shù]

***xiaochangshu* (BL27):** a point on the sacrum and on the level of the 1st posterior sacral foramen, 1.5 *cun* lateral to the median sacral crest (Fig. 24)

膀胱俞 [páng guāng shù]

***pangguanshu* (BL28):** a point on the sacrum and on the level of the 2nd posterior sacral foramen, 1.5 *cun* lateral to the median sacral crest (Fig. 24)

中膂俞 [zhōng lǚ shù]

***zhonglushu* (BL29):** a point on the sacrum and on the level of the 3rd posterior sacral foramen, 1.5 *cun* lateral to the median sacral crest (Fig. 24)

白环俞 [bái huán shù]

***baihuanshu* (BL30):** a point on the sacrum and on the level of the 4th posterior sacral foramen, 1.5 *cun* lateral to the median sacral crest (Fig. 24)

上髎 [shàng liáo]

***shangliao* (BL31):** a point on the sacrum, at the midpoint between the posteriosuperior iliac spine and the posterior midline, just at the 1st posterior sacral foramen (Fig. 24)

次髎 [cì liáo]

***ciliao* (BL32):** a point on the sacrum, medial and inferior to the posteriosuperior iliac spine, just at the 2nd posterior sacral foramen (Fig. 24)

中髎 [zhōng liáo]

***zhongliao* (BL33):** a point on the sacrum, medial and inferior to *ciliao* (GL 32), just at the 3rd posterior sacral foramen (Fig. 24)

下髎 [xià liáo]

***xialiao* (BL34):** a point on the sacrum, medial and inferior to *zhongliao*

(BL33), just at the 4th posterior sacral foramen (Fig. 24)

会阳 [huì yáng]

***huiyang* (GL 35):** a point on the sacrum, 0.5 *cun* lateral to the tip of the coccyx (Fig. 24)

承扶 [chéng fú]

***chengfu* (BL36):** a point on the posterior side of the thigh, at the midpoint of the inferior gluteal crease (Fig. 22)

殷门 [yīn mén]

***yinmen* (BL37):** a point on the posterior side of the thigh and on the line connecting *chengfu* (BL36) and *weizhong* (BL40), 6 *cun* below *chengfu* (BL36) (Fig. 22)

浮郄 [fú xì]

***fuxi* (BL38):** a point at the lateral end of the popliteal crease, 1 *cun* above *weiyang* (BL39), medial to the tendon of the biceps muscle of the thigh (Fig. 22)

委阳 [wěi yáng]

***weiyang* (BL39):** a point at the lateral end of the popliteal crease, medial to the tendon of the biceps muscle of the thigh (Fig. 22)

委中 [wěi zhōng]

***weizhong* (BL40):** a point at the midpoint of the popliteal crease, between the tendon of the biceps muscle of the thigh and the semitendinous muscle (Fig. 22)

附分 [fù fēn]

***fufen* (BL41):** a point on the back, below the spinous process of the 2nd thoracic vertebra, 3 *cun* lateral to the posterior midline (Fig. 24)

魄户 [pò hù]

***pohu* (BL42):** a point on the back, below the spinous process of the 3rd thoracic vertebra, 3 *cun* lateral to the posterior midline (Fig. 24)

膏肓 [gāo huāng]

***gaohuang* (BL43):** a point on the back, below the spinous process of the 4th thoracic vertebra, 3 *cun* lateral to the posterior midline (Fig. 24)

神堂 [shén táng]

***shentang* (BL44):** a point on the back, below the spinous process of the 5th thoracic vertebra, 3 *cun* lateral to the posterior midline (Fig. 24)

譩譆 [yī xī]

***yixi* (BL45):** a point on the back, below the spinous process of the 6th thoracic vertebra, 3 *cun* lateral to the posterior midline (Fig. 24)

膈关 [gé guān]

***geguan* (BL46):** a point on the back, below the spinous process of the 7th thoracic vertebra, 3 *cun* lateral to the posterior midline (Fig. 24)

魂门 [hún mén]

***hunmen* (BL47):** a point on the back, below the spinous process of the 9th thoracic vertebra, 3 *cun* lateral to the posterior midline (Fig. 24)

阳纲 [yáng gāng]

***yanggang* (BL48):** point on the back, below the spinous process of the 10th thoracic vertebra, 3 *cun* lateral to the posterior midline (Fig. 24)

意舍 [yì shè]

***yishe* (BL49):** point on the back, below the spinous process of the 11th thoracic vertebra, 3 *cun* lateral to the posterior midline (Fig. 24)

胃仓 [wèi cāng]

***weicang* (BL50):** point on the back, below the spinous process of the 12th thoracic vertebra, 3 *cun* lateral to the posterior midline (Fig. 24)

肓门 [huāng mén]

***huangmen* (BL51):** point on the lower back, below the spinous process of the 1st lumbar vertebra, 3 *cun* lateral to the posterior midline (Fig. 24)

志室 [zhì shì]

***zhishi* (BL52):** point on the lower back, below the spinous process of the 2nd lumbar vertebra, 3 *cun* lateral to the posterior midline (Fig. 24)

胞肓 [bāo huāng]

***baohuang* (BL53):** point on the buttock and on the level of the 2nd posterior sacral foramen, 3 *cun* lateral to the median sacral crest (Fig. 24)

秩边 [zhì biān]

***zhibian* (BL54):** point on the buttock and on the level of the 4th posterior sacral foramen, 3 *cun* lateral to the median sacral crest (Fig. 24)

合阳 [hé yáng]

***heyang* (BL55):** point on the posterior side of the leg and on the line connecting *weizhong* (BL40) and *chengshan* (BL57), 2 *cun* below *weizhong* (BL40) (Fig. 22)

承筋 [chéng jīn]

***chengjin* (BL56):** point on the posterior side of the leg and on the line connecting *weizhong* (BL40) and *chengshan* (BL57), at the center of the gastrocnemius muscle belly, 5 *cun* below *weizhong* (BL40) (Fig. 22)

承山 [chéng shān]

***chengshan* (BL57):** point on the posterior midline of the leg, between *weizhong* (BL40) and *kunlun* (BL60), in a pointed depression formed below the gastrocnemius muscle belly when the leg is stretched or the heel is lifted (Fig. 22)

飞阳 [fēi yáng]

***feiyang* (BL58):** point on the posterior side of the leg, 7 *cun* directly above *kunlun* (BL60) and 1 *cun* lateral and inferior to *chengshan* (BL57) (Fig. 22)

跗阳 [fū yáng]

***fuyang* (BL59):** point on the posterior side of the leg, posterior to the lateral malleolus, 3 *cun* directly above *kunlun* (BL60) (Fig. 22)

昆仑 [kūn lún]

***kunlun* (BL60):** point posterior to the external malleolus, in the depression between the tip of the external malleolus and the Achilles tendon (Fig. 22)

仆参 [pú cān]

***pucan* (BL61):** point on the lateral side of the foot, posterior and inferior to the external malleolus, directly below *kunlun* (BL60), lateral to the calcaneum, at the junction of the red and white skin (Fig. 22)

申脉 [shēn mài]

***shenmai* (BL62):** point on the lateral side of the foot, in the depression directly below the external malleolus (Fig. 22)

金门 [jīn mén]

***jinmen* (BL63):** point on the lateral side of the foot, directly below the anterior border of the external malleolus, on the lower border of the cuboid bone (Fig. 22)

京骨 [jīng gǔ]

***jinggu* (BL64):** point on the lateral side of the foot, below the tuberosity of the 5th metatarsal bone, at the junction of the red and white skin (Fig. 22)

束骨 [shù gǔ]

***shugu* (BL65):** point on the lateral side of the foot, posterior to the 5th metatarsophalangeal joint, at the junction of the red and white skin (Fig. 22)

足通谷 [zú tōng gǔ]

***zutonggu* (BL66):** point on the lateral side of the foot, anterior to the 5th metatarsophalangeal joint, at the junction of the red and white skin

(Fig. 22)

至阴 [zhì yīn]

***zhiyin* (BL67):** point on the lateral side of the distal segment of the little toe, 0.1 *cun* from the corner of the toenail (Fig. 22)

足少阴肾经穴 [zú shào yīn shèn jīng xué]

points of kidney meridian: acupuncture-moxibustion points distributed on the kidney meridian (KI)

涌泉 [yǒng quán]

***yongquan* (KI1):** point on the sole, in the depression at the junction of the anterior third and posterior two-thirds of the line connecting the base of the 2nd and 3rd toes and the heel (Fig. 14)

然谷 [rán gǔ]

***rangu* (KI2):** point on the medial border of the foot, below the tuberosity of the navicular bone, and at the junction of the red and white skin (Fig. 22)

太溪 [tài xī]

***taixi* (KI3):** point on the medial side of the foot, posterior to the medial malleolus, in the depression between the tip of the medial malleolus and the Achilles tendon (Fig. 22)

大钟 [dà zhōng]

***dazhong* (KI4):** point on the medial side of the foot, posterior and inferior to the medial malleolus, in the depression medial and anterior to the attachment of the Achilles tendon (Fig. 22)

水泉 [shuǐ quán]

***shuiquan* (KI5):** point on the medial side of the foot, posterior and inferior to the medial malleolus, 1 *cun* directly below *taixi* (KI3), in the depression of the medial side of the tuberosity of the calcaneum (Fig. 22)

照海 [zhào hǎi]

***zhaohai* (KI6):** point on the medial side of the foot, in the depression below the tip of the medial malleolus (Fig. 22)

复溜 [fù liù]

***fuliu* (KI7):** point on the medial side of the leg, 2 *cun* directly above taixi (KI3), anterior to the Achilles tendon (Fig. 22)

交信 [jiāo xìn]

***jiaoxin* (KI8):** point on the medial side of the leg, 2 *cun* above *taixi* (KI3) and 0.5 *cun* anterior to *fuliu* (KI7), posterior to the medial border of the tibia (Fig. 22)

筑宾 [zhù bīn]

***zhubin* (KI9):** point on the medial side of the leg and on the line connecting *taixi* (KI3) and *yingu* (KI10), 5 *cun* above *taixi* (KI3), medial and inferior to the gastrocnemius muscle belly (Fig. 22)

阴谷 [yīn gǔ]

***yingu* (KI10):** point on the medial side of the popliteal fossa, between the tendons of the semitendinous and semimembranous muscles when the knee is flexed (Fig. 22)

横骨 [héng gǔ]

***henggu* (KI11):** point on the lower abdomen, 5 *cun* below the center of the umbilicus and 0.5 *cun* lateral to the anterior midline (Fig. 24)

大赫 [dà hè]

***dahe* (KI12):** point on the lower abdomen, 4 *cun* below the center of the umbilicus and 0.5 *cun* lateral to the anterior midline (Fig. 24)

气穴 [qì xué]

***qixue* (KI13):** point on the lower abdomen, 3 *cun* below the center of the umbilicus and 0.5 *cun* lateral to the anterior midline (Fig. 24)

四满 [sì mǎn]

***siman* (KI14):** point on the lower abdomen, 2 *cun* below the center of the umbilicus and 0.5 *cun* lateral to the anterior midline (Fig. 24)

中注 [zhōng zhù]

***zhongzhu* (KI15):** point on the lower abdomen, 1 *cun* below the center of the umbilicus and 0.5 *cun* lateral to the anterior midline (Fig. 24)

肓俞 [huāng shù]

***huangshu* (KI16):** point on the middle abdomen, 0. 5 *cun* lateral to the center of the umbilicus (Fig. 24)

商曲 [shāng qū]

***shangqu* (KI17):** point on the upper abdomen, 2 *cun* above the center of the umbilicus, and 0.5 *cun* lateral to the anterior midline (Fig. 24)

石关 [shí guān]

***shiguan* (KI18):** point on the upper abdomen, 3 *cun* above the center of the umbilicus, and 0.5 *cun* lateral to the anterior midline (Fig. 24)

阴都 [yīn dū]

***yindu* (KI19):** point on the upper abdomen, 4 *cun* above the center of the umbilicus and 0.5 *cun* lateral to the anterior midline (Fig. 24)

腹通谷 [fù tōng gǔ]

***futonggu* (KI20):** point on the upper abdomen, 5 *cun* above the center of the umbilicus and 0.5 *cun* lateral to the anterior midline (Fig. 24)

幽门 [yōu mén]

***youmen* (KI21):** point on the upper abdomen, 6 *cun* above the center of the umbilicus and 0.5 *cun* lateral to the anterior midline (Fig. 24)

步廊 [bù láng]

***bulang* (KÍ):** point on the chest, in the 5th intercostal space, 2 *cun* lateral to the anterior midline (Fig. 24)

神封 [shén fēng]

***shenfeng* (KI23):** point on the chest, in the 4th intercostal space, 2 *cun* lateral to the anterior midline (Fig. 24)

灵墟 [líng xū]

***lingxu* (KI24):** point on the chest, in the 3rd. intercostal space, 2 *cun* lateral to the anterior midline (Fig. 24)

神藏 [shén cáng]

***shencang* (KI25):** point on the chest, in the 2nd intercostal space, 2 *cun* lateral to the anterior midline (Fig. 24)

彧中 [yù zhōng]

***yuzhong* (KI26):** point on the chest, in the 1st intercostal space, 2 *cun* lateral to the anterior midline (Fig. 24)

俞府 [shù fǔ]

***shufu* (KI27):** point on the chest, below the lower border of the clavicle, 2 *cun* lateral to the midline (Fig. 24)

手厥阴心包经穴 [shǒu jué yīn xīn bāo jīng xué]

points of pericardium meridian: acupuncture-moxibustion points distributed on the pericardium meridian (PC)

天池 [tiān chí]

***tianchi* (PC1):** point on the chest, in the 4th intercostal space, 1 *cun* lateral to the nipple and 5 *cun* lateral to the anterior midline (Fig. 15)

天泉 [tiān quán]

***tianquan* (PC2):** point on the medial side of the arm, 2 *cun* below the anterior end of the axillary fold, between the long and short heads of the biceps muscle of the arm (Fig. 21)

曲泽 [qū zé]

***quze* (PC3):** point at the midpoint of the cubital crease, on the ulnar side of the tendon of the biceps muscle of the arm (Fig. 21)

郄门 [xì mén]

***ximen* (PC4):** point on the palmar side of the forearm and on the line connecting *quze* (PC3) and *daling* (PC7), 5 *cun* above the crease of the wrist (Fig. 21)

间使 [jiān shǐ]

***jianshi* (PC5):** point on the palmar side of the forearm and on the line connecting *quze* (PC3) and *daling* (PC7) , 3 *cun* above the crease of the wrist, between the tendons of the long palmar muscle and radial flexor muscle of the wrist (Fig. 21)

内关 [nèi guān]

***neiguan* (PC6):** point on the palmar side of the forearm and on the line connecting *quze* (PC3) and *daling* (PC7), 2 *cun* above the crease of the wrist, between the tendons of the long palmar muscle and radial flexor muscle of the wrist (Fig. 21)

大陵 [dà líng]

***daling* (PC7):** point at the midpoint of the crease of the wrist, between the tendons of the long palmar muscle and radial flexor muscle of the wrist (Fig. 21)

劳宫 [láo gōng]

***laogong* (PC8):** point at the center of the palm, between the 2nd and 3rd metacarpal bones, but close to the latter, and on the part touching the tip of the middle finger when a fist is made (Fig. 21)

中冲 [zhōng chōng]

***zhongchong* (PC9):** point at the center of the tip of the middle finger (Fig. 21)

手少阳三焦经穴 [shǒu shào yáng sān jiāo jīng xué]

points of triple energizer meridian: acupuncture-moxibustion points distributed on the triple energizer meridian (TE)

关冲 [guān chōng]

***guanchong* (TE1):** point on the ulnar side of the distal segment of the ring finger, 0.1 *cun* from the corner of the nail (Fig. 21)

液门 [yè mén]

***yemen* (TE2):** point on the dorsum of the hand, between the ring and littlel fingers, at the junction of the red and white skin, proximal to the margin of the web (Fig. 21)

中渚 [zhōng zhǔ]

***zhongzhu* (TE3):** point on the dorsum of the hand, proximal to the 4th metacarpophalangeal joint, in the depression between the 4th and 5th metacarpal bones (Fig. 21)

阳池 [yáng chí]

***yangchi* (TE4):** point at the midpoint of the dorsal crease of the wrist, in the depression on the ulnar side of the tendon of the extensor muscle of the fingers (Fig. 21)

外关 [wài guān]

***waiguan* (TE5):** point on the dorsal side of the forearm and on the line connecting *yangchi* (TE4) and the tip of the olecranon, 2 *cun* proximal to the dorsal crease of the wrist, between the radius and the ulna (Fig. 21)

支沟 [zhī gōu]

***zhigou* (TE6):** point on the dorsal side of the forearm and on the line connecting *yangchi* (TE4) and the tip of the olecranon, 3 *cun* proximal to the dorsal crease of the wrist, between the radius and the ulna (Fig. 21)

会宗 [huì zōng]

***huizong* (TE7):** point on the dorsal side of the forearm, 3 *cun* proximal to the dorsal crease of the wrist, on the ulnar side of *zhigou* (TE6) and on the radial border of the ulna (Fig. 21)

三阳络 [sān yáng luò]

***sanyangluo* (TE8):** point on the dorsal side of the forearm, 4 *cun* proximal to the dorsal crease of the wrist, between the radius and the ulna (Fig. 21)

四渎 [sì dú]

***sidu* (TE9):** point on the dorsal side of the forearm and on the line connecting *yangchi* (TE4) and the tip of the olecranon, 5 *cun* distal to the tip of the olecranon, between the radius and ulna (Fig. 21)

天井 [tiān jǐng]

***tianjing* (TE10):** point on the lateral side of the upper arm, in the depression 1 *cun* proximal to the tip of the olecranon when the elbow is flexed (Fig. 21)

清冷渊 [qīng lěng yuān]

***qinglengyuan* (TE11):** point with the elbow flexed, on the lateral side of the upper arm, 2 *cun* above the tip of the olecranon and 1 *cun* above *tianjing* (TE10) (Fig. 21)

消泺 [xiāo luò]

***xiaoluo* (TE12):** point on the lateral side of the upper arm, at the midpoint of the line connecting *qinglengyuan* (TE11) and *naohui* (TE13) (Fig. 21)

臑会 [nào huì]

***naohui* (TE13):** point on the lateral side of the upper arm and on the line connecting the tip of the olecranon and *jianliao* (TE14), 3 *cun* below *jianliao* (TE14), and on the posterioinferior border of the deltoid muscle (Fig. 21)

肩髎 [jiān liáo]

***jianliao* (TE14):** point on the shoulder, posterior to *jianyu* (LI15), in the depression inferior and posterior to the acromion when the arm is abducted (Fig. 21)

天髎 [tiān liáo]

***tianliao* (TE15):** point on the scapula, at the midpoint between *jianjing* (GB21) and *quyuan* (SI13), at the superior angle of the scapula (Fig. 23a)

天牖 [tiān yǒu]

***tianyou* (TE16):** point on the lateral side of the neck, directly below the posterior border of the mastoid process, on the level of the mandibular angle, and on the posterior border of the sternocleidomastoid muscle (Fig. 23a,b)

翳风 [yì fēng]

***yifeng* (TE17):** point posterior to the ear lobe, in the depression between the mastoid process and mandibular angle (Fig. 23a,b)

瘛脉 [chì mài]

***chimai* (TE18):** point on the head, at the center of the mastoid process, and at the junction of the middle third and lower third of the line connecting *jiaosun* (TE20) and *yifeng* (TE17) along the curve of the ear helix (Fig. 23a,b)

颅息 [lú xī]

***luxi* (TE19):** point on the head, at the junction of the upper third and middle third of the line connecting *jiaosun* (TE20) and *yifeng* (TE17) along the curve of the ear helix (Fig. 23a,b)

角孙 [jiǎo sūn]

***jiaosun* (TE20):** point on the head, above the ear apex within the hairline (Fig. 23a,b)

耳门 [ěr mén]

***ermen* (TE21):** point on the face, anterior to the supratragic notch, in the depression behind the posterior border of the condyloid process of the mandible (Fig. 23b)

耳和髎 [ěr hé liáo]

***erheliao* (TE22):** point on the lateral side of the head, on the posterior margin of the temples, anterior to the anterior border of the root of the ear auricle and posterior to the superficial temporal artery (Fig. 23b)

和髎 [hé liáo]

***heliao* (TE22),** same as 耳和髎 [ěr hé liáo]

丝竹空 [sī zhú kōng]

***sizhukong* (TE23):** point on the face, in the depression of the lateral end of the eyebrow (Fig. 23a,b)

足少阳胆经穴 [zú shào yáng dǎn jīng xué]

points of gallbladder meridian: acupuncture-moxibustion points distributed on the gallbladder meridian (BL)

瞳子髎 [tóng zǐ liáo]

***tongziliao* (GB1):** point on the face, lateral to the outer canthus, on the lateral border of the orbit (Fig. 23a,b)

听会 [tīng huì]

***tinghui* (GB2):** point on the face, anterior to the intertragic notch, in the depression posterior to the condyloid process of the mandible when the mouth is open (Fig. 23b)

上关 [shàng guān]

***shangguan* (GB3):** point anterior to the ear, directly above *xiaguan* (ST7), in the depression above the upper border of the zygomatic arch (Fig. 23b)

颔厌 [hàn yàn]

***hanyan* (GB4):** point on the head, in the hair above the temples, at the junction of the upper fourth and lower three fourths of the curved line connecting *touwei* (ST8) and *qubin* (GB7) (Fig. 23b)

悬颅 [xuán lú]

***xuanlu* (GB5):** point on the head, in the hair above the temple, at the midpoint of the curved line connecting *touwei* (ST8) and *qubin* (GB7) (Fig. 23b)

悬厘 [xuán lí]

***xuanli* (GB6):** point on the head, in the hair above the temples, at the junction of the upper three fourths and lower fourth of the curved line connecting *touwei* (ST8) and *qubin* (GB7) (Fig. 23b)

曲鬓 [qū bìn]

***qubin* (GB7):** point on the head, at a crossing point of the vertical posterior border of the temples and horizontal line through the ear apex (Fig. 23b)

率谷 [shuài gǔ]

***shuaigu* (GB8):** point on the head, directly above the ear apex, 1.5 *cun* above the hairline, directly above *jiaosun* (TE20) (Fig. 23b)

天冲 [tiān chōng]

***tianchong* (GB9):** point on the head, directly above the posterior border of the ear root, 2 *cun* above the hairline and 0. 5 *cun* posterior to *shuaigu* (GB8) (Fig. 23a,b)

浮白 [fú bái]

***fubai* (GB10):** point on the head, posterior and superior to the mastoid process, at the junction of the middle third and upper third of the curved line connecting *tianchong* (GB9) and *wangu* (GB12) (Fig. 23a,b)

头窍阴 [tóu qiào yīn]

***touqiaoyin* (GB11):** point on the head, posterior and superior to the mastoid process, at the junction of the middle third and lower third of the curved line connecting *tianchong* (GB9) and *wangu* (GB12) (Fig. 23a,b)

完骨 [wán gǔ]

***wangu* (GB12):** point on the head, in the depression posterior and inferior to the mastoid process (Fig. 23b)

本神 [běn shén]

***benshen* (GB13):** point on the head, 0.5 *cun* above the anterior hairline, 3 *cun* lateral to *shenting* (GV24), at the junction of the medial two thirds and lateral third of the line connecting *shenting* (GV24) and *touwei* (ST8) (Fig. 23a,b)

阳白 [yáng bái]

***yangbai* (GB14):** point on the forehead, directly above the pupil, 1 *cun* above the eyebrow (Fig. 23a,b)

头临泣 [tóu lín qì]

***toulinqi* (GB15):** point on the head, directly above the pupil and 0.5 *cun* above the anterior hairline, at the midpoint of the line connecting *shenting* (GV24) and *touwei* (ST8) (Fig. 23a,b)

目窗 [mù chuāng]

***muchuang* (GB16):** point on the head, 1.5 *cun* above the anterior hairline and 2.25 *cun* lateral to the midline of the head (Fig. 23a,b)

正营 [zhèng yíng]

***zhengying* (GB17):** point on the head, 2.5 *cun* above the anterior hairline and 2.25 *cun* lateral to the midline of the head (Fig. 23b)

承灵 [chéng líng]

***chengling* (GB18):** point on the head, 4 *cun* above the anterior hairline and 2.25 *cun* lateral to the midline of the head (Fig. 23a,b)

脑空 [nǎo kōng]

***naokong* (GB19):** point on the head and on the level of the upper border of the external occipital protuberance or *naohu* (GV17) , 2. 25 *cun* lateral to the midline of the head (Fig. 23a,b)

风池 [fēng chí]

***fengchi* (GB20):** point on the nape, below the occipital bone, on the level of *fengfu* (GV16), in the depression between the upper ends of the sternocleidomastoid and trapezius muscles (Fig. 23a,b)

肩井 [jiān jǐng]

***jianjing* (GB21):** point on the shoulder, directly above the nipple, at the midpoint of the line connecting *dazhui* (GV14) and the acromion (Fig. 23a and 24)

渊液 [yuān yè]

***yuanye* (GB22):** point on the lateral side of the chest, on the midaxillary line when the arm is raised, 3 *cun* below the axilla, in the 4th intercostal space

辄筋 [zhé jīn]

***zhejin* (GB23):** point on the lateral side of the chest, 1 *cun* anterior to *yuanye* (GB22), on the level of the nipple, and in the 4th intercostal space

日月 [rì yuè]

***riyue* (GB24):** point on the upper abdomen, directly below the nipple, in the 7th intercostal space, 4 *cun* lateral to the anterior midline (Fig. 24)

京门 [jīng mén]

***jingmen* (GB25):** point on the lateral side of the waist, 1.8 *cun* posterior to *zhangmen* (LR13), below the free end of the 12th rib (Fig. 24)

带脉 [dài mài]

***daimai* (GB26):** point on the lateral side of the abdomen, 1.8 *cun* below *zhangmen* (LR13), at the crossing point of a vertical line through the free end of the 11th rib and a horizontal line through the umbilicus (Fig. 24)

五枢 [wǔ shū]

***wushu* (GB27):** point on the lateral side of the abdomen, anterior to the anteriosuperior iliac spine, 3 *cun* below the level of the umbilicus (Fig. 24)

维道 [wéi dào]

***weidao* (GB28):** point on the lateral side of the abdomen, anterior and inferior to the anteriosuperior iliac spine, 0. 5 *cun* anterior and inferior to *wushu* (GB27) (Fig. 24)

居髎 [jū liáo]

***juliao* (GB29):** point on the hip, at the midpoint of the line connecting the anteriosuperior iliac spine and the prominence of the great trochanter

环跳 [huán tiào]

***huantiao* (GB30):** point on the lateral side of the thigh, at the junction of the middle third and lateral third of the line connecting the prominence of the great trochanter and the sacral hiatus when the patient is in a lateral recumbent position with the thigh flexed (Fig. 22)

风市 [fēng shì]

***fengshi* (GB31):** point on the lateral midline of the thigh, 7 *cun* above the popliteal crease, or at the place touching the tip of the middle finger when the patient stands erect with the arms hanging down freely (Fig. 22)

中渎 [zhōng dú]

***zhongdu* (GB32):** point on the lateral side of the thigh, 2 *cun* below *fengshi* (GB31), or 5 *cun* above the popliteal crease, between the lateral vastus muscle and biceps muscle of the thigh (Fig. 22)

膝阳关 [xī yáng guān]

***xiyangguan* (GB33):** point on the lateral side of the knee, 3 *cun* above *yanglingquan* (GB34) , in the depression above the external epicondyle of the femur (Fig. 22)

阳陵泉 [yáng líng quán]

***yanglingquan* (GB34):** point on the lateral side of the leg, in the depression anterior and inferior to the head of the fibula (Fig. 22)

阳交 [yáng jiāo]

***yangjiao* (GB35):** point on the lateral side of the leg, 7 *cun* above the tip of the external malleolus, on the posterior border of the fibula (Fig. 22)

外丘 [wài qiū]

***waiqiu* (GB36):** point on the lateral side of the leg, 7 *cun* above the tip of the external malleolus, on the anterior border of the fibula and on the level of *yangjiao* (GB 35) (Fig. 22)

光明 [guāng míng]

***guangming* (GB37):** point on the lateral side of the leg, 5 *cun* above the tip of the external malleolus, on the anterior border of the fibula (Fig. 22)

阳辅 [yáng fǔ]

***yangfu* (GB38):** point on the lateral side of the leg, 4 *cun* above the tip of the external malleolus, slightly anterior to the anterior border of the fibula (Fig. 22)

悬钟 [xuán zhōng]

***xuanzhong* (GB39):** point on the lateral side of the leg, 3 *cun* above the tip of the external malleolus, on the anterior border of the fibula (Fig. 22)

丘墟 [qiū xū]

***qiuxu* (GB40):** point anterior and inferior to the external malleolus, in the depression lateral to the tendon of the long extensor muscle of the toes (Fig. 22)

足临泣 [zú lín qì]

***zulinqi* (GB41):** point on the lateral side of the instep of the foot, posterior to the 4th metatarsophalangeal joint, in the depression lateral to the tendon of the extensor muscle of the little toe (Fig. 22)

地五会 [dì wǔ huì]

***diwuhui* (GB42):** point on the lateral side of the instep of the foot, posterior to the 4th metatarsophalangeal joint, between the 4th and 5th metatarsal bones, medial to the tendon of the extensor muscle of the little toe (Fig. 22)

侠溪 [xiá xī]

***xiaxi* (GB43):** point on the lateral side of the instep of the foot, between the 4th and 5th toes, at the junction of the red and white skin, proximal to the margin of the web (Fig. 22)

足窍阴 [zú qiào yīn]

***zuqiaoyin* (GB44):** point on the lateral side of the distal segment of the 4th toe, 0.1 *cun* from the corner of the toenail (Fig. 22)

足厥阴肝经穴 [zú jué yīn gān jīng xué]

points of liver meridian: acupuncture-moxibustion points distributed on the liver meridian (LR)

大敦 [dà dūn]

***dadun* (LR1):** point on the lateral side of the distal segment of the great toe, 0.1 *cun* proximal to the corner of the nail (Fig. 22)

行间 [xíng jiān]

***xingjian* (LR2):** point on the instep of the foot, between the 1st and 2nd toes, at the junction of the red and white skin proximal to the margin of the web (Fig. 22)

太冲 [tài chōng]

***taichong* (LR3):** point on the instep of the foot, in the depression of the posterior end of the 1st interosseous metatarsal space (Fig. 22)

中封 [zhōng fēng]

***zhongfeng* (LR4):** point on the instep of the foot, anterior to the medial malleolus, on the line connecting *shangqiu* (SP5) and *jiexi* (ST41), in the depression medial to the tendon of the anterior tibial muscle (Fig. 22)

蠡沟 [lí gōu]

***ligou* (LR5):** point on the medial side of the leg, 5 *cun* above the tip of the medial malleolus, on the midline of the medial surface of the tibia (Fig. 22)

中都 [zhōng dū]

***zhongdu* (LR6):** point on the medial side of the leg, 7 *cun* above the tip of the medial malleolus, on the midline of the medial surface of the tibia (Fig. 22)

膝关 [xī guān]

***xiguan* (LR7):** point on the medial side of the leg, posterior and inferior to the medial epicondyle of the tibia, 1 *cun* posterior to *yinlingquan* (SP9), at the upper end of the medial head of the gastrocnemius muscle (Fig. 22)

曲泉 [qū quán]

***ququan* (LR8):** point on the medial side of the knee, at the medial end of the popliteal crease when the knee is flexed, posterior to the medial epicondyle of the tibia, in the depression of the anterior border of the insertion of the semimemebranous and semitendinous muscles (Fig. 22)

阴包 [yīn bāo]

***yinbao* (LR9):** point on the medial side of the thigh, 4 *cun* above the medial epicondyle of the femur, between the medial vastus muscle and sartorius muscle (Fig. 22)

足五里 [zú wǔ lǐ]

***zuwuli* (LR10):** point on the medial side of the thigh, 3 *cun* directly below *qichong* (ST30), at the proximal end of the thigh, below the pubic tubercle and on the lateral border of the long abductor muscle of the thigh (Fig. 22)

阴廉 [yīn lián]

***yinlian* (LR11):** point on the medial side of the thigh, 2 *cun* directly below *qichong* (ST30), at the proximal end of the thigh, below the pubic tubercle and on the lateral border of the long abductor muscle of the thigh (Fig. 22)

急脉 [jí mài]

***jimai* (LR12):** point lateral to the pubic tubercle, lateral and inferior to *qichong* (ST30), in the inguinal groove where the pulsation of the femoral artery is palpable, 2.5 *cun* lateral to the anterior midline (Fig. 24)

章门 [zhāng mén]

***zhangmen* (LR13):** point on the lateral side of the abdomen, below the free end of the 11th rib (Fig. 24)

期门 [qī mén]

***qimen* (LR14):** point on the chest, directly below the nipple, in the 6th intercostal space, 4 *cun* lateral to the anterior midline (Fig. 24)

督脉穴 [dū mài xué]

points of governor vessel: acupuncture-moxibustion points distributed on the governor vessel (GV)

长强 [cháng qiáng]

***changqiang* (GV1):** point below the tip of the coccyx, at the midpoint of the line connecting the tip of the coccyx and anus (Fig. 24)

腰俞 [yāo shù]

***yaoshu* (GV2):** point on the sacrum and on the posterior midline, just at the sacral hiatus (Fig. 24)

腰阳关 [yāo yáng guān]

***yaoyangguan* (GV3):** point on the low back and on the posterior midline, in the depression below the spinous process of the 4th lumbar vertebra (Fig. 24)

命门 [mìng mén]

***mingmen* (GV4):** point on the lower back and on the posterior midline, in the depression below the spinous process of the 2nd lumbar vertebra (Fig. 24)

悬枢 [xuán shū]

***xuanshu* (GV5):** point on the lower back and on the posterior midline, in the depression below the spinous process of the 1st lumbar vertebra (Fig. 24)

脊中 [jǐ zhōng]

***jizhong* (GV6):** point on the back and on the posterior midline, in the depression below the spinous process of the 11th thoracic vertebra

(Fig. 24)

中枢 [zhōng shū]

***zhongshu* (GV7):** point on the back and on the posterior midline, in the depression below the spinous process of the 10th thoracic vertebra (Fig. 24)

筋缩 [jīn suō]

***jinsuo* (GV8):** point on the back and on the posterior midline, in the depression below the spinous process of the 9th thoracic vertebra (Fig. 24)

至阳 [zhì yáng]

***zhiyang* (GV9):** point on the back and on the posterior midline, in the depression below the spinous process of the 7th thoracic vertebra (Fig. 24)

灵台 [líng tái]

***lingtai* (GV10):** point on the back and on the posterior midline, in the depression below the spinous process of the 6th thoracic vertebra (Fig. 24)

神道 [shén dào]

***shendao* (GV11):** point on the back and on the posterior midline, in the depression below the spinous process of the 5th thoracic vertebra (Fig. 24)

身柱 [shēn zhù]

***shenzhu* (GV12):** point on the back and on the posterior midline, in the depression below the spinous process of the 3rd thoracic vertebra (Fig. 24)

陶道 [táo daò]

***taodao* (GV13):** point on the back and on the posterior midline, in the depression below the spinous process of the 1st thoracic vertebra (Fig. 23a and 24)

大椎 [dà zhuī]

***dazhui* (GV14):** point on the posterior midline, in the depression below the 7th cervical vertebra (Fig. 23a and 24)

哑门 [yǎ mén]

***yamen* (GV15):** point on the nape, 0.5 *cun* directly above the midpoint of the posterior hairline, below the 1st cervical vertebra (Fig. 23a,b)

风府 [fēng fǔ]

***fengfu* (GV16):** point on the nape, 1 *cun* directly above the midpoint of the posterior hairline, directly below the external occipital protuberance, in the depression between the trapezius muscle of both sides (Fig. 23a,b)

脑户 [nǎo hù]

***naohu* (GV17):** point on the head, 2.5 *cun* directly above the midpoint of the posterior hairline, in the depression on the upper border of the external occipital protuberance (Fig. 23a,b)

强间 [qiáng jiān]

***qiangjian* (GV18):** point on the head, 4 *cun* directly above the midpoint of the posterior hairline and 1.5 *cun* above *naohu* (GV17) (Fig. 23a,b)

后顶 [hòu dǐng]

***houding* (GV19):** point on the head, 5.5 *cun* directly above the midpoint of the posterior hairline and 3 *cun* above *naohu* (GV17) (Fig. 23a,b)

百会 [bǎi huì]

***baihui* (GV20):** point on the head, 5 *cun* directly above the midpoint of the anterior hairline, at the midpoint of the line connecting the apexes of both ears (Fig. 23a,b)

前顶 [qián dǐng]

***qianding* (GV21):** point on the head, 3.5 *cun* directly above the midpoint of the anterior hairline and 1.5 *cun* anterior to *baihui* (GV20) (Fig. 23a,b)

囟会 [xìn huì]

***xinhui* (GV22):** point on the head, 2 *cun* directly above the midpoint of the anterior hairline and 3 *cun* anterior to *baihui* (GV20) (Fig. 23a,b)

上星 [shàng xīng]

***shangxing* (GV23):** point on the head, 1 *cun* directly above the midpoint of the anterior hairline (Fig. 23a,b)

神庭 [shén tíng]

***shenting* (GV24):** point on the head, 0.5 *cun* directly above the midpoint of the anterior hairline (Fig. 23a,b)

素髎 [sù liáo]

***suliao* (GV25):** point at the center of the nose apex (Fig. 23a,b)

水沟 [shuǐ gōu]

***shuigou* (GV26):** point at the junction of the upper third and middle third of the philtrum (Fig. 23a,b)

兑端 [duì duān]

***duiduan* (GV27):** point on the labial tubercle of the upper lip, on the vermilion border between the philtrum and upper lip (Fig. 23a,b)

龈交 [yín jiāo]

***yinjiao* (GV28):** point inside the upper lip, at the junction of the labial frenum and upper gum (Fig. 23a,b)

任脉穴 [rèn mài xué]

points of conception vessel: acupuncture-moxibustion points distributed on the conception vessel (CV)

会阴 [huì yīn]

***huiyin* (CV1):** point on the perineum, at the midpoint between the posterior border of the scrotum and anus in male, and between the posterior commissure of the large labia and anus in female (Fig. 20)

曲骨 [qū gǔ]

***qugu* (CV2):** point on the lower abdomen and on the anterioir midline, at the midpoint of the upper border of the pubic symphysis (Fig. 24)

中极 [zhōng jí]

***zhongji* (CV3):** point on the lower abdomen and on the anterior midline, 4 *cun* below the center of the umbilicus (Fig. 24)

关元 [guān yuán]

***guanyuan* (CV4):** point on the lower abdomen and on the anterior midline, 3 *cun* below the center of the umbilicus (Fig. 24)

石门 [shí mén]

***shimen* (CV5):** point on the lower abdomen and on the anterior midline, 2 *cun* below the center of the umbilicus (Fig. 24)

气海 [qì haǐ]

***qihai* (CV6):** point on the lower abdomen and on the anterior midline, 1.5 *cun* below the center of the umbilicus (Fig. 24)

阴交 [yīn jiāo]

***yinjiao* (CV7):** point on the lower abdomen and on the anterior midline, 1 *cun* below the center of the umbilicus (Fig. 24)

神阙 [shén què]

***shenque* (CV8):** point on the middle abdomen and at the center of the umbilicus (Fig. 24)

水分 [shuǐ fēn]

***shuifen* (CV9):** point on the upper abdomen and on the anterior midline, 1 *cun* above the center of the umbilicus (Fig. 24)

下脘 [xià wǎn]

***xiawan* (CV10):** point on the upper abdomen and on the anterior midline, 2 *cun* above the center of the umbilicus (Fig. 24)

建里 [jiàn lǐ]

***jianli* (CV11):** point on the upper abdomen and on the anterior midline, 3 *cun* above the center of the umbilicus (Fig. 24)

中脘 [zhōng wǎn]

***zhongwan* (CV12):** point on the upper abdomen and on the anterior midline, 4 *cun* above the center of the umbilicus (Fig. 24)

上脘 [shàng wǎn]

shangwan **(CV13):** point on the upper abdomen and on the anterior midline, 5 *cun* above the center of the umbilicus (Fig. 24)

巨阙 [jù què]

juque **(CV14):** point on the upper abdomen and on the anterior midline, 6 *cun* above the center of the umbilicus (Fig. 24)

鸠尾 [jiū wěi]

jiuwei **(CV15):** point on the upper abdomen and on the anterior midline, 1 *cun* below the xiphosternal synchondrosis (Fig. 24)

中庭 [zhōng tíng]

zhongting **(CV16):** point on the chest and on the anterior midline, on the level of the 5th intercostal space, on the xiphosternal synchondrosis (Fig. 24)

膻中 [dàn zhōng]

danzhong **(CV17):** point on the chest and on the anterior midline, on the level of the 4th intercostal space, at the midpoint of the line connecting both nipples (Fig. 24)

玉堂 [yù táng]

yutang **(CV18):** point on the chest and on the anterior midline, on the level of the 3rd. intercostal space (Fig. 24)

紫宫 [zǐ gōng]

zigong **(CV19):** point on the chest and on the anterior midline, on the level of the 2nd intercostal space (Fig. 24)

华盖 [huá gài]

huagai **(CV20):** point on the chest and on the anterior midline, on the level of the 1st intercostal space (Fig. 24)

璇玑 [xuán jī]

xuanji **(CV21):** point on the chest and on the anterior midline, 1 *cun* below *tiantu* (CV22) (Fig. 24)

天突 [tiān tū]

tiantu **(CV22):** point on the neck and on the anterior midline, at the center of the suprasternal fossa (Fig. 24)

廉泉 [lián quán]

lianquan **(CV23):** point on the neck and on the anterior midline, in the depression above the upper border of the hyoid bone (Fig. 24)

承浆 [chéng jiāng]

***chengjiang* (CV24):** point on the face, in the depression at the midpoint of the mentolabial sulcus (Fig. 24)

特定穴 [tè dìng xué]

specific points: points on the meridians with specific therapeutic effects, hence, specific names. They are the five transport points, source points, connecting points, alarm points, back transport points, eight influential points, cleft points, crossing points, eight confluence points, and lower sea points

五输穴 [wǔ shù xué]

five transport points: five points on each of the twelve meridians distributing distal to the elbow and knees, varying in their condition of the flow of *qi* and blood. They are the well points, spring points, stream points, river points and sea points.

井穴 [jǐng xué]

well points: transport points located at the end of the fingers or toes. Each of the twelve meridians has a well point. They are *shaoshang* (LU11), *shangyang* (LI1), *zhongchong* (PC9), *guanchong* (TE1), *shaochong* (HT9), *shaoze* (SI1), *yinbai* (SP1), *lidui* (ST45), *dadun* (LR1), *zuqiaoyin* (GB44), *yongquan* (KI1), and *zhiyin* (BL67). They are mainly used for emergency revival.

荥穴 [yíng xué]

spring points: transport points located at the distal ends of the limbs mainly in the metacarpal and metatarsal regions. Each of the twelve meridians has a spring point, namely, *yuji* (LU10), *erjian* (LI2), *laogong* (PC8), *yeman* (TE2), *shaofu* (HT8), *qiangu* (SI2), *dadu* (SP2), *neiting* (ST44), *xingjian* (LR2), *xiaxi* (GB43), *rangu* (KI2), and *tonggu* (BL66). They are mainly used for treating febrile diseases.

俞穴 [shù xué]

(1)acupoints: acupuncture points in general; **(2) stream points:** transport points located on the hands or feet. Each of the twelve meridians has a stream point, namely, *taiyuan* (LU9), *sanjian* (LI3), *daling* (PC7), *zhongzhu* (TE3), *shenmen* (HT7), *houxi* (SI3), *taibai* (SP3), *xiangu* (ST43), *taichong* (LR3), *zulinqi* (GB41), *taixi* (KI3), and *shugu* (BL65). They are mainly used for treating rheumatism.

经穴 [jīng xué]

(1) meridian points: points on the fourteen meridians, 361 in all; **(2) river**

points: transport points mostly located on the legs and forearms. Each of the twelve meridians has a spring point, namely, *jingqu* (LU8), *yangxi* (LI5), *jianshi* (PC5), zhigou (TE6), *lingdao* (HT4), *yanggu* (SI5), *shangqiu* (SP5), *jiexi* (ST41), *zhongfeng* (LR4), *yangfu* (GB38), fuliu (KI7), and *kunlun* (BL60). They are mainly used for treating cough, asthma, and disorders of the throat

合穴 [hé xué]

sea points: transport points mostly located on the elbow or the knee. Each of the twelve meridians has a sea point, namely, *chize* (LU5), *quchi* (LI11), *quze* (PC3), *tianjing* (TE10), shaohai (HT3), *xiaohai* (SI8), *yinlingquan* (SP9), *zusanli* (ST36), *ququan* (LR8), *yanglingquan* (GB34), *yingu* (KI10), and *weizhong* (BL40). They are mainly used for treating diseases of the *fu* organs such as the stomach and intestines.

原穴 [yuán xué]

source points: points where the original *qi* of *zang-fu* organs passes or stays. Each of the twelve meridians has a source point, namely, *taiyuan* (LU9), *jinggu* (UB64), *hegu* (LI4), *taixi* (KI3), *chongyang* (ST42), *daling* (PC7), *taibai* (SP3), *yangchi* (TE4), *shenmen* (HT7), *qiuxu* (GB40), *wangu* (SI4), *and taichong* (LR3).

络穴 [luò xué]

connecting points: points for the fourteen meridians to connect the respective yin and yang meridians interior-exteriorly. The spleen meridian has two connecting points, hence fifteen in all. They are *pianli* (LI6), dazhong (KI4), lieque (LU7), feiyang (BL58), gongsun (SP4), *waiguan* (TE5), *fenglong* (ST40), *neiguan* (PC6), *zhizheng* (SI7), *ligou* (LR5), *tongli* (HT5), *guangming* (GB37), *dabao* (SP21), *changqiang* (GV1), and *jiuwei* (CV15).

郄穴 [xì xué]

cleft point: point where the meridian *qi* accumulates deeply. Each of the twelve meridians, together with the yin heel, yang heel, yin link, and yang link vessels, has a cleft point, hence sixteen in all. They are *kongzui* (LU6), *huizong* (TE7), *ximen* (PC4), *yanglao* (SI6), *yinxi* (HT6), *liangqiu* (ST34), *wenliu* (LI7), *waiqiu* (GB36), *jinmen* (UB63), *fuyang* (UB59), *diji* (SP8), *jiaoxin* (KI8), *zhongdu* (LR6), *yangjiao* (GB35), *shuiquan* (KI5), and *zhubin* (KI9). The cleft point is mainly used to treat acute disorders and pains in the area related to its respective meridian, and diseases of the corresponding internal organ.

募穴 [mù xué]

alarm point: point located on the chest or abdomen, where the *qi* of the respective internal organ is concentrated, and so pathological reactions such as tenderness will be found if the internal organ is diseased. *Zhongfu* (LU1), *zhongwan* (CV12), *danzhong* (CV17), *shimen* (CV5), *juque* (CV14), *jingmen* (GB25), *qimen* (LR14), *tianshu* (ST25), *riyue* (GB24), *huanyuan* (CV4), *zhangmen* (LR13), and *zhongji* (CV3) are alarm points.

背俞穴 [bèi shù xué]

back transport points: specific points located along the bladder meridian on the back, whither the *qi* of the *zang-fu* organs flows, and pain upon pressure is often found when the corresponding *zang-fu* organ is diseased. The points and their corresponding organs are: *feishu* (BL13)—lung; *jueyin*shu (BL14)—pericardium; *xinshu* (BL15)—heart; *ganshu* (BL18)—liver; *danshu* (BL19)—gallbladder; *pishu* (BL20)—spleen; *sanjiaoshu* (BL22)— triple energizer; *shenshu* (BL23)—kidney; *dachangshu* (BL25)—large intestine; *xiaochangshu* (BL27)—small intestine; *pangguanshu* (BL28)—urinary bladder.

八会穴 [bā huì xué]

eight influential points: eight important points which are closely related to the *zang, fu, qi*, blood, bone, marrow, tendons and blood vesesl respectively, namely, zhangmen (LR13) to the *zang*-organs, *zhongwan* (CV12) to the *fu*-organs, *danzhong* (CV17) to *qi*, *geshu* (BL17) to blood, *dazhu* (BL11) to the bones, *xuanzhong* (GB39) to the marrow, *yanglingquan* (GB34) to the tendons, and *taiyuan* (LU9) to the vessels

交会穴 [jiāo huì xué]

crossing point: point where two or more meridians intersect

八脉交会穴 [bā mài jiāo huì xué]

eight confluence points: points where the regular meridians communicate with the eight extra meridians, namely, *gongsun* (SP4), *neiguan* (PC6), *houxi* (SI3), *shenmai* (BL62), *waiguan* (TE 5), *zulinqi* (GB 41), *lieque* (LU7), and *zhaohai* (KI6)

下合穴 [xià hé xué]

lower confluent points; lower sea points: specific points on the three yang meridians of the foot where the *qi* of the six *fu*-organs flows into the meridian, namely, *zusanli* (ST36) for the stomach, *shangjuxu* (ST37) for the large intestine, *xiajuxu* (ST39) for the small intestine, *yanglingquan*

(GB34) for the gallbladder, *weizhong* (BL40) for the urinary bladder, and *weiyang* (BL39) for the triple energizer. Since three of them, i.e., ST36, GB34 and BL40, are the same as the sea points, they are also called the lower sea points.

经外穴 Extra Points

经外穴 [jīng wài xúe]

extra points: acupuncture-moxibustion points not distributed on the meridians

头颈部穴 [tóu jǐng bù xué]

points on the head and neck (HN): extra points located on the head and neck

四神聪 [sì shén cōng]

***sishencong* (EX-HN1):** four points on the head, 1 *cun* anterior, posterior and lateral to baihui (GV20) (Fig. 25)

当阳 [dāng yáng]

***dangyang* (EX-HN2):** point at the frontal part of the head, directly above the pupil, 1 *cun* above the anterior hairline (Fig. 25)

印堂 [yìn táng]

***yintang* (EX-HN3):** point on the forehead, at the midpoint between the eyebrows (Fig. 25)

鱼腰 [yú yāo]

***yuyao* (EX-HN4):** point on the forehead, directly above the pupil, in the eyebrow (Fig. 25)

太阳 [tài yáng]

***taiyang* (EX-HN5):** point at the temporal part of the head, between the lateral end of the eyebrow and the outer canthus, in the depression one finger breadth behind (Fig. 25)

耳尖 [ěr jiān]

***erjian* (EX-HN6):** point at the apex of the auricle when the ear is folded forward (Fig. 25)

球后 [qiú hòu]

***qiuhou* (EX-HN7):** point on the face, at the junction of the lateral fourth and medial three fourths of the infraorbital margin (Fig. 25)

上迎香 [shàng yíng xiāng]

***shangyingxiang* (EX-HN8):** point on the face, at the junction of the alar cartilage of the nose and the nasal concha, near the upper end of the nasolabial groove (Fig. 25)

内迎香 [nèi yíng xiāng]

***neiyingxiang* (EX-HN9):** point in the nostril, at the junction between the alar cartilage of the nose and the nasal concha (Fig. 25)

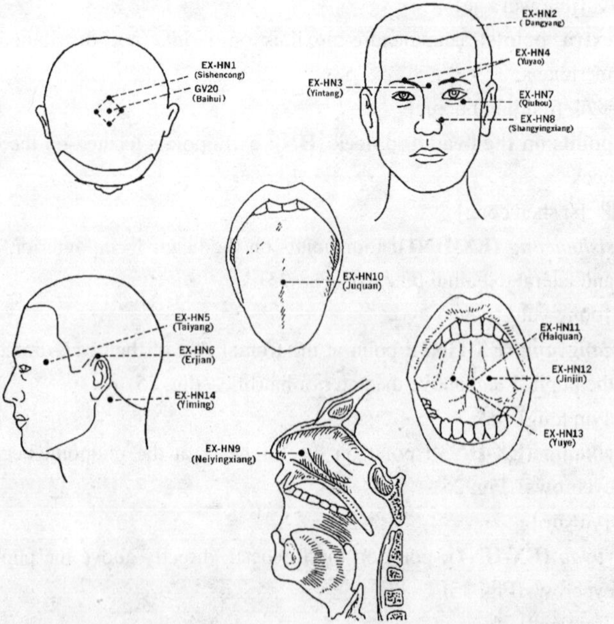

Fig.25 Extra points on the head and neck

聚泉 [jù quán]

***juquan* (EX-HN10):** point in the mouth, at the midpoint of the dorsal midline of the tongue (Fig. 25)

海泉 [hǎi quán]

***haiquan* (EX-HN11):** point in the mouth, at the midpoint of the frenulum of the tongue (Fig. 25)

金津 [jīn jīn]

***jinjin* (EX-HN12):** point in the mouth, on the vein on the left side of the frenulum of the tongue (Fig. 25)

玉液 [yù yè]

***yuye* (EX-HN13):** point in the mouth, on the vein on the right side of the frenulum of the tongue (Fig. 25)

翳明 [yì míng]

***yiming* (EX-HN14):** point on the nape, 1 *cun* posterior to *yifen* (TE17) (Fig. 25)

颈白劳 [jǐng bái láo]

***jingbailao* (EX-HN15):** point on the nape, 2 *cun* above *dazhui* (GV 14) and 1 *cun* lateral to the posterior midline (Fig. 25)

胸腹部穴 [xiōng fù bù xué]

points on the chest and abdomen (CA): extra points located on the chest and abdomen

子宫 [zǐ gōng]

***zigong* (EX-CA1):** point on the lower abdomen, 4 *cun* below the center of the umbilicus and 3 *cun* lateral to *zhongji* (CV3) (Fig. 26)

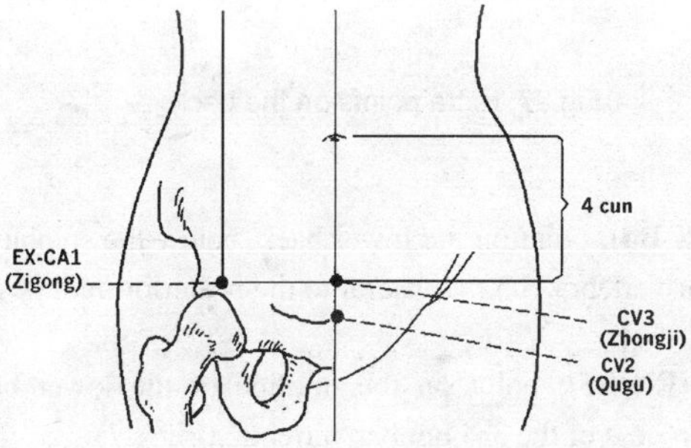

Fig.26 Extra points on the abdomen

背部穴 [bèi bù xué]

points on the back (B): extra points located on the back

定喘 [dìng chuǎn]

***dingchuan* (EX-B1):** point on the back, below the spinous process of the 7th cervical vertebra, 0.5 *cun* lateral to the posterior midline (Fig. 27)

夹脊 [jiá jǐ]

***jiaji* (EX-B2):** 17 points on each side of the back, below the spinous processes from the 1st thoracic to the 5th lumbar vertebrae, 0.5 *cun* lateral to the posterior midline (Fig. 27)

胃脘下俞 [wèi wǎn xià shù]

***weiwanxiashu* (EX-B3):** point on the back, below the spinous process of the 8th thoracic vertebra, 1.5 *cun* lateral to the posterior midline (Fig. 27)

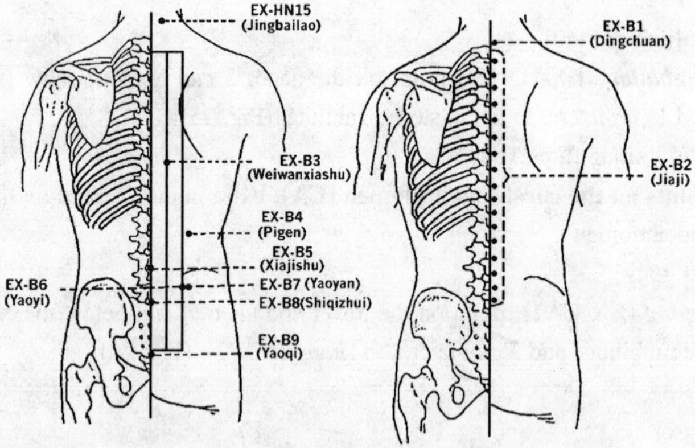

Fig.27 Extra points on the back

痞根 [pǐ gēn]

***pigen* (EX-B4):** point on the lower back, below the spinous process of the 1st lumbar vertebra, 3.5 *cun* lateral to the posterior midline (Fig. 27)

下极俞 [xià jí shù]

***xiajishu* (EX-B5):** point on the midline of the lower back, below the spinous process of the 3rd lumbar vertebra (Fig. 27)

腰宜 [yāo yí]

***yaoyi* (EX-B6):** point on the lower back, below the spinous process of the 4th lumbar vertebra, 3 *cun* lateral to the posterior midline (Fig. 27)

腰眼 [yāo yǎn]

***yaoyan* (EX-B7):** point on the lower back, below the spinous process of the 4th lumbar vertebra, in the depression 3.5 *cun* lateral to the posterior midline (Fig. 27)

十七椎 [shí qī zhuī]

***shiqizhui* (EX-B8):** point on the lower back and on the posterior midline, below the spinous process of the 5th lumbar vertebra (Fig. 27)

腰奇 [yāo qí]

***yaoqi* (EX-B9):** point on the lower back, 2 *cun* directly above the tip of the coccyx, in the depression between the sacral horns (Fig. 27)

上肢穴 [shàng zhī xué]

points on the upper extremities (UE): extra points located on the upper extremities

肘尖 [zhǒu jiān]

***zhoujian* (EX-UE1):** point on the posterior side of the elbow, at the tip of the olecranon when the elbow is flexed (Fig. 28)

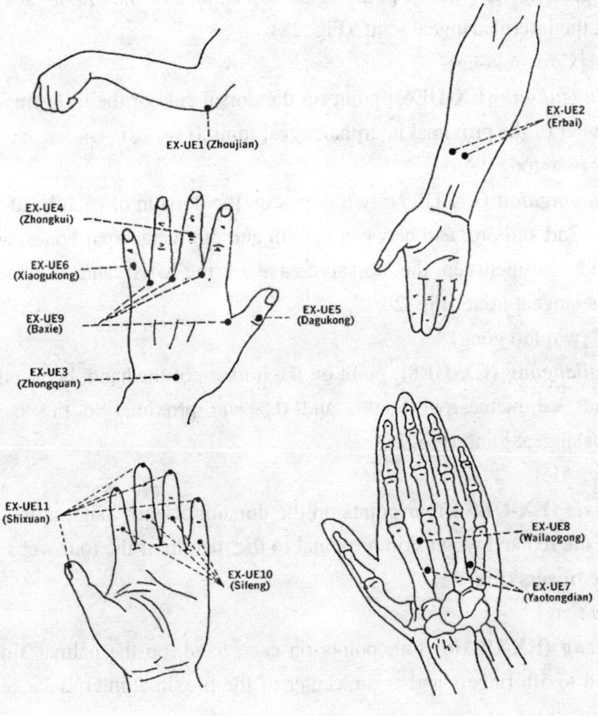

Fig.28 Extra points on the upper extremity

二白 [èr bái]

***erbai* (EX-UE2):** two points on the palmar side of each forearm, 4 *cun* proximal to the crease of the wrist, on each side of the tendon of the radial flexor muscle of the wrist (Fig. 28)

中泉 [zhōng quán]

***zhongquan* (EX-UE3):** point on the dorsal crease of the wrist, in the depression on the radial side of the tendon of the common extensor muscle of the fingers (Fig. 28)

中魁 [zhōng kuí]

***zhongkui* (EX-UE4):** point on the dorsal side of the middle finger, at the center of the proximal interphalangeal joint (Fig. 28)

大骨空 [dà gǔ kōng]

***dagukong* (EX-UE5):** point on the dorsal side of the thumb, at the center of the interphalangeal joint (Fig. 28)

小骨空 [xiǎo gǔ kōng]

***xiaogukong* (EX-UE6):** point on the dorsal side of the little finger, at the center of the proximal interphalangeal joint (Fig. 28)

腰痛点 [yāo tòng diǎn]

***yaotongdian* (EX-UE7):** two points on the dorsum of each hand, between the 2nd and 3rd, and between the 4th and 5th metacarpal bones, and at the midpoint between the dorsal crease of the wrist and the metacarpo-phalangeal joint (Fig. 28)

外劳宫 [wài láo gōng]

***wailaogong* (EX-UE8):** point on the dorsum of the hand, between the 2nd and 3rd metacarpal bones, and 0.5 *cun* proximal to the metacarpo-phalangeal joint (Fig. 28)

八邪 [bā xié]

***baxie* (EX-UE9):** four points on the dorsum of each hand, at the junction of the red and white skin proximal to the margin of the four webs between the fingers (Fig. 28)

四缝 [sì fèng]

***sifeng* (EX-UE10):** four points on each hand, on the palmar side of the 2nd to 5th fingers and at the center of the proximal interphalangeal joints (Fig. 28)

十宣 [shí xuān]

***shixuan* (EX-UE11):** ten points on both hands, at the tips of the 10 fingers, 0.1 *cun* from the free margin of the nails (Fig. 28)

下肢穴 [xià zhī xué]

points on the lower extremities (LE): extra points located on the lower extremities

髋骨 [kuān gǔ]

***kuangu* (EX-LE1):** two points on each thigh, in the lower part of the anterior surface of the thigh, 1.5 *cun* lateral and medial to *liangqiu* (ST34) (Fig. 29)

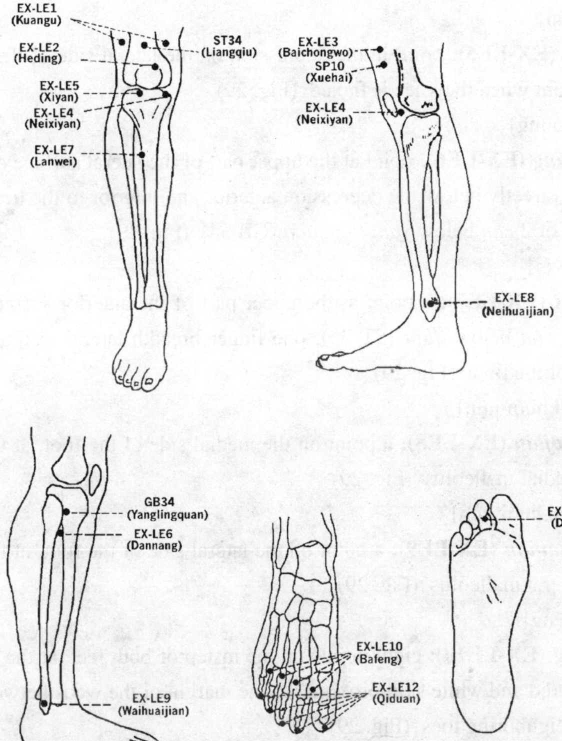

Fig.29 Extra points on the lower extremity

鹤顶 [hè dǐng]

***heding* (EX-LE2):** point above the knee, in the depression of the midpoint of the upper border of the patella (Fig. 29)

百虫窝 [bǎi chóng wō]

***baichongwo* (EX-LE3):** point 3 *cun* above the medial superior corner of the patella of the thigh with the knee flexed, i.e., 1 *cun* above *xuehai* (SP 10) (Fig. 29)

内膝眼 [nèi xī yǎn]

***neixiyan* (EX-LE4):** point in the depression medial to the patellar ligament when the knee is flexed (Fig. 29)

膝眼 [xī yǎn]

***xiyan* (EX-LE5):** point in the depression on the lateral side of the patellar ligament when the knee is flexed (Fig. 29)

胆囊 [dǎn náng]

***dannang* (EX-LE6):** point at the upper part of the lateral surface of the leg, 2 *cun* directly below the depression anterior and inferior to the head of the fibula or 2 *cun* below *yanglingquan* (GB 34) (Fig. 29)

阑尾 [lán wěi]

***lanwei* (EX-LE7):** a point at the upper part of the anterior surface of the leg, 5 *cun* below *dubi* (ST 35), one finger breadth lateral to the anterior crest of the tibia (Fig. 29)

内踝尖 [nèi huái jiān]

***neihuajian* (EX-LE8):** a point on the medial side of the foot, at the tip of the medial malleolus (Fig. 29)

外踝尖 [wài huái jiān]

***waihuaijian* (EX-LE9):** a point on the lateral side of the foot, at the tip of the lateral malleolus (Fig. 29)

八风 [bā fēng]

***bafeng* (EX-LE10):** eight points on the instep of both feet, at the junction of the red and white skin proximal to the margin of the webs between each two neighboring toes (Fig. 29)

独阴 [dú yīn]

***duyin* (EX-LE11):** a point on the plantar side of the 2nd toe, at the center of the distal interphalangeal joint (Fig. 29)

气端 [qì duān]

***qiduan* (EX-LE12):** ten points at the tips of the 10 toes of both feet, 0.1 *cun* from the free margin of each toenail (Fig. 29)

阿是穴 [ā shì xué]

***ashi*:** a category of points which have no fixed location and are found by eliciting tenderness at the diseased site

灸法及其他由针刺演变之疗法

Moxibustion and Other Techniques Derived from Acupuncture

艾 [ài]

moxa (Artemisia vulgaris): a plant from which moxa wool is prepared

艾绒 [ài róng]

moxa; moxa wool: a cottony material used, when ignited, as a counterirritant or cautery in moxibustion

艾炷 [ài zhù]

moxa cone: a cone-shaped mass made of moxa

艾条 [ài tiáo]

moxa stick: a round long stick made of moxa, also called moxa roll (艾卷 [ài juǎn])

艾卷 [ài juǎn]

moxa roll, same as moxa stick (艾条 [ài tiáo])

温灸器 [wēn jiǔ qì]

moxa burner: an instrument for moxibustion, usually a square or round box with a metallic network inside which contains ignited moxa

灸法 [jiǔ fǎ]

moxibustion: a therapeutic procedure involving ignited material (usually moxa) to apply heat to certain points or areas of the body surface for curing disease through regulation of the function of meridians and *zang-fu* organs

艾条灸 [ài tiáo jiǔ]

moxa-stick moxibustion; moxibustion using a moxa stick: moxibustion using an ignited moxa stick (Fig. 30)

艾卷灸 [ài juǎn jiǔ]

moxa-roll moxibustion: moxibustion with using an ignited moxa roll, also known as moxa-stick moxibustion (艾条灸 [ài tiáo jiǔ])

悬灸 [xuán jiǔ]

suspended moxibustion: a type of moxa-stick moxibustion, in which the ignited moxa stick is held above the skin, including mild moxibustion, pecking moxibustion, and revolving moxibustion

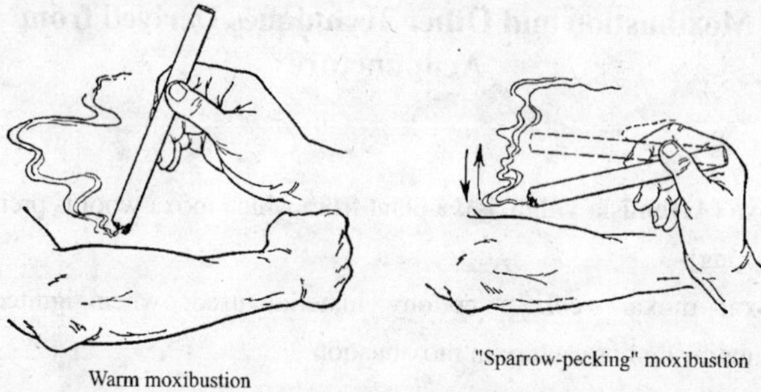

Fig.30 Moxa–stick moxibustion

温和灸 [wēn hé jiǔ]

mild moxibustion: a type of moxa-stick moxibustion, performed by holding an ignited moxa stick about an inch from the patient's skin, keeping the spot warm and making it reddened, but not burnt (Fig. 30)

雀啄灸 [què zhuó jiǔ]

"sparrow-pecking" moxibustion; pecking moxibustion: a type of moxa-stick moxibustion, performed by putting an ignited moxa stick near the patient's skin surface, and moving it up and down so as to give more heat than mild to the applied spot (Fig. 30)

回旋灸 [huí xuán jiǔ]

revolving moxibustion: a type of moxa-stick moxibustion, performed by keeping an ignited moxa stick at a fixed distance from the patient's skin, but moving it in a circular direction

艾炷灸 [ài zhù jiǔ]

moxa-cone moxibustion: moxibustion with an ignited moxa cone, which may be applied directly or indirectly

直接灸 [zhí jiē jiǔ]

direct moxibustion: moxibustion by applying an ignited moxa cone directly on the skin surface, also known as open moxibustion (明灸 [míng jiǔ]) or direct contact moxibustion (着肤灸[zháo fū jiǔ])

着肤灸 [zháo fū jiǔ]

direct contact moxibustion: another name for direct moxibustion (直接灸 [zhí jiē jiǔ])

明灸 [míng jiǔ]

open moxibustion: another name for direct moxibustion (直接灸 [zhí jiē jiǔ])

瘢痕灸 [bān hén jiǔ]

scarring moxibustion: a type of direct moxibustion with applying an ignited moxa cone till the skin is burned and then blisters and postulates, leaving a scar, also known as pustulating moxibustion (化脓灸 [huà nóng jiǔ])

化脓灸 [huà nóng jiǔ]

pustulating moxibustion: another name for scarring moxibustion (瘢痕灸 [bān hén jiǔ])

无瘢痕灸 [wú bān hén jiǔ]

non-scarring moxibustion: a type of direct moxibustion using an ignited moxa cone, which leaves the skin red but not injured, and so leaves no scar, also known as non-pustulating moxibustion (非化脓灸 [fēi huà nóng jiǔ])

非化脓灸 [fēi huà nóng jiǔ]

non-pustulating moxibustion: another name for non-scarring moxibustion (无瘢痕灸 [wú bān hén jiǔ])

间接灸 [jiàn jiē jiǔ]

indirect moxibustion: moxibustion using an ignited moxa cone, performed by placing something (e.g., a slice of ginger, garlic, some salt, or a cake of beaten drug) between the moxa cone and the skin, also known as interposed moxibustion (间隔灸 [jiān gé jiǔ])

间隔灸 [jiān gé jiǔ]

interposed moxibustion: another name for indirect moxibustion (间接灸 [jiān jiē jiǔ])

隔姜灸 [gé jiāng jiǔ]

ginger moxibustion: indirect moxibustion using a slice of fresh ginger, performed by placing beneath the moxa cone a piece of ginger about 3mm thick, with some pores made on it, used for treating vomiting, abdominal pain and diarrhea due to endogenous cold.

隔蒜灸 [gé suàn jiǔ]

garlic moxibustion: indirect moxibustion using a garlic slice, performed by placing a piece of fresh garlic about 3 mm thick with some pores made on it, used for treating sores and boils

隔盐灸 [gé yán jiǔ]

salt moxibustion: indirect moxibustion with salt, performed by filling the umbilical depression to the brim with salt and then putting a large ignited moxa cone on it, used for treating prostration, abdominal pain due to cold, acute vomiting and diarrhea

附子饼灸 [fù zǐ bǐng jiǔ]

aconite moxibustion: indirect moxibustion using a cake of *Radix Aconiti Lateralis* mixed with some wine placed on the point beneath the moxa cone, used for treating impotence or chronic diarrhea

温针灸 [wēn zhēn jiǔ]

moxibustion with warming needle: a practice used for treating rheumatic pains, performed by placing an ignited moxa stick on the handle of the needle after insertion

实按灸 [shí àn jiǔ]

pressing moxibustion: moxibustion performed by placing several layers of cloth or paper on the spot, and then pressing the ignited end of a moxa stick on the cloth or paper

雷火神针 [léi huǒ shén zhēn]

thunder-fire miraculous "needling": a type of pressing moxibustion performed by using a special kind of medicinal moxa roll containing mugwort, frankincense, wolfsbane, realgar, and other medicinal herbs

温灸器灸 [wēn jiǔ qì jiǔ]

moxa-burner moxibustion: moxibustion with a moxa burner

天灸 [tiān jiǔ]

natural moxibustion: a practice equivalent to moxibustion, performed by applying irritant medicine on certain spots on the skin to induce vesiculation or local congestion, also known as medicinal moxibustion (药物灸 [yào wù jiǔ]) or vesiculating moxibustion (发泡灸 [fā pào jiǔ])

药物灸 [yào wù jiǔ]

medicinal moxibustion: see natural moxibustion (天灸 [tiān jiǔ])

发泡灸 [fā pào jiǔ]

vesiculating moxibustion: see natural moxibustion (天灸 [tiān jiǔ])

一壮 [yī zhuàng]

one *zhuang*: the time for burning a moxa cone, taken as a unit in moxibustion

拔罐法 [bá guàn fǎ]

cupping therapy: to suck by placing a vacuumized, usually by fire, cup or jar onto the affected or any part of the body surface for therapeutic purposes

竹罐 [zhú guàn]

bamboo jar: a jar made of bamboo used for cupping therapy

陶罐 [táo guàn]

pottery jar: a jar made of pottery used for cupping therapy

玻璃罐 [bō lí guàn]

glass jar; glass cup: a cup or jar made of glass used for cupping therapy

抽气罐 [chōu qì guàn]

suction cup: a cup or jar with the air inside expelled by suction

火罐 [huǒ guàn]

cupping tool: a cup or jar vacuumized, usually by fire, used for cupping therapy

闪火法 [shǎn huǒ fǎ]

flash-fire cupping: a cupping procedure which involves flashing the fire of a piece of ignited alcohol-cotton once around the cup's interior and pressing the cup onto the treated area immediately after removing the ignited cotton

投火法 [tóu huǒ fǎ]

fire-insertion cupping: a cupping procedure which involves inserting a piece of ignited alcohol-cotton or paper into a cup and pressing the cup transversely onto the treated area of the lateral side of the body

架火法 [jià huǒ fǎ]

fire-rack cupping: a cupping procedure which involves placing at the site to be treated a piece of incombustible substance with a small alcohol-cotton ball on it, and covering with a cup after igniting the cotton ball

贴棉法 [tiē mián fǎ]

cotton-burning cupping: a cupping procedure involving a thin layer of alcohol-cotton on the wall of cup, and pressing the cup onto the treated area after igniting the cotton

滴酒法 [dī jiǔ fǎ]

alcohol fire cupping: a cupping procedure which involves spreading 1-3 drops of alcohol on the bottom of the cup and pressing the cup on the area to be treated after igniting the alcohol

抽气罐法 [chōu qì guàn fǎ]

suction cupping: cupping therapy using suction cups

煮罐法 [zhǔ guàn fǎ]

cup-boiling method: a cupping therapy method in which bamboo jars are used after being boiled in water or a herbal decoction for 1-2 minutes and turned upside down to be emptied

留罐 [liú guàn fǎ]

retained cupping: a common method of cupping in which the cup or jar is kept at the same site for 10-15 minutes

推罐 [tuī guàn]

glide-cupping: a cupping method in which the cup or jar is moved to and fro on the skin surface lubricated with vaseline in advance, also known as slide-cupping (走罐 [zǒu guàn])

走罐 [zǒu guàn]

slide-cupping, synonymous with glide-cupping (推罐 [tuī guàn])

留针拔罐 [liú zhēn bá guàn]

cupping with needle retention: a combined method of acupuncture and cupping in which cupping is applied to the acupuncture site with the needle retained after the arrival of *qi*

刺血拔罐 [cì xuè bá guàn]

bloodletting pricking and cupping: a combined method of pricking and cupping in which cupping is applied to the pricking site with a three-edged needle to increase bloodletting, also known as pricking-cupping bloodletting (刺络拔罐 [cì luò bá guàn])

刺络拔罐 [cì luò bá guàn]

pricking-cupping bloodletting, same as bloodletting pricking and cupping (刺血拔罐 [cì xuè bá guàn])

药罐 [yào guàn]

medicinal cupping: a type of suction cupping with cups containing a certain amount of medicinal fluid such as ginger juice or anti-rheumatic tincture

电针 [diàn zhēn]

electro-acupuncture; galvano-acupuncture: acupuncture with electric stimulation after the needle has been inserted and normal sensation is felt

电针仪 [diàn zhēn yí]

electric stimulator: an instrument that provides electric stimulation in electro-acupuncture

电测法 [diàn cè fǎ]

electro-exploratory method: a method for locating needling points in auriculo-acupuncture by testing the electric conductivity

穴位注射 [xué wèi zhù shè]

point injection: a treatment by which liquid medicine is injected into the point so as to obtain a therapeutic result through both needling stimulation and pharmaceutical reaction

水针 [shuǐ zhēn]

hydro-acupuncture, same as point injection (穴位注射 [xué wèi zhù shè])

穴位封闭 [xué wèi fēng bì]

acupoint block: block anesthesia accomplished by injecting anaesthetic into acupuncture points, a method for treating pains of various kinds

针刺麻醉 [zhēn cì má zuì]

acupuncture anesthesia: anaesthetic effect obtained through needling so that a surgical operation may be performed while the patient remains conscious

电针麻醉 [diàn zhēn má zuì]

electro-acupuncture anesthesia: anesthesia induced by electro-acupuncture

针麻诱导 [zhēn má yòu dǎo]

induction of acupuncture anesthesia: procedure of manual or electric stimulation to raise the pain threshold of the patient before a surgical operation

头针疗法 [tóu zhēn liáo fǎ]; 头皮针疗法 [tóu pí zhēn liáo fǎ]

scalp-acupuncture: a variety of acupuncture in which the corresponding functional areas of the cerebral cortex on the scalp are needled to treat encephalopathy of various kinds, such as cerebral embolism

头穴线 [tóu xué xiàn]

scalp acupuncture lines: lines used in scalp acupuncture, labeled with the alphabetic code MS (derived from "micro-system" and "scalp point")

额中线 [é zhōng xiàn]

middle line of forehead (MS1): the line 1 *cun* from GV24 straight down along the meridian

额旁1线 [é páng 1 xiàn]

lateral line 1 of forehead (MS2): the line 1 *cun* from BL3 straight down along the meridian

额旁中2线 [é páng zhōng 2 xiàn]

lateral line 2 of forehead (MS3): the line 1 *cun* from GB15 straight down along the meridian

额旁3线 [é páng 3 xiàn]

lateral line 3 of forehead (MS4): the line 1 *cun* from the point 0.75 *cun* medial to ST8 straight down

顶中线 [dǐng zhōng xiàn]

middle line of vertex (MS5): the line from GV20 to GV21 along the middle of the head

顶颞前斜线 [dǐng niè qián xié xiàn]

anterior oblique line of vertex-temporal (MS6): the line from *qianshencong* (one of the four acupuncture points collectively designated as EX-HN1, 1 *cun* anterior to GV20) obliquely to GB6

顶颞后斜线 [dǐng niè hòu xié xiàn]

posterior oblique line of vertex-temporal (MS7): the line from GV20 obliquely to GB7

顶旁1线 [dǐng páng 1 xiàn]

lateral line 1 of vertex: the line 1.5 *cun* lateral to the middle line of the vertex, 1.5 *cun* from BL6 backward along the meridian

顶旁2线 [dǐng páng 2 xiàn]

lateral line 2 of vertex (MS9): the line 2.25 *cun* lateral to the middle line of the vertex, 1.5 *cun* from GB17 backward along the meridian

颞前线 [niè qián xiàn]

anterior temporal line (MS10): the line from GB4 to GB5

颞后线 [niè hòu xiàn]

posterior temporal line (MS11): the line from GB8 to GB7

枕上正中线 [zhěn shàng zhèng zhōng xiàn]

upper-middle line of occiput (MS12): the line from GV18 to GV17

枕上旁线 [zhěn shàng páng xiàn]

upper-lateral line of occiput (MS13): the line 0.5 *cun* lateral and parallel to upper-middle line of the occiput

枕下旁线 [zhěn xià páng xiàn]

lower-lateral line of occiput (MS14): the line 2 *cun* from BL9 straight down

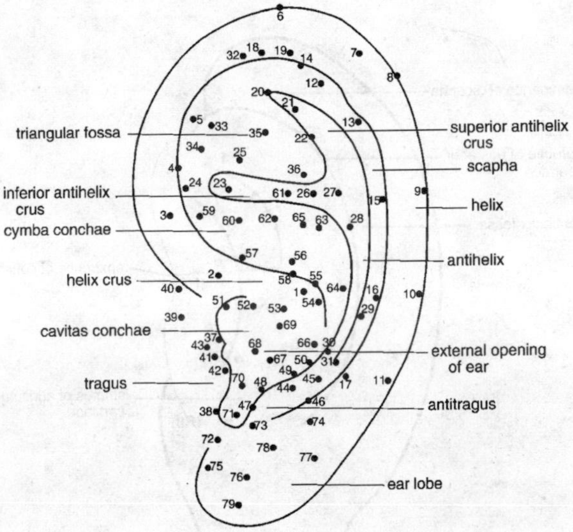

Fig.31 Points on the anterior aspect of the auricle

耳针疗法 [ěr zhēn liáo fǎ]

ear-acupuncture therapy; auriculo-therapy: a variety of acupuncture in which specific points on the ear are needled to treat a large variety of diseases, such as asthma, gastric troubles, neurasthenia, skin diseases, hypertension, enuresis, etc., and also for acupuncture anesthesia

耳轮 [ěr lún]

helix: prominent rim of the auricle

耳轮结节 [ěr lún jié jié]

helix tubercle: small tubercle at the posterosuperior aspect of the helix

耳轮脚 [ěr lún jiǎo]

helix crus: the transverse part of the helix that runs backward to the ear cavity

耳轮尾 [ěr lún wěi]

helix cauda: the inferior part of the helix, at the junction of the helix and earlobe

对耳轮 [duì ěr lún]

antihelix: elevated Y-shaped ridge opposite the helix, including the trunk, superior and inferior crura

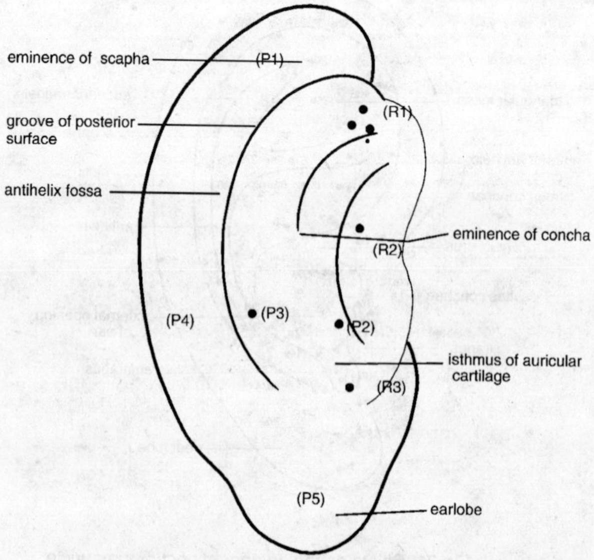

Fig.32 Points on the posterior aspect of the auricle

对耳轮体 [duì ěr lún tǐ]

trunk of antihelix: main vertical part of the antihelix

对耳轮上脚 [duì ěr lún shàng jiǎo]

superior crus of antihelix: upper (upward) branch of the antihelix

对耳轮下脚 [duì ěr lún xià jiǎo]

inferior crus of antihelix: lower (forward) branch of the antihelix

三角窝 [sān jiǎo wō]

triangular fossa: triangular depression between the two crura of the antihelix

耳舟 [ěr zhōu]

scapha: curved depression between the helix and antihelix

耳屏 [ěr píng]

tragus: cartilaginous projection anterior to external opening of the ear

对耳屏 [duì ěr píng]

antitragus: projection opposite the tragus

屏上切迹 [píng shàng qiē jì]

supratragic notch: depression between the helix crux and the upper border of the tragus

屏间切迹 [píng jiān qiē jì]

intertragic notch: depression between the tragus and antitragus

轮屏切迹 [lún píng qiē jì]

helix notch: depression between the antitragus and antihelix

耳垂 [ěr chuí]

earlobe: the lower part of the auricle where there is no cartilage

耳甲 [ěr jiǎ]

concha auricularis; concha: hollow of the auricle of the external ear, bounded anteriorly by the tragus and posteriorly by the antihelix

耳甲艇 [ěr jiǎ tǐng]

cymba conchae: upper part of the concha of the auricle, superior to the helix crus

耳甲腔 [ěr jiǎ qiāng]

cavity of concha; cavitas conchae: inferior part of the concha of the auricle, inferior to the helix crus

外耳门 [wài ěr mén]

external opening of the ear: orifice of the external auditory meatus

上耳根 [shàng ěr gēn]

superior auricular root: area where the upper border of the auricle is attached to the scalp

下耳根 [xià ěr gēn]

inferior auricular root: area where the earlobe is attached to the face

耳穴 [ěr xué]

ear acupoints: points used in ear acupuncture (see the table below and Figs. 31 and 32)

Chinese	Pinyin	English	Location
耳中	ěr zhōng	**ear center**	at the helix crus (1)
直肠	zhí cháng	**rectum**	at the helix anterosuperior to the helix crus (2)
尿道	niào dào	**urethra**	at the helix above the rectum area (3)
外生殖器	wài shēng zhī qì	**external genitals**	at the helix anterior to the inferior crus of the antihelix (4)
肛门	gāng mén	**anus**	at the helix anterior to the triangular fossa (5)
耳尖	ěr jiān	**ear apex**	at the tip of the auricle when the ear is folded toward the tragus (6)
结节	jié jié	**node**	at the helix tubercle (7)
轮 1	lún 1	**helix 1**	at the helix below the helix tubercle (8)
轮 2	lún 2	**helix 2**	at the helix below helix 1 (9)
轮 3	lún 3	**helix 3**	at the helix below helix 2 (10)
轮 4	lún 4	**helix 4**	at the helix below helix 3 (11)
指	zhǐ	**finger**	at the top of the scapha (12)
腕	wǎn	**wrist**	just below the finger area (13)
风溪	fēng xī	**wind stream**	at the junction of the finger and wrist areas, anterior to the helix tubercle (14)
肘	zhǒu	**elbow**	below the wrist area (15)
肩	jiān	**shoulder**	below the elbow area (16)
锁骨	suǒ hǔ	**clavicle**	below the shoulder area (17)
跟	gēn	**heel**	at the front part of the top of the superior crus of the antihelix (18)
趾	zhǐ	**toe**	at the back part of the top of the superior crus of antihelix, just below the ear apex (19)
踝	huái	**ankle**	below the heel and toe areas (20)
膝	xī	**knee**	at the middle 1/3 of the superior crus of the antihelix (21)
髋	kuān	**hip**	at the lower 1/3 of the superior crus of the antihelix (22)
坐骨神经	zuò gǔ shén jīng	**sciatic nerve**	at the front 2/3 of the inferior crus of the antihelix (23)
交感	jiāo gǎn	**sympathesis**	at the junction between the inferior crus of the antihelix and the inner border of the helix (24)
臀	tún	**gluteus**	at the back 1/3 of the inferior crus of the

			antihelix (25)
腹	fù	**abdomen**	at the upper 2/5 of the anterior part of the trunk of the antihelix (26)
腰骶椎	yāo dǐ zhuī	**lumbosacral vertebrae**	just behind the abdomen area (27)
胸	xiōng	**chest**	at the middle 2/5 of the front part of the antihelix (28)
胸椎	xiōng zhuī	**thoracic vertebrae**	just behind the chest area (29)
颈	jǐng	**neck**	at the lower 1/5 of the front part of the antihelix (30)
颈椎	jǐng zhuī	**cervical vertebrae**	just behind the neck area (31)
角窝上	jiǎo wō shàng	**superior triangular fossa**	in the upper part of the front 1/3 of the triangular fossa (32)
内生殖器	nèi shēng zhí qì	**internal genitals**	in the lower part of the front 1/3 of the triangular fossa (33)
角窝中	jiǎo wō zhōng	**middle triangular fossa**	at the middle 1/3 of the triangular fossa (34)
神门	shén mén	**shenmen**	in the upper part of the back 1/3 of the triangular fossa (35)
盆腔	pén qiāng	**pelvis**	in the lower part of the back 1/3 of the triangular fossa (36)
上屏	shàng píng	**upper tragus**	at the upper 1/2 of the outer side of the tragus (37)
下屏	xià píng	**lower tragus**	at the lower 1/2 of the outer side of the tragus (38)
外耳	wài ěr	**external ear**	in front of the supratragic notch, close to the helix (39)
屏尖	píng jiān	**apex of tragus**	at the upper end of the free border of the tragus (40)
外鼻	wài bí	**external nose**	at the middle of the outer side of the tragus (41)
肾上腺	shèn shàng xiàn	**adrenal gland**	at the lower end of the free border of the tragus (42)
咽喉	yān hóu	**throat**	at the upper 1/2 of the inner side of the tragus

			(43)
内鼻	nèi bí	**internal nose**	at the lower 1/2 of the inner side of the tragus
屏间前	ping jiān qián	**anterior intertragal notch**	in the lowest part of the tragus, in front of the intertragal notch
额	é	**forehead**	in the front part of the outer side of the antitragus (44)
屏间后	píng jiān hòu	**posterior intertragal notch**	in the anteroinferior part of the antitragus, behind the intertragal notch
颞	niè	**temple**	in the middle part of the outer side of the antitragus (45)
枕	zhěn	**occiput**	in the back part of the outer side of the antitragus (46)
皮质下	pí zhì xià	**subcortex**	in the inner side of the antitragus (47)
对屏尖	duì píng jiān	**apex of antitragus**	at the apex of the free border of the antitragus (48)
缘中	yuán zhōng	**central rim**	on the free border of the antitragus, at the mid-point between apex of the antitragus and the helix notch (49)
脑干	nǎo gàn	**brain stem**	at the helix notch (50)
口	kǒu	**mouth**	at the front 1/3 below the helix crus (51)
食道	shí dào	**esophagus**	at the middle 1/3 below the helix crus (52)
贲门	bēn mén	**cardia**	at the back 1/3 below the helix crus (53)
胃	wèi	**stomach**	at the place where the helix crus ends (54)
十二指肠	shī èr zhǐ cháng	**duodenum**	at the back 1/3 of the superior helix crux (55)
小肠	xiǎo cháng	**small intestine**	at the middle 1/3 of the superior helix crus (56)
大肠	dà cháng	**large intestine**	at the front 1/3 of the superior helix crus (57)
阑尾	lán wěi	**appendix**	between the small and large intestine areas (58)
艇角	tǐng jiǎo	**angle of superior concha**	at the front part below the inferior crus of the antihelix (59)
膀胱	páng	**bladder**	at the middle part below the inferior crus of

	guāng		the antihelix (60)
肾	shèn	**kidney**	at the back part below the inferior crus of the antihelix (61)
输尿管	shū niào guǎn	**ureter**	between the kidney and bladder areas (62)
胰胆	yí dǎn	**pancreas and gallbladder**	at the posterosuperior part of the cymba conchae (63)
肝	gān	**liver**	at the posteroinferior part of the cymba conchae (64)
艇中	tǐng zhōng	**center of superior concha**	between the small intestine and kidney areas (65)
脾	pí	**spleen**	at the posterosuperior part of the cavitas conchae (66)
心	xīn	**heart**	in the center of the cavitas conchae (67)
气管	qì guǎn	**trachea**	between the heart area and the external opening of the ear (68)
肺	fèi	**lung**	around the heart and trachea areas (69)
三焦	sān jiāo	**triple energizer**	posteroinferior to the external opening of the ear, between the lung and endocrine areas (70)
内分泌	nèi fēn mì	**endocrine**	inside the intertragic notch, at the anteroinferior part of the cavitas conchae (71)
牙	yá	**tooth**	in the anterosuperior part of the front side of the earlobe (72)
舌	shé	**tongue**	in the mediosuperior part of the front side of the earlobe (73)
颌	hé	**jaw**	in the posterosuperior part of the front side of the earlobe (74)
垂前	chuí qián	**anterior ear lobe**	in the anteromedial part of the front side of the earlobe (75)
眼	yǎn	**eye**	in the central part of the front side of the earlobe (76)
内耳	nèi ěr	**internal ear**	in the posteromedial part of the front side of the earlobe (77)
面颊	miàn jiá	**cheek**	at the junction between the internal ear and eye areas (78)
扁桃体	biǎn táo tǐ	**tonsil**	in the lower part of the front side of the

			earlobe (79)
耳背心	ěr bèi xīn	**heart of posterior surface**	in the upper part of the posterior surface of the auricle (P1)
耳背肺	ěr bèi fèi	**lung of posterior surface**	in the middle and inner part of the posterior surface of the auricle (P2)
耳背脾	ěr bèi pí	**spleen of posterior surface**	at the center of the posterior surface of the auricle (P3)
耳背肝	ěr bèi gān	**liver of posterior surface**	in the middle and outer part of the posterior surface of the auricle (P4)
耳背肾	ěr bèi shèn	**kidney of posterior surface**	in the lower part of the posterior surface of the auricle (P5)
耳背沟	ěr bèi gōu	**groove of posterior surface**	in the groove of the inferior crus of the antihelix
上耳根	shàng ěr gēn	**upper ear root**	at the upper border of the auricular root (R1)
耳迷根	ěr mí gēn	**root of ear vagus**	at the junction of the retroauricle and the mastoid, at the level of the helix crus (R2)
下耳根	xià ěr gēn	**lower ear root**	at the lower border of the auricular root (R3)

Note: The figures in parentheses refer to the points or areas shown in Figs. 31 and 32.

鼻针疗法 [bí zhēn liáo fǎ]

nose-acupuncture therapy: a variety of acupuncture in which specific points on the nose are needled for therapeutic purposes. The indications are the same as those for ear-acupuncture therapy.

面针疗法 [miàn zhēn liáo fǎ]

face-acupuncture therapy: a variety of acupuncture in which specific points on the face are needled to treat various disorders elsewhere in the body.

足针疗法 [zú zhēn liáo fǎ]

foot-acupuncture therapy: a variety of acupuncture in which specific points on the foot are needled to treat various disorders elsewhere in the body

埋线疗法 [mái xiàn liáo fǎ]

thread imbedding therapy: a form of acutherapy in which catgut is imbedded in the needle point to bring prolonged constant stimulation for treatment purposes. The indications are gastric and duodenal ulcer, asthma, pain in the loins and the back, etc.

磁珠疗法 [cí zhū liáo fǎ]

magnetic bead therapy: a form of acutherapy in which magnetized steel beads taped to the needle points are used as substitutes for needles and left in place for prolonged stimulation, indicated in treating chronic diseases

指压疗法 [zhǐ yā liáo fǎ]

finger-pressure therapy: a procedure performed by pressing and rubbing a given point with the finger(s) for treatment purposes. The indications are syncope, hysteria, epilepsy, toothache, etc.

指压麻醉 [zhǐ yā má zuì]

finger-pressure anesthesia: a method of inducing anesthesia by pressing definite point(s) with the fingers, usually for extracting teeth

金针拨障法 [jīn zhēn bō zhàng fǎ]

loop couching: a procedure for extracting cataracts using acupuncture technique. A special needle is inserted into the eye through an incision to remove the cataract from the pupil to restore eyesight.

其他疗法与保健

Other Therapies and Health Preservation

推拿按摩 *Tuina* and Medical Massage

按摩 [àn mó]

(1) massage: application of various manipulations to certain points or areas of the patient's body with movement of the patient's limbs in the prevention and treatment of disease, also called 推拿 [tuī ná]; **(2) pressing and rubbing:** two of the eight methods of bone-setting

推拿 [tuī ná]

(1) *tuina*: traditional Chinese medical massage, also called 按摩 [àn mó]; **(2) pushing and kneading:** two of the eight methods of bone-setting

推拿疗法 [tuī ná liáo fǎ]

***tuina* therapy:** treatment of disease by *tuina* [massage]

按摩科 [àn mó kē]

specialty of massage: one of the thirteen medical specialties during the Ming Dynasty (1368-1644)

按摩疗法 [àn mó liáo fǎ]

massotherapy: treatment of disease by massage

按蹻 [àn qiāo]

"limb-pressing": an ancient term for massage

按摩师 [àn mó shī]

masseur; masseuse: one who practices massage

按摩手法 [àn mó shǒu fǎ]

manipulation of massage: treatment on certain points or areas of the patient's body with the hand, elbow or other part of the body in a skillful manner

按法 [àn fǎ]

pressing: a manipulation of massage by pressing the point or affected part with the thumb, palm, or knuckle

按压法 [àn yā fǎ]

sustained pressing: pressing forcefully with sustained pressure by using the forearm or elbow

掐法 [qiā fǎ]

fingernail pressing: a manipulation of massage by pressing at a point on the body with a fingernail to produce a strong stimulation, usually used for treating syncope and convulsion

揉法 [róu fǎ]

kneading: a manipulation of massage applicable to all parts of the body by pressing and moving to and fro or circularly on an acupoint or affected area with the flat of the thumb, the tips of the index, middle and ring fingers, the thenar, or the root of the palm

捻法 [niǎn fǎ]

holding and twisting: a manipulation of massage performed by holding a digital joint or the skin with the thumb and index finger and twisting it as if twisting a thread, used to relieve rigidity of joints and ensure smooth flow of *qi* and blood

刮法 [guā fǎ]

scraping: a manipulation performed by scraping the part between the eyebrows, the nape, or the costal regions with the outer side of the thumb, the edge of a spoon or the rim of a coin downward or outward to cause local congestion

刮痧 [guā shā]

scraping to congestion: a popular treatment for excess-heat by scraping the patient's neck, chest or back to cause local congestion (cf 刮法 [guā fǎ])

拧法 [nǐng fǎ]

pinching and lifting: a manipulation performed by pinching and lifting a portion of the skin with the second segments of the flexed index and middle fingers like a vice to cause local congestion until the skin turns red and purple

点法 [diǎn fǎ]

point pressing: a manipulation by pressing with light, moderate or great force as required on a point with the middle finger while the index and ring fingers are slightly flexed, also called 捣法 [dǎo fǎ], 点击法 [diǎn jī fǎ], 捣击法 [dǎo jī fǎ] and 指针法 [zhǐ zhēn fǎ]

捣法 [dǎo fǎ]

pounding: a synonym for point pressing (点法 [diǎn fǎ])

捣击法 [dǎo jī fǎ]

pounding: a synonym for point pressing (点法 [diǎn fǎ])

点击法 [diǎn jī fǎ]

point-hitting: a synonym for point pressing (点法 [diǎn fǎ])

指针法 [zhǐ zhēn fǎ]

finger puncture: a synonym for point pressing (点法 [diǎn fǎ])

笃击法 [dǔ jī fǎ]

hitting with the knuckle: a manipulation performed by hitting a point on the patient's body with the knuckle of the operator's middle finger, applied chiefly to the head and upper limbs

抠法 [kōu fǎ]

digging: a manipulation performed by digging into a depressed part, such as the armpit, the groin of the cubital fossa with the thumb, middle or index finger with force to pluck a tendon and vessel for the treatment of numbness of the limb

滚法 [gǔn fǎ]

rolling: moving by turning a hollow fist with the thumb bent over the fingers over the skin back and forth continuously with moderate force and small amplitude

挠法 [náo fǎ]

scratching: making the index, middle and ring fingers of one hand hook shaped, pressing the fingertips onto the top of the patient's back and sliding them down to the lower back

挪法 [núo fǎ]

shifting: a manipulation performed by rubbing the body surface slowly but forcibly with the ulnar side of the palm up and down and to and fro, applied chiefly to the abdomen

摸法 [mō fǎ]

palpating: (1) palpating the body surface with the hand or fingers, chiefly for diagnosing; (2) one of the eight manipulations of bone setting, used to examine traumatic injury and adjacent soft tissues

擦法 [cā fǎ]

rubbing: a manipulation performed by rubbing with the flat of the fingers, the thenar or the palms to and fro over the skin continuously, applied to the forehead, limbs or back

捏法 [niē fǎ]

pinching: a manipulation performed by holding, lifting and releasing the tissue with the thumb opposing the radial middle segment of the crooked index finger, often applied to the back muscles along the spine

摩法 [mó fǎ]

circular rubbing: rubbing the affected part with the finger tips or the palm in a circular motion with moderate force and frequency

抹法 [mǒ fǎ]

wiping: a manipulation of massage performed by rubbing the skin with the palmar side of the operator's thumbs or the palms up and down, right and left, with moderate force to promote the flow of *qi* and blood

推法 [tuī fǎ]

pushing: pushing and squeezing the muscles with the fingers, palms, or elbow forward, apart, or spirally with force

一指禅推法 [yī zhǐ chán tuī fǎ]

single-finger meditation pushing: a manipulation of massage performed by pushing the tissue with the tip, the flat, or the outer side of the thumb, on which the operator's *qi* is concentrated by meditation, also called 一指禅功 [yī zhǐ chán gōng]

一指禅功 [yī zhǐ chán gōng]

single-finger meditation manipulation: synonym for single-finger meditation pushing (一指禅推法 [yī zhǐ chán tuī fǎ])

拳击法 [quán jī fǎ]

rapping: a manipulation performed by rapping with the back of the operator's fist, chiefly applied to the patient's back

拿法 [ná fǎ]

grasping: massage maneuver involving lifting and squeezing or lifting and rapidly releasing the affected muscles with three or five fingers of one or both of the operator's hands

抓法 [zhuā fǎ]

grasping with the whole hand: form of grasping by which the center of the palm is placed over the area, and the local tissue is grasped with the whole palm and fingers

拿捏法 [ná niē fǎ]

grasping and pinching: a combined manipulation of massage performed by grasping and pinching used together

捺法 [nà fǎ]

pressing down: a manipulation performed by pressing the body surface with the palm, grasping a piece of muscle, then releasing it and passing on for another grasp

梳法 [shū fǎ]

combing: a manipulation performed by combing the body surface, usually the abdomen, briskly with the fingertips of the two hands alternately

拂法 [fú fǎ]

whisking: a massage manipulation characterized by a quick light brushing movement

掸拂法 [dǎn fú fǎ]

brushing and whisking: a manipulation performed by brushing the patient's spine with the palms, finishing with a whisk

运法 [yùn fǎ]

circular kneading: a manipulation performed by kneading in a circular motion slowly and repeatedly with the thumb, juxtaposed fingers, or the base of the palm to promote circulation of *qi* and blood

扯法 [chě fǎ]

pulling: a manipulation performed by grasping the skin with the thumb and the middle segment of the index finger and giving it a pull before releasing it to cause local congestion, also called 揪法 [jīu fǎ]

揪法 [jīu fǎ]

dragging: a synonym for pulling manipulation (扯法 [chě fǎ])

拍法 [pāi fǎ]

patting: a manipulation to cause relaxation by patting gently with one or both palms, often performed at the beginning and end of massotherapy

托提法 [tuō tí fǎ]

supporting and lifting: a manipulation performed by putting the hands under the patient's armpits and lifting him or her up

挤法 [jǐ fǎ]

squeezing: a manipulation performed by squeezing the skin with the thumb and the index and middle fingers till the skin turns red and purple

搓法 [cuō fǎ]

twisting rubbing: manipulation performed by holding the limb or the chest with both palms and rubbing in opposite directions as if making a cord

撮法 [cuō fǎ]

taking up with fingers: a manipulation performed by grasping the skin with three fingers gently, then releasing it and moving on for another grasp

振法 [zhèn fǎ]

vibrating: a massage manipulation performed by placing a palm on the patient's body to make rapid local vibrations, also called 颤法 [chàn fǎ]

颤法 [chàn fǎ]

vibrating: a synonym for 振法 [zhèn fǎ]

扼法 [è fǎ]

holding tight: a manipulation performed by placing the palms on the body surface and then grasping and holding tight a piece of muscle with force for a moment, or doing the same with the thumbs and the remaining four fingers, chiefly applied to the back

扣[叩]法 [kòu fǎ]

tapping: a manipulation performed by tapping with the tips of the five fingers held together, chiefly applied to the top of the head, also called 啄击法 [zhuó jī fǎ]

啄击法 [zhuó jī fǎ]

pecking: a synonym for tapping manipulation (扣法 [kòu fǎ])

击法 [jī fǎ]

striking: a manipulation performed by striking the affected limb with the palm, fist or a specially made rod

弹击法 [tán jī fǎ]

flicking: a manipulation performed by hitting a point on the patient's body with the back of a fingertip by flicking it against the thumb

弹筋 [tán jīn]

tendon-plucking: a manipulation performed by repeatedly pulling up a tendon or muscle and immediately releasing it

捶法 [chuí fǎ]

stroking: a manipulation performed by stroking the patient's back with the ulnar side of the operator's hollow fist

棒击法 [bàng jī fǎ]

rod beating: beating the patient's head or loins gently with moderate force with a rod made of mulberry twigs bound together and wrapped in tough paper or cloth

扳法 [bān fǎ]

pulling: a massage manipulation performed by pulling, stretching and rotating the joints of the limbs or the waist to relieve rigidity, separate adhesion and help restore dislocated bones

扳腿推拿手法 [bān tuǐ tuī ná shǒu fǎ]

leg pulling: one of the three pulling manipulations of massage for lumbar hyperextension

拨法 [bō fǎ]

poking: a massage manipulation performed by poking or plucking a certain tendon with the fingers forcibly for movement and separation

摇法 [yáo fǎ]

rotating: a manipulation performed by turning the patient's head and neck, or shoulder, wrist, hip joint, knee joint or ankle to and fro to relieve rigidity

伸法 [shēn fǎ]

stretching: a massage manipulation performed by extending the disordered joints of the neck and limbs, including 引身法 [yǐn shēn fǎ] and 提伸法 [tí shēn fǎ]

引身法 [yǐn shēn fǎ]

pulling and stretching: one of the stretching manipulations combined with pulling

提伸法 [tí shēn fǎ]

lifting and stretching: one of the stretching manipulations combined with lifting

屈法 [qū fǎ]

flexing: a manipulation performed by bending the neck, loins, elbow, wrist, ankle, fingers or toes for relieving rigidity

拨络法 [bō luò fǎ]

collateral-poking: a manipulation performed by poking a certain collateral meridian involved and the affected musculature with the operator's fingers

踩法 [cǎi fǎ]

treading: a method of treating the affected lumbar or other areas by stepping on it with one foot or both feet , also called 跷法 [qiāo fǎ]

跷法 [qiāo fǎ]

stamping: a synonym for treading method (踩法 [cǎi fǎ])

踏跳法 [tà tiào fǎ]

rhythmic stepping method: a therapeutic technique performed by stepping on the patient's body rhythmically along the meridians, on acupoints, or on the affected part

拉腿手法 [lā tuǐ shǒu fǎ]

leg-pulling technique: a *tuina* manipulation for treating lumbago by pulling the leg

扭痧 [niǔ shā]

twisting to congestion: a manipulation by grasping, pulling and turning the skin with force to cause local congestion for the treatment of sunstroke and other related ailments, also called 扯痧 [chě shā] or 揪痧 [jiū shā]

扯痧 [chě shā]

pulling to congestion: a synonym for 扭痧 [niǔ shā]

揪痧 [jiū shā]

dragging to congestion: a synonym for 扭痧 [niǔ shā]

推扳手法 [tuī bān shǒu fǎ]

pushing-pulling: a type of manipulation in massotherapy performed by pressing tightly on the muscles with the fingers and pushing forward or pulling backward the muscle fibers in order to relax muscular spasm

三板推拿疗法 [sān bǎn tuī ná liáo fǎ]

tri-tabular *tuina*-therapy [massotherapy]: a type of massotherapy performed by using three kinds of boards, i.e., finger pushing board, leg board, and oblique board, for treating disorders of the spine and lower limbs

小儿推拿疗法 [xiǎo ér tuī ná liáo fǎ]

infantile *tuina*-therapy [massotherapy]: a kind of massage performed on a certain part of a baby's body to treat disease or induce passive movement of the limbs

捏脊 [niē jǐ]

pinching along the spine: a method for treating digestive disorders and malnutrition of children by pinching and kneading the skin and muscles along the spine, also called 捏积 [niē jī]

捏积 [niē jī]

synonym for pinching along the spine (捏脊 [niē jǐ])

自我按摩 [zì wǒ àn mō]

automassage: massage by oneself

栉头 [zhì tóu]

combing the head: an automassage manipulation performed by rubbing the head with the fingertips from the anterior to the posterior hairline to promote the flow of *qi* and blood

击头 [jī tóu]

tapping the head: an automassage manipulation performed by tapping the head with the tips of slightly bent fingers, for refreshment and improved flow of *qi* and blood

抹前额 [mǒ qián é]

wiping the forehead: an automassage manipulation performed by wiping the forehead with the flat of the index, middle and ring fingers of the right and left hands alternately till it feels hot, or with the thumbs pressing the temples and the remaining four fingers slightly bent, rubbing the forehead from the middle to the frontal eminences with the radial side of the index fingers repeatedly, for refreshment and sedation

存泥丸 [cún ní wán]

rubbing the forehead to the top: an automassage manipulation performed by rubbing the head from the forehead to the top with the right and left palms alternately, for refreshment

拧眉心 [nǐng méi xīn]

pinching the part between the eyebrows: an automassage manipulation performed by pinching the central part between the eyebrows with the tip of the thumb and index finger till red and purple spots appear, for treating headache, hypertension and insomnia

按太阳 [àn tài yáng]

pressing the temples: an automassage manipulation performed by pressing the temples with the tips of the thumbs or the middle fingers, for relieving headache, common cold and facial paralysis

摩面 [mó miàn]

rubbing the face: an automassage manipulation performed by rubbing the face with the palms till the whole face grows warm for promoting the local blood circulation

熨目 [yùn mù]

pressing the eyes with the hot palms: an automassage manipulation for improving eyesight, repeatedly performed for about 30 minutes by rubbing the palms till hot and then pressing them on the eyes

揉攒竹 [róu cuán zhú]

kneading *cuanzhu* (BL2): an automassage manipulation for relieving strain on the eye muscles, performed by pressing at the inner end of the eyebrows with the tip of the thumbs till local soreness and distension are felt

揉四白 [róu sì bái]

kneading sibai (ST2): an automassage manipulation to improve vision and prevent near-sightedness by kneading the points below the eyes with the tip of the middle fingers till local soreness and distension are felt

按目四眦 [àn mù sì zì]

pressing the four canthi: an automassage manipulation for improving the vision and prevent near-sightedness by pressing and rubbing the inner and outer canthus of the eyes with the knuckles of the bent thumbs over the fists till local soreness and distension are felt

刮眼眶 [guā yǎn kuàng]

scraping the orbital rims: antomassage manipulation for improving the vision and prevent near-sightedness by scraping with the radial side of the index fingers or the knuckles of the thumbs from the inner to the outer canthus along the upper and lower rims of the orbit alternately

旋耳 [xuán ěr]

revolving the ears: an automassage manipulation for improving acuity of hearing by pulling and twisting the ears with the fingers

按压耳穴 [àn yā ěr xué]

pressing the auricular points: antomassage manipulation for treating diseases by pressing certain points on the ear as a form of auriculo-acupuncture

按捺耳窍 [àn nà ěr qiào]

pressing the ear orifice: an automassage manipulation for improving the hearing by pressing the ears with the palms or stopping the opening of the external auditory canals with the tips of middle fingers on and off

按捏鼻梁 [àn niē bí liáng]

pressing and pinching the nose bridge: antomassage manipulation to prevent common cold by pressing and pinching the bridge of the nose

按迎香 [àn yíng xiāng]

pressing *yingxiang* (LI20): an automassage manipulation for treating common colds or rhinitis by pressing *yingxiang* (LI20) (the point beside the wing of nose) with the tip of the middle fingers till soreness and distension are felt

揉颊车 [róu jiá chē]

kneading *jiache* (ST6): an automassage manipulation for relieving toothache by kneading *jiache* (ST6), one finger breadth anterior and superior to the mandibular angle, with the tip of the middle fingers till soreness and distension are felt

叩[扣]齿 [kòu chǐ]

tapping the teeth: an automassage manipulation performed by tapping the upper and lower teeth on each other

搅舌 [jiǎo shé]

stirring the tongue: an automassage manipulation performed by moving the tongue right and left and up and down to massage the teeth and promote salivation

鸣天鼓 [míng tiān gǔ]

"sounding the celestial drum": an automassage manipulation performed by pressing the ears with the palms and beating the occiput with the fingers

摩颈项 [mó jǐng xiàng]

rubbing the neck: an automassage manipulation to prevent and treat stiff neck, performed by rubbing the neck with the right and left palm alternately till a hot sensation is experienced

按揉颈项 [àn róu jǐng xiàng]

pressing and kneading the neck and nape: an automassage manipulation performed by pressing and kneading the large muscles on the back of neck till local soreness and distension are experienced

拿颈项 [ná jǐng xiàng]

grasping the neck and nape: an automassage manipulation performed by grasping and rubbing the tendons of the large muscles on both sides of the neck with the thumbs and index and middle fingers downward with increasing force to cause soreness and pain

按揉风池 [àn róu fēng chí]

pressing and kneading *fengchi* (GB20): an automassage manipulation performed by pressing and kneading with the thumbs while the palms are placed over the ears till local soreness, distension and pain are experienced, for treating common cold, headache, stiff neck and hypertension

摩击上肢 [mó jī shàng zhī]

rubbing and stroking the upper arm: an automassage manipulation performed by rubbing and stroking the upper arm with the hands (left hand for the right arm and vice versa) to promote circulation of *qi* and blood for treating numbness and soreness

拿合谷 [ná hé gǔ]

grasping *hegu* (LI4): an automassage manipulation performed by grasping the region between the first and second metacarpal bones with the thumb and index finger of the other hand to cause local soreness and pain for relieving pain and curing headache, toothache, lockjaw and wry mouth

洗手 [xǐ shǒu]

wringing the hands: an automassage manipulation performed by rubbing and wringing the hands all over till they grow warm to promote circulation of *qi* and blood, and treat stiffness, numbness and frostbite of the hands

摩腹 [mó fù]

rubbing the abdomen: an automassage manipulation to promote digestion, performed by rubbing the abdomen with the hands in a clockwise motion

摩脐 [mó qí]

rubbing the navel: an automassage manipulation performed by rubbing the navel with the thenar eminence or the base of the palm slowly but forcibly till one feels comfortable, used for the treatment of gastralgia, belching, and abdominal distension and pain

捶腰背 [chuí yāo bèi]

striking the lower back: an automassage manipulation performed by striking the lower back with the back of the fists or with a wooden rod to relieve lower back pain

揉腰眼 [róu yāo yǎn]

kneading the sides of the small of the back: an automassage manipulation performed by kneading the sides of the small of the back with the knuckles of the bent thumbs to strengthen the kidney, and relieve lumbar aching and menstrual disorders

击下肢 [jī xià zhī]

striking the lower limb: an automassage manipulation performed by striking the lower limb with the root of the palms to promote the flow of *qi* and blood

按摩足三里 [àn mó zú sān lǐ]

massaging *zusanli* (ST36): an automassage manipulation performed by pressing and rubbing *zusanli* (ST36) with the tips of the thumbs while sitting till soreness and distension are felt, used for reinforcing *qi* and blood, and treating abdominal pain, indigestion, diarrhea, constipation, fatigue and insomnia

擦涌泉 [cā yǒng quán]

rubbing *yongquan* (KI1): an automassage manipulation performed by holding the left foot on the right leg with the left hand while sitting, and rubbing the center of its sole with the thenar of the right palm till the point grows warm and vice versa, for treatment of dizziness, blurring of vision, insomnia and hypertension

复合手法 [fù hé shǒu fǎ]

compound manipulation: combination of two or more manipulations used simultaneously, such as grasping-pinching and kneading-vibrating

一指禅推拿 [yī zhǐ chán tuī ná]

single-finger meditation massage: massotherapy with a single finger on which the operator's *qi* is concentrated by meditation

滚法推拿 [gǔn fǎ tuī ná]

rolling *tuina* [massage]: massotherapy with rolling as the chief manipulation, combined with kneading, pressing, grasping, holding and twisting, and twisting rubbing

内功推拿 [nèi gōng tuī ná]

internal exercise *tuina* [massage]: massotherapy chiefly based on palm pushing, with vigorous but soft manipulations

指压推拿 [zhǐ yā tuī ná]

finger-pressing *tuina* [massage]: massotherapy with digital point pressing as the chief manipulation

点穴疗法 [diǎn xué liáo fǎ]

digital point pressure therapy: therapy chiefly consisting in stimulating the points by various manipulations such as fingernail pressing, tapping, rapping, etc.

耳穴推拿疗法 [ěr xué tuī ná liáo fǎ]

ear-point *tuina* therapy [massotherapy]: branch of massotherapy performed by pressing and rubbing a vaccaria seed fixed to a tender point on the helix with a piece of adhesive plaster

保健球按摩 [bǎo jiàn qiú àn mó]

health-ball massage: type of massage performed by holding two walnuts or stone balls or steel balls about the same size in the hand and massaging them all the time with the fingers, a massotherapy not only beneficial to the hands, but also to one's general health, especially for the aged

药摩 [yào mó]

medicinal massage: massage performed with medicine as the medium chiefly in the form of balm or ointment, so also called ointment massage (膏摩 [gāo mó]) in ancient times, with hundreds of formulas prescribed for this purpose

膏摩 [gāo mó]

ointment massage: massage performed with ointment as the medium

推拿中的补泻手法 [tuī ná zhōng dè bǔ xiè shǒu fǎ]

reinforcement and reduction manipulations in *tuina* therapy [massotherapy]: reinforcing or reducing effect of the manipulations achieved in massotherapy, depending chiefly on the force, speed and direction

轻重徐疾补泻法 [qīng zhòng xú jí bǔ xiè fǎ]

reinforcement-reduction by varying the force and speed: Gentle and slow massage gives reinforcement, while quick and forcible massage causes reduction.

迎随顺逆补泻法 [yíng suí shùn nì bǔ xiè fǎ]

reinforcement-reduction by massaging along or against the meridian: Massaging in the same direction of the course of the meridian is reinforcement, while massaging in the direction opposed to that of the meridian is reduction.

择向补泻法 [zé xiàng bǔ xiè fǎ]

reinforcement-reduction by choosing direction: In general, afferent, upward, inward, or clockwise manipulation is regarded as reinforcement while efferent, downward, outward and counterclockwise manipulation is regarded as reduction; and for men, turning from the right to the left is reinforcement and from the left to the right is reduction, while for women, just the contrary.

徒手整复 [tú shǒu zhěng fù]

manual reduction: bare-handed restoration of the normal position of a body part

气功 *Qigong*

气功 [qì gōng]

***qigong*:** a system of exercise performed by taking a proper posture, adjusting the breathing and concentrating the mind to unite the essence, *qi* and mind as a whole for physical training, health preservation and prevention and treatment of diseases

导引 [dǎo yǐn]

***daoyin*; conducting (exercise):** an ancient Chinese physical exercise associated with respiratory movement and self-massage performed by conducting the mind and *qi*, used for health preservation and disease prevention and treatment

静功 [jìng gōng]

static *qigong*: *qigong* exercise without movement of the body and limbs, also called 内功 [nèi gōng]

内功 [nèi gōng]

internal exercise: a synonym for static *qigong* (静功 [jìng gōng])

动功 [dòng gōng]

dynamic *qigong*: *qigong* exercise with movement of the body and limbs, also called external exercise (外功 [wài gōng])

外功 [wài gōng]

external exercise: a synonym for dynamic *qigong* (动功 [dòng gōng])

硬气功 [yèng qì gōng]

hard *qigong*: *qigong* training for the hardening of muscles and joints and mobilizing the forces of the body for a concentrated blow, also called martial-art *qigong* (武术气功 [wǔ shù qì gōng])

武术气功 [wǔ shù qì gōng]

martial-art *qigong*: *qigong* as a kind of martial art, cultivated for self-defense, or as a form of physical training, also called hard *qigong* (硬

气功 [yèng qì gōng])

软气功 [ruǎn qì gōng]

soft *qigong*: *qigong* exercise for the training of enduring forces through posturization, breathing and mental concentration for preservation of health and prevention and treatment of diseases

医用气功 [yī yòng qì gōng]

medical *qigong*: *qigong* exercise performed for therapeutic purposes, especially for the treatment of functional and chronic diseases

气功疗法 [qì gōng liáo fǎ]

***qigong* therapy**: therapeutic treatment by practicing *qigong*

儒家气功 [rú jiā qì gōng]

Confucian *qigong*: that developed by the Confucian school, focused on the cultivation of quietude in mind and body and their coordination

道家气功 [dào jiā qì gōng]

Taoist *qigong*: that initiated and developed by Taoist priests, based on the principles of self-physiological alchemy and the microcosm of the universe with the goal of searching for the elixir of life and the fountain of perpetual youth

佛家气功 [fó jiā qì gōng]

Buddhist *qigong*: that developed by Buddhists based on the wisdom of liberation from reincarnation and self-observation to search for the perfection of purity of mind, and ultimately the union of the individual with the universe

动静相兼功 [dòng jìng xiāng jiān gōng]

static-dynamic combined *qigong*: a type of *qigong* characterized by combining static *qigong* with dynamic exercise

动中有静 [dòng zhōng yǒu jìng]

quiescence in motion: in a dynamic *qigong* exercise, keeping the mind quiet and highly concentrated

静中有动 [jìng zhōng yǒu dòng]

motion in quiescence: in a static *qigong* exercise, making the movements smoothly

内景 [nèi jǐng]

inner scene: image of the activities of the *zang-fu* organs, *qi* and blood formed in the mind

松 [sōng]

relaxation: a principle of *qigong* exercise, referring to relaxation of both the body and the mind

入静 [rù jìng]

entering quiescence; falling into static state: a restful state of the mind attained, with directional exercise of mental activity during the awakened state, in which the brain is aware of changes in physiological functions inside the body and maximally eliminates interference from both inside and outside

内视 [nèi shì]

inward vision: seeing inward at a certain part of the body to induce corresponding changes by means of the mind

调身 [tiáo shēn]; 身法 [shēn fǎ]

posture management: making the body suitable and convenient for *qigong* exercise to guarantee a smooth flow of internal *qi*, also called posturization (姿式 [zī shì])

姿式 [zī shì]

posturization: a synonym for management of posture (调身 [tiáo shēn])

调身要领 [tiáo shēn yào lǐng]

essentials of posture management: fundamental elements of adjusting the posture, viz loosening the clothing, keeping the head upright, drawing in the chest, straightening the back, drooping the shoulders, relaxing the waist and abdomen, contracting the buttocks, etc.

宽解衣带 [kuān jiě yī dài]

loosening the clothing: prerequisite for posture management

头如顶物 [tóu rú dǐng wù]

keeping the head upright as if carrying something on the top: one of the fundamental elements of posture management

头正 [zhèng tóu]

head upright: keeping the head upright as if the head were hung up at the vertex

颈松 [jìng sōng]

neck relaxed: keeping the neck relaxed so that the cervical vertebrae can be well spread out

沉肩 [chén jiān]

drooping shoulders: keeping the shoulders relaxed to prevent shrugging which causes muscular tension

坠肘 [zhuì zhǒu]

dropping elbows: having the elbows hanging down naturally when the shoulders are drooping, also called 垂肘 [chuí zhǒu]

垂肘 [chuí zhǒu]

down-hanging elbows, same as dropping elbows (坠肘 [zhuì zhǒu])

伸腰沉胯 [shēn yāo chén kuà]

stretching the waist and keeping the hips sunken: one of the fundamental elements of posture management

含胸拔背 [hán xiōng bá bèi]

drawing in the chest and straightening the back: one of the fundamental elements of posture management

舒腰松腹 [shū yāo sōng fù]

keeping the waist and abdomen relaxed: one of the fundamental elements of posture management

收臀松膝 [shōu tún sōng xī]

contracting the buttocks and relaxing the knees: one of the fundamental elements of posture management

五趾抓地 [wǔ zhǐ zhuā dì]

clutching the ground with the toes:. standing firmly

两目垂帘内视 [liǎng mù chuí lián nèi shì]

curtain-falling and inward vision: drooping the eyelids to create inward vision

塞兑反听 [sè duì fǎn tīng]

closing the mouth and stopping the ears

舌抵上腭 [shé dǐ shàng è]

sticking the tongue against the palate: licking the palate with the tongue just behind the upper gums in order to communicate with the conception and governor vessels, also called 舌柱上腭 [shé zhù shàng è], 柱舌 [zhù shé] or 搭鹊桥 [dā què qiáo]

舌柱上腭 [shé zhù shàng è]

tongue propping the palate, same as sticking the tongue against the palate (舌抵上腭 [shé dǐ shàng è])

柱舌 [zhù shé]

tongue propping: an abbreviation of tongue propping the palate (舌柱上腭 [shé zhù shàng è])

搭鹊桥 [dā què qiáo]

building the magpie bridge: another expression for sticking the tongue against the palate (舌抵上腭 [shé dǐ shàng è])

鹊桥 [què qiáo]

magpie bridge: specific name referring to two body portions in *qigong* exercise – the upper one is situated at the part between glabella and the nostrils, and the lower one between the coccyx and the anus

胎食 [tāi shí]

fetal feeding; saliva-swallowing: swallowing of refluxed saliva in *qigong* exercise

坐式 [zuò shì]

sitting posture: a variety of basic postures for *qigong* exercises, including plain sitting, leaning sitting and cross-legged sitting

平坐 [píng zuò]

plain sitting: sitting on a bench or in a chair with the shoulders relaxed, the palms resting on the thighs, and the feet on thr ground and set apart about the width of the shoulders

靠坐 [kào zuò]

leaning sitting: sitting on a bed with the back leaning against a cushion to make an angle of 120-140 degrees between the trunk and the thighs

盘坐 [pán zuò]

cross-legged sitting: sitting on a large bench, or a cushion spread on the ground with legs crossed and the hands grasped before the abdomen

单盘坐 [dān pán zuò]

single cross-legged sitting: sitting with one leg folded under the other, and the hands crossed on each other on or before the lower abdomen

双盘坐 [shuāng pán zuò]

double cross-legged sitting: sitting with the two feet folded to face each other on the medial aspects of the thighs with both soles facing upwards, and the hands placed before the lower abdomen

卧式 [wò shì]

lying posture: a variety of basic postures for *qigong* exercises, including supine, recumbent and reclining postures

仰卧式 [yǎng wò shì]

supine posture: lying on the back, with the legs stretched naturally and the hands stretched along the sides or grasped over the abdomen

侧卧式 [cè wò shì]

lateral recumbent posture: lying on one side, with the body slightly bent like a bow, the upper hand placed on the hip and the lower hand on the pillow, with fingers spread naturally

三接式 [sān jiē shì]

three-contact posture: lying on one side with the upper leg flexed and its sole placed on the knee of the other leg and the lower arm flexed with the palm placed on the elbow of the upper arm

半卧式 [bàn wò shì]

reclining posture: reclining on a couch or a bed with the upper part of the body and the head raised with pillows or cushions

站式 [zhàn shì]

standing posture: a variety of basic postures in *qigong* exercises, including natural stance, horseman's stance, ball-holding and downward-pressing postures

自然站式 [zì rán shì]

natural standing posture: standing naturally with the feet set apart about the width of the shoulders and the hands hanging naturally at the sides

骑马式 [qí mǎ shì]

horseman's stance: half squatting on two legs set aside and the heels turned outward, with the fists placed in front of the abdomen or at the sides

三圆式 [sān yuán shì]

three-circle posture: standing on the legs with the feet set apart about the width of the shoulders and the toes turned inward to form a circle with the knee slightly bent and the arms raised before the chest in a circle as if embracing a trunk and the fingers spread as if holding a basketball, also called ball-holding posture (抱球式 [bào qiú shì])

抱球式 [bào qiú shī]

ball-holding posture: another name for three-circle posture (三圆式 [sān yuán shì])

下按式 [xià àn shì]

downward-pressing posture: standing in the three-circle posture but with the arms hanging naturally at the sides, with the palms facing downward and the fingers pointing to the front, as if pressing a floating ball into water

走式 [zǒu shì]

walking posture: a variety of basic postures for *qigong* exercises, including *taiji* walking, eight-diagram walking, etc.

矮步 [ǎi bù]

half-squatting walking: walking with the upper part of the body and the head kept upright and eyes looking forward, smiling and performing various exercises at the same time

弓步 [gōng bù]

bow step: a step in which one leg is kept straight and the other bent with the body weight centered on the bent leg

太极步 [tài jí bù]

taiji walking: walking with the legs slightly bent and hands pressed to the sides or placed upon one another before the abdomen and the weight of the body shifting from side to side alternately

八卦步 [bā guà bù]

eight-diagram walking: walking with the toes of the feet turned slightly inward and clutching at the ground with the toes when stepping forward with the heels slightly elevated, the knees slightly bent, and the eyes looking forward smiling

上丹田 [shàng dān tián]

upper *dantian*; upper elixir field: the area between the eyebrows about 3 *cun* deeper than the point *yintang* (EX-HN3), which is the seat of mentality, also called mud ball (泥丸 [ní wán])

泥丸 [ní wán]

mud ball: another name for upper *dantian* (上丹田 [shàng dān tián])

中丹田 [zhōng dān tián]

middle *dantian*; middle elixir field: the area between the nipples in the chest about 3 *cun* deeper than the point *danzhong* (CV17) which is the seat of *qi* and a place where *qi* is trained and emitted to the outside of the body

下丹田 [xià dān tián]

lower *dantian*; lower elixir field: the area about 3 *cun* below the umbilicus with point *qihai* (CV6) as its center, where essence is transformed into *qi* and *qi* is trained and emitted to the outside of the body

丹田 [dān tián]

***dantian*; elixir field:** the place where *qi* is stored and the mind is focused in *qigong* exercises, compared by the Taoists in ancient China to the furnace in alchemy where elixir is tempered, hence the name

调息 [tiáo xī]

management of breath: training in breathing to bring the functions of *qi* into full play, also called 调气 [tiáo qì] and known as 吐纳 [tǔ nà] in ancient times

调气 [tiáo qì]

management of *qi*, same as management of breath (调息 [tiáo xī])

吐纳 [tǔ nà]

breathing in and out: a synonym for management of *qi* (调息 [tiáo xī])

自然呼吸 [zì rán hū xī]

natural breathing: breathing with no special attention paid to the breath at all, including thoracic breathing, abdominal breathing and mixed breathing

顺腹式呼吸 [shùn fù shì hū xī]

orthodromic abdominal breathing: that marked by dilating the abdomen while inhaling and contracting it while exhaling

逆腹式呼吸 [nì fù shì hū xī]

antidromic abdominal breathing: that marked by contracting the abdomen while inhaling and dilating it while exhaling

潜呼吸 [qiǎn hū xī]

latent breathing: abdominal breathing performed almost unnoticed, with a gentle rising and falling of the lower abdomen

脐呼吸 [qí hū xī]

navel breathing: finest abdominal breathing, with the abdomen remaining almost motionless, while the performer imagines that he is breathing through the umbilicus just as the fetus does in the womb, and hence also called fetal breathing (胎息 [tāi xī])

胎息 [tāi xī]

fetal breathing, synonymous with navel breathing (脐呼吸 [qí hū xī])

鼻吸鼻呼 [bí hū bí xī]

nasal breathing: inhaling and exhaling through the nose, a form of breathing usually adopted when static *qigong* is practiced

吐字呼吸 [tǔ zì hū xī]

word-articulating breathing: a form of breathing with articulation of some particular words while exhaling

提肛呼吸 [tí gāng hū xī]

anus-lifting breathing: a form of breathing with the anus contracted while inhaling, and relaxed while exhaling, used in the treatment of visceral prolapse and hemorrhoids

数吸 [shǔ xī]

breath counting: a means of combining mental concentration with breathing by counting the number of respirations

听息 [tīng xī]

breath listening: a means of combining mental concentration with breathing by listening to one's own respiration

意呼吸 [yì hū xī]

imaginary breathing: breathing coupled with certain thoughts and ideas that exchange of *qi* can be performed through the skin or pores to communicate with the universe

停息 [tíng xī]

breathing with pause: a form of respiration in which the breath is temporarily held at the end of inhalation or exhalation

随息 [suí xī]

following one's own breathing: a process in *qigong* exercises involving mentally following and feeling one's own breathing for the concentration of the mind

调心 [tiáo xīn]

management of the mind: a method of attaining mental concentration and guarding against distraction in *qigong* exercises, also called training of mind 练神 [liàn shén], preservation of mind 存神 [cún shén], and preservation of breath 存息 [cún xī] in ancient times

练神 [liàn shén]

training of the mind, same as management of the mind (调心 [tiáo xīn])

存神 [cún shén]

preservation of the mind, same as management of the mind (调心 [tiáo xīn])

存息 [cún xī]

preservation of the breath, same as management of the mind (调心

[tiáo xīn])

坐忘 [zuò wàng]

sitting forgetful: one of the Confucian techniques of self-cultivation, marked by sitting while forgetting the existence of the body, mind, and all subjects and objects

精、气、神 [jīng、qì、shén]

essence, *qi*, and mind: cultivation and training of the three as the basis and purpose of *qigong* exercises

炼丹 [liàn dān]

(1) alchemy: an ancient quasi-chemical art through which practitioners sought a formula to cure any disease and confer eternal youth; **(2) physiological alchemy:** a traditional Taoist static *qigong* exercise for training essence, *qi* and mentality, also known as inner elixir exercise (内丹功 [nèi dān gōng])

内丹 [nèi dān]

inner elixir: imaginary substance in the body, which was believed to make one live forever

内丹功 [nèi dān gōng]

inner elixir exercise: kind of static exercise in *qigong* for producing inner elixir, i.e., self-physiological cultivation

内丹术 [nèi dān shù]

inner elixir art, same as inner elixir exercise (内丹功 [nèi dān gōng])

炼己 [liàn jǐ]

training oneself: concentrating one's mind to get rid of mental distraction while doing *qigong* exercises

炼精 [liàn jīng]

training of essence: *qigong* exercise to reinforce the inborn essence

炼气 [liàn qì]

training of *qi*: strengthening vitality through breathing training

炼神 [liàn shén]

training of the mind: training the mental faculties through *qigong* exercises

炼精化气 [liàn jīng huà qì]

training essence into *qi*: *qigong* exercises for transforming essence into energy by conducting *qi* through the small complete cycle of circulation

炼气化神 [liàn qì huà shén]

training *qi* into mentality: *qigong* exercises for transforming energy into mental faculties by conducting *qi* through large complete cycle of circulation

练功 [liàn gōng]

practicing *qigong*: doing *qigong* exercises with appropriate posture, breathing and mental concentration

意守 [yì shǒu]

concentration of the mind: focusing one's concentration on one specific subject

排除杂念 [pái chú zá niàn]

getting rid of mental distractions: concentrating one's mind on one single subject to replace all other thoughts and ideas

意守自身 [yì shǒu zì shēn]

concentration on oneself: concentration of the mind on a certain part of the body, or a particular organ, meridian or point

意守丹田 [yì shǒu dān tián]

concentration on *dantian*: concentration of the mind on *dantian,* or the elixir field where *qi* is stored

意守体外 [yì shǒu tǐ wài]

concentration on something outside the body: concentration of the mind on an object, sign, sound or some past experience recalled

面壁 [miàn bì]

facing a wall: standing motionless as if facing a wall in order to get rid of all external disturbances and internal worries, also called looking at a wall (壁观 [bì guān])

壁观 [bì guān]

looking at a wall, same as facing a wall (面壁 [miàn bì])

存想 [cún xiǎng]

imaginary concentration: concentration on an imaginary object to get rid of distractions and induce a desired feeling

内气 [nèi qì]

inner *qi*: *qi* within the body that circulates through the meridians and induces *qi* sensation in the process of *qigong* exercise, also called 真气 [zhēn qì]

真气 [zhēn qì]

genuine *qi*, dynamic force of life activities of the human body, same as inner *qi* (内气 [nèi qì])

外气 [wài qì]

out-going *qi*: the *qi* that is emitted outside of a *qigong* master's body into a certain part of the patient for therapeutic purposes

周天 [zhōu tiān]

heavenly circuit; cosmic cycle: the complete cycle of *qi* circulation within the body

小周天 [xiǎo zhōu tiān]

small heavenly circuit; microcosmic cycle: a part of the complete cycle of *qi* circulation in the body, referring to the circulation through the conception and governor vessels

大周天 [dà zhōu tiān]

large heavenly circuit; macrocosmic cycle: the major part of the complete cycle of *qi* circulation, referring to the circulation through the regular and extra meridians (except conception and governor vessels)

离体周天 [lí tǐ zhōu tiān]

extracorporeal heavenly circuit; extracorporeal cosmic cycle: the part of the *qi* circulation cycle outside the body, either going out of the body through the coccyx and coming back into the body through *baihui* (GV20) or going out through the feet and coming back through the head

禅定 [chán dìng]

meditating fixation: one of the representative exercises of Buddhist *qigong* marked by meditation and fixation or stoppage of thinking

放松功 [fàng sōng gōng]

relaxation exercise: basic exercise in static *qigong* for rehabilitation by lessening tension of both the mind and body

内养功 [neì yǎng gōng]

inner nourishing exercise: a type of *qigong* characterized by combining silent reading of words or phrases with breathing training, taking a lying or sitting posture and abdominal breathing, for invigorating the functional activities of the digestive and respiratory systems

强壮功 [qiáng zhuàng gōng]

roborant exercise: type of *qigong* exercise by means of breathing and mind concentration on *dantian* to reinforce intrinsic *qi* and build up health

头面功 [tóu miàn gōng]

head-face exercise: exercise including bathing the face, combing the hair, kneading the temples and *fenchi* (GB20), and tapping the back of the head to regulate the meridians of the head and face, promote circulation of *qi* and blood, invigorate the brain and refresh the mind

眼功 [yǎn gōng]

eye exercise: exercise by focusing on the movements of the eye to regulate the flow of *qi* and blood through the liver meridian and improve acuity of vision

鼻齿功 [bí chǐ gōng]

nose-teeth exercise: exercise for clearing the nasal passage and consolidating the teeth

耳功 [ěr gōng]

ear exercise: exercise including pressing and "bathing" the ears and rubbing the helix to improve hearing

颈项功 [jìng xiàng gōng]

neck exercise: exercise for preventing and curing neck troubles

肩臂功 [jiān bì gōng]

shoulder-arm exercise: exercise for promoting circulation of *qi* and blood along the three yang and the three yin meridians of the hand

胸胁功 [xiōng xié gōng]

chest-hypochondrium exercise: exercise for preventing and treating diseases in the chest and hypochondriac regions

腹部功 [fù bù gōng]

abdomen exercise: a common *qigong* exercise of rubbing the abdomen and *dantian*, used to prevent and treat digestive disorders

腰部功 [yāo bù gōng]

waist exercise: exercise characterized by rubbing the waist to strengthen the lumbar muscles and replenish the kidney

下肢功 [xià zhī gōng]

lower limb exercise: exercise consisting of kneading the kneecaps and rubbing *yongquan* (KI1) to activate the flow of *qi* and blood, and to relax and strengthen the muscles and tendons of the lower limbs

理心功 [lǐ xīn gōng]

heart-regulation exercise: exercise for regulating *qi* and blood of the heart meridian and preventing and treating heart troubles

理脾功 [lǐ pí gōng]

spleen-regulation exercise: exercise for regulating *qi* and blood of the spleen meridian and promoting digestion

理肺功 [lǐ fèi gōng]

lung-regulation exercise: exercise for regulating *qi* and blood of the lung meridian

周天功 [zhōu tiān gōng]

heavenly circuit exercise: a type of *qigong* exercise in which *qi* is activated to travel in the small and large heavenly circuits for strengthening the mind and body, preserving health and prolonging life

小周天功 [xiǎo zhōu tiān gōng]

small heavenly circuit exercise: a type of *qigong* in which *qi* is activated to travel in the small heavenly circuit, i.e., through the conception and governor vessels

大周天功 [dà zhōu tiān gōng]

large heavenly circuit exercise: type of *qigong* in which *qi* is activated to travel in the large heavenly circuit, i.e., through the regular and extra meridians (except the conception and governor vessels)

周天自转功 [zhōu tiān zì zhuàn gōng]

automatic *qi* circulation exercise: exercise to conduct circulation of *qi*, with the navel as the center, by mental activities and breathing in coordination together with saying words silently

疏肝明目功 [shū gān míng mù gōng]

liver-soothing and vision-improving exercise: exercise which has the function of improving the eyesight, relaxing the neck and back muscles, and relieving muscular strain of the eye and promoting recovery from fatigue

铁裆功 [tiě dāng gōng]

iron-crotch exercise: an important exercise for increasing the physical strength and nimbleness of the lower part of the body in ancient times, now chiefly used for preserving health and reinforcing sexual competence of the male

虎步功 [hǔ bù gōng]

tiger-striding exercise: a kind of *qigong* exercise for training the waist and legs externally and the liver and kidney internally

叫化功 [jiào huā gōng]

beggar's exercise: a kind of *qigong* exercise for the poor people to ward off hunger and cold in ancient times and now to increase the resistance of the stomach and intestines to cold

五禽戏 [wǔ qín gōng]

five fauna-mimic frolics: movements in imitation of the movements of five types of wildlife — tiger, bear, monkey, deer, and bird, believed to have been initiated by Hua Tou (华佗 [huà tuó])

八段锦 [bā duàn jǐn]

eight-section brocade: a system of physical exercises in eight forms, widely practiced by people of all ages in ancient and modern times

站桩功 [zhàn zhuāng gōng]

stake-standing exercise: a category of *qigong* exercises characterized by taking a standing posture

自然站桩功 [zì rán zhàn zhuāng gōng]

natural stake-standing: type of standing exercise in which one stands upright with the knees slightly bent, the eyes looking straight ahead, and places both hands in front of the lower abdomen

三圆站桩功 [sān yuán zhàn zhuāng gōng]

tri-round stake-standing: a type of standing exercise in which one stands naturally, moves the hands up over the shoulders with the elbows and the palms facing each other as if holding a ball or up to the level of the chest with the elbows bent and palms facing the body as if embracing the trunk of a big tree

下按式站桩功 [xià àn shì zhàn zhuāng gōng]

hand-pressing stake-standing: a type of standing exercise in which one takes the natural stake-standing position with the knees bent, raises the hands to the level of the waist with the hands facing the ground, the fingers spread and pointing ahead, and the forearms kept horizontal as if pressing something downward

七星功 [qī xīng gōng]

seven-star exercise: simple, graceful and useful exercise with seven postures, beneficial to all parts of the body

易筋功 [yì jīn gōng]

sinew-transforming exercise: a dynamic exercise for training *qi* derived from the *Sinew Transforming Classic* credited to Dharma in the sixth century

九九阳功 [jiǔ jiǔ yáng gōng]

double-nine yang exercise: a dynamic exercise for training *qi*

运气 [yùn qì]

moving of *qi*: moving *qi* to a certain part of the body by mental concentration

练气 [liàn qì]

training of *qi*: the basic step of emitting *qi*

却谷食气 [què gǔ shí qì]

feeding on *qi* instead of food: the principle of a certain school of health preservation that the practitioner can be nourished by *qi* through *qigong* exercises instead of taking food

辟谷功 [bì gǔ gōng]

food-restricting exercise: a system of *qigong* exercises performed for the purpose of decreasing the practitioner's food-taking

减肥功 [jiǎn féi gōng]

slimming exercise: a system of *qigong* exercises performed for the purpose of reducing the body weight in an obese person

震桩式 [zhèn zhuāng shì]

pile-driving standing posture: standing on the feet with the knees slightly bent, the heels turned outward and the hands held apart in the front as if holding a ball, a basic posture commonly used for training *qi*

导气 [dǎo qì]

conducting of *qi*: guiding the *qi* flow to a portion or a point of the hand, to be emitted as out-going *qi*

合掌震桩导气 [hé zhǎng zhèn zhuāng dǎo qì]

conducting of *qi* with pile-driving standing and palms put together: form of conducting *qi* from *dantian* to the palms through the governor vessel and then back to *dantian* through the three yin meridians of the hands

一指禅导气 [yī zhǐ chán dǎo qì]

conducting of *qi* with single-finger meditation: taking a stake-standing posture with the left hand held at shoulder level and the right on the right side of the abdomen with the tips of the forefingers pointing to each other to conduct *qi*

对掌推拉导气 [duì zhǎng tuī lā dǎo qì]

palm-to-palm pushing-pulling conduction of *qi*: taking a standing posture and putting the palms together in the front and then rubbing the them against each other with *qi* emitted from *laogong* (PC8) of one palm to that of another

三点拉线导气 [sān diǎn lā xiàn dǎo qì]

three-point aligning conduction of *qi*: taking a standing posture and placing an ignited incense stick on a table in the front, with the right palm held on the left of the incense stick at a distance and the left hand on the right with its forefinger stretched to point to the ignited end of the incense stick and *laogong* (PC8) of the right palm to perform single-finger meditation to conduct *qi*

三点求圆导气 [sān diǎn qiú yuán dǎo qì]

three-point circle-drawing conduction of *qi*: taking a standing posture and making the ignited end of an incense stick and *laogong* (PC8) of the two palms an equilateral triangle and an imaginary circle to conduct *qi*

腾跃爆发导气 [téng yuè bào fā dǎo qì]

prancing to conduct *qi* in a burst: taking a standing posture with the knees slightly bent and making fists with both hands in front of the chest and then prancing and spreading the fingers suddenly to emit *qi* from *laogong* (PC8) in burst

发气 [fā qì]

emission of *qi*: sending *qi* out, also called 发功 [fā gōng] and 发放外气 [fā fàng wài qì], or 布气 [bù qì] in ancient times

发功 [fā gōng]

emission of trained *qi*, same as emission of *qi* (发气 [fā qì])

发放外气 [fā fàng wài qì]

emission of outgoing *qi*, same as emission of *qi* (发气 [fā qì])

布气 [bù qì]

distributing *qi*: an ancient term for emission of *qi* (发气 [fā qì])

发气手势 [fā qì shǒu shì]

***qi*-emitting hand gesture:** hand gesture for emitting the outgoing *qi*

一指禅式 [yī zhǐ chán shì]

single-finger meditation gesture: hand gesture for emitting *qi* with a single finger

平掌式 [píng zhǎng shì]

flat-palm gesture: hand gesture for emitting *qi* with an open palm

探爪式 [tàn zhuǎ shì]

spreading-claw gesture: hand gesture for emitting *qi* with the fingers slightly bent and shaped like a claw

剑决式 [jiàn jué shì]

sword-thrusting gesture: hand gesture for emitting *qi* with the index and middle fingers pointing forward

中指独立式 [zhōng zhǐ dú lì shì]

middle-finger-propping gesture: hand gesture for emitting *qi* with only the middle finger pointing forward

龙衔式 [lóng xián shì]

dragon-mouth gesture: hand gesture for emitting *qi*

气感 [qì gǎn]

sensation of *qi*: sensation of both genuine *qi* and evil *qi*

真气气感 [zhēn qì qì gǎn]

sensation of genuine *qi*: sensation of the direction, density, nature and volume of genuine *qi*, by which the body resistance can be judged

秽气气感 [huì qì qì gǎn]

sensation of evil *qi*: sensation experienced by the *qigong* master while treating a patient, by which the nature and severity of the patient's condition can be judged

收功 [shōu gōng]

closing form: (1) end or winding up of *qigong* exercise; (2) closing form of emission of *qi*, including that for the patient treated and that for the *qigong* master who gives treatment

气功偏差 [qì gōng piān chā]

deviation of *qigong*: adverse reactions in the course of *qigong* exercise, physical or mental, such as headache, dizziness, palpitations, shortness of breath, hand tremors, cold sweats, mental disorders and even schizophrenia

出偏 [chū piān]

deviation: an abbreviation of deviation of *qigong* (气功偏差 [qì gōng piān chā])

走火入魔 [zǒu huǒ rù mó]

evil reactions: a popular term for deviation of *qigong* (气功偏差 [qì gōng piān chā])

保健 Health Preservation

保健功 [bǎo jiàn gōng]

health-preserving exercise: exercise for preventing diseases and promote health

静坐 [jǐng zuò]

silent sitting: sitting silently with the eyes closed, the legs crossed, the tongue propped on the palate, and the mind concentrated on *dantian*, for cultivating the genuine *qi*

耳功 [ěr gōng]

ear exercise: while pressing the bilateral tragi with the palmar prominences to close the external auditory canals, flicking the occiput with the index fingers to cause a mild stimulation for regulating the brain function

叩齿 [kòu chǐ]

tapping the teeth: tapping the upper and lower teeth on each other to make the teeth firmer and improve digestion

舌功 [shé gōng]

tongue exercise: stirring the tongue in the mouth to produce saliva

赤龙搅海 [chì lóng jiǎo hǎi]

"red dragon stirring the sea": implicit and elegant expression for tongue exercise (舌功 [shé gōng])

漱津 [shù jīn]

gargling with saliva: gargling with the saliva produced by stirring of the tongue, swallowing and sending mentally to the lower *dantian*

擦鼻 [cā bí]

rubbing the nose: rubbing the sides of the nose with the backs of the thumbs up and down around *yingxiang* (LI20) for the prevention of colds and rhinitis

目功 [mù gōng]

eye exercise: gently rubbing the bilateral eyelids with the digital joints of the slightly bent thumbs and then rubbing the eyebrows, followed by rotating the eyeballs and looking into the distance, for improving vision

擦面 [cā miàn]

rubbing the face: rubbing the face with both palms from the top of the forehead down to the chin, and then from the chin up to the forehead, for improving one's looks

项功 [xiàng gōng]

nape exercise: placing the palms on the occiput with fingers crossed, repeatedly bending and lifting the head with force, for training the neck muscles and improving the local blood circulation

揉肩 [róu jiān]

kneading the shoulders: kneading the right shoulder with the left hand in a rotary motion and kneading the left shoulder with the right hand similarly, for improving the function of the shoulders

夹脊 [jiā jǐ]

pressing the spine: swinging the right and left arms to and fro alternately with the elbows bent 90 degrees and the hands making fists, for training the shoulders and pectoral muscles and preventing disorders of the spine

搓腰 [cuō yāo]

rubbing the waist: rubbing the waist with both palms up and down, and right and left, around the points *mingmen* (GV4) and *shenshu* (BL23)

搓内肾 [cuō nèi shèn]

rubbing the inner kidney: traditional term for rubbing the waist (搓腰 [cuo yao])

擦丹田 [cā dān tián]

kneading *dantian*: kneading the lower abdomen first with one hand and then the other in a circular motion around *dantian* for invigorating the spleen and tonifying the kidney

揉膝 [róu xī]

kneading the knees: kneading both knees with the hands simultaneously for soothing the tendons and strengthening the bones

擦涌泉 [cā yǒng quán]

rubbing *yongquan* (KI1): rubbing the left sole with the right index and middle fingers surrounding the point *yongquan* (KI1), and then the right sole with the left index and middle fingers, for the prevention of hypertension

天人相应 [tiān rén xiāng yìng]

correspondence between human beings and the natural environment

阴阳协调 [yīn yáng xié tiáo]

coordination between yin and yang

顺应四时 [shùn yīng sì shí]

adaptation to seasonal changes

养生十常 [yǎng shēng shí cháng]

doing ten things frequently for health preservation

齿常扣，津常咽 [chǐ cháng kòu, jīn cháng yàn]

tapping the teeth and swallowing the saliva frequently

面常搓，足常摩 [miàn cháng cuō, zú cháng mó]

rubbing the face and massaging the soles frequently

耳常弹，鼻常揉 [ěr cháng tán, bí cháng róu]

pricking the ears and rubbing the nose frequently

眼常运，腹常旋 [yǎn cháng yùn, fù cháng xuán]

moving the eyeballs and massaging the abdomen circularly frequently

肢常伸，肛常提 [zhī cháng shēn, gāng cháng tí]

stretching the limbs and contracting the anus frequently

睡眠十忌 [shuì mián shí jì]

ten items of avoidance for sleep: (1) avoid lying on the back while sleeping, (2) avoid anxiety, (3) avoid anger, (4) avoid overeating before going to bed, (5) avoid talking too much before going to sleep, (6) avoid sleeping facing the light, (7) avoid sleeping with the mouth open, (8) avoid sleeping with the head covered, (9) avoid sleeping in a draught, and (10) avoid sleeping with the head against the stove.

饮食有节 [yǐn shí yǒu jié]

temperance in eating and drinking

药膳 [yào shàn]

medicated diet: food cooked with medicinal substances for therapeutic purposes

药粥 [yào zhōu]

medicated porridge: porridge cooked with medicinal substances, such as lotus seeds, Chinese dates, etc.

药酒 [yào jiǔ]

medicated wine: wine containing medicinal substances to be taken regularly for therapeutic purposes, such as acanthopanax-bark wine for rheumatism

药茶 [yào chá]

medicated tea: herbal medicines mixed and prepared to be infused with boiling water and taken as tea or together with tea

常用引文与格言 Commonly Used Citations and Maxims

真气存内，邪不可干。 [zhēn qì cún nèi, xié bù kě gàn]

If body resisting forces prevail, attack of pathogens will not avail.

恬淡虚无，真气从之；精神内守，病从安来。 [tin dàn xū wú, zhēn qì cóng zhī; jīng shén nèi shǒu, bìng cóng ān lái]

Uncluttered mind preserves vitality, good spirit alienates fatality.

虚邪贼风，避之有时。 [xū xié zéi fēng, bì zhī yǒu shí]

Evil winds and draughts must be carefully avoided.

治未病。 [zhì wèi bìng]

Treat diseases before they get a hold.

勿药为中医。 [wù yào wéi zhōng yī]

No medication is better than wrong medication.

若要安，三里常不干。 [ruò yào ān, sān lǐ cháng bù gàn]

Moxibustion frequently applied to *zusanli* (ST36) makes one healthy.

背要常暖，胸要常护。 [bèi yào cháng nuǎn, yáo yào cháng hù]

Keep your back warm and your chest well covered all the time.

足要常搓，腹要常摩。 [zú yào cháng cuō, fù yào cháng mó]

Rub your soles and massage your abdomen frequently.

修性以保神，安心以全身。 [xiū xìng yǐ bǎo shén, ān xīn yǐ quán shēn]

Good character preserves one's soul, good temperament preserves one's life.

以动养形，以形养神。 [yǐ dòng yǎng xíng, yǐ xíng yǎng shén]

Exercise builds up the physique and the physique buoys up the spirit.

人欲劳于形，百病不能成。 [rén yù láo yú xíng, bǎi bìng bù néng chéng]

Physical labor keeps diseases away.

贪吃贪睡，添病减岁。 [tān chī tān shuì, tiān bìng jiǎn suì]

Overeating and oversleeping lead to disease and premature death.

食饱不可睡，睡则诸疾生。 [shí bǎo bù kě shuì, shuì zé zhū jí shēng]

One should not go to sleep immediately after having a heavy meal, otherwise disease will follow in no time.

饭后百步走，活到九十九。 [fàn hòu bǎi bù zǒu, huó dào jiǔ shí jiǔ]

If you wish to live to ninety-nine, walk one hundred steps after a meal each time.

先睡心，后睡眼。 [xiān shuì xīn, hòu shuì yǎn]

When going to sleep, ease your mind first and then close your eyes.

少思以养神，少欲以养精。 [shǎo sī yǐ yǎng shén, shǎo yù yǐ yǎng jīng]

Free of cares, your mind will be restful; free of inordinate desires, you will find yourself full of vigor.

多思则神殆，多念则智散。 [duō sī zé shén dài, duō niàn zé zhì sǎn]

Worries make one's spirit low, and cares make one's mind distracted.

多欲则智昏，多事则劳形。 [duō yù zé zhì hūn, duō shì zé láo xíng]

Lusts make one blind, and overwork makes one exhausted.

心胸宽，人快活；心胸窄，忧愁多。 [xīn xiōng kuān, rén kuài huó; xīn xiōng zǎi, yōu chóu duō]

A broad mind makes one happy while a narrow-mind makes one worry.

笑一笑，少一少；恼一恼，老一老。 [xiào yī xiào, shào yī shào; nǎo yī nǎo, lǎo yī lǎo]

Mirth makes one younger and fretting makes one older.

歌咏所以养性情，舞蹈所以养血脉。 [gē yǒng suǒ yǐ yǎng xìng qíng, wǔ dǎo suǒ yǐ yǎng xuè mài]

Singing can remold one's temperament, and dancing can promote one's blood flow.

诗书悦心，山林逸兴 ，可以延年。 [shī shū yuè xīn, shān lín yì xìng, kě yǐ yán nián]

Poetry pleases one's heart and scenery one's eye, both does life benefit by.

精神到处文章老，学问深处意气平。 [jīng shén dào chù wén zhāng lǎo, xué wèn shēn chù yì qì píng]

The best essay is written by the most concentrated mind, and a peaceful mood comes from a most learned head.

下棋可忘忧，慢跑可长寿。 [xià qí kě wàng yōu, màn pǎo kě cháng shòu]

Playing chess can relieve one's cares and leisurely running can make one live longer.

七情之病，看花解闷，听曲消愁，胜于服药。 [qī qíng zhī bìng, kàn huā jiě mèn, tīng qǔ xiāo chóu, shèng yú fú yào]

A flower show or a musical performance is a better cure for emotional disturbances than medicine.

欲不可纵，纵欲成灾；乐不可极，乐极生灾。 [yù bù kě zòng, zòng yù chéng zāi; lè bù kě jí, lè jí shēng zāi]

Sexual desire should be controlled, intemperance will bring harm, one should not seek sexual enjoyment to excess, otherwise disaster will follow.

起居有常，养其神也，不妄作劳，养其精也。 [qǐ jū yǒu cháng, yǎng qí shén yě, bù wàng zuò láo, yǎng qí jīng yě]

Regular daily life helps preserve vitality, temperance in sexual life helps preserve the reproductive essence.

衣着寒暖适体，勿侈华艳。 [yī zhuó hán nuǎn shì tǐ, wù chǐ huá yàn]

Dressing warmly and comfortably is better than dressing in luxurious and gaudy clothes.

晨起三百步，睡前一盆汤。 [chén qǐ sān bǎi bù, shuì qián yī pén tāng]

Walk three hundred steps after rising in the morning and bathe your feet in warm water before retiring at night.

立如松，坐如钟，卧如弓。 [lì rú sōng, zuò rú zhōng, wò rú gōng]

Stand upright like a pine, sit firm like a bell, and sleep on the side like a bow.

冬不欲极温，夏不欲极凉。 [dōng bù yù jí wēn, xià bù yù jī liáng]

Don't crave excessive coldness in summer, nor excessive warmth in winter.

饮食自倍，脾胃乃伤。 [yǐn shí zì bèi, pí wèi nǎi shāng]

Eating to excess injures the spleen and stomach.

烹调有方。 [pēng tiáo yǒu fāng]

Food should be cooked in the right way.

五谷为养，五果为助，五畜为益，五菜为充。 [wǔ gǔ wéi yǎng, wǔ guǒ wéi zhù, wǔ chù wéi yì,wǔ cài wéi chōng]

The five cereals are staple food, the fruits are auxiliary food, meats are beneficial and vegetables should be abundant.

菜饭宜清淡，少盐少疾患。 [cài fàn yì qīng dàn, shǎo yán shǎo jí huán]

Light food and not so salty, such a diet keeps one healthy.

乳贵有时，食贵有节。 [rǔ guì yǒu shí, shí guì yǒu jié]

Breast feeding should be given at regular hours, and food taken with temperance.

先饥而食，先渴而饮；食欲数而少，不欲顿而多。 [xiān jī ér shí, xiān kě ér yǐn; shí yù shuò ér shǎo, bù yù dùn ér duō]

Eat before becoming hungry and drink before becoming thirsty, frequent feeding with less food at a time is better than too much food taken at a single meal.

病从口入。 [bìng cóng kǒu rù]

Disease usually breaks in through the mouth.

药补不如食补。 [yào bǔ bù rú shí bǔ]

Taking nourishing food is better than taking tonics.

酒通血脉，消愁遣兴，少饮壮神，过多损命。 [jiǔ tōng xuè mài, xiāo chóu qiǎn xìng, shǎo yǐn zhuàng shén, guò duō sǔn mìng]

Wine is ready to enter the blood to quench one's sorrow and heighten one's merriment, it may keep up one's spirits if drunk in moderation, but endanger one's life if drunk to excess.

气大伤人，酒多伤身。 [qì dà shāng rén, jiǔ duō shāng shēn]

Both raving anger and overdrinking are harmful to health.

宁可三日无粮，不可一日无茶。 [nìng kě sān rì wú liáng, bù kě yī rì wú chá]

One should rather go three days without food than a single day without tea.

莫吃空心茶，休饮卯时酒，更兼戌后饭，禁之当谨守。 [mò chī kōng xīn chá, xiū yǐn mǎo shí jiǔ, gēng jiān xū hòu fàn, jìn zhī dāng jǐn shǒu]

Don't drink too much tea while fasting, don't drink too much wine in the early morning, and don't eat too much food in the late evening, the three don'ts should be observed closely.

饥不饱食，渴不狂饮。 [jī bù bǎo shí, kě bù kuáng yǐn]

Don't eat to excess when hungry or drink to excess when thirsty.

胃不和，卧不安。 [wèi bù hé, wò bù ān]

Indigestion disturbs sleep.

临床各科　CLINICAL MEDICINE

温病　Warm Diseases

天受 [tiān shòu]

(1) air-borne; (2) aerial infection: infection that is contracted by inhalation

传染 [chuán rǎn]

contagion: transmission of a disease by contact

时行 [shí xíng]

(1) epidemic: affecting a large number of individuals in the same place for a certain period of time; **(2) epidemicity:** state of being epidemic, also called 天行 [tiān xíng]

天行 [tiān xíng]

synonymous with 时行 [shí xíng]

时行戾气 [shí xíng lì qì]

epidemic pathogen: pathogen that causes an outbreak of epidemic disease

时毒 [shí dú]

seasonal toxin: pathogen that causes an infectious seasonal disease

温毒 [wēn dú]

warm toxin: pathogen that causes an infectious febrile disease

时病 [shí bìng]；**时令病** [shí lìng bìng]

seasonal diseases: diseases in the four seasons chiefly arising from the climatic influences

时疫 [shí yì]

(1) seasonal epidemic: epidemic of an acute infectious disease in a certain season; **(2) pestilence in summer**

天行时疫 [tiān xíng shí yì]

prevalent seasonal epidemic, synonymous with seasonal epidemic 时疫 [shí yì]

阴病 [yīn bìng]

yin disease: (1) a general designation for diseases with deficiency syndrome or of cold nature; (2) disease of yin meridian

阳病 [yáng bìng]

yang disease: (1) a general designation for diseases with excess syndrome and heat syndrome; (2) disease of yang meridian

卒病 [cù bìng]

abrupt illness: sudden onset of a disease

暴病 [bào bìng]

sudden illness: sudden attack of a serious disease

新病 [xīn bìng]

recent disease: disease occurring recently, usually referring to the onset of a new disease in addition to an old chronic illness

伤寒 [shāng hán]

(1) cold-induced disease: a general term for various externally contracted febrile diseases; **(2) cold affection:** a condition caused by cold, manifested as chills and fever, absence of sweating, headache, floating and tense pulse

热病 [rè bìng]

febrile disease: (1) disease due to exogenous pathogenic factors with fever as its main manifestation; (2) one of the cold-induced diseases; (3) febrile disease caused by summer heat

温病 [wēn bìng]

warm disease: acute externally contracted febrile disease caused by warm pathogens, clinically manifested chiefly as fever

伏气 [fú qì]

latent *qi*: (1) latent pathogen, another name for 伏邪 [fú xié]; (2) abbreviation of latent warm disease (伏气温病 [fú qì wēn bìng])

伏气温病 [fú qì wēn bìng]

latent warm disease: epidemic febrile disease caused by latent warm pathogen, marked by syndrome of internal heat with fever, thirst and fidgetiness at the onset

温[瘟]疫 [wēn yì]

pestilence: virulent infectious epidemic diseases

顺传 [shùn chuán]

sequential transmission: ordinary proceeding of a febrile disease from the exterior to the interior

逆传 [nì chuán]

non-sequential transmission: extraordinary proceeding of a febrile disease, for instance, directly from the superficies to the pericardium

感冒 [gǎn mào]

common cold; colds: affliction of the lung-superficies by pathogenic wind, mainly manifested as fever, chills, headache, general aching, congested nose, sneezing, itching throat and cough

时行感冒 [shí xíng gǎn mào]

influenza: invasion of the lung-superficies by a seasonal epidemic pathogen causing acute fever, sore throat, headache and general aching

风寒感冒 [fēng hán gǎn mào]

wind-cold affliction: illness caused by wind and cold, manifested as chilliness and mild fever, absence of sweating, headache, stuffed and running nose, sneezing, general aching, and floating and tense pulse

风热感冒 [fēng rè gǎn mào]

wind-heat affliction: illness caused by wind and heat, manifested as fever with mild chills, headache, sore throat, cough and expectoration of yellowish sputum, thirst, and rapid pulse

气虚感冒 [qì xū gǎn mào]

***qi*-deficiency colds:** colds in one with a constitution of *qi* deficiency

阳虚感冒 [yáng xū gǎn mào]

yang-deficiency colds: colds in one with a constitution of yang deficiency

血虚感冒 [xuè xū gǎn mào]

blood-deficiency colds: colds in one with a constitution of blood deficiency

阴虚感冒 [yīn xū gǎn mào]

yin-deficiency colds: colds in one with a constitution of yin deficiency

风温 [fēng wēn]

(1) wind-warm (disease): an acute externally contracted febrile disease caused by pathogenic wind-heat, marked by external heat syndrome at the onset; **(2) wind-warm (syndrome):** wind syndrome in acute febrile disease, usually occurring after diaphoresis, marked by high fever, spontaneous sweating, heaviness of the body and sleepiness

风温病 [fēng wēn bìng]

wind-warm disease: full name of wind-warm (风温 [fēng wēn]) as a disease

春温 [chūn wēn]

spring warm: an acute febrile disease caused by latent warm-heat pathogen, marked by presence of internal heat at the onset

春温病 [chūn wēn bìng]

spring warm disease: full name of spring warm (春温 [chūn wēn]) as a disease

冒暑 [mào shǔ]

summer-heat affliction: ailment of the nose and throat with catarrh, sneezing and coughing in summer

暑秽 [shǔ huì]

summer filth: a type of heat stroke occurring in summer, marked by sudden syncope

暑秽病 [shǔ huì bìng]

summer filth disease: full name of summer filth (暑秽 [shǔ huì])

暑湿流注 [shǔ shī liú zhù]

multiple abscesses of summer-dampness: multiple abscesses deep in muscles occurring in summer and autumn, ascribed to the invasion of summer-dampness

暑病 [shǔ bìng]

summer-heat disease: a collective term for acute diseases caused by summer heat

阳暑 [yáng shǔ]

yang summer affliction: affliction by heat in summer, usually referring to heatstroke

阴暑 [yīn shǔ]

yin summer affliction: affliction by cold in summer, e.g., affliction due to exposure to cold draught or excessive cold drinks

伤暑 [shāng shǔ]

summer-heat affliction: a general term for various conditions caused by summer-heat, especially for mild cases of heatstroke and sunstroke

感暑 [gǎn shǔ]

summer-heat affection, same as 伤暑 [shāng shǔ]

中暑 [zhòng shǔ]

sunstroke; heatstroke: an acute disease caused by summer-heat, marked by sudden loss of consciousness or high fever with restlessness, trismus, and even convulsions

暑厥 [shǔ jué]

summer-heat syncope: severe case of sunstroke marked by loss of consciousness and cold limbs

暑厥证 [shǔ jué zhèng]

summer-heat syncope syndrome: full name of summer-heat syncope (暑厥 [shǔ jué]) as a syndrome

暑痉 [shǔ jìng]

summer convulsion: a convulsive disease in children caused by pathogenic summer warm, a type of summer-wind (暑风 [shǔ fēng])

暑痫 [shǔ xián]

summer convulsive seizure: a type of severe heat-stroke in summer with sudden loss of consciousness and convulsions

暑温 [shǔ wēn]

summer warm: an acute externally contracted febrile disease caused by heat pathogen in summer, marked by heat syndrome of the stomach meridian at the onset

暑温病 [shǔ wēn bìng]

summer warm disease: full name of summer warm (暑温 [shǔ wēn]) as a disease

暑瘵 [shǔ zhài]

summer phthisis: sudden onset of cough and hemoptysis caused by summer-heat, resembling phthisis

暑风 [shǔ fēng]

summer-wind: a disease marked by sudden onset of opisthotonos and convulsions caused by summer-heat

暑风证 [shǔ fēng zhèng]

summer-wind syndrome: a syndrome marked by sudden onset of opisthotonos and convulsions caused by summer-heat

暑入阳明 [shǔ rù yáng míng]

summer-heat into *yangming*: a syndrome occurring in the initial stage of summer warm disease, manifested by high fever, profuse sweating, thirst, fidgetness, dry yellow tongue coating, and surging rapid pulse

暑入阳明证 [shǔ rù yāng míng zhèng]

syndrome of summer-heat into *yangming*: full name of summer- heat into *yangming* 暑入阳明 (shǔ rù yáng míng) as a syndrome

湿病 [shī bìng]

dampness disease: any disease caused by dampness, usually with symptoms such as distending pain and swelling of joints, heaviness sensation of the body, watery diarrhea, or edema

湿阻 [shī zǔ]

dampness impediment: an externally contracted disease characterized by impairment of the lung and defense system by pathogenic dampness, with such manifestations as aching and heavy sensation in the head and body, anorexia, and epigastric stuffiness, also known as dampness affliction (伤湿 [shāng shī]) or dampness ailment (冒湿 [mào shī])

冒湿 [mào shī]

dampness ailment: a synonym for dampness impediment (湿阻 [shī zǔ])

伤湿 [shāng shī]

dampness affliction: a synonym for dampness impediment (湿阻 [shī zǔ])

湿温 [shī wēn]

damp-warm: an infectious febrile disease caused by damp-heat, prevalent in summer and autumn, marked by prolonged fever, general aches and pains with heaviness, stuffiness in the chest and distension in the abdomen, and greasy coating of the tongue, usually referring to typhoid and paratyphoid fever

湿温病 [shī wēn bìng]

damp-warm disease: full name of damp-warm (湿温 [shī wēn])

伏暑 [fú shǔ]

latent summer-heat: acute febrile disease caused by latent summer-heat or summer-damp pathogen, occurring in autumn or winter

伏暑病 [fú shǔ bìng]

latent summer-heat disease: full name of latent summer-heat (伏暑 [fú shǔ]) as a disease

秋燥 [qiū zào]

autumn-dryness (disease): an externally contracted febrile disease caused by dryness-heat in autumn, marked by fever with dry throat, dry cough, dry skin, and other symptoms of dryness

秋燥病 [qiū zào bìng]

autumn dryness disease: full name of autumn-dryness (秋燥 [qiū zào]) as a disease

凉燥 [liáng zào]

cool-dryness: a seasonal disease caused by coolness and dryness in autumn, marked by chills, headache, fever, absence of sweating, dryness of the nasal cavity and mouth, dry cough, and thin whitish tongue coating

凉燥病 [liáng zào bìng]

cool-dryness disease: full name of cool-dryness (凉燥 [liáng zào])

温燥 [wēn zào]

warm-dryness: a seasonal disease caused by warmth and dryness in autumn, marked by fever, headache, absence of sweating, dry cough, dryness of the throat, thirst, reddened tongue tip and margin, and rapid floating pulse

温燥病 [wēn zào bìng]

warm-dryness disease: full name of warm-dryness (温燥[wēn zào])

冬温 [dōng wēn]

winter warm: febrile disease in winter

外感 [wài gǎn]

external affection: affection caused by exogenous pathogenic factors

潮热 [cháo rè]

tidal fever: fever recurring daily, in most cases in the afternoon, like the regular rise and fall of the tide

阴虚潮热 [yīn xū cháo rè]

tidal fever of yin deficiency: tidal fever due to consumption of essence, as seen in tuberculosis

日晡潮热 [rī bū cháo rè]

late afternoon (tidal) fever: tidal fever in the afternoon, especially that caused by accumulation of pathogenic heat in the intestine (cf. 阳明腑证 [yáng míng fǔ zhèng])

上火 [shàng hǔo]

up-rising of fire: a condition caused by excessive internal heat, manifested by constipation, inflammation of the nasal and oral cavity, conjunctival congestion, etc.

结胸 [jié xiōng]

thoracic accumulation: accumulation of pathogenic factors (such as heat or cold in combination with retained fluid or phlegm or stagnant blood) in the chest, often manifested by tenderness and fullness sensation in the costal region with fever and sweating, or by pain and tenderness from the epigastrium to the lower abdomen with constipation and thirst

大结胸 [dà jié xiōng]

major thoracic accumulation: massive accumulation of phlegm-heat in the chest, a serious disease characterized by fullness, pain and tenderness of the chest and abdomen

小结胸 [xiǎo jié xiōng]

minor thoracic accumulation: mild case of accumulation of phlegm- heat in the chest, marked by epigastric distension, stuffiness and tenderness

寒结胸 [hán jié xiōng]

thoracic accumulation of cold: accumulation of pathogenic cold in the chest, marked by thoracic fullness and tenderness, constipation, absence of fever and thirst, whitish slippery coating of the tongue, and deep and slow pulse

血结胸 [xuè jié xiōng]

thoracic accumulation of blood: accumulation of stagnant blood in the chest, marked by thoracic distension, pain and tenderness

大头瘟 [dà tóu wēn]

"swollen-head infection"; erysipelas facialis: an acute infection of the face marked by high fever and local redness, swelling, hotness and pain.

虾蟆瘟 [há ma wēn]

"toad-like infection": another name for erysipelas facialis (大头瘟 [dà tóu wēn])

烂喉痧 [làn hóu shā]

scarlatina: an acute infectious disease caused by toxic warm-heat and marked by swelling and erosion of the throat, with an erythematous rash, also called 疫喉痧 [yì hóu shā] or simply 疫痧 [yì shā], 烂喉丹痧[làn hóu dān shā] or simply 丹痧 [dān shā]

疫喉痧 [yì hóu shā]

scarlet fever: another name for scarlatina (烂喉痧 [làn hóu shā])

疫痧 [yì shā]

scarlet fever, same as scarlatina (烂喉痧 [làn hóu shā])

烂喉丹痧 [làn hóu dān shā]

scarlatina angionosa: scarlet fever with painful pharyngitis, another name for 烂喉痧 [làn hóu shā]

丹痧 [dān shā]

another name for scarlatina (烂喉痧 [làn hóu shā])

瘴气 [zhàng qì]

miasma: noxious effluvium that is alleged to cause malaria

瘴疟 [zhàng nüè]

miasmic malaria: severe malaria with loss of consciousness or jaundice

疟疾 [nüè jì]

malaria: an externally contracted disease caused by malarial parasites, marked by paroxysms of shivering chills, high fever and sweating, also called 疟病 [nüè bìng], and abbreviated as 疟 [nüè]

疟病 [nüè bìng]

same as 疟疾 [nüè jì]

疟 [nüè]

an abbreviation for 疟疾 [nüè jì]

正疟 [zhèng nüè]

ordinary malaria: malaria with regular attacks of chills, fever and sweating

温疟 [wēn nüè]

warm malaria: malaria with higher fever and lower chills than an ordinary attack

暑疟 [shǔ nüè]

summer-heat malaria: malaria with manifestations of summer heat with damp

湿疟 [shī nüè]

damp malaria: malaria marked by internal damp-heat, manifested as un-surfaced fever, inhibited sweating, nausea and vomiting

寒疟 [hán nüè]

cold malaria: malaria with higher chills and lower fever than in an ordinary attack

热瘴 [rè zhàng]

heat miasmic malaria: miasmic malaria with marked heat symptoms

冷瘴 [lěng zhàng]

chilly miasmic malaria: miasmic malaria with trembling chills, also called 寒瘴 [hán zhàng]

寒瘴 [hán zhàng]

cold miasmic malaria: a synonym for chilly miasmic malaria (冷瘴 [lěng zhàng])

瘴毒 [zhàng dú]

miasmic toxin: the pathogenic factor that causes miasmic malaria

瘴疟 [zhàng nüè]

miasmic malaria: malignant malaria

劳疟 [láo nüè]

debilitating malaria: chronic malaria with general debility

疟母 [nüè mǔ]

malarial mass: splenomegaly in chronic malaria, also called 疟痞 [nüè pǐ] or 疟积 [nüè jī]

疟痞 [nüè pǐ]

malarial lump, synonymous with malarial mass (疟母 [nüè mǔ])

疟积 [nüè jī]

malarial accumulation, synonymous with malarial mass (疟母 [nüè mǔ])

牝疟 [pìn nüè]

yin malaria: chronic malaria in a debilitated patient with severe shivering chills but low-grade fever

痢疾 [lì jí]

dysentery: an infectious disease of the intestines, marked by abdominal pain, frequent stools containing blood and mucus, and tenesmus

白痢 [bái lì]

white dysentery: a type of dysentery with whitish mucous purulent stool

湿热痢 [shī rè lì]

damp-heat dysentery: a type of dysentery with frequent bloody mucoid stools, tenesmus, and burning sensation in the anus

寒湿痢 [hán shī lì]

cold-damp dysentery: a type of dysentery characterized by passage of whitish, thin mucoid stools, absence of fever and thirst, distending distress of the epigastrium and dull pain in the abdomen, tenesmus, poor appetite, pale tongue with whitish coating, and slow pulse

时疫痢 [shí yì lì]

epidemic dysentery: a variety of dysentery that becomes epidemic, also known as 疫痢 [yì lì]

疫痢 [yì lì]

epidemic dysentery, same as 时疫痢 [shí yì lì]

疫毒痢 [yì dú lì]

epidemic toxic dysentery: dysentery with acute onset of high fever, vomiting and frequent passage of bloody-mucoid stools, severe tenesmus, and even impaired consciousness

噤口痢 [jìn kǒu lì]

food-denial dysentery: severe case of dysentery with utter loss of appetite and vomiting upon eating and drinking

休息痢 [xiū xī lì]

intermittent dysentery: dysentery occurring at intervals

迁延痢 [qiān yán lì]

protracted dysentery: dysentery lasting a long time

久痢 [jiǔ lì]

chronic dysentery: dysentery marked by long duration

虚寒痢 [xū hán lì]

deficiency-cold dysentery: chronic dysentery due to deficiency-cold of the spleen and kidney, characterized by passage of thin mucous stools accompanied by dull pain in the lower abdomen, poor appetite, lassitude, coolness of the limbs, weakness of the loins and aversion to cold

赤痢 [chì lì]

red dysentery: dysentery with bloody stool

赤白痢 [chì bái lì]

red-white dysentery: dysentery with frequent passage of stools containing blood and mucus

寒泻 [hán xiè]

cold diarrhea: diarrhea due to accumulation of pathogenic cold in the interior, marked by passage of watery stools with undigested food, dull abdominal pain, whitish slippery coating of the tongue, deep and slow pulse

热泻 [rè xiè]

heat diarrhea: diarrhea due to accumulated heat in the large intestine, with malodorous, yellow stools accompanied by abdominal pain, and burning sensation in the anus

干霍乱 [gān huò luàn]

dry choleraic turmoil: an acute illness marked by severe abdominal pain associated with an urgent but ineffectual desire to vomit and defecate, also called colicky intestinal turmoil 绞肠痧 [jiǎo cháng shā] or 搅肠痧 [jiǎo cháng shā]

绞肠痧 [jiǎo cháng shā]

colicky intestinal turmoil: another name for dry choleraic turmoil (干霍乱 [gān huò luàn])

搅肠痧 [jiǎo cháng shā]

colicky intestinal turmoil, same as 绞肠痧 [jiǎo cháng shā]

寒霍乱 [hán huò luàn]

cold choleraic turmoil: choleraic turmoil with severe loss of yin fluid

热霍乱 [rè huò luàn]

heat choleraic turmoil: choleraic turmoil with high fever and other heat symptoms

霍乱 [huò luàn]

(1) cholera: an acute infectious disease caused by *Vibrio cholerae* (as defined in recent years); **(2) choleraic turmoil:** any disease characterized by sudden and drastic vomiting and diarrhea, including acute gastroenteritis, food poisoning and cholera (as defined before 1820)

霍乱病 [huò luàn bìng]

cholera: an acute infectious disease caused by *Vibrio cholerae*

霍乱转筋 [huò luàn zhuǎn jīn]

systremma in choleraic turmoil: cramp in the muscles of the calf of the leg following drastic vomiting and diarrhea

转筋霍乱 [zhuǎn jīn huò luàn]

choleraic turmoil with systremma: sudden and drastic vomiting and diarrhea causing cramps in the calf muscles of the leg

胃家实 [wèi jiā shí]

excessiveness of the stomach (and intestines): accumulation of pathogenic heat in the stomach and intestines, which often results in the damage of fluid and brings on such symptoms as high fever, persistent thirst, profuse sweating, full and gigantic pulse, constipation or discharge of hard fecal masses, and abdominal pain

发黄 [fā huáng]

yellow discoloration: a yellowish pigmentation of the skin and sclera

黄疸 [huáng dǎn]

jaundice: a syndrome characterized by yellow discoloration of the skin and sclera

阳黄 [yáng huáng]

yang jaundice: a type of jaundice characterized by bright yellow discoloration of the skin and sclera, usually acute at the onset and accompanied by damp-heat symptoms

阴黄 [yīn huáng]

yin jaundice: a type of jaundice characterized by dim yellow discoloration of the skin and sclera, usually chronic in progress and accompanied by cold-dampness or deficiency-cold symptoms

急黄 [jí huáng]

fulminant jaundice: a critical case of jaundice with sudden onset, rapid deterioration and poor prognosis, accompanied by high fever, impairment of consciousness, abdominal distension, ascites, and hematemesis

内科 Internal Medicine

内科杂病 [zá bìng]

miscellaneous internal diseases: various internal diseases excluding cold-induced diseases and warm diseases

宿疾 [sù jí]

old chronic disease: a disease that has a long history and is not cured

固(痼)疾 [gù jí]

stubborn chronic disease: chronic disease difficult to cure

隐疾 [yǐn jí]

occult disease: euphemism for venereal disease or impotence

失音 [shī yīn]

aphonia: loss of voice

失音病 [shī yīn bìng]

aphonia: a diseased state characterized by loss of voice

咳嗽 [ké sòu]

cough: Strictly speaking, the two Chinese characters have different meanings. 咳 [ké] means the expelling of air from the lungs suddenly with an explosive noise but no expectoration, while 嗽 [sòu] refers to the expectoration of sputum without an explosive noise. Generally, the two Chinese characters are used together to denote "cough", regardless of noise or expectoration.

干咳 [gān ké]

dry cough: cough with no or scanty expectoration, also called 干咳嗽 [gān ké sòu]

干咳嗽 [gān ké sòu]

cough with no expectoration: cough indicating consumption of fluid in the lung, also abbreviated as dry cough 干咳 [gān ké]

外感咳嗽 [wài gǎn ké sòu]

externally contracted cough: cough in exogenous affections, characterized by an acute onset and often accompanied by chills and fever

风寒咳嗽 [fēng hán ké sòu]

wind-cold cough: cough caused by wind-cold, marked by association with frothy expectoration, stuffed-up nose, chills or aversion to cold, general aching and no sweating

风热咳嗽 [fēng rè ké sòu]

wind-heat cough: cough caused by wind-heat, marked by association with sticky expectoration, fever, thirst, and sore throat

风燥咳嗽 [fēng zào ké sòu]

wind-dryness cough: cough caused by wind-dryness, marked by dry cough with itching of the throat and other symptoms of dryness

内伤咳嗽 [nèi shāng ké sòu]

internally damaged cough: cough due to internal damage, characterized by a chronic course, often accompanied by dyspnea or shortness of breath

痰湿咳嗽 [tán shī ké sòu]

phlegm-damp cough: cough due to accumulation of phlegm-damp in the lung, marked by association with copious expectoration, relieved when phlegm is discharged, also known as 痰咳 [tán ké]

痰咳 [tán ké]

phlegmatic cough: a synonym for phlegm-damp cough (痰湿咳嗽 [tán shī ké sòu])

肺虚咳嗽 [fèi xū ké sòu]

lung-insufficiency cough: cough due to insufficiency (mostly yin deficiency) of the lung, marked by dry cough or blood-stained sputum, accompanied by emaciation, fidgetiness, insomnia, night sweats, malar flush and afternoon fever

气虚咳嗽 [qì xū ké sòu]

***qi*-deficient cough:** cough due to deficiency of lung *qi*, marked by chronic cough with feeble sound, profuse thin expectoration, lassitude, spontaneous sweating, and vulnerability to colds

五更咳 [wǔ gēng ké]

fifth-watch cough: cough occurring or exaggerated daily before dawn, usually due to spleen insufficiency with profuse production of phlegm in the early morning

劳咳 [láo ké]

phthisical cough: chronic cough due to phthisis or consumption by overfatigue or sexual intemperance, also called 劳嗽 [láo sòu]

劳嗽 [láo sòu]

another name for phthisical cough (劳咳 [láo ké])

短气 [duǎn qì]

shortness of breath: rapid labored breathing

少气 [shǎo qì]

asthenic breathing: weak or faint breathing

上气 [shàng qì]

adverse ascent of *qi*; dyspnea: a state characterized by reversed upward flow of *qi* in the lung, usually seen in an external affliction when the airway is obstructed by phlegm

咳逆上气 [ké nì shàng qì]

cough with dyspnea

喘 [chuǎn]

dyspnea: difficult and labored breathing

喘证 [chuǎn zhèng]

dyspnea (syndrome): a morbid state characterized by difficult and labored breathing

喘病 [chuǎn bìng]

dyspnea (disease): a synonym for 喘证 [chuǎn zhèng]

实喘 [shí chuǎn]

dyspnea of excess type: dyspnea caused by excessive pathogenic factors marked by rapid, forceful and coarse breathing with acute onset and short duration

虚喘 [xū chuǎn]

dyspnea of deficiency type: dyspnea due to insufficient functioning of the lung and kidney, marked by shortness of breath and dyspnea upon exertion

哮 [xiào]

wheezing: difficult and labored breathing with a whistling sound

哮病 [xiào bìng]

wheezing (disease): a morbid state characterized by difficult and labored breathing with a whistling sound

哮喘 [xiào chuǎn]

asthma: a general term for dyspnea with wheezing

寒哮 [hán xiào]

cold wheezing: a type of asthma due to invasion of pathogenic cold, marked by dyspnea with wheezing, cough with thin mucous expectoration, stuffiness in the chest, whitish and slippery tongue coating, floating and tense pulse, also known as 冷哮 [lěng xiào]

冷哮 [lěng xiào]

asthma of cold type, synonymous with cold wheezing

热哮 [rè xiào]

heat wheezing: a type of asthma due to retention of heat-phlegm which causes obstruction of the respiratory tract, marked by dyspnea, wheezing, thick and yellowish sputum, distress in the chest, flushed face, thirst and desire to drink, reddened tongue with yellow and greasy coating, slippery and rapid pulse

痰喘 [tán chuǎn]

phlegm dyspnea: dyspnea caused by excessive phlegm in the lung, marked by tachypnea with phlegmatic sound, cough, and stuffiness of the chest

寒痰 [hán tán]

cold phlegm: a type of phlegm syndrome characterized by expectoration of thin and foamy sputum, usually due to cold

水饮 [shuǐ yǐn]

fluid exudate: the fluid that comes from the internal organs as a result of pathological change

饮证 [yǐn zhèng]

fluid-retention syndrome: a collective term for various diseases resulting from fluid retention in the body, generally including 痰饮 [tán yǐn], 悬饮 [xuán yǐn], 溢饮 [yì yǐn], and 支饮 [zhī yǐn]

痰饮 [tán yǐn]

phlegm-fluid retention: (1) a general term for retention of phlegm and fluid in any part of the body; (2) a particular designation for retention of fluid in the gastrointestinal tract, e.g., gastric retention in pyloric stenosis

悬饮 [xuán yǐn]

pleural fluid retention: excess fluid retained in the side of the thorax with stretching pain during respiration

溢饮 [yì yǐn]

subcutaneous fluid retention: excessive fluid of the body flooding the body surface and muscles

支饮 [zhī yǐn]

thoracic fluid retention: retention of excessive fluid in the lung and chest

伏饮 [fú yǐn]

recurrent fluid retention: a disease marked by frequent attacks of backache, feeling of fullness and distension of the chest and hypochondrium, cough, vomiting, chills and fever

热痰 [rè tán]

heat-phlegm: (1) a morbid condition caused by phlegm in combination with heat; (2) phlegm lingering in the heart meridian, joined and aggravated by heat, giving rise to mania and palpitation

火痰 [huǒ tán]

fire-phlegm: a synonym for heat-phlegm (热痰 [rè tán])

顽痰 [wán tán]

stubborn fluid retention: chronic case of phlegm retention difficult to cure, e.g., bronchial asthma with repeated attacks, mania, and epilepsy

肺痈 [fèi yōng]

lung abscess: abscess occurring in the lung, marked by fever, cough, chest pain, expectoration of foul turbid or bloody purulent sputum

肺胀 [fèi zhàng]

lung distension: a disease of the lung characterized by persistent accumulation of air in the lung, resulting from chronic cough or asthma, manifested by distension sensation in the chest, profuse expectoration, shortness of breath upon mild exertion, cyanosis or even edema of limbs, including pulmonary emphysema and pulmonary heart disease

肺萎 [fèi wěi]

lung atrophy: a disease of the lung due to chronic cough, marked by atrophy of the lung with shortness of breath and expectoration

虚劳(病) [xū láo (bìng)]

consumptive disease: a disease characterized by consumption, either infectious or non-infectious, the latter also known as 虚损 [xū sǔn], and the former 劳(痨)瘵 [láo zhài]

虚损 [xū sǔn]

consumption: deficiency and impairment of yin, yang, *qi* or blood in *zang-fu* organs, usually due to non-infectious factors

劳(痨)瘵 [láo zhài]

phthisis: chronic infectious consumptive diseases such as pulmonary tuberculosis

痨病 [láo bìng]

phthisis (disease): old name for pulmonary tuberculosis

骨蒸 [gǔ zhēng]

bone steaming: a term for hectic fever with night sweats, as seen in consumptive diseases

劳倦 [láo juàn]

overexertion syndrome: a morbid state caused by overexertion, manifested by fatigue, lassitude, fidgetiness, shortness of breath upon exertion, and spontaneous sweating

劳伤 [láo shāng]

overstrain consumption, synonymous with 劳倦 [láo juàn]

五劳 [wǔ láo]

(1) five kinds of strain: protracted looking, lying, sitting, standing or walking for too long a time; **(2) five kinds of consumptive diseases:** consumption of the lung, liver, heart, spleen, and kidney

肺痨 [fèi láo]

lung phthisis: wasting away of the lung, old name for pulmonary tuberculosis

肺劳 [fèi láo]

(1) lung consumption: a consumptive disease of the lung due to overstrain, manifested by cough, shortness of breath, back pain, lassitude and emaciation; **(2) lung phthisis,** also known as 肺痨 [fèi láo]

肝劳 [gān láo]

liver consumption: a disease due to impairment of the liver by emotional upset, manifested by blurred vision, pain in the chest and hypochondrium, flaccid muscles and tendons, and difficulty in movement

心劳 [xīn láo]

heart consumption: a consumptive disease of the heart marked by exhaustion of the heart blood due to overstrain, manifested by fidgetiness, insomnia, palpitation, and liability to be affected by panic

脾劳 [pí láo]

spleen consumption: a consumptive disease of the spleen due to improper diet or mental stress, marked by muscular wasting, weakness of limbs, anorexia, abdominal distension, and loose stools

肾劳 [shèn láo]

kidney consumption: a consumptive disease of the kidney due to excessive sexual activity, marked by lumbago, spermatorrhea or menoxenia, night sweats, hectic fever, and weakness in the legs

虚烦 [xū fán]

fidgetiness of deficiency type: fidgetiness due to deficiency of yin which brings on endogenous heat

虚热 [xū rè]

fever of deficiency type: fever due to deficiency of yin, yang, *qi* or blood

内伤发热 [nèi shāng fā rè]

internally damaged fever: fever due to disorder of internal organs caused by emotional stress, improper diet, overwork, sexual intemperance, etc.

阴虚发热 [yīn xū fā rè]

yin-deficiency fever: fever due to yin deficiency, marked by appearance of fever in the afternoon or at night, sensation of heat in the chest, palms and soles, accompanied by night sweats, dryness in the mouth, reddened tongue, and thready rapid pulse

阳虚发热 [yáng xū fā rè]

yang-deficiency fever: fever due to yang deficiency, marked by appearance of fever in the morning, accompanied by spontaneous sweating, intolerance of wind, lassitude, anorexia, and feeble pulse

血虚发热 [xuè xū fā rè]

blood-deficiency fever: fever due to blood deficiency, marked by low fever with dizziness, lassitude, palpitations, pallor, pale tongue, and thin weak pulse

劳蒸 [láo zhēng]

consumptive steaming fever: hectic fever due to consumption

干血痨 [gān xuè láo]

consumption with blood deficiency and stasis: a consumptive disease seen mostly in women, often accompanied by menopenia or amenorrhea

心悸 [xīn jì]

palpitation: a subjective feeling of unduly rapid or violent heart beat

惊悸 [jīng jì]

fright palpitation: palpitation ascribed to being frightened

怔忡 [zhèng zhòng]

fearful throbbing: a severe case of palpitation

胸痛 [xiōng tòng]

chest pain

胸痹 [xiōng bì]

chest *qi*-blockage: pectoral pain, sometimes accompanied by a feeling of suffocation

胸痹心痛 [xiōng bì xīn tòng]

***qi*-blocked heartache:** angina pectoris

真心痛 [zhēn xīn tòng]

true heartache: angina pectoris, so named to distinguish it from gastralgia which was also called heartache in ancient times

厥心痛 [jué xīn tòng]

heartache with cold limbs: (1) extreme pain in the heart leading to collapse with cold limbs; (2) heartache caused by cold that blocks the *qi* flow, manifested as cold limbs

冷心痛 [lěng xīn tòng]

cold heartache: severe pain in the region over the heart, accompanied by cold limbs and cold sweats

肝郁胁痛 [gān yù xié tòng]

hypochondriac pain due to liver stagnation: a type of hypochondriac pain mostly caused by emotional upset, accompanied by stuffiness feeling in the chest, poor appetite and wiry pulse, also known as 肝气胁痛 [gān qì xié tòng]

肝气胁痛 [gān qì xié tòng]

hypochondriac pain due to liver *qi*: a synonym for hypochondriac pain due to liver stagnation (肝郁胁痛 [gā yù xié tòng])

汗证 [hàn zhèng]

sweating syndrome: a state characterized by abnormal sweating due to yin-yang disharmony or infirmity of the subcutaneous interstices and pores, also known as sweating disease (汗病 [hàn bìng])

汗病 [hàn bìng]

sweating disease: a synonym for sweating syndrome (汗证 [hàn zhèng])

自汗 [zì hàn]

spontaneous sweating: abnormal sweating in the daytime aggravated by mild exertion and unconnected with environmental factors

盗汗 [dào hàn]

night sweats: sweating during sleep which stops upon awakening

脱汗 [tuō hàn]

sweating in shock: profuse sweating associated with listlessness, cold limbs, and hardly perceivable pulse, usually occurring in a critical case

战汗 [zhàn hàn]

sweating following rigors: a type of sweating occurring in cases of acute febrile diseases, characterized by sudden occurrence of shivering chills and then generalized sweating, indicating a sharp struggle of normal *qi* against the pathogen

黄汗 [huáng hàn]

yellow sweat: yellow-colored sweat associated with bitterness and stickiness in the mouth, thirst but no desire to drink, yellow and greasy tongue coating, ascribed to the interior accumulation of damp-heat

气虚自汗 [qì xū zì hàn]

spontaneous sweating in *qi* deficiency: spontaneous sweating resulting from deficiency of defensive *qi*, usually accompanied by fatigue, weakness and aversion to wind

阳虚自汗 [yáng xū zì hàn]

spontaneous sweating in yang deficiency: an abnormal state characterized by spontaneous sweating accompanied by aversion to cold

阴虚盗汗 [yīn xū dào hàn]

night sweats in yin deficiency: night sweats resulting from deficiency of yin with exuberant yang which stimulates the discharge of sweat while sleeping when the defensive *qi* goes inward

眩晕 [xuàn yùn]

(1) dizziness: the disordered state characterized by a sensation of unsteadiness with a feeling of movement within the head; **(2) vertigo:** more serious state characterized by a sensation that either the environment or one's own body is revolving

风寒眩晕 [fēng hán xuàn yùn]

wind-cold dizziness [vertigo]: dizziness or vertigo due to exogenous affection by wind-cold, usually accompanied by headache, joint pain or general aching, and aversion to wind and cold

风热眩晕 [fēng rè xuàn yùn]

wind-heat dizziness [vertigo]: dizziness or vertigo due to upward drive of pathogenic wind-heat, often accompanied by distress in the chest and vomiting, and even fainting

肝阳眩晕 [gān yáng xuàn yùn]

liver yang dizziness [vertigo]: intermittent dizziness or vertigo due to up-rising of liver yang, often accompanied by headache, insomnia, irritability and wiry pulse

肝火眩晕 [gān huǒ xuàn yùn]

liver fire dizziness [vertigo]: dizziness or vertigo due to liver fire induced by an emotional upset, usually accompanied by headache, blood-shot eyes, irritability, bitter taste in the mouth, reddened tongue with yellowish coating, wiry and rapid pulse

风痰眩晕 [fēng tán xuàn yùn]

wind-phlegm dizziness [vertigo]: dizziness or vertigo ascribed to wind-phlegm, usually accompanied by headache, blurred vision, tightness of the chest, palpitations, vomiting, and expectoration of sticky sputum

肾虚眩晕 [shèn xū xuàn yùn]

kidney-insufficiency dizziness [vertigo]: dizziness or vertigo due to inadequate kidney essence for nourishing the brain, usually accompanied by tinnitus, listlessness, forgetfulness and weakness of the loins and legs

血虚眩晕 [xuè xū xuàn yùn]

blood-deficiency dizziness [vertigo]: dizziness or vertigo ascribed to blood deficiency, marked by aggravation on exertion, pallor, insomnia, pale tongue and thready pulse

气虚眩晕 [qì xū xuàn yùn]

***qi*-deficiency dizziness [vertigo]:** dizziness or vertigo ascribed to *qi* deficiency, marked by aggravation upon exertion, listlessness, poor appetite, pale tongue and weak pulse

感暑眩晕 [gǎn shǔ xuàn yùn]

summer-heat dizziness [vertigo]: dizziness or vertigo due to affection by summer-heat, also known as 中暑眩晕 [zhòng shǔ xuàn yùn]

中暑眩晕 [zhòng shǔ xuàn yùn]

heat-stroke dizziness [vertigo]: a synonym for summer-heat dizziness [vertigo] (感暑眩晕 [gǎn shǔ xuàn yùn])

头痛 [tóu tòng]

headache: pain in the head either due to external contraction or internal injury

真头痛 [zhēn tóu tòng]

real headache: severe pain in the head

头风 [tóu fēng]

recurrent headache: chronic headache with repeated recurrence

偏头风 [piān tóu fēng]

migraine: unilateral headache

雷头风 [léi tóu fēng]

thunder-headache: pain with loud noise in the head

外感头痛 [waì gǎn tóu tòng]

externally contracted headache: various types of headache ascribed to exogenous afflictions

风寒头痛 [fēng hán tóu tòng]

wind-cold headache: headache due to attack of external wind-cold, marked by pain in the head extending to the nape and back, aversion to cold and wind, soreness and pain in the joints, watery nasal discharge, thin and whitish tongue coating and floating tense pulse

风热头痛 [fēng rè tóu tòng]

wind-heat headache: headache due to attack of external wind-heat, usually associated with fever, thirst, constipation, floating and rapid pulse

风湿头痛 [fēng shī tóu tòng]

wind-damp headache: headache due to attack of external wind-damp, marked by pain in the head as if it were tightly bound, accompanied by heaviness in the limbs, stuffiness in the chest, anorexia, white greasy tongue coating, and soft pulse

痰浊头痛 [tán zhuó tóu tòng]

phlegm-turbidity headache: headache resulting from turbid phlegm, marked by pain and distension of the head associated with stuffiness in the chest, nausea, expectoration, white greasy tongue coating, and slippery pulse

内伤头痛 [nèi shāng tóu tòng]

internal damage headache: headache marked by slow onset and intermittent recurrence, accompanied by deficiency syndromes of *qi*, blood, or *zang-fu* organs, or with manifestations indicating presence of endogenous pathogenic factors

肝阳头痛 [gān yáng tóu tòng]

liver yang headache: headache ascribed to exuberant liver yang, usually accompanied by dizziness, irritability, irascibility, disturbed sleep and wiry pulse

风痰头痛 [fēng tán tóu tòng]

wind-phlegm headache: headache ascribed to wind-phlegm, usually accompanied by dizziness, heaviness of the body, distress in the chest and expectoration of sticky sputum

气虚头痛 [qì xū tóu tòng]

***qi*-deficiency headache:** headache ascribed to *qi* deficiency, usually aggravated during exertion, accompanied by anorexia and lassitude

瘀血头痛 [yū xuè tóu tòng]

stagnant-blood headache: chronic headache, stabbing in character and fixed in location, often occurring after a traumatic injury

血虚头痛 [xuè xū tóu tòng]

blood-deficiency headache: headache ascribed to blood deficiency, marked by dull pain in the head, usually accompanied by dizziness, pallor and palpitation

百合病 [bǎi hé bìng]

"lily disease": ancient term for neurosis with mental strain, listlessness, sleeplessness, anorexia, sham heat and sham cold, bitterness in the mouth, yellow urine, rapid pulse, etc. It is so called because it can be effectively treated by administering *Bulbus Lilii*.

癫狂 [diān kuáng]

depressive-manic psychosis: a term referring to depression and mania in combination

癫病 [diān bìng]

depressive psychosis: a mental disorder characterized by severe depression, often abbreviated as depression in the strict and serious sense (癫 [diān])

癫 [diān]

depression: that used in the strict and serious sense, a synonym for depressive psychosis

狂病 [kuáng bìng]

manic psychosis: a psychotic disorder characterized by mental and physical hyperactivity, disorganization of behavior, and elevation of mood, often abbreviated as mania (狂 [kuáng])

狂 [kuáng]

mania: abbreviation for manic psychosis (狂病 [kuáng bìng])

痫病 [xián bìng]

epilepsy (disease): a disease or syndrome characterized by paroxysmal transient loss of consciousness with generalized tonic-clonic seizures, up-staring of the eyes and stertorous breathing, often preceded by an aura, also called 痫证 [xián zhèng], 癫痫 [diān xián] and 羊痫风 [yang xián fēng]

痫证 [xián zhèng]

epilepsy (syndrome), same as 痫病 [xián bìng]

癫痫 [diān xián]

epilepsy: a synonym for 痫病 [xián bìng]

羊痫风 [yáng xián fēng]

"bleating convulsion": a popular name for epilepsy

阳痫 [yáng xián]

yang epilepsy: epilepsy associated with a yang syndrome

阴痫 [yīn xián]

yin epilepsy: epilepsy associated with a yin syndrome

惊痫 [jīng xián]

fright epilepsy: (1) epilepsy induced by fright; (2) infantile convulsion

脏躁 [zàng zào]

hysteria: a morbid condition characterized by violent emotional paroxysms, anxiety, and disturbances of the sensory and motor functions

梅核气 [méi hé qì]

"plum-stone" syndrome; globus hystericus: disturbing subjective sensation of a lump in the throat commonly experienced in hysteria

奔豚 [bēn tún]

"running piglet": an ancient name for the morbid condition characterized by a feeling of masses of gas ascending within the abdomen like running piglets

嗜睡 [shì shuì]

somnolence: excessive sleepiness

失眠 [shī mián]

insomnia: prolonged inability to obtain normal sleep, also known as 不得卧 [bù dé wò]

不得卧 [bù dé wò]

inability to sleep: a synonym for insomnia (失眠 [shī mián])

肝火不得卧 [gān huǒ bù dé wò]

liver fire insomnia: insomnia with dream-disturbed sleep and irritability due to exuberant liver fire

心血虚不得卧 [xīn xuè xū bù dé wò]

heart blood deficiency insomnia: insomnia with abnormal wakefulness and forgetfulness due to deficiency of heart blood

心气虚不得卧 [xīn qì xū bù dé wò]

heart *qi* deficiency insomnia: insomnia with fidgetiness, lassitude, spontaneous sweating due to deficiency of heart *qi*

健忘 [jiàn wàng]

amnesia: loss of memory, also known as forgetfulness (善忘 [shàn wàng])

善忘 [shàn wàng]

forgetfulness: a synonym for amnesia (健忘 [jiàn wàng])

痴呆 [chī dāi]

dementia: a condition of deteriorated mentality characterized by marked decline of the intellectual function and emotional apathy

卒中 [cù zhōng]

stroke: a sudden and severe attack, as of cerebral apoplexy

中风 [zhòng fēng]

wind-stroke; apoplexy: a sudden and severe attack affecting the brain due to blockage of or hemorrhage from the cerebral vessel

中风病 [zhòng fēng bìng]

stroke syndrome: a synonym for wind-stroke (中风 [zhòng fēng])

中风闭证 [zhòng fēng bì zhèng]

block pattern of wind-stroke: a pattern of wind-stroke characterized by blockage of the orifices manifested by loss of consciousness, trismus, spastic tonus of the limbs, pertaining to an excess condition which can be further classified into yin block and yang block

中风阴闭 [zhòng fēng yīn bì]

yin block of wind-stroke: blocking of the orifices by damp-phlegm in wind-stroke, manifested by pallor, lying in quiescence, cool limbs, excessive secretion in the mouth, and white greasy tongue coating

中风阳闭 [zhòng fēng yáng bì]

yang block of wind-stroke: blocking of the orifices by phlegm-heat in wind-stroke, manifested by fever, flushing face, coarse breathing, foul breath, restlessness and yellow greasy tongue coating

中风脱证 [zhòng fēng tuō zhèng]

prostration pattern of stroke: a pattern of wind-stroke characterized by prostration of yang *qi* during the attack, manifested by loss of consciousness, closed eyes with opened mouth, flaccid paralysis of the limbs, profuse cold sweats, incontinence of urine and feces, and faint breathing

真中风 [zhēn zhòng fēng]

true wind-stroke: apoplexy caused by exogenous pathogenic wind marked by sudden loss of consciousness, wry mouth, hemiplegia and aphasia, often abbreviated as true stroke (真中 [zhēn zhòng])

真中 [zhēn zhòng]

true stroke: abbreviation of true wind-stroke (真中风 [zhēn zhòng fēng])

类中风 [lèi zhòng fēng]

apoplectoid wind-stroke: apoplexy caused by endogenous pathogenic wind, usually ascribed to internal stirring of liver wind or transformation of damp-phlegm into heat and wind, also abbreviated as apoplectoid stroke (类中 [lèi zhòng])

类中 [lèi zhòng]

apoplectoid stroke: abbreviation of apoplectoid wind-stroke (类中风 [lèi zhòng fēng])

中脏 [zhòng zàng]

***zang*-(organ) stroke:** very serious form of apoplexy with sudden loss of consciousness, aphasia, and paralysis of lips with salivation

中腑 [zhòng fǔ]

fu-(organ) stroke: serious form of apoplexy with onset of fainting, hemiplegia, distortion of the face and dysphasia

中经 [zhòng jīng]

meridian stroke: mild form of apoplexy with paralysis of the face and limbs, dysphasia, but no impairment of consciousness

中络 [zhòng luò]

collateral stroke: mildest form of apoplexy with slight distortion of the face and numbness of limbs

口噤 [kǒu jìn]

trismus: lockjaw with difficulty in opening the mouth

失语 [shī yǔ]

aphasia: loss of the ability of expression by speech

偏枯 [piān kū]

hemiplegia: paralysis of one side of the body

半身不遂 [bàn shēn bù suí]

hemiplegia, same as 偏枯 [piān kū]

口呙僻不遂 [wāi pì bù suí]

hemiplegia with wry mouth: paralysis of one side of the body with retraction of the angle of the mouth, which often occurs after stroke

口僻 [kǒu pì]

deviation of the mouth: retraction of the angle of the mouth in unilateral facial paralysis, also known as wry mouth 口呙 [kǒu wāi]

口呙 [kǒu wāi]

wry mouth: a synonym for deviation of the mouth 口僻 [kǒu pì]

麻木 [má mù]

numbness: reduced sensibility to touch. Strictly speaking, 麻 [má] and 木 [mù] have different meanings, the former referring to a tingling sensation, while the latter to loss of the ability to feel and move; but the term composed of the two characters in combination often means loss of sensation or numbness.

中风昏迷 [zhòng fēng hūn mí]

apoplectic coma: coma occurring in wind-stroke

厥 [jué]

(1) syncope: temporary loss of consciousness; **(2) cold limbs**

厥证 [jué zhèng]

syncope: a morbid state characterized by temporary loss of consciousness with cold limbs resulting from disordered flow of *qi* and blood

食厥 [shí jué]

crapulent syncope: syncope due to eating and drinking too much at one sitting

气厥 [qì jué]

qi **syncope:** syncope induced by emotional upset or spiritual stimulation, marked by sudden fainting, loss of consciousness, cold limbs, trismus, thin white tongue coating

血厥 [xuè jué]

blood syncope: syncope following a fit of rage that causes an upward reverse flow of *qi* and blood, marked by flushed face and stringy forceful pulse

痰厥 [tán jué]

phlegm syncope: syncope occurring after a fit of serious coughing in one with chronic cough, asthma and expectoration, marked by gurgling sounds in the throat, white greasy tongue coating and deep slippery pulse

昏厥 [hūn jué]

fainting: sudden loss of consciousness

手足厥冷 [shǒu zú jué lěng]

cold limbs in syncope: cold limbs up to above the knees and elbows with sudden loss of consciousness, occurring in syncope or shock, also called reversed cold limbs 手足逆冷 [shǒu zú nì lěng] and abbreviated as 四逆 [sì nì]

手足逆冷 [shǒu zú nì lěng]

reversed cold limbs: a synonym for cold limbs in syncope 手足厥冷 [shǒu zú jué lěng]

四逆 [sì nì]

abbreviation of 手足厥冷 [shǒu zú jué lěng]

蛔厥 [huí jué]

ascariasis syncope: syncope due to acute abdominal pain caused by ascarides, as seen in cases of biliary ascariasis

热厥 [rè jué]

heat collapse: collapse due to excessive pathogenic heat in the interior of the body, a symptom of syncope or shock in cases of acute febrile diseases

痉病 [jìng bìng]

convulsive disease: a diseased state characterized by rigidity of the nape, convulsion of the limbs and opisthotonos

热甚发痉 [rè shèn fā jìng]

febrile convulsion: convulsion induced by high fever

抽搐 [chōu chù]

convulsion: a violent involuntary contraction or series of contractions

痿 [wěi]

atrophy-flaccidity: flaccid paralysis with muscular atrophy

痿病 [wěi bìng]

atrophy-flaccidity (disease): a diseased condition characterized by flaccid paralysis with muscular atrophy of a limb

痿证 [wěi zhèng]

atrophy-flaccidity (syndrome): a syndrome characterized by flaccid paralysis with muscular atrophy of a limb

痿躄 [wěi bì]

atrophic crippling: crippling with muscular atrophy of a lower limb

脚弱 [jiǎo ruò]

leg weakness: lack of strength with muscular atrophy of a lower limb

脚气 [jiǎo qì]

(1) leg flaccidity; (2) beriberi

脚气冲心 [jiǎo jì chōng xīn]

beriberi involving the heart: a serious case of beriberi with heart failure, manifested by palpitation and shortness of breath

筋痿 [jīn wěi]

tendon atrophy-flaccidity: one of the atrophy-flaccidity syndromes ascribed to the exuberant liver heat which wilts the tendons with contracture of the limbs, also called liver atrophy-flaccidity (肝痿 [gān wěi])

肝痿 [gān wěi]

liver atrophy-flaccidity: another name for tendon atrophy-flaccidity (筋痿 [jīn wěi])

脉痿 [mài wěi]

vessel atrophy-flaccidity: one of the atrophy-flaccidity syndromes ascribed to the up-flaming of heart fire with emptiness of blood vessels in the lower part that makes the legs extremely flaccid and unable to support the body's weight, also called heart atrophy-flaccidity (心痿 [xīn wěi])

心痿 [xīn wěi]

heart atrophy-flaccidity: another name for vessel atrophy-flaccidity (脉痿 [mài wěi])

肉痿 [ròu wěi]

muscle atrophy-flaccidity: one of the atrophy-flaccidity syndromes ascribed to heat or damp in the spleen that causes damage to the muscles and leads to numbness or even immobility of the limbs, also called spleen atrophy-flaccidity (脾痿 [pí wěi])

脾痿 [pí wěi]

spleen atrophy-flaccidity: another name for muscle atrophy-flaccidity (肉痿 [ròu wěi])

骨痿 [gǔ wěi]

bone atrophy-flaccidity: one of the atrophy-flaccidity syndromes ascribed to impairment of the kidney with consumption of essence, manifested by limpness of the loins and flaccidity of the legs with inability to walk, also called kidney atrophy-flaccidity (肾痿 [shèn wěi])

肾痿 [shèn wěi]

kidney atrophy-flaccidity: another name for bone atrophy-flaccidity (骨痿 [gǔ wěi])

颤震[振] [chàn zhèn]

tremor: a diseased state characterized by involuntary shaking or trembling of the head or hands, also called 振掉 [zhèn diào]

振掉 [zhèn diào]

a synonym for 颤震 [chàn zhèn]

痹(病) [bì (bìng)]

(1) blockage disease: a diseased state characterized by invasion of the pathogenic factors that cause stagnation of *qi* and blood and blockage of the collateral meridians ; **(2) arthralgia:** blockage disease in the narrow sense involving the joints of the limbs, marked by joint pain with difficulty in movement

历节风 [lì jié fēng]

arthritis: swollen and painful joints with limitation in motion, including acute rheumatic arthritis, rheumatoid arthritis and gout

三痹 [sān bì]

three kinds of arthralgia: arthralgia caused by wind, cold and damp, respectively

热痹 [rè bì]

heat arthralgia: arthritis due to heat, marked by pain, heat, redness and swelling of the joints, usually accompanied by fever

尫痹(病) [wāng bì (bìng)]

ankylosing arthralgia: a disease characterized by arthralgia with joint deformities

骨痹(病) [gǔ bì (bìng)]

bone blockage (disease): a disease characterized by the invasion of pathogenic wind-cold-dampness to the bones that produces severe joint pain with cold sensation and difficulty in moving, synonymous with cold arthralgia (寒痹 [hán bì]) and agonizing arthralgia (痛痹 [tòng bì])

肌痹(病) [jī bì (bìng)]

muscle blockage (disease): a disease characterized by invasion of the joints and superficial muscles by cold-damp, synonymous with damp arthralgia (湿痹 [shī bì]) and detained arthralgia (着痹 [zhuó bì])

风痹 [fēng bì]

wind arthralgia: arthralgia ascribed to invasion by wind, marked by migratory joint pains, also called migratory arthralgia (行痹 [xíng bì])

行痹 [xíng bì]

migratory arthralgia: another name for wind arthralgia (风痹 [fēng bì])

寒痹 [hán bì]

cold arthralgia: severe joint pain exaggerated by cold, also known as agonizing arthralgia (痛痹 [tòng bì])

痛痹 [tòng bì]

agonizing arthralgia: a synonym for cold arthralgia (寒痹 [hán bì])

湿痹 [shī bì]

damp arthralgia: arthralgia ascribed to invasion by dampness, marked by swelling with heavy sensation in the joints with fixed or localized pain, also known as detained arthralgia (着痹 [zhuó bì])

着痹 [zhuó bì]

detained arthralgia: another name for damp arthralgia (湿痹 [shī bì])

肝胃气痛 [gān wèi qì tòng]

liver *qi* gastralgia: pain in the stomach ascribed to the perverted flow of liver *qi*, usually related to emotional disturbance

胃痛 [wèi tòng]

gastralgia: pain in the stomach

胃脘痛 [wèi wǎn tòng]

epigastric pain: a state characterized by pain in the epigastric region

痞满 [pǐ mǎn]

stuffiness: an abnormal state characterized by a tight and full sensation due to impairment of *qi* movement or retention of *qi*, often in the middle energizer, and sometimes in the chest

实痞 [shí pǐ]

stuffiness (syndrome) of excess type: stuffiness caused by accumulation of pathogenic factors

虚痞 [xū pǐ]

stuffiness (syndrome) of deficiency type: stuffiness without accumulation of pathogenic factors

胃痞 [wèi pǐ]

stomach stuffiness: stuffiness in the stomach region, also called epigastric stuffiness (心下痞 [xīn xià pǐ])

心下痞 [xīn xià pǐ]

epigastric stuffiness: a synonym for stomach stuffiness (胃痞 [wèi pǐ])

呕吐 [ǒu tù]

vomiting: forcible expulsion of the stomach contents through the mouth. Making sounds of vomiting while casting up the matter from the stomach is called 呕 [ǒu], and vomiting without sound is 吐 [tù]

热呕 [rè ǒu]

heat vomiting: vomiting immediately after taking food due to accumulated heat in the stomach or attack on the stomach by evil heat

寒呕 [hán ǒu]

cold vomiting: vomiting due to invasion of the stomach by cold or deficiency-cold of the stomach, characterized by vomiting upon exposure to cold or long after eating, cyanotic complexion and coolness of limbs

泛酸 [fàn suān]

acid regurgitation: flow of the acid gastric contents in the opposite direction – from the stomach to the mouth

吐酸 [tù suān]

acid vomiting: vomiting of the acid gastric contents in the reverse flow — from the stomach to the mouth

吞酸 [tūn suān]

acid swallowing: swallowing of the acid gastric contents flowing backward — from the stomach to the mouth

嘈杂 [cáo zá]

gastric upset: disturbed feeling in the stomach, often accompanied by acid regurgitation

呃逆 [è nì]

hiccup; hiccough: upward reversion of stomach *qi* with an involuntary movement of the diaphragm, causing a characteristic sound

反胃 [fǎn wèi]

regurgitation: flowing back of the stomach contents into the mouth

噎嗝 [yē gé]

dysphagia: difficulty in swallowing caused by narrowing or obstruction of the esophagus, also called 膈噎 [gé yē] or 鬲咽 [gé yān]

膈噎 [gé yē]

dysphagia: same as 噎嗝 [yē gé]

鬲咽 [gé yān]

aphagopraxia: another name for dysphagia (噎嗝 [yē gé])

上膈 [shàng gé]

upper obstruction: obstruction in the upper portion, characterized by vomiting instantly after intake of food

下膈 [xià gé]

lower obstruction: obstruction in the lower portion, characterized by vomiting in the evening of undigested food taken during the day

伤食 [shāng shí]

dyspepsia: indigestion caused by improper diet or overeating

伤食证 [shāng shí zhèng]

dyspepsia (syndrome): a syndrome characterized by indigestion ascribed to improper diet or overeating

宿食 [sù shí]

food retention: a synonym for food stagnation (食滞 [shí zhì])

食滞 [shí zhì]

food stagnation: retention of undigested food in the stomach and intestines, also known as food stagnancy (停食 [tíng shí]) and food retention (宿食 [sù shí])

食积 [shí jī]

food aggregation: a diseased state characterized by the piling up of undigested food in the stomach and intestines, bringing about abdominal distension and pain, vomiting, diarrhea and anorexia

停食 [tíng shí]

food stagnancy, same as food stagnation (食滞 [shí zhì])

关格 [guān gé]

block-rejection: (1) anuria and vomiting occurring simultaneously; (2) simultaneous retention of urine and stool; (3) very strong pulse indicating divorce of yin and yang

关格(病) [guān gé (bìng)]

anuria with vomiting: diseased state characterized by anuria and incessant vomiting

吐矢 [tù shǐ]

vomiting of fecal matter: a symptom seen in intestinal obstruction

便秘 [biàn mì]

constipation: infrequent or difficult evacuation of the feces

脾约 [pí yuē]

splenic constipation: infrequent passage of dry hardened feces as a consequence of dysfunction of the spleen

实秘 [shí mì]

constipation of excess type: a collective term referring to various types of constipation ascribed to pathogenic factors such as heat, cold, stagnant *qi* and phlegm

虚秘 [xū mì]

constipation of deficiency type: a collective term for various types of constipation related to deficiency conditions, such as deficiency of *qi*, yang or yin, usually seen in aged or debilitated subjects or postpartum cases

热秘 [rè mì]

heat constipation: a type of constipation accompanied by fever, flushed face, thirst, abdominal distension, yellow and dry tongue coating

气秘 [qì mì]

***qi* constipation:** (1) constipation due to stagnation of *qi*, accompanied by frequent eructation, stuffiness in the chest, impaired appetite, and even abdominal pain; (2) constipation due to deficiency of *qi*, marked by difficulty in defecation while the feces are neither dry nor hard, usually accompanied by other symptoms of *qi* deficiency

痰秘 [tán mì]

phlegm constipation: a type of constipation accompanied by stuffy sensation in the chest, dyspnea, and sweating from the head, ascribed to accumulation of phlegm and damp-heat in the intestines

冷秘 [lěng mì]

cold constipation: a type of constipation ascribed to the binding of yin cold in the intestines, also known as yin binding (阴结 [yīn jié]) or cold binding (寒结 [hán jié]), manifested by difficulty in passage of feces with abdominal colic, distension, tenderness and cold limbs

寒结 [hán jié]

cold binding: a synonym for cold constipation (冷秘 [lěng mì])

阴结 [yīn jié]

yin binding: a synonym for cold constipation (冷秘 [lěng mì])

泄泻(病) [xiè xiè (bìng)]

diarrhea (disease): a diseased condition characterized by abnormal frequency and liquidity of fecal discharge

暴泻(病) [bào xiè (bìng)]

sudden diarrhea (disease): a diseased condition characterized by sudden onset of diarrhea

久泄 [jiǔ xiè]

chronic diarrhea: diarrhea lasting for a long time or continually recurring

五更泻 [wǔ gēng xiè]

fifth-watch diarrhea: diarrhea occurring daily before dawn, usually due to deficiency of vital gate fire (kidney yang) to warm the spleen

下利清谷 [xià lì qīng gǔ]

diarrhea with undigested food: frequent discharge of fluid stools containing undigested food

滑泄 [huá xiè]

(1) **incessant diarrhea:** chronic diarrhea with fecal incontinence;

(2) **spermatorrhea,** same as 滑精 [huá jīng]

飧泄 [sūn xiè]

lienteric diarrhea: diarrhea due to spleen insufficiency induced by stagnancy of liver *qi*, marked by watery stool containing undigested food, borborygmi and abdominal pain

脾虚泄泻 [pí xū xiè xiè]

spleen-insufficiency diarrhea: recurrent diarrhea with stools containing undigested food, aggravated by eating fatty food, and marked by sallow complexion, lassitude, pale tongue with whitish coating, and weak pulse

肾虚泄泻 [shèn xū xiè xiè]

kidney-insufficiency diarrhea: chronic diarrhea occurring before dawn daily, accompanied by abdominal pain and borborygmi, aversion to cold and cold limbs

湿热泄泻 [shī rè xiè xiè]

damp-heat diarrhea: diarrhea due to accumulation of pathogenic damp-heat in the intestines, usually accompanied by burning sensation in the anus, scanty deep-colored urine, and yellowish greasy tongue coating

伤食泄泻 [shāng shí xiè xiè]

indigestion diarrhea: diarrhea occurring as a result of impairment of the stomach and spleen by immoderate eating and drinking, usually accompanied by belching with fetid odor, abdominal distension and pain, and thick greasy tongue coating

虚寒泄泻 [xū hán xiè xiè]

deficiency-cold diarrhea: chronic diarrhea accompanied by abdominal pain and borborygmi, aversion to cold, cold limbs, pale tongue with white coating, deep and thready pulse

腹痛 [fù tòng]

abdominal pain: pain in the abdomen below the epigastrium and above the pubic hair

气滞腹痛 [qì zhì fù tòng]

***qi*-stagnation abdominal pain:** abdominal pain unfixed in location, usually aggravated by emotional changes and accompanied by distension, eructation, and wiry pulse

血瘀腹痛 [xuè yū fù tòng]

blood-stasis abdominal pain: persistent abdominal pain fixed in location, accompanied by tenderness, purplish tongue and choppy pulse

寒冷腹痛 [hán lěng fù tòng]

cold abdominal pain: lingering abdominal pain due to the presence of pathogenic cold, which may be aggravated by exposure to cold and alleviated by warmth, also known as 寒气腹痛 [hán qì fù tòng]

寒气腹痛 [hán qì fù tòng]

cold-*qi* abdominal pain: a synonym for cold abdominal pain (寒冷腹痛 [hán lěng fù tòng])

虚寒腹痛 [xū hán fù tòng]

deficiency-cold abdominal pain: a state ascribed to deficiency-cold of the spleen and stomach characterized by lingering abdominal pain on and off, aggravated by hunger and exposure to cold and alleviated by warmth and pressing, often accompanied by lassitude, aversion to cold, loose bowels, pale tongue with whitish coating, and deep thready pulse

食积腹痛 [shí jī fù tòng]

food-retention abdominal pain: abdominal pain due to retention of undigested food

虫积腹痛 [chóng jī fù tòng]

parasitic abdominal pain: abdominal pain due to intestinal parasitosis

胃缓 [wèi huǎn]

relaxed stomach: gastroptosis

肠痈 [cháng yōng]

(1) acute appendicitis; (2) periappendicular abscess

胁痛(病) [xié tong (bìng)]

lateropectoral or **hypochondriac pain:** a diseased state characterized by unilateral or bilateral pain in the lateropectoral or hypochondriac region. It more definitely refers to hypochondriac pain according to its old names 胁下痛 [xié xià tòng] or 季肋痛 [jì lèi tòng].

胁下痛 [xié xià tòng]

hypochondriac pain: pain of the lower part of the lateropectoral region

季肋痛 [jì lèi tòng]

hypochondriac pain: pain over the region of the last few ribs

胆胀(病) [dǎn zhàng (bìng)]

gallbladder distension: a diseased state characterized by obstruction of the gallbladder with right hypochondriac distension and pain

臌胀(病) [gǔ zhàng (bìng)]

abdominal distension: diseased state characterized by distension of the abdomen with gas or fluid

单腹胀 [dān fù zhàng]

simple abdominal distension: abdominal distension without edema of the limbs

气臌 [qì gǔ]

tympanites: abdominal distension with gas

水臌 [shuǐ gǔ]

ascites: abdominal distension with fluid

血臌 [xuè gǔ]

ascites with engorgement: abdominal distension with fluid with varicose veins and vascular spiders

萎黄 [wěi huáng]

sallowness: yellowish and withered complexion often seen in such chronic cases as anemia

萎黄病 [wěi huáng bìng]

sallow disease: a diseased state characterized by yellowish and withered complexion associated with general weakness, lassitude, and loose stools, often seen in such chronic cases as anemia

黄胖 [huáng pàng]

yellowish puffiness: a yellowish puffy complexion often seen in ankylostomiasis, malnutrition and other chronic diseases

黄胖病 [huáng pàng bìng]

yellowish puffy disease: a chronic diseased state characterized by yellowish and puffy complexion, often seen in ankylostomiasis, malnutrition and other chronic diseases

虫积 [chóng jī]

parasitic worm aggregation: painful mass ascribed to the aggregation of parasitic worms in the intestines

狐惑 [hú huò]

"foxy bewitching" ; throat-anus-genital syndrome: an ancient term for a disease resembling Behçet's syndrome

痞块 [pǐ kuài]

stuffy lump: lump in the abdomen with a sensation of stuffiness and fullness, usually caused by undigested food, stagnant blood and retained phlegm

癥瘕积聚 [zhēng jiǎ jī jù]

aggregation-accumulation masses: a collective term for various masses formed in the abdomen

积聚 [jī jù]

aggregation-accumulation: a term referring to mass formation in the abdomen with distension or pain due to *qi* stagnation, blood stasis or retention of phlegm

积证 [jī zhèng]

aggregation syndrome: a syndrome characterized by mass formation in the abdomen, immovable with definite shape and fixed local pain, ascribed to aggregation of pathogenic factors, particularly stagnant blood and turbid phlegm

聚证 [jù zhèng]

accumulation syndrome: syndrome characterized by mass formation in the abdomen, with no definite shape and easily movable accompanied by distending pain, usually ascribed to accumulation of stagnant *qi*

癥瘕 [zhēng jiǎ]

abdominal mass: mass formed in the abdomen, called 癥 [zhēng] if it is an aggregation of stagnant blood with definite shape and fixed pain, and called 瘕 [jiǎ] if it is an accumulation of *qi* that has no fixed shape and is easily movable, or appears and disappears from time to time, with a migratory pain, if ever present

水肿 [shuǐ zhǒng]

edema: (1) an abnormal excess accumulation of fluid in the body, usually ascribed to dysfunction of the lung, spleen, kidney and bladder; (2) any of the morbid states with abnormal excess accumulation of fluid in the body

水肿病 [shuǐ zhǒng bìng]

edematous disease, same as edema (水肿 [shuǐ zhǒng])

水气 [shǐ qì]

water *qi*: (1) an ancient term for edema (水肿 [shuǐ zhǒng]); (2) another name for retained fluid (水饮 [shuǐ yǐn])

水胀 [shuǐ zhàng]

watery distension: a kind of edema marked initially by abdominal distension, and then swelling of the extremities

虚肿 [xū zhǒng]

edema of deficiency: edema occurring in deficiency conditions of the spleen, of the liver and kidney, or of the lung

阳水 [yáng shuǐ]

yang edema: edema due to attack of wind or immersion of water-damp involving the lung and the spleen, respectively, usually with an acute onset and a short course accompanied by heat and excess symptoms

风水 [fēng shuǐ]

wind edema: a type of edema especially of the face and head, ascribed to attack on the lung by pathogenic wind, manifested by sudden onset of edema accompanied by aching joints, fever, chills, and floating pulse

阴水 [yīn shuǐ]

yin edema: edema due to dysfunction of the spleen and the kidney, usually with a gradual onset and a long course, associated with cold and deficiency symptoms

五水 [wǔ shuǐ]

five kinds of edema: edema due to dysfunction of the heart, liver, spleen, lung and kidney, respectively

心水 [xīn shuǐ]

heart edema: edema due to dysfunction of the heart, a variety of edema marked by anasarca, orthopnea and difficulty in lying flat

肝水 [gān shuǐ]

liver edema: edema due to dysfunction of the liver, a variety of edema marked by enlarged abdomen and hypochondriac pain

脾水 [pí shuǐ]

spleen edema: edema due to dysfunction of the spleen, a variety of edema marked by abdominal distension, heaviness of the limbs, lassitude and oliguria

肺水 [fèi shuǐ]

lung edema: edema due to dysfunction of the lung, a variety of edema marked by general anasarca, oliguria, and loose stools

肾水 [shèn shuǐ]

kidney edema: edema due to dysfunction of the kidney, a variety of edema marked by swelling and distension of the abdomen, accompanied by lumbago, oliguria and cold feet

郁病 [yù bìng]

depression; depressive disease: a diseased state characterized by a depressed mood with feelings of despair or uneasiness, caused by emotional factors with stagnant *qi*

血证 [xuè zhèng]

(1) hemorrhagic syndrome: a general term for various hemorrhages; **(2) blood troubles:** group of disorders involving the blood, including bleeding, blood stasis and blood heat

失血 [shī xuè]

loss of blood: a general term for various kinds of profuse bleeding

夺血 [duó xuè]

(1) loss of blood, same as 失血 [shī xuè]; **(2) dehydration of blood:** decrease of the blood volume resulting from massive sweating

鼻衄 [bí nǜ]

epistaxis: hemorrhage from the nose irrelevant to trauma, or vicarious menstruation

齿衄 [chǐ nǜ]

gingival hemorrhage: bleeding from the gums irrelevant to trauma

咳血 [ké xuè]

hemoptysis with coughing: expectoration of blood or blood-stained sputum together with coughing

咯血 [kǎ xuè]

hemoptysis without coughing: spontaneous expectoration of blood without coughing

吐血 [tù xuè]

hematemesis: vomiting of blood

尿血 [niào xuè]

hematuria: discharge of bloody urine or blood streaks in the urine, but with no pain during urination

血尿 [xuè niào]

bloody urine: urine containing blood

便血 [biàn xuè]

hematochezia: bleeding per rectum, including bloody stool and passage of pure blood through the anus

近血 [jìn xuè]

nearby bleeding: bleeding into the alimentary tract near the anus, the discharged blood being fresh red

远血 [yuǎn xuè]

distant bleeding: bleeding into the alimentary tract distant from the anus, the discharged blood being dark or black

蓄血 [xù xuè]

blood accumulation: a disease caused by stagnated blood accumulated in a meridian or an organ, e.g., in the uterus (manifested by distension and pain in the lower abdomen, chills and fever, delirium or other mental disorders at night), or in the middle energizer (manifested by pain, tenderness and resistance to touch over the epigastrium)

紫斑 [zǐ bān]

purpura: (1) any of a group of conditions characterized by ecchymoses or small hemorrhages in the skin and mucous membrane; (2) the purplish discoloration resulting from extravasation of blood in the skin and mucous membrane

血脱 [xuè tuō]

blood prostration: diseased state characterized by pale and withered complexion, dizziness, blurred vision or accompanied by bleeding, usually ascribed to consumption of genuine yin and emptiness of the blood chamber

液脱 [yè tuō]

fluid prostration: a diseased state characterized by extreme consumption of body fluids

消渴(病) [xiāo kě (bìng)]

wasting thirst; diabetes: a general term for diseases characterized by excessive thirst, polyuria, polyphagia with emaciation, but chiefly referring to diabetes mellitus

三消 [sān xiāo]

three types of diabetes: a collective term for diabetes marked by three polys, namely polydipsia, polyphagia and polyuria

上消 [shàng xiāo]

upper wasting-thirst; upper diabetes: diabetes characterized by polydipsia, also called 肺消 [fèi xiāo]

肺消 [fèi xiāo]

lung diabetes: a synonym for upper diabetes (上消 [shàng xiāo])

中消 [zhōng xiāo]

middle wasting-thirst; middle diabetes: diabetes characterized by polyphagia, emaciation, and constipation, also called stomach diabetes (胃消 [wèi xiāo]) or spleen diabetes (脾消 [pí xiāo])

胃消 [wèi xiāo]

stomach diabetes: a synonym for middle diabetes (中消 [zhōng xiāo])

脾消 [pí xiāo]

spleen diabetes: a synonym for middle diabetes (中消 [zhōng xiāo])

下消 [xià xiāo]

lower wasting-thirst; lower diabetes: diabetes characterized by polyuria with thick suspension in the urine, also called kidney diabetes (肾消 [shèn xiāo])

肾消 [shèn xiāo]

kidney diabetes: a synonym for lower diabetes (下消 [xià xiāo])

尿浊 [niào zhuó]

turbid urination: discharge of turbid urine with no difficulty or pain in urination, a condition different from stranguria turbidity or chylous stranguria

淋证 [lìn zhèng]

stranguria: a variety of diseases characterized by frequent, painful and dripping urination

淋浊 [lìn zhuó]

(1) stranguric turbidity: frequent painful discharge of turbid urine and sometimes pus-like fluid, ascribed to the down-pouring of damp-heat and phlegm-turbidity to the bladder; **(2) gonorrhea:** sexually transmitted infection marked by inflammation of the urethral orifice and frequent painful dripping of turbid urine

五淋 [wǔ lìn]

five kinds of stranguria: (1) urolithic stranguria, *qi* stranguria, chylous stranguria, strain stranguria, and heat stranguria; (2) *qi* stranguria, blood stranguria, chylous stranguria, urolithic stranguria, and strain stranguria

石淋 [shí lìn]

urolithic stranguria: painful and difficult urination due to the passage of urinary calculi

气淋 [qì lìn]

***qi* stranguria:** stranguria due to *qi* disorders, either stagnation or deficiency

劳淋 [láo lìn]

strain stranguria: stranguria ascribed to overstrain, marked by dripping of urine with dull pains, usually seen in chronic cases

膏淋 [gāo lìn]

chylous stranguria: painful discharge of turbid, milky urine like rice-water

血淋 [xuè lìn]

blood stranguria: painful discharge of bloody urine

热淋 [rè lìn]

heat stranguria: stranguria ascribed to heat, marked by discharge of reddened urine with acute onset, and accompanied by burning pain and generalized fever

癃闭 [lóng bì]

uroschesis and ischuria: difficulty in urination (癃 [lóng]) or anuria (闭 [bì]), seen in diseases of the urinary bladder and urethra with retention of urine, or in renal failure with extreme suppression of urine secretion

遗精 [yí jīng]

seminal emission: involuntary emission of semen

梦遗 [mèng yí]

nocturnal emission: involuntary emission of semen during sleep

滑精(病) [huá jīng (bìng)]

spermatorrhea: (the diseased state characterized by) involuntary and frequent discharge of semen without copulation

早泄(病) [zǎo xiè (bìng)]

premature ejaculation: (the diseased state characterized by) ejaculation of semen immediately after or even prior to penetration

阳痿(病) [yáng wěi (bìng)]

impotence: an abnormal state of a male characterized by inability to initiate or maintain an erection in sexual intercourse

血精 [xuè jīng]

hemospermia: presence of blood in the semen

不育 [bù yù]

sterility: inability to produce offspring

精冷 [jīng lěng]

frigid semen: diseased state characterized by thin seminal fluid with inadequate spermatozoa due to decline of the life gate fire, which often leads to sterility, also called 精寒 [jīng hán]

精寒 [jīng hán]

cold semen: a synonym for frigid semen 精冷 [jīng lěng]

精少 [jīng shǎo]

scanty semen: (1) defective ejaculation; (2) oligospermia

遗尿(病) [yí niào (bìng)]

enuresis: (the diseased state characterized by) involuntary discharge of urine

腰痛 [yāo tòng]

lumbago: pain in the lumbar region caused by disordered *qi* and blood flow in the related collateral vessels in exogenous afflictions, traumatic injuries or kidney insufficiency

外感腰痛 [wài gǎn yāo tòng]

externally contracted lumbago: pain in the lumbar region ascribed to affection by external factors, such as living in a damp place, exposure to wind after sweating, or rain-drenching

寒湿腰痛 [hán shī yāo tòng]

cold-damp lumbago: lumbago ascribed to attack of cold-damp, manifested by severe pain in the lumbar region together with cold and heavy sensation, aggravated on lying down and on rainy days

湿热腰痛 [shī rè yāo tòng]

damp-heat lumbago: stretching lumbar pain ascribed to attack of damp-heat, usually accompanied by local hotness, thirst but no desire to drink, reddened tongue with yellow greasy coating

风寒腰痛 [fēng hán yāo tòng]

wind-cold lumbago: lumbago ascribed to attack of wind-cold, manifested as the presence of pain together with a cold sensation, ameliorated by warmth and aggravated by cold weather

风热腰痛 [fēng rè yāo tòng]

wind-heat lumbago: pain and heat sensation in the lumbar region, usually accompanied by sore throat, mild sweating and rapid floating pulse

风湿腰痛 [fēng shī yāo tòng]

wind-damp lumbago: lumbar pain ascribed to attack of wind-damp, usually occurring after exposure to wind while sleeping in a damp place, marked by contracture, heaviness and pain in the lower back with limited motility or accompanied by fever and aversion to wind

内伤腰痛 [nèi shāng yāo tòng]

internally injured lumbago: lumbago ascribed to internal injury, such as chronic overstrain, general debility in the aged, overindulgence in sex, and emotional depression

肾虚腰痛 [shèn xū yāo tòng]

kidney-insufficiency lumbago: lumbar pain ascribed to deficiency of kidney *qi* and essence, usually aggravated on exertion and ameliorated upon lying down, and accompanied by weakness of the loins and legs

血虚腰痛 [xuè xū yāo tòng]

blood-deficiency lumbago: pain in the lumbar region ascribed to blood deficiency, usually occurring in women with metrorrhagia

气滞腰痛 [qì zhì yāo tòng]

***qi*-stagnation lumbago:** lumbar pain ascribed to *qi* stagnation, stabbing in character but not fixed in location, often accompanied by distension of the abdomen and hypochondriac regions

血瘀腰痛 [xuè yū yāo tòng]

blood-stasis lumbago: lumbago ascribed to blood stasis, marked by pain with fixed location, ameliorated in the daytime and aggravated at night

腰软 [yāo ruǎn]

lumbar limpness: lack of strength in the lower back, due to either invasion of wind-damp or kidney insufficiency

疝 [shàn]

(1) hernia: protrusion of a part of an organ or tissue from the body cavity through an abnormal opening; **(2) genital disease:** a collective term for diseases of the male and female genitalia; **(3) lower abdominal colic:** severe colicky pain in the lower abdomen usually accompanied by constipation and ischuria

疝气 [shàn qì]

a synonym for 疝 [shàn]

小肠气 [xiǎo cháng qì]

hernia: another name for 疝 [shàn]

妇产科 Gynecology and Obstetrics

胞 [bāo]

(1) uterus; (2) placenta; (3) bladder

玉门 [yù mén]

virginal vaginal orifice: external opening of the vagina in a virgin

龙门 [lóng mén]

nulliparous vaginal orifice: external opening of the vagina in a nulliparous married woman

胞门 [bāo mén]

parous vaginal orifice: external opening of the vagina in a para

产门 [chǎn mén]

parturient vaginal orifice: external opening of the vagina of a parturient

子门 [zǐ mén]

cervical orifice: external opening of the cervix of the uterus into the vagina

人胞 [rén bāo]

placenta: an organ lining the uterus during pregnancy by which the fetus is nourished through the umbilical cord, and which is expelled after birth

胞衣 [bāo yī]

afterbirth: placenta and the membranes, delivered from the uterus after the birth of the child, also called 胎衣 [tāi yī]

胎衣 [tāi yī]

another name for afterbirth (胞衣 [bāo yī])

血室 [xuè shì]

blood chamber: another name for the uterus (胞宫 [bāo gōng])

阴户 [yīn hù]

vulva: region of the external female genital organs including the labia majora, labia minora, mons pubis, clitoris, and vestibule of the vagina

阴道 [yīn dào]

vagina: genital canal in the female, leading from the uterus to the vulva, also called 子肠 [zǐ cháng]

子肠 [zǐ cháng]

another name for the vagina (阴道 [yīn dào])

胞宫 [bāo gōng]

uterus: female organ in which menstruation is formed and the developing fetus is nourished

经带胎产 [jīng dài tāi chǎn]

menstrual disorders, leukorrheal diseases, gravid troubles and parturition problems: the four general categories of gynecological and obstetrical diseases

月经 [yuè jīng]

menstruation: cyclic discharge from the genital tract of a woman, usually at approximately one-month intervals, also called menstrual discharge (经水 [jīng shuǐ]), monthly discharge (月水 [yuè shuǐ]), or "monthly matter" (月事 [yuè shì])

经血 [jīng xuè]

menstrual blood: blood discharged through the vagina during menstruation

经水 [jīng shuǐ]

menstrual discharge: another term for menstruation, also called monthly discharge (月水 [yuè shuǐ])

月水 [yuè shuǐ]

monthly discharge: another term for menstruation, same as menstrual discharge (经水 [jīng shuǐ])

月事 [yuè shì]

"monthly matter": another term for menstruation

并月 [bìng yuè]

bimonthly menstruation: menstruation occurring once every two months

居经 [jū jīng]

tri-monthly menstruation: menstruation occurring once every three months, also called quarterly menstruation (季经 [jì jīng])

季经 [jì jīng]

quarterly menstruation: menstruation occurring once each season, same as tri-monthly menstruation (居经 [jū jīng])

避年 [bì nián]

annual menstruation: menstruation occurring once a year

暗经 [àn jīng]

latent menstruation: absence of menstrual discharge, life-long, but with the potentiality of pregnancy

天癸 [tiān guǐ]

(1) *tiangui;* sex-stimulating essence: a substance that promotes growth, development and reproduction in both sexes; **(2) menstruation**

天癸竭 [tiān guǐ jié]

(1) exhaustion of the sex-stimulating essence; (2) cease of menstruation; menopause

月经病 [yuè jīng bìng]

emmeniopathy: any disorder of menstruation, including abnormal cycles, intervals and amount of discharge as well as accompanying symptoms

月经不调 [yuè jīng bù tiáo]

menstrual irregularities: irregular menstruation and other menstrual complaints

月经先期 [yuè jīng xiān qī]

early periods; polymenorrhea: periods that come one week or more ahead of due time, also known as 经行先期 [jīng xíng xiān qī] or 经早 [jīng zǎo]

经行先期 [jīng xíng xiān qī]

early periods; shortened menstrual cycles: same as 月经先期 [yuè jīng xiān qī]

经早 [jīng zǎo]

abbreviated term for early periods (月经先期 [yuè jīng xiān qī])

血热经行先期 [xuè èr jīng xíng xiān qī]

early periods due to blood heat: periods coming before due time, with massive discharge deep red in color, accompanied by irritability, reddened tongue with yellow coating, and slippery, rapid and forceful pulse

气虚经行先期 [qì xū jīng xíng xiān qī]

early periods due to *qi* deficiency: periods coming before due time, with thin and pinkish discharge, accompanied by lassitude, pallor, pale tongue, and weak pulse

月经后期 [yuè jīng hòu qī]

late periods; oligomenorrhea: periods that come one week or more after due time, also called 经行后期 [jīng xíng hòu qī], 经期错后 [jīng qī cuò hòu], 经迟 [jīng chí]

经行后期 [jīng xíng hòu qī]

late periods: same as 月经后期 [yuè jīng hòu qī]

经期错后 [jīng qī cuò hòu]

lengthened menstrual cycles: same as 月经后期 [yuè jīng hòu qī]

经迟 [jīng chí]

an abbreviated term for 月经后期 [yuè jīng hòu qī]

血寒经行后期 [xuè hán jīng xíng hòu qī]

late periods due to blood cold: periods coming after due time with scanty discharge of dark-colored blood, accompanied by aversion to cold, cold limbs, and lower abdominal pain which is alleviated by warmth

血虚经行后期 [xuè xū jīng xíng hòu qī]

late periods due to blood deficiency: periods coming after due time with scanty discharge of light colored blood, accompanied by sallow complexion, dizziness, pale tongue, and weak, thready pulse

气滞经行后期 [qì zhì jīng xíng hòu qī]

late periods due to *qi* stagnation: periods coming after due time with scanty discharge of normal-colored blood, accompanied by mammary distension, discomfort in the chest, hypochondriac pain and distending pain in the lower abdomen

月经先后无定期 [yuè jīng xiān hòu wú dìng qī]

irregular periods; irregular menstrual cycle: periods that come with an irregular cycle, more than one week early or later, also called 经乱 [jīng luàn]

经乱 [jīng luàn]

a shortened term for irreguair periods (月经先后无定期 [yuè jīng xiān hòu wú dìng qī])

月经过少 [yuè jīng guò shǎo]

scanty menorrhea; hypomenorrhea: menstrual discharge of less than the normal amount occurring at regular intervals, the period of flow being less than usual duration, also known as 月经涩少 [yuè jīng sè shǎo]

月经涩少 [yuè jīng sè shǎo]

scanty inhibited menorrhea: same as scanty menorrhea; hypomenorrhea (月经过少[yuè jīng guò shǎo])

血虚月经过少 [xuè xū yuè jīng guò shǎo]

hypomenorrhea due to blood deficiency: menstrual discharge of abnormally small amount, pinkish in color, accompanied by sallow complexion, dizziness, palpitation, pale tongue, and thready weak pulse

肾虚月经过少 [shèn xū yuè jīng guò shǎo]

hypomenorrhea due to kidney insufficiency: menstrual discharge of abnormally small amount, bright red in color, accompanied by aching of loins and knees, dizziness, tinnitus, and deep pulse

血滞月经过少 [xuè zhì yuè jīng guò shǎo]

hypomenorrhea due to blood stagnation: menstrual discharge of abnormally small amount, purple-red in color or containing blood clots, accompanied by distending pain in the lower abdomen

停经 [tíng jīng]

ceasing of menstruation: a general term for the stoppage of the menses, including abnormal stoppage in a diseased state or normal stoppage during pregnancy and lactation, or even referring to the ending of a period with no more menstrual discharge

闭经 [bì jīng]; **经闭** [jīng bì]

amenorrhea: failure of menstruation to occur at puberty or abnormal stoppage of the menses for more than three months after menarche

火邪经闭 [huǒ xié jīng bì]

evil-fire amenorrhea: a type of amenorrhea ascribed to endogenous heat and fire, usually accompanied by cough and shoulder pain if the lung is involved, by restlessness at night if the heart is involved, by hypochondriac pain if the liver is involved, and by constipation if the spleen is involved.

虫积经闭 [chóng jī jīng bì]

helminthic amenorrhea: a type of amenorrhea caused by intestinal worms that consume yin and blood

血瘀经闭 [xuè yū jīng bì]

blood-stasis amenorrhea: a type of amenorrhea caused by stagnation of *qi* or accumulation of cold which leads to blood stasis in the thoroughfare and conception vessels, usually accompanied by lower abdominal pain and tenderness

血亏经闭 [xuè kuī jīng bì]

blood-deficiency amenorrhea: a type of amenorrhea caused by chronic loss of blood, multiple deliveries, or intemperate sexual life which leads to deficiency of yin and blood, usually accompanied by anorexia, emaciation, pallor or sallow complexion

血枯经闭 [xuè kū jīng bì]

blood-exhaustion amenorrhea: severe case of anemorrhea due to blood deficiency

心虚经闭 [xīn xū jīng bì]

heart-insufficiency amenorrhea: a type of amenorrhea caused by depression or anxiety that involves the heart in the function of governing blood

脾虚经闭 [pí xū jīng bì]

spleen-insufficiency amenorrhea: a type of amenorrhea usually accompanied by anorexia, stuffiness in the abdomen, and loose bowels

肾虚经闭 [shèn xū jīng bì]

kidney-insufficiency amenorrhea: a type of amenorrhea caused by congenital defect, marrying too early, intemperate sexual life or multiple deliveries, usually marked by tinnitus, dizziness, aching in the loins, and weakness of the legs

经期延长 [jīng qī yán cháng]

menostaxis: excessively prolonged menstruation in regular cycles

经间期出血 [jīng jiān qī chū xuè]

intermenstrual bleeding: periodic uterine bleeding occurring between the two menstrual periods at the ovulatory time

痛经 [tòng jīng]

dysmenorrhea; painful menstruation: lower abdominal pain with referring pain to the lower back occurring around or during the menstrual period, also called abdominal pain during menstruation (经行腹痛 [jīng xíng fù tòng])

经行腹痛 [jīng xíng fù tòng]

abdominal pain during menstruation, synonymous with dysmenorrhea (痛经 [tòng jīng])

气滞痛经 [qì zhì tòng jīng]

***qi*-stagnation dysmenorrhea:** a type of dysmenorrhea caused by emotional depression, and marked by distending pain in the lower abdomen accompanied by distention and discomfort in the chest and breasts before or during menstruation

血瘀痛经 [xuè yū tòng jīng]

blood-stasis dysmenorrhea: a type of dysmenorrhea characterized by stabbing pain in the lower abdomen with tenderness, occurring before or during menstruation with little menstrual discharge. The pain is usually alleviated after discharge of blood clots.

寒凝痛经 [hán níng tòng jīng]

cold-congealing dysmenorrhea: a type of dysmenorrhea marked by sluggish menstrual flow with cold feeling and pain in the lower abdomen, which can be alleviated by warmth

湿热痛经 [shī rè tòng jīng]

damp-heat dysmenorrhea: a type of dysmenorrhea accompanied by leukorrhagia with yellowish discharge

气血虚弱痛经 [qì xuè xū ruò tòng jīng]

***qi*-blood-deficiency dysmenorrhea:** a type of dysmenorrhea marked by reduced amount of thin and pink-colored menstrual flow associated with persistent dull pain in the lower abdomen which usually occurs during the late period of menstruation and can be alleviated by pressing

肾虚痛经 [shèn xū tòng jīng]

kidney-insufficiency dysmenorrhea: a type of dysmenorrhea caused by congenital defect, marrying too early, intemperate sexual life or multiple deliveries, and usually accompanied by dizziness, aching in the loins and weakness of the legs

倒经 [dǎo jīng]

vicarious menstruation: menstrual flow from some part other than the vagina, especially from the nose, also called 逆经 [nì jīng]

逆经 [nì jīng]

a synonym for 倒经 [dǎo jīng]

月经过多 [yuè jīng guò duō]

menorrhagia; hypermenorrhea: excessive uterine bleeding occurring at regular intervals, also called 经水过多 [jīng shuǐ guò duō] or 月水过多 [yuè shuǐ guò duō]

经水过多 [jīng shuǐ guò duō]

same as 月经过多 [yuè jīng guò duō]

月水过多 [yuè shuǐ guò duō]

same as 月经过多 [yuè jīng guò duō]

崩漏 [bēng lòu]

metrorrhagia and metrostaxis: excessive uterine bleeding with a sudden onset occurring not in the regular menstruation period (崩 [bēng]) or incessant dripping of blood (漏 [lòu])

血崩 [xuè bēng]

blood flooding; metrorrhagia: sudden massive uterine bleeding, also called 崩中 [bēng zhōng]

崩中 [bēng zhōng]

uterine flooding: synonym for blood flooding or metrorrhagia (血崩 [xuè bēng])

漏下 [lòu xià]

uterine dripping; metrostaxis: slight but persistent escape of blood from the uterus

崩证 [bēng zhèng]

metrorrhagic syndrome: a syndrome marked by sudden profuse uterine bleeding

经崩 [jīng bēng]

menstrual flooding; menorrhagia: profuse uterine bleeding in a prolonged menstrual period of more than two weeks

经漏 [jīng lòu]

menstrual dripping: incessant escape of small amounts of blood from the uterus in a prolonged menstrual period of more than two weeks

血热崩漏 [xuè rè bēng lòu]

blood-heat metrorrhagia and metrostaxis: excessive uterine bleeding, deep red in color, usually occurring in women with constitution of exuberant yang or after an emotional upset, accompanied by flushed face, dryness of the mouth, insomnia, deep red tongue, and full and rapid pulse

血瘀崩漏 [xuè yū bēng lòu]

blood-stasis metrorrhagia and metrostaxis: excessive uterine bleeding containing blood clots, accompanied by lower abdominal pain with tenderness, dark red tongue, and choppy pulse

气虚崩漏 [qì xū bēng lòu]

***qi*-deficiency metrorrhagia and metrostaxis:** excessive uterine bleeding or incessant dripping of thin and pinkish blood, accompanied by lassitude, anorexia, loose stools, and weak pulse

肾虚崩漏 [shèn xū bēng lòu]

kidney-insufficiency metrorrhagia and metrostaxis: excessive uterine bleeding accompanied by weakness of the loins and knees, usually caused by intemperance in sexual life, multiple deliveries, or marrying too early

气陷血崩 [qì xiàn xuè bēng]

***qi*-sinking metrorrhagia:** excessive uterine bleeding due to spleen insufficiency with sunken *qi*, marked by thin and pinkish discharge accompanied by lassitude and shortness of breath, and aggravated upon exertion

气郁血崩 [qì yù xuè bēng]

***qi*-stagnation metrorrhagia:** excessive uterine bleeding after a fit of rage, marked by sudden onset of profuse discharge of purplish-red blood with clots, accompanied by irritability, and discomfort in the hypochondriac region

经行发热 [jīng xíng fā rè]

fever during menstruation: fever occurring during or around each menstrual period, also known as 经来发热 [jīng lái fā rè]

经来发热 [jīng lái fā rè]

a synonym for 经行发热 [jīng xíng fā rè]

经期水肿 [jīng qī shǐ zhǒng]

edema during menstruation: edema of the face and limbs occurring during or prior to each menstrual period either due to yang deficiency of the spleen and kidney or due to *qi* stagnation with damp retention

经行浮肿 [jīng xíng fú zhǒng]

same as 经期水肿 [jīng qī shuǐ zhǒng]

经行头痛 [jīng xíng tóu tòng]

headache during menstruation: headache occurring during or around each menstrual period

经行眩晕 [jīng xíng xuán yūn]

dizziness during menstruation: dizziness occurring during or around each menstrual period

经行身痛 [jīng xíng shēn tòng]

general aching during menstruation: generalized aching over the body occurring during or prior to each menstrual period, usually accompanied by fever and aversion to cold

经行吐衄 [jīng xíng tù nǜ]

hematemesis and epistaxis during menstruation: a type of vicarious or supplementary menstruation

经行衄血 [jīng xíng nǜ xuè]

epistaxis during menstruation: a type of vicarious or supplementary menstruation

经行吐血 [jīng xíng tù xuè]

hematemesis during menstruation: a type of vicarious or supplementary menstruation

经行便血 [jīng xíng biàn xuè]

ano-urethral bleeding during menstruation: discharge of blood through the anus and urethra during each menstrual period, also called 错经 [cuò jīng]

错经 [cuò jīng]

"erroneous menstruation": a synonym for ano-urethral bleeding during menstruation (经行便血 [jīng xíng biàn xuè])

经行泄泻 [jīng xíng xiè xiè]

diarrhea during menstruation: diarrhea occurring during each menstruation and stopping spontaneously when the period is over, also called 经来泄泻 [jīng lái xiè xiè]

经来泄泻 [jīng lái xiè xiè]

a synonym for 经行泄泻 [jīng xíng xiè xiè]

经行乳房胀痛 [jīng xíng rǔ fáng zhàng tòng]

distending pain in the breasts during menstruation: distention or sensation of fullness and pain in the breasts during or prior to each menstrual period

经行情志异常 [jīng xíng qíng zhì yì cháng]

moodiness during menstruation; premenstrual syndrome: depression, gloominess, irritability and other changes of mood occurring prior to or during each menstrual period and returning to normal after the period

经行口糜 [jīng xíng kǒu mí]

oral ulcer during menstruation: ulceration in the mouth or on the tongue occurring prior to or during each menstrual period

经行痦瘰 [jīng xíng bèi lěi]

urticaria during menstruation: raised red patches of skin with intense itching occurring prior to or during each menstrual period, also called hives during menstruation (经行风疹块 [jīng xíng fēng zhěn kuài])

经行风疹块 [jīng xíng fēng zhěn kuài]

hives during menstruation, same as urticaria during menstruation 经行痦瘰 [jīng xíng bèi lěi]

断经前后诸证 [duàn jīng qián hòu zhū zhèng]

menopausal syndromes: syndromes related to menopause, such as hot flushes, excessive sweating, lassitude, irritability, dizziness, tinnitus, palpitations, insomnia, amnesia, back ache, heat sensation in the palms and soles

绝经前后诸病 [jué jīng qián hòu zhū bìng]

menopausal diseases, same as menopausal syndromes (断经前后诸证 [duàn jīng qián hòu zhū zhèng])

经断复来 [jīng duàn fù lái]

postmenopausal hemorrhage: uterine bleeding occurring two years or more after menopause

带下 [dài xià]

vaginal discharge; leukorrhea: (1) normal vaginal discharge in physiological conditions or abnormal discharge in morbid conditions;

(2) a collective term used in ancient times for various kinds of gynecological diseases, for all of them occur below the belt vessel. (The Chinese character 带 refers to the belt vessel and 下 means below.)

白带 [bái dài]

leukorrhea: whitish discharge from the vagina

黄带 [huáng dài]

yellowish leukorrhea: yellowish viscid discharge from the vagina, usually indicating the presence of pathogenic damp

赤白带 [chì bái dài]

reddish leukorrhea: profuse leukorrhea mixed with reddish discharge, usually indicating the presence of damp-heat

带下病 [dài xià bìng]

leukorrheal diseases: a group of morbid states characterized by excessive leukorrhea with abnormal color, quality and smell, accompanied by general or local symptoms

脾虚带下 [pí xū dài xià]

spleen-insufficiency leukorrhagia: that due to deficiency of spleen yang, marked by incessant profuse leukorrhea, thin and whitish or pale yellow with no unpleasant smell, accompanied by lassitude, anorexia, loose bowels, edema of the legs, pale tongue with white greasy coating, and relaxed pulse

肾虚带下 [shèn xū dài xià]

kidney-insufficiency leukorrhagia: that due to deficiency of kidney yang, marked by continuous profuse watery leukorrhea, accompanied by dizziness, tinnitus, lumbar pain, aversion to cold, cold limbs, cold sensation in the lower abdomen, frequent micturition, dim complexion, and deep, thready and slow pulse

湿热带下 [shī rè dài xià]

damp-heat leukorrhagia: that caused by down-pouring of damp-heat, marked by profuse, sticky yellow leukorrhea with an unpleasant odor, usually accompanied by bitterness in the mouth, dryness of the throat, lower abdominal pain, reddened tongue with yellow greasy coating, and soggy rapid pulse

湿毒带下 [shī dú dài xià]

toxic-damp leukorrhagia: that caused by the invasion of toxic damp, marked by excessive purulent and bloody leukorrhea with an offensive odor, accompanied by lower abdominal pain, lumbar aching, bitterness in the mouth, dryness of the throat, reddened tongue with yellow greasy coating, and slippery rapid pulse

交接出血 [jiāo jiē chū xuè]

copulative bleeding: vaginal bleeding during sexual intercourse

阴挺 [yīn tǐng]

prolapse of uterus: downward displacement of the uterus, even with the entire uterus outside the vaginal orifice

妊娠 [rèn shēn]

pregnancy: the condition of having a developing embryo or fetus in the body from conception to delivery

重身 [chóng shēn]

same as 妊娠 [rèn shēn]

不孕 [bù yùn]

infertility: lack of capacity to produce offspring

全不产 [quán bù chǎn]

ancient name for primary infertility, i.e., infertility occurring in those who have never conceived

断绪 [duàn xù]

an ancient name for secondary infertility, i.e., infertility occurring in those who have previously conceived

肾虚不孕 [shèn xū bù yùn]

kidney-insufficiency infertility: that ascribed to deficiency of the kidney *qi*, yin or yang

宫冷不孕 [gōng lěng bù yùn]

uterus-coldness infertility: that ascribed to deficiency-cold of the kidney which fails to warm the uterus, usually marked by coldness in the lower abdomen, aversion to cold, cold limbs, retarded menstruation, and even frigidity

胞寒不孕 [bāo hán bù yùn]

same as 宫冷不孕 [gōng lěng bù yùn]

血虚不孕 [xuè xū bù yùn]

blood-deficiency infertility: that caused by insufficiency of the spleen and stomach or chronic loss of blood, marked by general weakness, lassitude, and sallow complexion

血滞不孕 [xuè zhì bù yùn]

blood-stagnation infertility: that due to impeded blood flow, often accompanied by lower abdominal pain and retarded menstruation

肝郁不孕 [gān yù bù yùn]

liver-depression infertility: that due to depression of the liver, often accompanied by irregularity of menstrual cycles, distention and pain in the breasts before the periods, hypochondriac discomfort, depression and irritability

嫉妒不孕 [jì dù bù yùn]

infertility due to jealousy: a type of infertility in women with depression of the liver caused by emotional factors such as jealousy

痰湿不孕 [tán shī bù yùn]

phlegm-damp infertility: that caused by the accumulation of phlegm-damp, marked by late periods or even amenorrhea, profuse leukorrhea, dizziness, palpitations and discomfort in the chest

湿痰不孕 [shī tán bù yùn]

same as 痰湿不孕 [tán shī bù yùn]

血瘀不孕 [xuè yū bù yùn]

blood stasis infertility: that caused by blood stasis, usually marked by retarded menstruation, presence of blood clots in the menstrual discharge, and pain in the lower abdomen with tenderness

肥胖不孕 [féi pàng bù yùn]

obesity infertility: a type of infertility occurring in obese women who eat too much fat which turns to phlegm-damp blocking the conception vessel, often accompanied by palpitation, shortness of breath, and leukorrhagia

脂塞不孕 [zhī hán bù yùn]

fat infertility: that due to excessive fat which blocks the uterine vessel

胎元 [tāi yuán]

(1) embryo within the mother's womb; **(2) essence that feeds the fetus;** **(3) placenta**

脐带 [qí dài]

umbilical cord: structure by which the fetus is attached to the placenta

激经 [jī jīng]

"stimulated menses": regular menstruation during early pregnancy, which stops spontaneously when the fetus is fully grown, also known as 盛胎 [shèng tāi] or 垢胎 [gòu tāi]

盛胎 [shèng tāi]

another name for menstruation during pregnancy (激经 [jī jīng])

垢胎 [gòu tāi]

another name for menstruation during pregnancy (激经 [jī jīng])

妊娠病 [rèn shēn bìng]

diseases of pregnancy: diseases that occur in the period of pregnancy and are related to pregnancy

妊娠恶阻 [rèn shēn è zǔ]

morning sickness: nausea and vomiting during early pregnancy, also abbreviated as 恶阻 [è zǔ]

恶阻 [è zǔ]

morning sickness: abbreviation for 妊娠恶阻 [rèn shēn è zǔ]

妊娠呕吐 [rèn shēn ǒu tù]

hyperemesis gravidarum: vomiting during pregnancy, synonym for morning sickness (妊娠恶阻 [rèn shēn è zǔ])

妊娠腹痛 [rèn shēn fù tòng]

abdominal pain of pregnancy: lower abdominal pain occurring in pregnancy, usually due to the fetal impediment to the circulation of *qi* and blood, also called 胞阻 [bāo zǔ]

胞阻 [bāo zǔ]

fetal impediment: a synonym for abdominal pain of pregnancy (妊娠腹痛 [rèn shēn fù tòng])

妊娠眩晕 [rèn shē xuán yūn]

vertigo in pregnancy: vertigo or even fainting occurring in pregnancy, also called 子晕 [zǐ yūn]

子晕 [zǐ yūn]

gravid vertigo: a synonym for vertigo during pregnancy (妊娠眩晕 [rèn shēn xuán yūn])

妊娠痫证 [rèn shēn xián zhèng]

eclampsia of pregnancy: convulsions occurring during pregnancy, also known as 子痫 [zǐ xián]

子痫 [zǐ xián]

same as 妊娠痫证 [rèn shēn xián zhèng]

子冒 [zǐ mào]

same as 子痫 [zǐ xián]

妊娠小便淋痛 [rèn shēn xiǎo biàn lìn tòng]

stranguria during pregnancy: difficult and painful discharge of urine during pregnancy, also known as 子淋 [zǐ lìn]

子淋 [zǐ lìn]

gravid stranguria: a synonym for stranguria during pregnancy (妊娠小便淋痛 [rèn shēn xiǎo biàn lìn tòng])

胎气上逆 [tāi qì shàng nì]

upward reversal of fetus *qi*: feeling of oppression in the abdomen and thorax, even with dyspnea, during pregnancy, also known as 子悬 [zǐ xuán]

子悬 [zǐ xuán]

gravid oppression: a synonym for upward reversal of fetus *qi* (胎气上逆 [tāi qì shàng nì])

胎死不下 [tāi sǐ bù xià]

missed labor: retention of a dead fetus in the uterus beyond the normal period of pregnancy

鬼胎 [guǐ tāi]

hydatidiform mole: abnormal pregnancy with a mass in the uterus resembling a hydatid ("resembling a ghost" in Chinese)

胎水肿满 [tāi shuǐ zhǒng mǎn]

excess of amniotic fluid: that causing abnormally enlarged abdomen, sensation of fullness and dyspnea, also known as 子满 [zǐ mǎn]

子满 [zǐ mǎn]

hydramnios: a synonym for excess of amniotic fluid (胎水肿满 [tāi shuǐ zhǒng mǎn])

妊娠心烦 [rèn shēn xīn fán]

vexation during pregnancy: state of being annoyed or worried during pregnancy, also called 子烦 [zǐ fán]

子烦 [zǐ fán]

gravid vexation: vexation occurring during pregnancy, same as 妊娠心烦 [rèn shēn xīn fán]

妊娠咳嗽 [rèn shēn ké sòu]

cough during pregnancy: persistent cough during pregnancy, also called gravid cough 子嗽 [zǐ sòu]

子嗽 [zǐ sòu]

gravid cough: a synonym for cough during pregnancy (妊娠咳嗽 [rèn shēn ké sòu])

妊娠失音 [rèn shēn shī yīn]

aphonia of pregnancy: loss of voice due to pregnancy, also called 子喑 [zǐ yīn]

子喑 [zǐ yīn]

gravid aphonia: a synonym for aphonia of pregnancy (妊娠失音 [rèn shēn shī yīn])

妊娠肿胀 [rèn shēn zhǒng zhàng]

edema of pregnancy: edema of the face and limbs occurring in the late stage of pregnancy, also called 子肿 [zǐ zhǒng]

子肿 [zǐ zhǒng]

gravid edema: a synonym for edema of pregnancy (妊娠肿胀 [rèn shēn zhǒng zhàng])

胎寒 [tāi hán]

(1) cold syndrome of gravida: a disorder in pregnant women due to immoderate eating of raw and cold food, or exposure to wind during pregnancy, manifested by excessive movements of the fetus, increased borborygmi, diarrhea, distending pain of the chest and abdomen and contraction of the limbs; **(2) fetal cold:** cold syndrome in the newborn

胎热 [tāi rè]

(1) heat syndrome of gravida: a disorder in pregnant women marked by blood-shot eyes with crusting at the margins of the eyelids, resulting from upward attack of pathogenic heat along the liver meridian; **(2) fetal heat:** heat syndrome in the newborn

胎动不安 [tāi dòng bù ān]

threatened miscarriage: continuous moving of the fetus causing pain in the lower abdomen

分娩 [fēn miǎn]

labor: the physical activities involved in parturition

临产 [lín chǎn]

parturition: the process of giving birth to offspring

试胎 [shì tāi]

testing labor: abdominal pain that goes on for a short time and then stops during the eighth or ninth month of pregnancy

弄胎 [nòng tāi]

false labor: intermittent abdominal pain that occurs toward the end of the term of pregnancy without backache

试月 [shì yuè]

a synonym for testing labor (试胎 [shì tāi])

试水 [shì shuǐ]

early leakage of amniotic fluid: the condition characterized by leakage of the amniotic fluid which is not followed by childbirth

堕胎 [duò tāi]

early abortion: spontaneous abortion occurring within the first twelve weeks of pregnancy

小产 [xiǎo chǎn]

late abortion: spontaneous abortion occurring after the twelfth week and before the twenty-eighth week of pregnancy

胎漏 [tāi lòu]

vaginal bleeding during pregnancy: a sign of threatened miscarriage

胎元不固 [tāi yuán bù gù]

insecurity of fetus: provision of inadequate support for the fetus, which leads to liability to abortion

临产病 [lín chǎn bìng]

parturient diseases: diseases related to labor, occurring in the birth process and within four hours after delivery

难产 [nán chǎn]

dystocia: difficult labor, also called 产难 [chǎn nán]

产难 [chǎn nán]

difficult labor: same as 难产 [nán chǎn]

胞衣先破 [bāo yī xiān pò]

early rupture of the fetal membrane: rupture of the fetal membrane at the end of the term of pregnancy but not followed by childbrith

沥浆产 [lì jiāng chǎn]

premature amniotic rupture, also known as 沥浆生 [lì jiāng shēng]

沥浆生 [lì jiāng shēng]

a synonym for premature amniotic rupture (沥浆产 [lì jiāng chǎn])

滑胎 [huá tāi]

habitual abortion: spontaneous abortion in three or more consecutive pregnancies

气虚滑胎 [qì xū huá tāi]

***qi*-deficiency habitual abortion:** habitual abortion due to deficiency of *qi*

血虚滑胎 [xuè xū huá tāi]

blood-deficiency habitual abortion: habitual abortion due to deficiency of blood

血热滑胎 [xuè rè huá tāi]

blood-heat habitual abortion: habitual abortion due to heat in blood

肾虚滑胎 [shèn xū huá tāi]

kidney-insufficiency habitual abortion: habitual abortion due to deficiency of kidney *qi*

交骨不开 [jiāo gǔ bù kāi]

fixation of pubic cartilage: that which impedes the passage of the fetus during parturition

胞衣不下 [bāo yī bù xià]

detention of afterbirth: retarded delivery of afterbirth

息胞 [xī bāo]

same as 胞衣不下 [bāo yī bù xià]

恶露 [è lù]

lochia: vaginal discharge in the puerperium

恶露不下 [è lù bù xià]

retention of lochia: retarded discharge of lochia

恶露不绝 [è lù bù jué]

lochiorrhea: abnormally prolonged discharge of lochia

恶露不止 [è lù bù zhǐ]

incessant discharge of lochia: a synonym for lochiorrhea (恶露不绝 [è lù bù jué])

产后恶露不绝 [chǎn hòu è lù bù jué]

(postpartum) lochiorrhea, same as 恶露不绝 [è lù bù jué]

产后病 [chǎn hòu bìng]

diseases following childbirth: diseases occurring in the puerperal period and related to labor and puerperium

产后三病 [chǎn hòu sān bìng]

three postpartum illnesses: convulsive disease, depression-drowsiness, and dyschezia following delivery

产后三急 [chǎn hòu sān jí]

three postpartum emergencies: continuous vomiting, profuse sweating and diarrhea following delivery

产后三脱 [chǎn hòu sān tuō]

three kinds of postpartum exhaustion: exhaustion of blood, *qi* (vital energy) and mental power after delivery

产后三冲 [chǎn hòu sān chōng]

three postpartum crises: three critical conditions caused by putrid blood derived from lochioschesis following childbirth, namely the heart crisis, the lung crisis, and the stomach crisis

败血冲心 [bài xuè chōng xīn]

heart crisis due to putrid blood: a critically diseased state following childbirth characterized by impaired consciousness and mania ascribed to invasion of the heart by putrid blood derived from lochioschesis

败血冲肺 [bài xuè chōng fèi]

lung crisis due to putrid blood: a critically diseased state following childbirth characterized by stuffiness in the chest, shortness of breath, and epistaxis ascribed to the invasion of the lung by putrid blood derived from lochioschesis

败血冲胃 [bài xuè chōng wèi]

stomach crisis due to putrid blood: a critically diseased state following childbirth characterized by nausea, vomiting, and abdominal distention and pain ascribed to invasion of the stomach by putrid blood derived from lochioschesis

产后血晕 [chǎn hòu xuè yūn]

postpartum fainting: fainting occurring following childbirth due to excessive loss of blood

产后血崩 [chǎn hòu xuè bēng]

postpartum metrorrhagia: sudden profuse uterine bleeding following childbirth

产后郁冒 [chǎn hòu yù mào]

(1) postpartum depression with dizziness: that usually ascribed to excessive blood loss, profuse sweating, or affection by external pathogens; **(2) postpartum fainting:** a synonym for 产后血晕 [chǎn hòu xuè yūn]

产后身痛 [chǎn hòu shēn tòng]

postpartum general aching: general aching involving the trunk, limbs and joints in the puerperal period

产后小便不通 [chǎn hòu xiǎo biàn bù tōng]

postpartum retention of urine: retention of urine occurring following childbirth, usually accompanied by distention and pain in the lower abdomen

产后小便失禁 [chǎn hòu xiǎo biàn shī jìn]

postpartum incontinence of urine: incontinence of urine occurring following childbirth

产后大便难 [chǎn hòu dà biàn nán]

postpartum dyschezia: difficult evacuation of feces from the rectum occurring following childbirth

产后发热 [chǎn hòu fā rè]

postpartum fever: fever following childbirth due to various causes, particularly puerperal infection

产后头痛 [chǎn hòu tóu tòng]

postpartum headache: headache following childbirth, often due to excessive blood loss and sometimes due to blood stasis

产后怔忡 [chǎn hòu zhèng chōng]

postpartum palpitation: palpitation occurring following childbirth, usually due to excessive blood loss

产后自汗 [chǎn hòu zì hàn]

spontaneous sweating following childbirth: an abnormal condition of sweating occurring following childbirth usually due to weak constitution and consumption of *qi* and blood during labor

产后盗汗 [chǎn hòu dào hàn]

night sweats following childbirth: an abnormal condition of sweating occurring following childbirth usually due to consumption of blood and yin during labor

产后病温 [chǎn hòu bìng wēn]

puerperal epidemic febrile disease: a general term for various epidemic febrile diseases occurring following delivery

产后尿血 [chǎn hòu niào xuè]

postpartum hematuria: hematuria following childbirth, usually due to affection by heat in a state of deficiency of *qi* and blood

产后腰痛 [chǎn hòu yāo tòng]

postpartum lumbago: dull pain in the lower back following childbirth, usually due to injury to the kidney *qi* and stagnation of blood in the belt vessel

产后腹痛 [chǎn hòu fù tòng]

postpartum abdominal pain: pain in the lower abdomen following childbirth, accompanied by dizziness, lassitude, palpitation and shortness of breath if it is due to deficiency of blood with impaired blood supply to the uterine vessels, and accompanied by mass formation and tenderness in the lower abdomen and purplish tongue if it is due to stagnation of blood and cold in the uterine vessels

产后胁痛 [chǎn hòu xié tòng]

postpartum hypochondriac pain: pain in the hypochondriac region occurring following childbirth, usually due to stagnation of *qi* and blood or excessive blood loss impairing the liver meridian

产后腹胀 [chǎn hòu fù zhàng]

postpartum abdominal distention: abdominal distention due to stagnated blood which impairs the flow of *qi* with involvement of the spleen and stomach or due to improper diet

产后水肿 [chǎn hòu shuǐ zhǒng]

postpartum edema: edema occurring following childbirth, usually seen in one with spleen and kidney yang deficiency which is further impaired by labor in pregnant women with weak spleen and kidney, a condition which is aggravated by childbirth

产后痹证 [chǎn hòu bì zhèng]

postpartum arthralgia: arthralgia occurring following childbirth, usually due to invasion of pathogenic wind-cold-damp in a deficiency condition of *qi* and blood

产后痉证 [chǎn hòu jīng zhèng]

postpartum convulsion: sudden onset of rigidity, convulsions, trismus and opisthotonos in the puerperal period, also called 产后痉病 [chǎn hòu jīng bìng]

产后痉病 [chǎn hòu jīng bìng]

postpartum convulsive disease: a synonym for postpartum convulsion (产后痉证 [chǎn hòu jīng zhèng])

产后病痉 [chǎn hòu bìng jīng]

postpartum convulsion, same as postpartum convulsive disease (产后痉病 [chǎn hòu jīng bìng])

蓐劳 [rù láo]

puerperal phthisis: a state of general weakness following childbirth accompanied by cough, dyspnea, stuffiness in the chest, chills and fever

缺乳 [quē rǔ]

oligogalactia; hypogalactia: deficiency of milk secretion

产后缺乳 [chǎn hòu quē rǔ]

postpartum oligogalactia; postpartum hypogalactia: deficiency of milk secretion following childbirth

乳汁不行 [rǔ zhī bù xíng]

agalactia: no milk secretion following childbirth, also called 乳汁不通 [rǔ zhī bù tōng]

乳汁不通 [rǔ zhī bù tōng]

same as 乳汁不行 [rǔ zhī bù xíng]

乳汁自出 [rǔ zhī zì chū]

galactorrhea: spontaneous flow of milk irrespective of nursing

产后乳汁自出 [chǎn hòu rǔ zhī zì chū]

postpartum galactorrhea: spontaneous flow of milk irrespective of nursing following childbirth

乳溢 [rǔ yì]

same as galactorrhea (乳汁自出 [rǔ zhī zì chū])

儿科 Pediatrics

龆龀 [tiáo chèn]

seven- or eight-year-old children

稚子 [zhì zǐ]

ten-year-old children

纯阳之体 [chún yáng zhī tǐ]

pure-yang constitution: constitution of infants and children characterized by fullness of vitality while healthy and exuberance of yang (e.g., liability to high fever and impairment of fluid) while ill

稚阴稚阳 [zhì yīn zhì yáng]

immature yin and yang: yin and yang that have not yet fully developed in young children

易虚易实 [yì xū yì shí]

liability to change from excess to deficiency and vice versa: a distinctive characteristic of children's diseases in the transformation between excess and deficiency

易寒易热 [yì hán yì rè]

liability to change from heat to cold and vice versa: a distinctive characteristic of children's diseases in the transformation between cold and heat natures

初生不啼 [chū shēng bù tí]

failure to cry in the newborn; asphyxia neonatorum: perinatal asphyxia in the newborn

初生不乳 [chū shē bù rǔ]

failure to suck in the newborn: a condition marked by inability of the newborn to suck milk, often due to inadequacy of genuine *qi*, deficiency-cold of the spleen and stomach, or accumulation of filthy heat

惊风 [jīng fēng]

infantile convulsion: series of muscular contractions associated with opisthotonus, loss of consciousness, occurring in infants and young children

惊风病 [jīng fēng bìng]

infantile convulsive disease: full name of infantile convulsion (惊风 [jīng fēng]) as a disease

惊风八候 [jīng fēng bā hòu]

eight signs of infantile convulsion: signs of infantile convulsion – clonic contraction of the hands, twitching of the fingers, forward bending of the back, hyperextension of the body, turning of the head, stretching of the arms, up-staring of the eyes, and immobility of the eyeballs

急惊风 [jí jīng fēng]

acute infantile convulsion: infantile convulsion of acute onset accompanied by high fever and loss of consciousness, mostly due to exogenous contraction, sometimes caused by fright

慢惊风 [màn jīng fēng]

chronic infantile convulsion: repeated infantile convulsion of gradual onset associated with loss of consciousness or paralysis and poor prognosis

慢脾风 [màn pí fēng]

chronic convulsion with spleen insufficiency: a type of chronic infantile convulsion usually occurring after protracted vomiting and diarrhea with spleen *qi* deficiency

慢惊夹痰 [màn jīng jiā tán]

chronic convulsion with phlegm: chronic convulsion complicated by heat-phlegm, manifested by afternoon fever, thirst, epigastric distention, shortness of breath, expectoration, insomnia, and convulsions on and off

慢惊自汗 [màn jīng zì hàn]

chronic convulsion with incessant sweating: a critical case of chronic convulsion with impending shock

惊厥 [jīng jué]

(1) faint from fright; (2) convulsion

瘛疭 [chì zòng]

clonic convulsion: convulsion marked by alternating contraction and relaxation of the muscles

婴儿瘛疭 [yīng ér chì zòng]

infantile clonic convulsion: clonic convulsion occurring in infants

天钓 [tiān diào]

upward-staring convulsion: infantile convulsion usually due to accumulation of heat in the heart and lung, marked by convulsion with tossed head and upward staring eyes, high fever, cyanosis and salivation

内钓 [nèi diào]

visceral convulsion: infantile convulsion mainly manifested as visceral contraction and colic

脐风 [qí fēng]

neonatal tetanus: a severe form of infectious tetanus occurring during the first few days after birth, mostly due to unhygienic practice in dressing the umbilical stump

脐风三证 [qí féng sān zhèng]

three signs of neonatal tetanus: "pursed mouth", lockjaw, and "locked abdomen"

撮口 [cuō kǒu]

"pursed mouth": a sign of neonatal tetanus marked by spasm of the buccal muscles with difficulty in opening the mouth

噤风 [jìn fēng]

lockjaw: a sign of neonatal tetanus marked by spasm of the muscles of mastication resulting in inability to cry and to suck milk

锁肚 [suǒ dù]

"locked abdomen": a sign of neonatal tetanus marked by protruding of the swollen umbilicus and distention of the abdomen with stoppage of bowel movements

惊风抽搐 [jīng fēng chōu chù]

convulsive seizure: series of involuntary contractions of muscles

惊风腹痛 [jīng fēng fù tòng]

convulsion with abdominal pain: a morbid condition often caused by accumulation of undigested food with heat and phlegm associated with wind affliction

惊风烦渴 [jīng fēng fán kě]

convulsion with vexing thirst: vexing thirst due to consumption of body fluids occurring after convulsion

硬肿症 [yìng zhǒng zhèng]

sclerederma: chronic hardening and thickening of the skin

胎赤 [tāi chì]

fetal redness; erythroderma neonatorum: abnormal redness of the skin in a newborn, often due to affection by toxic heat at the fetal stage

胎禀 [tāi bǐng]

fetal endowment: quality derived from the parents

胎弱 [tāi ruò]

fetal weakness: congenital weak constitution, also known as 胎怯 [tāi qiè]

胎怯 [tāi qiè]

fetal feebleness: synonym for fetal weakness (胎弱 [tāi ruò])

胎寒 [tāi hán]

(1) fetal cold: a cold syndrome of the newborn, marked by abdominal pain with cold huddling extremities, shivering, incessant crying or lockjaw; **(2) cold syndrome of gravida** (cf. 胎寒 [tāi hán] on p.613)

胎热 [tāi rè]

(1) fetal heat: a febrile disease of the newborn attributed to the mother's improper diet and medication during pregnancy; **(2) heat syndrome of gravida** (cf. 胎热 [tāi rè] on p.613)

胎毒 [tāi dú]

fetal toxicosis: boils, blisters, eczema, etc. in newborns which were considered in ancient times to result from endogenous toxicity of the pregnant mother before birth

胎黄 [tāi huáng]

neonatal jaundice; icterus neonatorum: jaundice seen in the newborn, also called 胎疸 [tāi dǎn]

胎疸 [tāi dǎn]

fetal jaundice: a synonym for neonatal jaundice (胎黄 [tāi huáng])

胎黄病 [tāi huáng bìng]

neonatal jaundice (disease); icterus neonatorum: full name of neonatal jaundice (胎黄 [tāi huáng]) as a disease

囟填 [xìn tián]

bulging fontanel: outward swelling of the fontanel in an infant, often seen in cases of infectious disease with excessive internal heat or indigestion with retention of undigested food, and also as a prodromal sign of infantile convulsion if accompanied by high fever and vomiting

囟陷 [xìn xiàn]

sunken fontanel: depressed fontanel in an infant, often due to consumption of yin fluid in cases of acute febrile disease or diarrhea, and sometimes due to congenital defect

解颅 [jiě lú]

hydrocephalus: abnormal accumulation of excess fluid within the skull marked by enlargement of the head and persistent non-closure of the skull sutures

解颅病 [jiě lú bìng]

hydrocephalus (disease): a disease characterized by accumulation of excess fluid within the skull

百晬内嗽 [bǎi zuì nèi sòu]

neonatal cough: cough occurring in a newborn within one hundred days after its birth, often due to common cold or respiratory infection

夜啼 [yè tí]

night crying: morbid night crying in babies, in most cases due to cold in the spleen or heat in the heart, and sometimes due to being frightened

热夜啼 [rè yè tí]

night crying due to heat: night crying in babies caused by heart heat, marked by flushed face, fever, and irritability

寒夜啼 [hán yè tí]

night crying due to cold: night crying in babies caused by spleen cold, marked by pallor, hands and abdomen cold to the touch, and coiled posture suggesting abdominal pain

客忤 [kè wǔ]

fright seizure: a seizure of fright

客忤夜啼 [kè wǔ yè tí]

night crying due to fright: night crying in babies caused by fright

伤乳 [shāng rǔ]

infantile dyspepsia: that caused by improper breast feeding

溢乳 [yì rǔ]

milk regurgitation: that resulting from overfeeding or improper way of nursing, also called 呕乳 [ǒu rǔ]

呕乳 [ǒu rǔ]

vomiting of milk: a synonym for milk regurgitation (溢乳 [yì rǔ])

五迟 [wǔ chí]

five kinds of retardation: retarded development in infants covering standing, walking, hair-growing, tooth eruption and speaking

立迟 [lì chí]

retardation of standing: inability to stand in children till several years of age

行迟 [xíng chí]

retardation of walking: chronic inability to walk in children

发迟 [fà chí]

retardation of hair-growing: retarded growth of hair in children

齿迟 [chǐ chí]

retardation of tooth-eruption: retarded eruption of teeth in children

语迟 [yǔ chí]

retardation of speaking: inability to speak in children till 4 - 5 years of age

五硬 [wǔ yìng]

five types of stiffness: stiffness of the hand, foot, waist, flesh and neck in children

五软 [wǔ ruǎn]

five types of flaccidity: flaccidity of the neck, nape, extremities, muscles and mastication as striking features of delayed growth and mental retardation in infants

鸡胸 [jī xiōng]

chicken breast; pigeon chest: deformity of the chest in which the sternum is prominent, usually due to rickets, also called "tortoise chest"

(龟胸 [guī xiōng])

龟胸 [guī xiōng]

"tortoise chest": a synonym for pigeon chest (鸡胸 [jī xiōng])

龟背 [guī bèi]

kyphosis; humpback: back shaped like a tortoise-shell, kind of deformity in children due to underdevelopment and malnutrition, as seen in cases of rickets

脐疮 [qí chuāng]

omphalelcosis: ulceration of the umbilicus

脐湿 [qí shī]

omphalorrhea: effusion at the navel

脐血 [qí xuè]

omphalorrhagia: hemorrhage or oozing of blood from the umbilicus

脐疝 [qí shàn]

umbilical hernia: a type of abdominal hernia in which part of the intestine protrudes at the umbilicus and is covered with skin, also called 脐突 [qí tū]

脐突 [qí tū]

protrusion of the navel: another name for umbilical hernia (脐疝 [qí shàn])

差颓 [cī tuí]

unilateral enlargement of the testis

流涎 [liú xián]

salivation; ptyalism: excessive flow of saliva

小儿多涎 [xiǎo ér duō xián]

salivation in infant: excessive discharge of thick saliva due to heat in the spleen or excessive discharge of thin saliva due to deficiency-cold of the spleen and stomach

滞颐 [zhì yí]

drooling with wet cheek: another expression for salivation in an infant

齘齿 [xiè chǐ]

teeth grinding: grinding of teeth during sleep, often due to exuberant fire in the heart and stomach or due to deficiency of *qi* and blood

马牙 [mǎ yá]

gingival eruption: sporadic eruption of small round nodules on the gums in the newborn, causing difficulty in sucking milk

螳螂子 [táng láng zǐ]

corpus adiposum bucca: encapsulated mass of fat (looking like a mantis egg, and hence the Chinese name) in the cheek of an infant, causing difficulty in sucking, also called 颊脂垫 [jiá zhī diàn]

颊脂垫 [jiá zhī diàn]

buccal fat pad: another name for corpus adiposum bucca (螳螂子 [táng láng zǐ])

木舌 [mù shé]

wooden tongue: swollen, hardened tongue, seen in glossitis of the newborn

地图舌 [dì tú shé]

geographic tongue: irregular shedding of the tongue coating indicating deficiency of stomach *qi* and yin

连舌 [lián shé]

ankyloglossia: restricted movement of the tongue that causes difficulty in sucking

结舌 [jié shé]

tongue tie: a synonym for ankyloglossia (连舌 [lián shé])

鹅口疮 [é kǒu chuāng]

thrush: a disease of infants and young children of poor health, characterized by the presence of white patches of soft material on the buccal mucosa and tongue, looking like the mouth of a goose, also known as "snow-white mouth" (雪口 [xuě kǒu])

雪口 [xuě kǒu]

"snow-white mouth": another name for thrust (鹅口疮 [é kǒu chuāng])

口疮 [kǒu chuāng]

aphtha: small oral ulcer

口糜 [kǒu mí]

ulcerative stomatitis: stomatitis characterized by the appearance of shallow ulcers on the cheeks, tongue, gums and palate

燕口疮 [yàn kǒu chuāng]

angular stomatitis: single or multiple fissures at the corners of the mouth

口疳 [kǒu gān]

oral sore: aphthous ulcer, usually occurring in malnourished children

疳 [gān]

(infantile) malnutrition: an infantile disease due to improper feeding, digestive disorders or intestinal parasitosis with symptoms of wasting, pallor or sallow complexion, potbelly, and chronic diarrhea

疳证 [gān zhèng]

malnutrition syndrome: a syndrome characterized by malnutrition in infants

疳病 [gān bìng]

malnutrition disease, synonymous with malnutrition (疳 [gān])

疳气 [gān qì]

malnutrition *qi*: infantile malnutrition at the early stage, characterized by leanness, lusterless complexion, and anorexia

疳气证 [gān qì zhèng]

malnutrition *qi* syndrome: a syndrome characterized by early-stage malnutrition in infants

疳积 [gān jī]

malnutrition with accumulation: infantile malnutrition at the intermediate stage, characterized by marked leanness, sallow complexion, distended abdominal, and listlessness

疳积证 [gān jī zhèng]

malnutrition-accumulation syndrome: syndrome of malnutrition in infants at the intermediate stage with marked leanness and distended abdomen

干疳 [gān gān]

dryness malnutrition: infantile malnutrition at the extreme stage with drying up of *qi* and blood, marked by a dry and shriveled body worn to a shadow

干疳证 [gān gān zhèng]

dryness malnutrition syndrome: a syndrome of malnutrition in infants at the extreme stage with a dry and shriveled body worn to a shadow

丁奚疳 [dīng xī gān]

T-shaped malnutrition: severe case of infantile malnutrition with an emaciated T-shaped figure

五疳 [wǔ gān]

five malnutrition syndromes: an ancient classification of infantile malnutrition, namely, malnutrition involving the spleen, liver, heart, lung, and kidney, respectively

脾疳 [pí gān]

spleen malnutrition: basic syndrome of infantile malnutrition due to accumulation of damp-heat in the spleen, marked by sallow complexion, fever, distended abdomen, emaciation, anorexia, compulsive eating of dirt and mud, and loose bowels, also called feeding malnutrition (食疳 [shi gan])

食疳 [shí gān]

feeding malnutrition: another name for spleen malnutrition (脾疳 [pí gān])

肺疳 [fèi gān]

lung malnutrition: one of the five malnutrition syndromes named in ancient times, characterized by damage to the lung meridian by accumulated heat in cases of malnutrition, manifested as oral and nasal sores and dyspnea, also called *qi* malnutrition (气疳 [qì gān])

气疳 [qì gān]

***qi* malnutrition:** another name for lung malnutrition (肺疳 [fèi gān])

心疳 [xīn gān]

heart malnutrition: one of the five malnutrition syndromes according to an ancient classification, which is caused by improper feeding with sweetstuff that produces heat affecting the heart, manifested as flushed face, fever with sweats, frightened restlessness, grinding of the teeth, oral sores, anorexia and leanness, also called fright malnutrition (惊疳 [jīng gān])

惊疳 [jīng gān]

fright malnutrition: another name for heart malnutrition (心疳 [xīn gān])

肝疳 [gān gān]

liver malnutrition: one of the five malnutrition syndromes according to an ancient classification, which is caused by improper feeding with damage to the liver by heat, manifested by cyanotic complexion, night-blindness, emaciation with a distended abdomen, also called tendon malnutrition (筋疳 [jīn gān])

筋疳 [jīn gān]

tendon malnutrition: another name for liver malnutrition (肝疳 [gān gān])

肾疳 [shèn gān]

kidney malnutrition: one of the five malnutrition syndromes according to an ancient classification, which is ascribed to congenital defect with weak constitution and excessive eating of sweetstuff that produces heat to consume the kidney yin, manifested as heat in the upper portion and cold in the lower portion, vomiting and diarrhea, rectal prolapse, genital sores, and night crying, also known as bone malnutrition (骨疳 [gǔ gān])

骨疳 [gǔ gān]

bone malnutrition: another name for kidney malnutrition (肾疳 [shèn gān])

眼疳 [yǎn gān]

eye malnutrition: attack of liver fire to the eyes in a malnourished child, manifested as inflammation of the eyes first, and then corneal opacity associated with emaciation

蛔疳 [huí gān]

ascaris malnutrition: malnutrition due to ascaris infestation

虫积 [chóng jī]

intestinal parasitosis: infestation of parasitic worms in the intestines, marked by sallow complexion, emaciation, potbelly, and fits of umbilical pain

哺乳疳 [bǔ rǔ gān]

breast-feeding malnutrition: malnutrition of an infant due to improper breast-feeding

乳积 [rǔ jī]

milk indigestion: indigestion due to improper milk feeding

食积 [shí jī]

dyspepsia; indigestion: retention of undigested food, manifested by abdominal distention and pain, vomiting, diarrhea, and impaired appetite

厌食 [yàn shí]

anorexia: a diseased state in children characterized by loss of appetite for food

苦夏 [kǔ xià]

summer affliction: a children's disease occurring in summer, marked by anorexia and loss of weight

疰夏 [zhù xià]

summer consumption: children's disease usually occurring in summer, with symptoms of dyspepsia, dizziness, lassitude and wasting, or with persistent fever

疰夏病 [zhù xià bìng]

summer consumptive disease: full name of summer consumption (疰夏 [zhù xià]) as a disease

夏季热 [xià jì rè]

summer fever: a disease of young children, characterized by prolonged fever in summer owing to lack of adaptability to hot weather

夏季热病 [xià jì rè bìng]

summer fever disease: full name of summer fever (夏季热 [xià jì rè] as a disease

小儿暑温 [xiǎo ér shǔ wēn]

epidemic summer fever in children: an epidemic disease in children caused by toxic warm pathogen in summer and characterized clinically by high fever, convulsions and coma with sudden onset, usually referring to encephalitis B

小儿诸热 [xiǎo ér zhū rè]

various kinds of fever in children

夜热 [yè rè]

fever at night: that usually due to improper feeding or exogenous affection which impairs the function of the spleen and lung

惊热 [jīng rè]

fever due to fright: fever in children induced by fright

客热 [kè rè]

irregular recurrent fever: fever which comes and goes from time to time

血热 [xuè rè]

(1) blood fever: a type of fever which recurs daily at noon and subsides in the evening; **(2) fever at blood stage:** fever accompanied by bleeding symptoms

癖热 [pǐ rè]

fever with splenohepatomegaly: irregular fever accompanied by abdominal distension, vomiting, and enlarged liver and spleen

骨蒸热 [gǔ zhēng rè]

"bone-steaming" fever; consumptive fever: hectic fever accompanied by emaciation, night sweats or mass formation in the abdomen, usually due to improper feeding without timely treatment or remnant heat after a severe disease which consumes the vital essence and body fluid

食积寒热 [shí jī hán rè]

indigestion with chills and fever: indigestion with accumulation of undigested food accompanied by chills and fever

小儿虚热 [xiǎo ér xū rè]

asthenic fever in children: low or tidal fever caused by excessive diaphoresis or purgation or after a serious disease

变蒸 [biàn zhēng]

developmental fever: fever due to the growth and development of the child

痧 [shā]

(1) rash: skin eruption, generally referring to fine, sand-like papules; **(2) noxious attack:** sudden attack of impaired consciousness or vomiting and diarrhea in children in summer, attributed to the invasion of a noxious factor which can often be driven out by scraping the skin

小儿发痧 [xiǎo ér fā shā]

(1) eruptive disease in children; **(2) noxious attack in children:** a popular name for sudden attack of acute vomiting and diarrhea or heat stroke in children

闷痧 [mèn shā]

noxious drowsiness attack: a noxious attack with mental confusion

寒痧 [hán shā]

cold noxious attack: a noxious attack in children marked by tidal fever, cool fingertips, and aversion to cold

热痧 [rè shā]

heat noxious attack: a noxious attack in children marked by fever with restlessness, flushed face, and dire thirst

风疹 [fēng zhěn]

rubella: an infectious eruptive disease caused by a wind-heat pathogen and manifested by low fever, cough, enlargement of the postauricular and suboccipital lymph nodes and generalized pink skin rash, also called 风痧 [fēng shā]

风痧 [fēng shā]

"wind rash", same as rubella (风疹 [fēng zhěn])

麻疹 [má zhěn]

measles: a highly contagious disease caused by a specific seasonal pathogen, clinically marked by skin eruption preceded by coryza, characteristic spots on the buccal mucosa, palpebral conjunctivitis and fever, also called 痧子 [shā zǐ]

痧子 [shā zǐ]

another term for measles (麻疹 [má zhěn])

麻毒内攻 [má dú nèI gōng]

inward invasion of measles: severe case of measles with inadequate eruption to expel the toxins

麻毒入营 [má dú rù yíng]

measles involving constructive system: measles with the toxin penetrating into the constructive system, manifested by high fever, delirium, convulsion, or loss of consciousness

麻毒闭肺 [má dú bì fèi]

measles toxin blocking the lung: measles complicated by pneumonia, also known as measles toxin into lung (麻毒陷肺 [má dú xiàn fèi])

麻毒陷肺 [má dú xiàn fèi]

measles toxin into the lung: measles complicated by pneumonia

麻毒攻目 [má dú gōng mù]

measles attacking the eyes: measles complicated by keratoconjunctivitis

麻疹顺证 [má zhěn shùn zhèng]

improving case of measles: a case of measles with favorable prognosis

麻疹逆证 [má zhěn nì zhèng]

deteriorating case of measles: a case of measles with complications

麻疹闭证 [má zhěn bì zhèng]

measles block syndrome: measles without adequate eruption to expel toxins

麻疹险证 [má zhěn xiǎn zhèng]

critical case of measles

奶麻 [nǎi má]

roseola infantum; exathema subitum: an acute eruptive disease in infants, characterized by sudden subsidence of a high fever of 3-4 days duration with a simultaneous appearance of a macular rash

痘 [dòu]

pox: pea-like skin sores, as seen on the skin of smallpox and chickenpox patients

水痘 [shuǐ dòu]

chickenpox; varicella: an acute contagious disease caused by an epidemic pathogen, marked by fever and formation of vesicles, also called 水疱 [shuǐ pào], 水花 [shuǐ huā], or 水疮 [shuǐ chuāng]

水疱 [shuǐ pào]

another name for chickenpox (水痘 [shuǐ dòu])

水花 [shuǐ huā]

another name for chickenpox (水痘 [shuǐ dòu])

水疮 [shuǐ chuāng]

another name for chickenpox (水痘 [shuǐ dòu])

天花 [tiān huā]

smallpox: an acute contagious febrile disease characterized by skin eruption with pustules, sloughing, and scar formation, also known as 痘疮 [dòu chuāng]

痘疮 [dòu chuāng]

variola: another name for smallpox (天花 [tiān huā])

疫喉 [yì hóu]

epidemic throat diseases: a general term for diphtheria and scarlatina

白喉 [bái hóu]

diphtheria: an acute febrile contagious disease marked by the formation of false membrane in the throat, also called 白缠喉 [bái chán hóu]

白缠喉 [baí chán hóu]

another name for diphtheria (白喉 [bái hóu])

丹痧 [dān shā]

scarlatina: an infection characterized by inflammation of the throat with erythematous rash, also called 喉痧 [hóu shā], 疫痧 [yì shā], or 烂喉丹痧[làn hóu dān shā]

疫痧 [yì shā]

"epidemic erythema": another name for scarlatina (丹痧 [dān shā])

烂喉丹痧 [làn hóu dān shā]

"erosion of the throat with erythema": another name for scarlatina (丹痧 [dān shā])

喉痧 [hóu shā]

"throat infection with erythema": another name for scarlatina (烂喉痧 [làn hóu shā])

杨莓舌 [yáng méi shé]

strawberry-tongue: a crimson, prickly tongue with peeled coating, resembling a strawberry, a sign of scarlatina when the toxin enters the constructive system

痄腮 [zhà sāi]

mumps; epidemic parotitis: an epidemic disease caused by toxic wind-heat and characterized by painful swelling of one or both parotid glands, also called swollen cheek (腮肿 [sāi zhǒng])

腮肿 [sāi zhǒng]

swollen cheek: another name for mumps (痄腮 [zhà sāi])

肺风痰喘 [fèi fēng tán chuǎn]

lung wind with phlegmatic dyspnea: dyspnea in children due to obstruction of *qi* by phlegm in a wind-cold affection of the lung meridian

肺炎喘嗽 [fèi yán chuǎn sòu]

lung inflammation with dyspnea and cough: an external contraction with obstruction of the lung collaterals by the pathogen and manifested mainly by fever, cough, dyspnea and flaring nares

马脾风 [mǎ pí fēng]

sudden asthmatic attack: critical case of asthma in children with a sudden attack due to inflammation of the throat

百日咳 [bǎi rì ké]

pertussis: an acute contagious infection of the respiratory system with characteristic paroxysmal cough, consisting of a deep inspiration, followed by a series of quick, short coughs which end with a long shrill, whooping inspiration, also known as 鹭鸶咳 [lù sī ké], 顿咳 [dùn ké]

顿咳 [dùn ké]

whooping cough: same as pertussis (百日咳 [bǎi rì ké])

鹭鸶咳 [lù sī ké]

"egret's cough": another name for pertussis (百日咳 [bǎi rì ké])

食积盗汗 [shí jī dào hàn]

night sweats accompanying indigestion: sweating during sleep due to retention of food

胃虚汗 [wèi xū hàn]

stomach-insufficiency sweating: abnormal spontaneous sweating due to decreased function of the stomach, distributed from the head to the umbilicus, and accompanied by pallor and lassitude

气鬲 [qì gé]

***qi* dysphagia:** dysphagia due to *qi* disorder

小儿呕吐 [xiǎo ér ǒu tù]

infantile vomiting: vomiting in infants usually due to excess nursing

寒吐 [hán tù]

cold vomiting: vomiting in infants due to deficiency-cold in the stomach

热吐 [rè tù]

heat vomiting: vomiting in infants due to heat in the stomach

胃热呕吐 [wèi rè ǒu tù]

stomach-heat vomiting: same as heat vomiting (热吐 [rè tù])

伤食吐 [shāng shí tù]

vomiting due to improper feeding

伤乳吐 [shāng rǔ tù]

vomiting of milk due to overfeeding, also known as 溢乳 [yì rǔ]

溢乳 [yì rǔ]

milk vomiting: a simplified expression for vomiting of milk due to overfeeding (伤乳吐 [shāng rǔ tù])

积吐 [jī tù]

retention vomiting: vomiting due to retention of food, cold, *qi* or parasitic worms

虫吐 [chóng tù]

ascaris vomiting: vomiting due to intestinal ascariasis when the ascarides enter the stomach

惊吐 [jīng tù]

fright vomiting: vomiting due to being frightened, usually accompanied by fever in the morning and evening, with disturbed sleep and restlessness

小儿卒利 [xiǎo ér cù lì]

sudden infantile diarrhea: sudden occurrence of diarrhea in infants, also called 小儿暴泻 [xiǎo ér bào xiè]

小儿暴泻 [xiǎo ér bào xiè]

same as 小儿卒利 [xiǎo ér cù lì]

小儿泄泻 [xiǎo ér xiè xiè]

infantile diarrhea: the diseased state in infants characterized by abnormally frequent passage of thin, watery stools

小儿寒湿泻 [xiǎo ér hán shī xiè]

infantile cold-damp diarrhea: a type of infantile diarrhea caused by cold-dampness which impairs the spleen, marked by frequent discharge of watery stools with abdominal pain, cold limbs, pallor, and no desire to drink

小儿湿热泻 [xiǎo ér shī rè xiè]

infantile damp-heat diarrhea: a type of infantile diarrhea caused by damp-heat which invades the stomach and intestines, usually occurring in summer, marked by frequent discharge of watery stools with abdominal pain, fever and thirst

小儿热泻 [xiǎo ér rè xiè]

infantile heat diarrhea: a type of infantile diarrhea caused by invasion of the large intestine by summer-heat, marked by frequent discharge of blood-tinged or foamy stools, accompanied by spells of borborygmi, abdominal pain and restlessness

小儿火泻 [xiǎo ér huǒ xiè]

infantile fire diarrhea: a type of infantile diarrhea caused by accumulation of intense heat in the large intestine, marked by spouting discharge of large amounts of watery stools, accompanied by a burning sensation in the anus, abdominal pain, fever and flushed face

脐寒泻 [qí hán xiè]

umbilical cold diarrhea: a type of infantile diarrhea due to wind-cold invasion of the cut end of the umbilicus which has not been properly treated, marked by discharge of thin stools accompanied by abdominal pain and borborygmi

脾虚泻 [pí xū xiè]

spleen-insufficiency diarrhea: a type of chronic infantile diarrhea marked by discharge of loose stools containing undigested food soon after meals, accompanied by emaciation, sallow complexion and listlessness

中寒泻 [zhòng hán xiè]

cold-stroke diarrhea: a type of infantile diarrhea caused by direct attack of cold to the spleen and stomach, marked by discharge of thin stools, anorexia, abdominal pain, cold limbs, and pallor

伤食泻 [shāng shí xiè]

indigestion diarrhea: a type of infantile diarrhea due to indigestion either as a result of improper feeding or due to decreased function of the stomach, marked by discharge of loose stools containing undigested food with sour fetid odor

飧水泻 [sūn shuǐ xiè]

watery lienteric diarrhea: a type of infantile diarrhea characterized by discharge of watery stools containing undigested food

肾虚泻 [shèn xū xiè]

kidney-insufficiency diarrhea: a type of infantile diarrhea due to deficiency of kidney yang as a result of a congenital defect or after a protracted disease, marked by discharge of liquid stools daily before dawn

小儿腹痛 [xiǎo ér fù tòng]

abdominal pain in children

盘肠气痛 [pán cháng qì tòng]

intestinal *qi* colic: a type of abdominal pain often occurring in children with a weak spleen after exposure to cold

气积腹痛 [qì jī fù tòng]

***qi*-stagnation abdominal pain:** abdominal pain due to *qi* stagnation, marked by dull pain accompanied by abdominal distension and belching

虫积腹痛 [chóng jī fù tòng]

worm-accumulating abdominal pain: that usually referring to abdominal pain due to intestinal ascariasis

食积腹痛 [shí jī fù tòng]

food-retention abdominal pain: abdominal pain due to retention of food

小儿腹胀 [xiǎo ér fù zhàng]

abdominal distension in children

虚胀 [xū zhàng]

abdominal distension of deficiency type: a type of abdominal distension due to *qi* deficiency or blood deficiency

实胀 [shí zhàng]

abdominal distension of excess type: a type of abdominal distension due to food retention, damp stagnation, damp-heat accumulation, or blood stasis

伤食腹胀 [shāng shí fù zhàng]

abdominal distension accompanying indigestion: abdominal distension due to overeating with indigestion

小儿瘿气 [xiǎo ér yǐng qì]

endemic goiter in children

小儿消渴 [xiǎo ér xiāo kě]

diabetes in children

消上 [xiāo shàng]

upper diabetes: diabetes marked by polydipsia

消肌 [xiāo jī]

muscle-wasting diabetes: diabetes marked by polyphagia and emaciation

消浊 [xiāo zhuó]

turbid diabetes: diabetes marked by turbid urine

癫痫 [diān xián]

epilepsy: paroxysmal transient disturbance of the mind manifested as episodic loss of consciousness with generalized tonic-clinic seizures, also called 颠疾 [diān jí] or 痫证 [xián zhèng]

颠疾 [diān jí]

epilepsy in older children: epilepsy occurring in children over ten years of age

痫证 [xián zhèng]

epilepsy in younger children: epilepsy occurring in children under ten years of age

阴痫 [yīn xián]

(1) yin epilepsy: epilepsy accompanied by yin symptoms such as cold limbs, pallor and feeble voice; **(2) yin convulsions,** same as chronic infantile convulsions (慢惊风 [màn jīng fēng])

阳痫 [yáng xián]

(1) yang epilepsy: epilepsy accompanied by yang symptoms such as fever, sweating, flushed face, trismus or incessant crying; **(2) yang convulsions,** same as acute infantile convulsions (急惊风 [jí jīng fēng])

暴痫 [bào xián]

sudden epilepsy: sudden occurrence of epilepsy with no predisposing factor

食痫 [shí xián]

dietary epilepsy: epileptic seizure induced by overfeeding

风痫 [fēng xián]

wind epilepsy: (1) epilepsy with aphasia after seizure; (2) convulsive seizure induced by affection of exogenous wind

惊痫 [jīng xián]

fright epilepsy: epileptic seizure induced by fright

痰痫 [tán xián]

phlegm epilepsy: epileptic seizure due to phlegm, marked by salivation, phlegmatic sounds in the throat, mental confusion with eyes staring straight ahead

寒痫 [hán xián]

cold epilepsy: epileptic seizure predisposed by cold

热痫 [rè xián]

heat epilepsy: epileptic seizure induced by internally accumulated heat

虫痫 [chóng xián]

parasitic epilepsy: epilepsy caused by parasitosis, e.g., cysticercosis

胎痫 [tāi xián]

fetal epilepsy: epilepsy in newborn due to injury of the fetus before delivery

瘀血痫 [yū xuè xián]

blood-stasis epilepsy: epilepsy in children caused by trauma or birth injury

小儿麻痹 [xiǎo ér má bì]

infantile paralysis; poliomyelitis: an acute infectious disease characterized clinically by fever, sore throat, and paralysis of the limbs, subsequently with permanent disability and deformity

小儿浮肿 [xiǎo ér fú zhǒng]

edema in children: edema occurring in children mostly 2-7 years old, also called 小儿水肿 [xiǎo ér shuǐ zhǒng]

小儿水肿 [xiǎo ér shuǐ zhǒng]

edema in children: same as 小儿浮肿 [xiǎo ér fú zhǒng]

小儿水气肿 [xiǎo ér shuǐ qì zhǒng]

anasarca in children: generalized edema occurring in children

小儿遗尿 [xiǎo ér yí niào]

enuresis in children; bed-wetting: urinating while asleep, ascribed to inadequacy of genuine *qi* and immaturity of the internal organs in children

遗尿 [yí niào]

enuresis; bed-wetting: urinary incontinence during sleep, mostly occurring in children

兔唇 [tù chún]

harelip: congenital cleft or defect of the upper lip

腭裂 [é liè]

cleft palate: congenital fissure of the palate

侏儒 [zhū rú]

dwarfism: unusually shortness of stature

外科 External Medicine

外证 [wài zhèng]

external disease: a collective term for diseases with lesions visible or palpable from without, mostly referring to skin diseases and some surgical conditions

疹 [zhěn]

rash: temporary eruption on the skin, mostly referring to papula

斑 [bān]

macula: a general term for any spot or area distinguishable by color from its surroundings

疱疹 [pào zhěn]

vesicle: small circumscribed elevation of the outer layer of skin enclosing a watery liquid

痂 [jiá]

crust: outer layer formed by the drying of a bodily exudate

丘疹 [qiū zhěn]

papule: small conical elevation of the skin

脓疱 [nóng pào]

pustule: small circumscribed elevation of the skin containing pus

肿疡 [zhǒng yáng]

swelling (sore): any swelling in external diseases that has not ruptured

溃疡 [kuì yáng]

ulcer: any lesion in external diseases with a local defect of the surface produced by the sloughing of the necrotic tissue

结核 [jié hé]

subcutaneous node: a general term for any round mass formed under the skin

疮疡 [chuāng yáng]

sore and ulcer: any pyogenic infection on the body surface

疡 [yáng]

(1) ulcer; (2) surgical conditions

疮 [chuāng]

(1) sore; (2) wound

肿毒 [zhǒng dú]

toxic swelling: swelling in a pyogenic inflammation

漏 [lòu]

fistula: an abnormal passage leading from an abscess or hollow organ to the body surface

疖 [jiē]

furuncle; boil: a localized swelling and inflammation of the skin, having a hard central core, and forming pus

暑疖 [shǔ jiē]

summer boil: boil secondary to miliaria or small furuncle, occurring in summer

蝼蛄疖 [lóu gū jiē]

folliculitis abscedens et suffodiens: multiple abscesses of the scalp

发际疮 [fà jì chuāng]

hairline boil: boil occurring at the back of the neck close to the hairline

疖病 [jiē bìng]

furunculosis: the condition of tending to develop multiple furuncles

坐板疮 [zuò bǎn chuāng]

gluteal boil: boil on the buttock

疔 [dīng]

deep-rooted boil: a boil with its central core deeply rooted

蛇眼疔 [shé yǎn dīng]

snake-eye whitlow [felon]: paronychia with inflammation of both sides of the fingernail, resembling the eyes of a snake

蛇头疔 [shé tóu dīng]

snake-head whitlow [felon]: digital pyogenic inflammation with a swollen fingertip resembling the head of a snake

蛇肚疔 [shé dù dīng]

snake-body whitlow [felon]: digital pyogenic inflammation with swelling of the middle segment of the finger, resembling the body of a snake

托盘疔 [tuō pán dīng]

palmar pustule: acute pyogenic inflammation of the central part of the palm, with a pustule formation like a pearl placed on a tray, also called 掌心毒 [zhǎng xīn dú]

掌心毒 [zhǎng xīn dú]

palmar pustule, synonymous with 托盘疔 [tuō pán dīng]

足底疔 [zú dǐ dīng]

plantar pustule: acute pyogenic inflammation of the sole with pustule formation

红丝疔 [hóng sī dīng]

(1) "red-streaked boil": a boil complicated by acute inflammation of the adjacent lymph vessel or vessels, forming a painful red streak or streaks under the skin; **(2) acute lymphangitis:** acute inflammation of the lymph vessel

疫疔 [yì dīng]

cutaneous anthrax: an infectious zoonotic disease transmitted to humans by contact with infected animals, manifested as a small, painless, pruritic papular lesion that enlarges, ulcerates, and becomes crusted with a dense black eschar

烂疔 [làn dīng]

gas gangrene: an acute, severe infection, often occurring in a dirty, lacerated wound, in which the lesion is filled with thin purulent fluid and gas, followed by sloughing of a large amount of necrotic tissue

颜面疔疮 [yán miàn dīng chuāng]

deep-rooted boil on the face: deep-rooted furuncle or carbuncle occurring on the face, which may easily progress to pyosepticemia

痈 [yōng]

abscess: a pyogenic infection with localized collection of pus buried in tissues or organs

内痈 [nèi yōng]

internal abscess: abscess formed in an internal organ

外痈 [wài yōng]

superficial abscess: abscess occurring in the subcutaneous tissue

颈痈 [jǐng yōng]

suppurative lymphadenitis of neck: a condition characterized by enlarged, inflamed and tender cervical lymph nodes

腋痈 [yè yōng]

axillary abscess: acute suppurative axillary lymphadenitis with abscess formation

胯腹痈 [kuà fǔ yōng]

inguinal lymphadenitis; inguinal abscess: acute pyogenic inflammation in the inguinal region with enlarged painful lymph node and difficulty in walking

委中毒 [wěi zhōng dú]

popliteal lymphadenitis: acute pyogenic inflammation in the popliteal region with localized stiffness and pain which causes difficulty in bending and extending the leg

脐痈 [qí yōng]

(1) omphalitis: inflammation of the umbilicus; **(2) umbilical abscess:** acute pyogenic inflammation in the umbilical region with pus collection, usually easy to heal after rupture

脐疮 [qí chuāng]

umbilical sore: an acute inflammation in the umbilical region

脐漏 [qí lòu]

umbilical fistula: an abnormal passage communicating with the gut or with the urachus at the umbilicus

锁喉痈 [suǒ hóu yōng]

throat-blocking phlegmon: (1) phlegmon of the neck, which causes obstruction of the throat and difficulty in swallowing; (2) abscess on the laryngeal protuberance

丹毒 [dān dú]

erysipelas: an acute infection of the skin marked by intense local redness

火丹 [huǒ dān]

erysipelas, same as 丹毒 [dān dú]

抱头火丹 [pào tóu huǒ dān]

head erysipelas; facial erysipelas: erysipelas that affects the head or face

流火 [liú huǒ]

shank erysipelas: erysipelas that affects the leg

赤游丹 [chì yóu dān]

wandering erysipelas: a type of erysipelas in children characterized by changing the location of the lesion either from the trunk to the extremities or from the extremities to the trunk

无名肿毒 [wú míng zhǒng dú]

nameless toxic swelling: a kind of local inflammation on the body surface, often hard, red and painful

发 [fā]

(1)cellulitis: acute, diffuse and suppurative inflammation of the deep subcutaneous tissue; **(2) phlegmon:** purulent inflammation and infiltration of connective tissue

发背 [fā bèi]

dorsal carbuncle: carbuncle occurring on the back

搭手 [dā shǒu]

laterodorsal carbuncle: carbuncle occurring on the lateral back

手部疔疮 [shǒu bù dīng chuāng]

pustule of the hand

手发背 [shǒu fā bèi]

phlegmon of dorsum of hand: an acute pyogenic infection of the dorsum of the hand, characterized by diffuse swelling and inflammation which forms a suppurative or gangrenous lesion that may extend into deep subcutaneous tissues and muscles

足发背 [zú fā bèi]

phlegmon of the dorsum of foot: acute pyogenic infection of the dorsum of the foot with diffuse swelling and inflammation

臀痈 [tún yōng]

gluteal abscess: cellulitis of the buttocks with abscess formation

疽 [jū]

phlegmon: purulent inflammation and infiltration of connective tissue

有头疽 [yǒu tóu jū]

carbuncle: a necrotizing infection of skin and subcutaneous tissue with multiple openings for the discharge of pus and sloughing of dead tissue

瘭疽 [biāo jū]

whitlow; felon: an extremely painful abscess on the palmar aspect of the fingertip

发颐 [fā yí]

suppurative parotitis: inflammation of the parotid gland associated with suppuration

肩胛疽 [jiān jiǎ jū]

scapular carbuncle: carbuncle occurring in the scapular region

股阴疽 [gǔ yīn jū]

thigh yin cellulitis: cellulitis on the medial aspect of the thigh

股阳疽 [gǔ yáng jū]

thigh yang cellulitis: cellulitis on the lateral aspect of the thigh

流注 [liú zhù]

metastatic abscess: a secondary abscess, usually multiple, deeply located, and distant from the primary lesion

髂窝流注 [qià wō liú zhù]

metastatic abscess of iliac fossa: a type of metastatic abscess occurring in the iliac fossa

无头疽 [wú tóu jū]

deep abscess: a pyogenic inflammation located deeply with no color change of the skin surface, usually difficult to rupture and heal

附骨疽 [fù gǔ jū]

lateral suppurative osteomyelitis: a suppurative inflammatory bone disease, marked by local death and separation of tissue, occurring on the lateral side of the thigh

咬骨疽 [yǎo gǔ jū]

medial suppurative osteomyelitis: a suppurative inflammatory bone disease, marked by local death and separation of tissue, occurring on the medial side of thigh

环跳疽 [huán tiào jū]

suppurative coxitis: suppurative inflammation of the hip joint

臁疮 [lián chuāng]

shank sore: chronic ulcer on the shank

脱疽 [tuō jū]

finger-toe gangrene: gangrene of the extremities, especially referring to thromboangiitis, also called 脱骨疽 [tuō gǔ jū]

脱骨疽 [tuō gǔ jū]

gangrene of the extremities, synonymous with 脱疽 [tuō jū]

走黄 [zǒu huáng]

pyosepticemia: a general septicemia in which secondary foci of suppuration occur and multiple abscesses are formed

疔疮走黄 [dīng chuāng zǒu huáng]

deep-rooted boil with pyosepticemia

内陷 [nèi xiàn]

inward invasion: penetration (of pyogenic toxin) into the blood and internal organs

干陷 [gān xiàn]

non-festering inward invasion: a type of inward invasion marked by scanty suppuration of the pyogenic lesion with impaired consciousness and collapse

火陷 [huǒ xiàn]

inward invasion of fire: a type of inward invasion with penetration of fire toxin into the nutrient system, manifested by high fever, thirst, restlessness and delirium associated with dark-colored and dehydrated inflamed lesion

疮毒内陷 [chuāng dú nèi xiàn]

inward invasion of pyogenic toxin: penetration of pyogenic toxin into the blood and internal organs, resulting in generalized pyogenic infection

瘰疬 [luǒ lì]

scrofula: tuberculosis of the cervical lymph node

流痰 [liú tán]

tuberculosis of bone and joint, also known as 骨痨 [gǔ láo], 疮痨 [chuāng láo]

骨痨 [gǔ láo]

bone phthisis, synonymous with tuberculosis of bone and joint (流痰 [liú tán])

疮痨 [chuāng láo]

same as 流痰 [liú tán]

乳头破碎 [rǔ tóu pò suì]

cracked nipple, also called 乳头风 [rǔ tóu fēng]

乳头风 [rǔ tóu fēng]

cracked nipple, synonymous with 乳头破碎 [rǔ tóu pò suì]

乳痈 [rǔ yōng]

acute mastitis: acute pyogenic inflammation of the breast

内吹乳痈 [nèi chuī rǔ yōng]

pregnant mastitis: mastitis occurring during pregnancy

外吹乳痈 [wài chuī rǔ yōng]

puerperal mastitis: mastitis occurring after delivery

乳发 [rǔ fā]

phlegmonous mastitis: inflammation of the breast leading to necrosis and abscess formation

乳疽 [rǔ jū]

intramammary abscess: a variety of acute mastitis characterized by early formation of abscess and rupture

乳痨 [rǔ láo]

mammary phthisis: tuberculosis of the breast, also called mammary phlegm (乳痰 [rǔ tán])

乳痰 [rǔ tán]

mammary phlegm: another name for mammary phthisis (乳痨 [rǔ láo]), so called because of the thin pus discharged resembling phlegm

乳漏 [rǔ lòu]

mammary fistula: an abnormal passage between the lacteal duct of the gland and the cutaneous surface of the breast or areola of the nipple

乳癖 [rǔ pǐ]

hyperplasia of the mammary gland: presence of nodular masses in the breast, painful, movable and not firm, often related to the menstrual cycle and emotional change

乳中结核 [rǔ zhōng jié hé]

nodule in the breast: same as breast nodule (乳核 [rǔ hé])

乳核 [rǔ hé]

breast nodule: benign tumor of the breast, usually referring to fibro-adenoma of the mammary gland, also known as nodule in the breast (乳中结核 [rǔ zhōng jié hé])

乳疬 [rǔ lì]

(1) gynecomastia: excessive development of the breast in the male; **(2) mastauxy** (in children): enlargement of the breast in children

乳衄 [rǔ nǜ]

thelorrhagia: bleeding from the nipple

瘿 [yǐng]

goiter: enlargement of the thyroid gland, causing a swelling in the front part of the neck

气瘿 [qì yǐng]

***qi* goiter:** goiter due to emotional depression or geographical factors, mainly referring to simple goiter or endemic goiter

肉瘿 [ròu yǐng]

fleshy goiter: soft or beefy goiter, often accompanied by irritability, palpitation, discomfort in the chest, or menstrual disorder, mostly referring to the thyroid enlargement in Graves' disease or adenoma of the thyroid gland

石瘿 [shí yǐng]

stony goiter: enlarged thyroid, nodulated and as hard as stone, mostly referring to carcinoma of the thyroid

筋瘿 [jīn yǐng]

varicose goiter: goiter with prominent varicose veins

瘿痈 [yǐng yōng]

acute thyroiditis: acute inflammation of the thyroid gland, with mass formation, swelling, heat and pain

瘤 [liú]

tumor: a neoplasm which persists and has no physiological use, often caused by stagnant blood, retained phlegm, and lingering turbid *qi*

气瘤 [qì liú]

***qi* tumor:** a term for multiple pedunculated soft tumors arising superficially under the skin, becoming flat on pressing and bulging again when the pressure is removed as if they were filled with air (*qi*), mostly referring to neurofibroma

血瘤 [xuè liú]

blood tumor; hemangioma: a vascular tumor composed of dilated blood vessels in the skin or subcutaneously, including capillary hemangioma and carvernous hemangioma

肉瘤 [ròu liú]

fat tumor: lipoma

筋瘤 [jīn liú]

varix: an enlarged and tortuous vein, usually in the leg

骨瘤 [gǔ liú]

bone tumor: osteoma

脂瘤 [zhī liú]

sebaceous cyst: a cyst derived from the sebaceous gland, filled with lipid-rich debris, also called 粉瘤 [fěn liú]

粉瘤 [fěn liú]

sebaceous cyst, same as 脂瘤 [zhī liú]

岩 [yán]

cancer; carcinoma

舌菌 [shé jūn]

carcinoma of the tongue, also called 舌岩 [shé yán]

舌岩 [shé yán]

carcinoma of the tongue, same as 舌菌 [shé jūn]

茧唇 [jiǎn chún]

carcinoma of the lip

失荣 [shī róng]

cervical malignancy with cachexia: advanced case of malignant tumor of the cervical lymph node, either primary or metastatic, accompanied by cachexia

乳岩 [rǔ yán]

mammary cancer

肾岩 [shèn yán]

carcinoma of the penis, also known as 肾癌 [shèn ái]

肾癌 [shèn ái]

carcinoma of the penis, same as 肾岩 [shèn yán]

肾岩翻花 [shèn yán fān huā]

carcinoma of the penis with ulceration

痔 [zhì]

hemorrhoid; pile: varicose dilatation of a vein of the superior or inferior hemorrhoidal plexus

内痔 [nèi zhì]

internal hemorrhoid: varicose dilatation of a vein of the superior hemorrhoidal plexus, situated above the pectinate line

外痔 [wài zhì]

external hemorrhoid: varicose dilatation of a vein of the inferior hemorrhoidal plexus, situated distal to the pectinate line

内外痔 [nèi wài zhì]

mixed hemorrhoid: varicose dilatation of a vein connecting the superior and inferior hemorrhoidal plexuses, forming an external and an internal hemorrhoid in continuity

血箭痔 [xuè jiàn zhì]

blood-spurting hemorrhoids: internal hemorrhoids with massive bleeding

脱肛 [tuō gāng]

prolapse of the rectum: protrusion of the rectal mucous membrane through the anus

肛漏 [gāng lòu]

anal fistula: a fistula opening on the cutaneous surface near the anus, which may communicate with the rectum, also called 肛瘘 [gāng lòu]

肛瘘 [gāng lòu]

anal fistula, same as 肛漏 [gāng lòu]

肛裂 [gāng liè]

anal fissure: a painful linear ulcer at the margin of the anus

肛痈 [gāng yōng]

anorectal abscess: abscess arising in the anorectum

息肉痔 [xī ròu zhì]

rectal polyp: polyp of the rectum

肠痔 [cháng zhì]

perianal abscess: a superficial abscess occurring beneath the perianal skin

交肠 [jiāo cháng]

rectovesical fistula: fistula between the rectum and the urinary bladder

子痈 [zǐ yōng]

epididymitis and orchitis

囊痈 [náng yōng]

scrotal abscess

子痰 [zǐ tán]

tuberculosis of epididymis: tuberculosis involving the epididymis which gradually increases in size, suppurates, and ruptures to discharge thin purulent fluid resembling phlegm

水疝 [shuǐ shàn]

hydrocele: an accumulation of fluid in the testicle

精浊 [jīng zhuó]

prostatitis: inflammation of the prostate marked by frequent overflow of seminal fluid from the urethral orifice

精癃 [jīng lóng]

prostatic hypertrophy: hypertrophy of the prostate that causes difficulty in urination or retention of urine

睾丸萎缩 [gāo wán wěi suō]

atrophy of testis

睾丸肿痛 [gāo wán zhǒng tòng]

painful and swollen testis

偏坠 [piān zhuì]

unilateral swelling of testis: that which is often accompanied by a bearing-down pain

热疮 [rè chuāng]

herpes febrilis: herpes simplex usually occurring as a concomitant of fever

蛇串疮 [shé chuàn chuāng]

herpes zoster: an acute eruptive disease characterized by severe pain along the girdled distribution of clustered vesicles, also called 缠腰火丹 [chán yāo huǒ dān], 缠腰蛇丹 [chán yāo shé dān] and 火带疮 [huǒ dài chuāng]

缠腰火丹 [chán yāo huǒ dān]

another name for 蛇串疮 [shé chuàn chuāng]

缠腰蛇丹 [chán yāo shé dān]

another name for 蛇串疮 [shé chuàn chuāng]

火带疮 [huǒ dài chuāng]

another name for 蛇串疮 [shé chuàn chuāng]

蛇丹 [shén dān]

another name for 蛇串疮 [shé chuàn chuāng]

疣 [yóu]

verruca; wart: a horny projection on the skin

瘊子 [hóu zǐ]

wart: popular name for verruca (疣 [yóu])

疣目 [yóu mù]

verruca vulgaris: a lobulated hyperplastic epidermal lesion with a horny surface, usually occurring on the back of the hand, fingers or scalp

扁瘊 [biǎn hóu]

verruca plana; flat wart: a small, smooth, slightly raised wart, occurring on the face, back of the hands, or wrists

跖疣 [zhí yóu]

verruca plantaris; plantar wart: wart on the sole of the foot

鼠乳 [shǔ rǔ]

infectious wart: small papular, umbilicated skin lesion transmitted by contact, containing white cheese-like substance, and usually occurring on the trunk or face

丝状疣 [sī zhuàng yóu]

verruca filiformis: a wart with soft, thin, threadlike projections on its surface, also called 线瘊 [xiàn hóu]

线瘊 [xiàn hóu]

filiform wart: another name for verruca filiformis (丝状疣 [sī zhuàng yóu])

趼子 [jiǎn zǐ]

callus: popular name for 胼胝 [piàn zhī]

胼胝 [piàn zhī]

(1) callus: hard thickened area on the skin ; **(2) callosity:** state of being callous

鸡眼 [jī yǎn]

clavus: corn

皲裂 [jūn liè]

crack: that occurring on the skin

皲裂疮 [jūn liè chuāng]

rhagades: linear cracks or fissures on the skin, especially such lesions around the mouth or other regions subjected to frequent movement

痱（子） [fèi (zǐ)]

miliaria; prickly heat: an inflammatory disorder of the skin characterized by redness, eruption, and itching due to blockage of sweat ducts

粉刺 [fěn cì]

acne: an inflammatory disease of the follicles and sebaceous glands, occurring on the face, chest and back, also known as 酒刺 [jiǔ cì]

酒刺 [jiǔ cì]

acne, same as 粉刺 [fěn cì]

雀斑 [què bān]

freckle: small brown spot on the skin

血缕 [xuè lǚ]

vascular spider: spider nevus

酒皶鼻 [jiǔ zhā bí]

rosacea: chronic hyperemic disease of the skin, usually involving the middle part of the face, particularly the nose, also known as 赤鼻 [chì bí]

赤鼻 [chì bí]

"red nose": another name for rosacea (酒皶鼻 [jiǔ zhā bí])

猫眼疮 [māo yǎn chuāng]

erythema multiforme: an acute self-limited inflammatory skin disease characterized by sudden onset of erythematous macular, bullous, papular, nodose, or vesicular eruption

瓜藤缠 [guā téng chán]

erythema nodosum: a type of panniculitis which most often affects young women and is characterized by the development of crops of transient, inflammatory nodules that are usually tender, multiple, and bilateral, most commonly located on the shins

红蝴蝶疮 [hóng hú dié chuāng]

lupus erythematosus: a systemic or non-systemic disease marked by butterfly rash

皮痹 [pí pì]

"skin blockage": scleroderma

白癜风 [bái diàn fēng]

vitiligo: a skin disease manifested as smooth white spots on various parts of the body, also called 白驳风 [bái bó fēng]

白驳风 [bái bó fēng]

same as (白癜风 [bài diàn fēng])

白屑风 [bái xiè fēng]

seborrhea sicca: scaly seborrheic dermatitis

牛皮癣 [niú pí xuǎn]

neurodermatitis: chronic disorder of the skin characterized by patches of itching lichenoid eruption resembling cattle hide, also known as stubborn lichen (顽癣 [wán xuǎn]) because of its chronicity

摄领疮 [shè lǐng chuāng]

cervical neurodermatitis: neurodermatitis occurring on the nape and neck

顽癣 [wán xuǎn]

"stubborn lichen": another name for neurodermatitis (牛皮癣 [niú pí xuǎn])

风热疮 [fēng rè chuāng]

pityriasis rosea: an acute or subacute, self-limited exanthematous disease, the onset of which is marked by the presence of a solitary rose-colored herald plaque, most often seen on the trunk, followed by the development of papular or macular lesions which have vesicular borders subsequently that tend to peel and produce a scaly collarette, also known as "wind itch" (风痒 [fēng yǎng])

风痒 [fēng yǎng]

"wind itch": another name for pityriasis rosea (风热疮 [fēng rè chuāng])

白疕 [bái bì]

psoriasis: a chronic skin disease marked by rounded, circumscribed, erythematous, dry, scaling patches, covered by silvery white, lamellar scales, resembling the bark of a pine tree

松皮癣 [sōng pí xuǎn]

"pine-bark lichen": another name for psoriasis (白疕 [bái bì])

面游风 [miàn yóu fēng]

seborrhea; seborrheic dermatitis: a chronic inflammation of the skin marked by excessive secretion of sebum

发落 [fà luò]

alopecia: a disease causing the hair to fall

发蛀脱发 [fà zhù tuō fà]

alopecia seborrheica: alopecia associated with seborrheic dermatitis

斑秃 [bān tū]

alopecia areata: patchy loss of hair, occurring in sharply defined areas

油风 [yóu fēng]

alopecia: a disease marked by sudden patchy loss of hair, which usually occurs in sharply defined areas, referring to alopecia areata (斑秃 [bān tū]), but may involve the whole scalp and the beard

疥疮 [jiè chuāng]

scabies: contagious dermatitis caused by mite, also called 疥癞 [jiè lài]

疥癞 [jiè lài]

same as 疥疮 [jiè chuāng]

风团 [fēng tuán]

wheal: suddenly formed itching elevation of the skin surface

风瘙痒 [fēng sào yǎng]

pruritus cutis: itching of the skin

隐(瘾)疹 [yǐn zhěn]

urticaria; hives: an allergic disorder of the skin, marked by red or pale wheals, on and off, and usually by intense itching, also known as 风瘾疹 [fēng yǐn zhěn]

风瘾疹 [fēng yǐn zhěn]

same as 隐疹 [yǐn zhěn]

虫咬皮炎 [chóng yǎo pí yán]

insect dermatitis: a dermatitis caused by insect bite or the toxin-containing irritant hairs of certain insects

接触性皮炎 [jiē chù xìng pí yán]

contact dermatitis: dermatitis caused by substances coming in contact with the skin

漆疮 [qī chuāng]

lacquer dermatitis: a type of contact dermatitis produced by lacquer

膏药风 [gāo yào fēng]

adhesive-plaster dermatitis: a type of contact dermatitis caused by the application of adhesive plaster

药毒 [yào dú]

dermatitis medicamentosa: drug eruption

湿疮 [shī chuāng]

eczema: an inflammatory skin disease characterized by symmetrical distribution, itching, vesiculation, watery discharge, and the development of scales and crusts, also called 湿疹 [shī zhěn]

湿疹 [shī zhě]

same as 湿疮 [shī chuāng]

旋耳疮 [xuán ěr chuāng]

auricular eczema: eczema occurring in the auricular region

四弯风 [sì wān fēng]

cubito-popliteal eczema: eczema occurring in the cubital and popliteal fossae

肾囊风 [shèn náng fēng]

scrotal eczema: eczema of the scrotum

脐疮 [qí chuāng]

umbilical eczema: eczema occurring in the umbilical region

浸淫疮 [jìn yín chuāng]

exudative eczema: eczema in the acute stage characterized by erythema, edema associated with serous exudate

婴儿湿疮 [yīng ér shī chuāng]

infantile eczema: a form common in infants, which usually occurs on the cheeks and then may extend to other areas, also called 奶癣 [nǎi xuǎn]

奶癣 [nǎi xuǎn]

"milk dermatitis": another name for infantile eczema (婴儿湿疮 [yīng ér shī chuāng])

湿癣 [shī xuǎn]

exudative dermatitis: a variety of dermatitis marked by itching and exudation, mostly referring to acute eczema

脚湿气 [jiǎo shī qì]

tinea pedis: tinea involving the feet, also known as 脚气疮 [jiǎo qì chuāng]

脚气疮 [jiǎo qì chuāng]

same as 脚湿气 [jiǎo shī qì]

黄水疮 [huáng shuǐ chuāng]

impetigo: a contagious pyoderma which is usually seen in children and is characterized by discrete fragile vesicles that become pustular, and rupture to discharge a thin yellow seropurulent fluid

癣 [xuǎn]

ringworm; tinea: any superficial fungal infection caused by a dermatophyte and involving the skin, hair and nails

秃疮 [tū chuāng]

scabby scalp: usually referring to white ringworm

白秃疮 [bái tū chuāng]

tinea alba; white ringworm: a type of ringworm of the scalp, manifested by multiple whitish or gray scaly lesions

肥疮 [féi chuāng]

tinea favosa; favus: a type of ringworm characterized by formation of yellow cup-shaped crusts

风癣 [fēng xuǎn]

tinea corporis, synonymous with tinea circinata (圆癣 [yuán xuǎn])

股癣 [gǔ xuǎn]

tinea cruris: tinea in the groin or perineal area

鹅掌风 [é zhǎng fēng]

tinea manuum: ringworm affecting the hands

鹅爪风 [é zhuǎ fēng]

tinea unguium: ringworm affecting the nails and making them opaque, white, thickened and brittle

干癣 [gān xuǎn]

(1) chronic eczema; (2) neurodermatitis

圆癣 [yuán xuǎn]

tinea circinata: tinea involving glabrous skin areas other than the hands and feet, characterized by one or more well-demarcated erythematous, scaly macules with raised borders and central healing, producing annular outlines

紫白癜风 [zǐ bái diàn fēng]

tinea versicolor: a skin disorder characterized by multiple macular patches, of all sizes and shapes, varying from white in pigmented skin to tan or brown in pale skin

腋臭 [yè chòu]

hircismus: strong odor of the axillae caused by apocrine sweat

麻风 [má fēng]

leprosy: a chronic infectious disease characterized by the formation of nodules on the surface of the body and especially on the face, accompanied by loss of sensation, also called 大风 [dà fēng], 疠风 [lì fēng], 癞病 [lài bìng]

大风 [dà fēng]

another name for 麻风 [má fēng]

疠风 [lì fēng]

another name for 麻风 [má fēng]

癞病 [lài bìng]

another name for 麻风 [má fēng]

烧伤 [shāo shāng]

burn: injury to tissue caused by contact with fire, also called 火伤 [huǒ shāng]

火伤 [huǒ shāng]

burn, same as 烧伤 [shāo shāng]

金疮 [jīn chuāng]

incised wound

破伤风 [pò shāng fēng]

tetanus: an acute, often fatal, disease caused by toxic wind pathogen introduced through a wound, manifested as lockjaw, glottal spasm, generalized muscle spasm, opisthotonos and respiratory spasm, also called 金疮痉 [jīn chuāng jìng]

金疮痉 [jīn chuāng jìng]

tetanus: another name for 破伤风 [pò shāng fēng]

冻疮 [dòng chuāng]

chilblain: an inflammatory swelling or sore caused by exposure to cold, also called 冻风 [dòng fēng]

冻风 [dòng fēng]

same as 冻疮 [dòng chuāng]

褥疮 [rù chuāng]

bedsore: decubitus ulcer

青蛇毒 [qīng shé dú]

superficial thrombophlebitis: inflammation of a superficial vein associated with thrombus formation

股肿 [gǔ zhǒng]

deep thrombophlebitis: thrombus formation and inflammation of a deep-located vein

毒蛇咬伤 [dú shé yǎo shāng]

venomous snake bite

毒虫咬伤 [dú chóng yǎo shāng]

insect bite

眼科 Ophthalmology

五轮 [wǔ lún]

five orbiculi: a collective term for the eyelid, canthus, white of the eye, black of the eye and pupil. A theory of ophthalmology holds that each of the *zang* organs is physio-pathologically related to one of the orbiculi respectively. (cf. 肉轮 [ròu lún], 血轮 [xuè lún], 气轮 [qì lún], 风轮 [fēng lún], 水轮 [shuǐ lún])

肉轮 [ròu lún]

"flesh orbiculus": eyelid, one of the five orbiculi, which is believed to be closely related to the spleen

血轮 [xuè lún]

"blood orbiculus": canthus, one of the five orbiculi, which is believed to be closely related to the heart

气轮 [qì lún]

"*qi* orbiculus": white of the eye, one of the five orbiculi, which is believed to be closely related to the lung

风轮 [fēng lún]

"wind orbiculus": black of the eye, one of the five orbiculi, which is believed to be closely related to the liver

水轮 [shuǐ lún]

"water orbiculus": pupil, one of the five orbiculi, which is believed to be closely related to the kidney

八廓 [bā kuò]

eight regions of the eye: an ancient hypothesis of dividing the eye into eight regions, each of which is thought to be related to a particular internal organ pathologically. This hypothesis is obsolete because of controversies on the location of the regions and their relationship to the internal organs.

胞睑 [bāo jiǎn]

palpebra: eyelid

目眦 [mù zì]

canthus (of the eye): corner of the eye formed by the meeting of the upper and lower eyelids

眦 [zì]

an abbreviation for 目眦 [mù zì]

目锐眦 [mù ruì zì]

lateral canthus (of the eye): lateral corner of the eye, also called 锐眦 [ruì zì]

锐眦 [ruì zì]

same as 目锐眦 [mù ruì zì]

外眦 [wài zì]

outer canthus, same as lateral canthus (目锐眦 [mù ruì zì])

目内眦 [mù nèi zì]

inner canthus (of the eye): medial corner of the eye, also called 内眦 [neì zì]

内眦 [nèi zì]

inner canthus; medial canthus, same as inner canthus of the eye (目内眦 [mù nèi zì])

大眦 [dà zì]

big canthus: another name for inner canthus (内眦 [neì zì])

小眦 [xiǎo zì]

small canthus: another name for outer canthus (外眦 [wài zì])

目眶 [mù kuàng]

eye socket; orbit: the bony cavity that encloses and protects the eye

目眶骨 [mù kuàng gǔ]

orbit bone: bone forming the eye socket

目上网 [mù shàng wǎng]

(1) margin of the upper eyelid; (2) upper palpebral musculature

目下网 [mù xià wǎng]

(1) margin of the lower eyelid; (2) lower palpebral musculature

目纲 [mù gāng]

tarsi of eyelid: plates forming the framework of the eyelid

睑弦 [jiǎn xián]

palpebral margin: edge of free margin of the eyelid, from which the eyelashes arise

目弦 [mù xián]

margin of the eyelid, same as palpegral margin (睑弦 [jiǎn xián])

目上胞 [mù shàng bāo]

upper eyelid: the superior of the paired movable folds that protect the anterior surface of the eyeball

目上弦 [mù shàng xián]

margin of the upper eyelid

目下胞 [mù xià bāo]

lower eyelid: the inferior of the paired movable folds that protect the anterior surface of the eyeball

目下弦 [mù xià xián]

margin of the lower eyelid

睑内 [jiǎn nèi]

palpebral conjunctiva: the membrane that lines the inner side of the eyelid

白睛 [bái jīng]

white of the eye: white part of the eyeball, also called 白仁 [bái rén]

白仁 [bái rén]

"white kernel": another name for white of the eye (白睛 [bái jīng])

泪泉 [lèi quán]

lacrimal gland: the gland that secretes tears

泪窍 [lèi qiào]

lacrimal punctum: opening of the lacrimal duct at the inner canthus of the eye, also called 泪堂 [lèi táng] or 泪点 [lèi diǎn]

泪堂 [lèi táng]

same as lacrimal punctum (泪窍 [lèi qiào])

泪点 [lèi diǎn]

same as lacrimal punctum (泪窍 [lèi qiào])

黑睛 [hēi jīng]

black of the eye: black part of the eyeball, referring to the cornea

瞳神 [tóng shén]

(1) pupil: opening at the center of the iris of the eye; **(2) pupil and intra-ocular tissues**

瞳子 [tóng zǐ]

same as 瞳神 [tóng shén]

瞳人 [tóng rén]

same as 瞳神 [tóng shén]

瞳仁 [tóng rén]

same as 瞳神 [tóng shén]

黄仁 [huáng rén]

"yellow kernel": a traditional name for the iris

睛帘 [jīng lián]

iris: muscular membrane suspended in front of the lens of the eye

虹彩 [hóng cǎi]

iris: another name for 睛帘 [jīng lián]

神水 [shén shuǐ]

aqueous humor: the fluid produced in the eye, occupying the space between the crystalline lens and the cornea

晶珠 [jīng zhū]

crystalline lens: lens of the eye

精珠 [jīng zhū]

lens: transparent lens-shaped body in the eye, also called crystalline lens (晶珠 [jīng zhū])

神膏 [shén gāo]

vitreous: clear colorless transparent jelly that fills the eyeball

视衣 [shì yī]

coats of the eyeball; chorioretina: choroid and retina

目珠 [mù zhū]

eyeball: the round part of the eye within the eyelids and socket

眼带 [yǎn dài]

muscles of the eyeball: extraocular muscles

目系 [mù xì]

ocular connector: the cord connecting the eye with the brain, including the ocular nerve and blood vessels associated with the eye

羞明 [xīu míng]]

photophobia: abnormal fear of light

目痛 [mù tòng]

eye pain: pain of the eye, one of the common symptoms indicating eye diseases

目眵 [mù chī]

eye secretion: secretion of the eye, thin or mucilaginous or even pus-like, often occurring in external ocular diseases

眵泪 [chī lèi]

eye secretion and tears

眵泪胶粘 [chī lèi jiāo nián]

tears with mucopurulent secretion

遇风流泪 [yù fēng liú lèi]

lacrimation induced by wind: secretion and discharge of tears induced by exposure to wind

不时泪溢 [bù shí lèi yì]

epiphora: abnormal overflow of tears from time to time

白睛红赤 [bái jīng hóng chì]

redness of the white of the eye; hyperemia of the bulbar conjunctiva, also called 白睛混赤 [bái jīng hún chì]

白睛混赤 [bái jīng hún chì]

hyperemia of the bulbar conjunctiva, same as 白睛红赤 [bái jīng hóng chì]

白睛暴赤 [bái jīng bào chì]

sudden redness of the bulbar conjunctiva: sudden onset of hyperemia of the bulbar conjunctiva

白睛浮壅 [bái jīng fú yōng]

chemosis: excessive edema of the bulbar conjunctiva

白睛赤肿 [bái jīng chì zhǒng]

redness and swelling of the bulbar conjunctiva: hyperemia with swelling of the bulbar conjunctiva

白睛涩痛 [bái jīng sè tòng]

irritation and pain of the bulbar conjunctiva

抱轮红赤 [bào lún hóng chì]

ciliary hyperemia: redness of the bulbar conjunctiva surrounding the ciliary body, also called 白睛抱红 [bái jīng bào hóng] or 赤带抱轮 [chì dài bào lún]

白睛抱红 [bái jīng bào hóng]

same as 抱轮红赤 [bào lún hóng chì]

赤带抱轮 [chì dài bào lún]

same as 抱轮红赤 [bào lún hóng chì]

赤脉贯睛 [chì mài guàn jīng]

hyperemia of the bulbar conjunctiva: a condition marked by hyperemic vessels passing across the bulbar conjunctiva

结膜红赤 [jié mó hóng chì]

conjunctival hyperemia: redness of the palpebral conjunctiva

障 [zhàng]

ophthalmopathy: a general term for any eye disease

外障 [wài zhàng]

external ophthalmopathy: any of the external ocular diseases

内障 [nèi zhàng]

internal ophthalmopathy: any of the inner eye diseases

目盲 [mù máng]

blindness: lack or loss of the ability to see

赤膜 [chì mó]

congestive membrane: a red membranous vascular tissue

翳 [yì]

nebula: cloudy opacity of the cornea which may impair the vision to different degrees according to the location of the opaque area

新翳 [xīn yì]

fresh nebula: newly developed opacity of the cornea with a coarse surface and indistinct margins, tending to further development

宿翳 [sù yì]

chronic corneal opacity: opacity of the cornea with a smooth surface and clear-cut margins, usually due to scar formation

星翳 [xīng yì]

dotted nebula: small opaque dots on the cornea

蛛丝飘浮 [zhū sī piāo fú]

muscae volitantes: threads or spots before the eyes due to filaments in the vitreous body

针眼 [zhēn yǎn]

stye; hordeolum: a small furuncle occurring on the eyelid, also known as 偷针 [tōu zhēn], 土疡 [tǔ yáng]]

偷针 [tōu zhēn]

another name for stye or hordeolum (针眼 [zhēn yǎn])

土疡 [tǔ yáng]

another name for stye or hordeolum (针眼 [zhēn yǎn])

胞生痰核 [bāo shēng tán hé]

chalazion: a small lump formed on the eyelid, without redness or pain, also called 胞睑肿核 [bāo jiǎn zhǒng hé] or 睥生痰核 [pì shēng tán hé]

胞睑肿核 [bāo jiǎn zhǒng hé}

another name for chalazion (胞生痰核 [bāo shēng tán hé])

睥生痰核 [pì shēng tán hé]

another name for chalazion (胞生痰核 [bā shēng tán hé])

椒疮 [jiāo chuāng]

trachoma: an eye disease marked by innumerable granulations, red and hard, shaped like Chinese prickly ash (and hence the Chinese name "prickly-ash sore"), accumulating on the conjunctival surfaces

倒睫 [dào jié]

trichiasis: a condition of ingrowing eyelashes

睫毛倒入 [jié máo dào rù]

trichiasis, same as 倒睫 [dào jié]

倒睫拳毛 [dào jié quán máo]

trichiasis and entropion: inversion of the margin of the eyelid with ingrowing eyelashes, one of the sequelae of trachoma

睥翻粘睑 [pì fān zhān jiǎn]

cicatrical ectropion of eyelid: eversion of the margin of an eyelid caused by scar tissue

睥肉粘轮 [pì ròu zhān lún]

symblepharon: adhesion between the tarsal conjunctiva and bulbar conjunctiva

粟疮 [sù chuāng]

"millet sore"; follicular conjunctivitis: an eye disease marked by formation on the conjunctival surface of numerous follicles in the shape and size of millet

睑弦赤烂 [jiǎn xián chì làn]

tarsitis; marginal blepharitis: inflammation and ulceration of the margin of the eyelid, also called 眼缘赤烂 [yǎn yuán chì làn] or 风弦赤烂 [fēng xián chì làn]

眼缘赤烂 [yǎn yuán chì làn]

same as 睑弦赤烂 [jiǎn xián chì làn]

风弦赤烂 [fēng xián chì làn]

another name for marginal blepharitis (眼缘赤烂 [yǎn yuán chì làn])

睑弦糜烂 [jiǎn xián mí làn]

ulcerative marginal blepharitis: ulceration of the margin of the eyelid

眦帷赤烂 [zì wéi chì làn]

blepharitis angularis: inflammation of the eyelid affecting the inner canthus

风赤疮痍 [fēng chì chuāng yí]

eczematous dermatitis of the eyelid: disease of the eyelid characterized by redness of the palpebral skin with vesicles or even local erosion, also called 风赤疮疾 [fēng chì chāung jí]

风赤疮疾 [fēng chì chāung jí]

another name for eczematous dermatitis of the eyelid (风赤疮痍 [fēng chì chuāng yí])

胞肿 [bāo zhǒng]

swelling of the eyelid; palpebral edema

胞肿如桃 [bāo zhǒng rú táo]

"peach-like eyelid swelling"; inflammatory swelling of the eyelid: severe swelling of the eyelid with redness resembling a ripe peach

胞虚如球 [bāo xū rú qiú]

non-inflammatory edema of the eyelid: severe swelling of the eyelid, but with no change in the local skin color, also called 睥虚如球 [pì xū rú qiú]

睥虚如球 [pì xū rú qiú]

another name for inflammatory swelling of the eyelid (胞虚如球 [bāo xū rú qiú])

上胞下垂 [shàng bāo xià chuí]

blepharoptosis: drooping of the upper eyelid, also called 睑皮垂缓[jiǎn pí chuí huǎn]

睑皮垂缓 [jiǎn pí chuí huǎn]

another name for blepharoptosis (上胞下垂 [shàng bāo xià chuí])

睑废 [jiǎn fèi]

"invalid eyelid": serious blepharoptosis

胞轮振跳 [bāo lún zhèn tiào]

tic of the eyelid: involuntary twitching of the eyelid, also called 睥轮振跳 [pì lún zhèn tiào]

睥轮振跳 [pì lún zhèn tiào]

tic of the eyelid: same as 胞轮振跳 [bāo lún zhèn tiào]

目连劄 [mù lián zhá]

frequent nictitation: frequent winking that cannot be controlled, often abbreviated as 目劄 [mù zhá]

目劄 [mù zhá]

an abbreviation of frequent nictitation (目连劄 [mù lián zhá])

睑内结石 [jiǎn nèi jié shí]

calculus of conjunctiva: formation of single or multiple granules in the palpebral conjunctiva, fine, firm, hard and yellowish in color

流泪证 [liú lèi zhèng]

dacryorrhea syndrome: a general term for various conditions characterized by overabundant flow of tears, also called 流泪病症 [liú lèi bìng zhèng]

流泪病症 [liú lèi bìng zhèng]

dacryorrhea disease, same as 流泪证 [liú lèi zhèng]

热泪 [rè lèi]

heat dacryorrhea: dacryorrhea occurring in inflammatory eye diseases as a symptom

冷泪 [lěng lèi]

cold dacryorrhea: dacryorrhea with no redness, pain or opacity of the eyes

漏睛 [lòu jīng]

chronic dacryocystitis: chronic inflammation of the lacrimal sac with frequent outflow of fluid or pus from the inner canthus, also known as 眦漏 [zì lòu]

眦漏 [zì lòu]

canthus pyorrhea: synonym for 漏睛 [lòu jīng]

窍漏 [qiào lòu]

orifice pyorrhea: another name for 漏睛 [lòu jīng]

漏睛脓出 [lòu jīng nóng chū]

dacryopyorrhea: frequent discharge of tears mixed with pus

大眦脓漏 [dà zì nóng lòu]

inner-canthus dacryopyorrhea: a synonym for 漏睛脓出 [lòu jīng nóng chū]

漏睛疮 [lòu jīng chuāng]

acute dacryocystitis: an acute inflammation of the lacrimal sac with purulent discharge

赤脉传睛 [chì mài chuán jīng]

angular conjunctivitis: conjunctivitis with reddening at the canthus and spreading to the white of the eye

胬肉攀睛 [nǔ ròu pān jīng]

pterygium: triangular fleshy mass occurring at the canthus and covering art of the cornea, even causing disturbance of vision

流金凌木 [liú jīn líng mù]

pseudopterygium: conjunctival scar attached to the cornea, resembling a ptyergyum but not firmly adherent to the underlying tissue. (The literal meaning of the Chinese name is a flow of metal invading wood, in which the bulbar conjunctiva pertains to metal and the cornea to wood)

风火眼 [fēng huǒ yǎn]

wind-fire attack on the eye; acute conjunctivitis: acute attack of wind-fire on the eye, marked by acute onset of redness and pain in the eye accompanied by photophobia and lacrimation, usually abbreviated as 火眼 [huǒ yǎn]

风火眼痛 [fēng huǒ yǎn tòng]

wind-fire painful eye, same as acute conjunctivitis 风火眼 [fēng huǒ yǎn]

风热眼 [fēng rè yǎn]

wind-heat attack on the eye, same as acute conjunctivitis 风火眼 [fēng huǒ yǎn]

火眼 [huǒ yǎn]

inflamed eye; conjunctivitis, also called 赤眼 [chì yǎn]

赤眼 [chì yǎn]

reddened eye: same as conjunctivitis (火眼 [huǒ yǎn])

暴发火眼 [bào fā huǒ yǎn]

epidemic conjunctivitis: acute contagious inflammation of the conjunctiva occurring in an epidemic

暴风客热 [bào fēng kè rè]

sudden attack of wind-heat on the eye: acute inflammatory eye disease with sudden onset, due to external contraction of wind-heat, also called 伤寒眼 [shāng hán yǎn]

伤寒眼 [shāng hán yǎn]

cold-induced affection of the eye: a popular name for acute conjunctivitis (暴风客热 [bào fēng kè rè])

天行赤眼 [tiān xíng chì yǎn]

epidemic conjunctivitis: a highly infectious eye disease characterized by sudden onset of inflammation of the white of the eye, usually bilateral, and quickly spreading among many people, also called 天行赤目 [tiān xíng chì mù] or 天行暴赤 [tiān xíng bào chì]

天行赤目 [tiān xíng chì mù]

same as 天行赤眼 [tiān xíng chì yǎn]

天行暴赤 [tiān xíng bào chì]

same as 天行赤眼 [tiān xíng chì yǎn]

暴赤生翳 [bào chì shēng yì]

acute keratoconjunctivitis: acute inflammation of the conjunctiva and cornea

天行赤眼暴翳 [tiān xíng chì yǎn bào yì]

epidemic kerato-conjunctivitis: a highly infectious disease that may turn into an epidemic, characterized by simultaneous inflammation of the cornea and conjunctiva

天行赤目暴翳 [tiān xíng chì mù bào yì]

epidemic keratoconjunctivitis: same as 天行赤眼暴翳[tiān xíng chì yǎn bào yì]

金疳 [jīn gān]

phlyctenular conjunctivitis: a variety of conjunctivitis marked by the presence of small vesicles, also called 金疡 [jīn yáng]

金疡 [jīn yáng]

same as 金疳 [jīn gān]

火疳 [huǒ gān]

episcleritis: an eye disease caused by excessive fire which invades the inner surface of the white of the eye, resulting in bulging of localized dark violet patches, also called 火疡 [huǒ yáng]

火疡 [huǒ yáng]

same as 火疳 [huǒ gān]

白膜侵睛 [bái mó qīn jīng]

invasion of white membrane into the cornea: ocular disease generally referring to phlyctenular kerato-conjunctivitis

白膜蔽睛 [bái mó bì jīng]

pannus: a membranous tissue causing a superficial opacity of the cornea, usually occurring in cases of trachoma

白睛青蓝 [bái jīng qīng lán]

blue whites of the eye: bluish discoloration of the bulbar conjunctiva surrounding the cornea after recurrent inflammation of the sclera with violet bulging

白睛溢血 [bái jīng yì xuè]

subconjunctival ecchymosis: extravasation beneath the conjunctiva

白涩症 [bái sè zhèng]

white xerotic syndrome: an eye disease characterized by uncomfortable feeling of dryness and roughness but with no apparent redness or swelling, generally referring to chronic conjunctivitis or superficial punctate keratitis

白涩病 [bái sè bìng]

white xerotic disease: a synonym for white xerotic syndrome (白涩症 [bái sè zhèng])

赤丝虬脉 [chì sī qiú mài]

hyperemia of subconjunctival capillaries, also called 白睛虬脉 [bái jīng qiú mài]

白睛虬脉 [bái jīng qiú mài]

same as 赤丝虬脉 [chì sī qiú mài]

黄油障 [huáng yóu zhàng]

pinguecula: a yellowish triangular patch of proliferation on the bulbar conjunctiva close to the inner canthus

聚星障 [jù xīng zhàng]

punctate keratitis: an eye disease characterized by the appearance of multiple fine drops of opacity on the cornea

花翳白陷 [huā yì bái xiàn]

ulcerative keratitis: keratitis with ulceration of the corneal surface

凝脂翳 [níng zhī yì]

purulent keratitis: severe keratitis with purulent disintegration of the cornea

黄液上冲 [huáng yè shàng chōng]

hypopyon: accumulation of pus between the cornea and the iris (i.e., the anterior chamber)

蟹睛症 [xiè jīng zhèng]

"crab's eye" disease: a severe eye disease marked by perforation of cornea with prolapse of the iris, looking like a crab's eye, also called 蟹睛病 [xiè jīng bìng]

蟹睛病 [xiè jīng bìng]

same as 蟹睛症 [xiè jīng zhèng]

混睛障 [hún jīng zhàng]

interstitial keratitis: an eye disease with visual disturbance marked by deep deposits in the substance of the cornea, which becomes grayish and opaque, also called 混睛外障 [hún jīng wài zhàng] or 气翳 [qì yì]

气翳 [qì yì]

***qi* nebula:** a synonym for interstitial keratitits (混睛障 [hún jīng zhàng])

混睛外障 [hún jīng wài zhàng]

same as 混睛障 [hún jīng zhàng]

风轮赤豆 [fēng lún chì dòu]

corneal "red-bean": a corneal lesion of the granular vesicle surrounded by small blood vessels, shaped like a red bean, which leaves a scar after recurrent attacks, causing disturbance of vision, mostly referring to fascicular keratitis

赤膜下垂 [chì mó xià chuí]

drooping pannus: a membranous vascular tissue extending downward into the cornea, most frequently occurring in cases of trachoma

垂帘翳 [chuí lián yì]

drooping nebula, same as drooping pannus (赤膜下垂 [chì mó xià chuí]), usually referring to trachomatous pannus

血翳包睛 [xuè yì bāo jīng]

keratic pannus: superficial vascularization covering the entire cornea

瞳神紧小 [tóng shén jǐn xiǎo]

miosis: contracted pupil, often caused by iridocyclitis or panuveitis

瞳神散大 [tóng shén sǎn dà]

mydriasis: dilation of the pupil

瞳神干缺 [tóng shén gān quē]

pupillary metamorphosis: loss of the normal round shape of the pupil, usually seen in chronic iridocyclitis, also called 瞳人干缺 [tóng rén gān quē] or 瞳神缺陷 [tóng shén quē xiàn]

瞳人干缺 [tóng rén gān quē]

same as 瞳神干缺 [tóng shén gān quē]

瞳神缺陷 [tóng shén quē xiàn]

same as 瞳神干缺 [tóng shén gān quē]

绿风内障 [lǜ fēng nèi zhàng]

(greenish) glaucoma: a group of eye diseases characterized by hardening of the eyeball, impaired vision, and dilation of the pupil with greenish discoloration

青风内障 [qīng fēng nèi zhàng]

bluish glaucoma: mild case of simple glaucoma

黄风内障 [huáng fēng nèi zhàng]

yellowish glaucoma: advanced stage of glaucoma with the pupil discolored to yellow

圆翳内障 [yuán yì nèi zhàng]

cataract: a chronic eye disease marked by opacity in the lens, impairing vision or causing blindness

惊震内障 [jīng zhèn nèi zhàng]

traumatic cataract: cataract resulting from injury to the eye

胎患内障 [tāi huàn nèi zhàng]

congenital cataract: any of various types of usually bilateral ocular opacity present at birth

云雾移睛 [yún wù yí jīng]

hyalosis: presence of cloudy or star-shaped opacities in the vitreous humor

暴盲 [bào máng]

sudden blindness: sudden loss of vision while no abnormal appearance of the eye can be found

视瞻昏渺 [shì zhān hūn miǎo]

blurring of vision: impaired vision with no abnormality of the external eye

青盲 [qīng máng]

bluish blindness: a group of eye diseases characterized by increasing impairment of vision to total blindness with no abnormal appearance of the external eye, usually referring to optic atrophy

高风内障 [gāo fēng nèi zhàng]

pigmentary retinopathy: a hereditary progressive degenerative disease characterized by night blindness, constriction of the visual field, and eventual blindness

高风雀目 [gāo fēng què mù]

same as 高风内障 [gāo fēng nèi zhàng]

异物入目 [yì wù rù mù]

foreign body in the eye: small foreign body attached to or embedded in the surface of the eyeball

撞击伤目 [zhuàng jī shāng mù]

collision eye injury: eye injury due to a knock with no ruptured wound

真睛破损 [zhēn jīng pò sǔn]

ruptured wound of the eyeball: penetrating injury to the eyeball or other eye injury with a ruptured wound

物损真睛 [wù sǔn zhēn jīng]

traumatic injury to the eyeball: a synonym for ruptured wound of the eyeball (真睛破损 [zhēn jīng pò sǔn])

电光伤目 [diàn guāng shāng mù]

electric ophthalmia; flash ophthalmia: inflammation of the eye caused by a flash

疳积上目 [gān jī shàng mù]

(malnutritional) keratomalacia: softening and ulceration of the cornea of the eye resulting from malnutrition, also called 疳眼 [gān yǎn]

疳眼 [gān yǎn]

keratomalacia: same as 疳积上目 [gān jī shàng mù]

近视 [jìn shì]

myopia: a condition in which one is only able to see clearly things that are close to the eyes

能近怯远症 [néng jìn qiè yuǎn zhèng]

nearsightedness: another expression for myopia (近视 [jìn shì])

远视 [yuǎn shì]

hyperopia: condition in which vision is better for distant than for near objects

能远怯近症 [néng yuǎn qiè jìn zhèng]

farsightedness: another expression for hyperopia (远视 [yuǎn shì])

视物易色 [shì wù yì sè]

chromatopsia: disturbance of vision in which the color of the objects appear unnaturally colored or colorless objects appear colored

视直为曲 [shì zhí wéi qū]

metamorphopsia: disturbance of vision in which objects are seen distorted in shape

雀盲 [què máng]

nyctalopia; night blindness: failure of vision at night or in a dim light, also called 雀目 [què mù], 雀目内障 [què mù nèi zhàng]

雀目 [què mù]

sparrow's vision: another name for night blindness (雀盲 [qù máng])

雀目内障 [què mù nèi zhàng]

same as 雀盲 [què máng]

目偏视 [mù piān shì]

squint; strabismus: a condition in which the eyes do not move together but look in different directions at once, also called 偏斜瞻视 [piān xié zhān shì]

偏斜瞻视 [piān xié zhān shì]

strabismus: another name for 目偏视 [mù piān shì]

风牵偏视 [fēng qiān piān shì]

paralytic strabismus: squint caused by attack of wind to the collateral meridian

突起睛高 [tū qǐ jīng gāo]

sudden protrusion of the eyeball: eye disease characterized by painful protrusion and distension of the eyeball, often referring to purulent ophthalmia

睛高突起 [jīng gāo tū qǐ]

same as 突起睛高 [tū qǐ jīng gāo]

睛胀 [jīng zhàng]

distension of the eyeball: a synonym for 突起睛高 [tū qǐ jīng gāo]

目痒 [mù yǎng]

eye itching: a condition characterized by intense itching of the eye, often referring to catarrhal conjunctivitis

瞽症 [gǔ zhèng]

blindness in ophathalmosteresis: blindness with loss of both eyes

耳鼻喉科 Diseases of the Ear, Nose and Throat

耳科 [ěr kē]

otology: a branch of medicine that deals with the ear and its diseases

完骨 [wán gǔ]

mastoid bone: mastoid part of the temporal bone

耳疔 [ěr dīng]

ear boil: boil of the external auditory meatus, also called 耳疖 [ěr jiē]

耳疖 [ěr jiē]

ear furuncle: a synonym for 耳疔 [ěr dīng]

耳疮 [ěr chuāng]

ear sore: diffuse inflammation of the external auditory meatus

旋耳疮 [xuán ěr chuāng]

peri-auricular eczema: redness, itching, exudation and oozing vesicular lesions surrounding the ear, also known as 月蚀疮 [yuè shí chuāng]

月蚀疮 [yuè shí chuāng]

eclipsed lunar eczema: another name for peri-auricular eczema (旋耳疮 [xuán ěr chuāng])

耳壳流痰 [ěr qiào liú tán]

auricular pseudocyst: cystic collection of fluid on the auricle, soft with no hotness or tenderness, nor change in skin color, referring to exudative perichondritis of the auricle

耳胀 [ěr zhàng]

ear distension: feeling of distension with pain in the ear, symptom often occurring in acute non-suppurative otitis media

耳闭 [ěr bì]

ear block: feeling of blocking in the ear developed after a long course of ear distension, often occurring in chronic non-suppurative otitis media

脓耳 [nóng ěr]

otopyorrhea; suppurative otitis media: a disease of the ear characterized by perforation of the tympanic membrane and discharge of pus

脓耳变证 [nóng ěr biàn zhèng]

deteriorated otopyorrhea: complications of suppurative otitis media, including postauricular infection (耳根毒 [ěr gēn dú]), postauricular abscess (耳根痈 [ěr gēn yōng]), otopyorrhea with facial paralysis (脓耳口眼㖞斜 [nóng ěr kǒu yǎn wāi xié]) and otogenic intracranial infection (黄耳伤寒 [huáng ěr shāng hán])

耳根毒 [ěr gēn dú]

postauricular infection: a disease marked by pain and tenderness at the mastoid region, local swelling and even rupture with discharge of pus, also known as postauricular abscess (耳根痈 [ěr gēn yōng]) or subperiosteal abscess of the mastoid (耳后附骨痈 [ěr hòu fù gǔ yōng])

耳根痈 [ěr gēn yōng]

postauricular abscess: postauricular infection with formation of abscess

耳后附骨痈 [ě hòu fù gǔ yōng]

subperiosteal abscess of the mastoid: a synonym for postauricular abscess (耳根痈 [ěr gēn yōng])

脓耳口眼㖞斜 [nóng ěr kòu yǎn wāi xié]

otopyorrhea with facial paralysis: suppurative otitis media with wry eye and mouth as complications

黄耳伤寒 [huáng ěr shāng hán]

otogenic intracranial infection: suppurative otitis media complicated by mental derangement or convulsion

耳鸣 [ěr míng]

tinnitus: ringing in the ear

风热耳鸣 [fēng rè ěr míng]

wind-heat tinnitus: low-pitched ringing in the ear, usually unilateral, occurring in a wind-heat affliction

肝火耳鸣 [gān huǒ ěr míng]

liver fire tinnitus: rumbling in the ear, usually unilateral with sudden onset, accompanied by hypochondriac distension, irritability, and wiry rapid pulse

痰火耳鸣 [tán huǒ ěr míng]

phlegm-fire tinnitus: soft sound in the ear, usually unilateral, accompanied by local pain and distension, or even discharge of pus from the ear

脏腑虚损耳鸣 [zàng fǔ xū sǔn ěr míng]

***zang-fu* insufficiency tinnitus:** high-pitched ringing in the ear, usually bilateral, accompanied by deficiency syndrome of the corresponding organ

肾虚耳鸣 [shèn xū ěr míng]

kidney-insufficiency tinnitus: high-pitched ringing in the ear, usually bilateral, accompanied by dizziness, aching loins and weak legs

重听 [chóng tīng]

hearing impairment: decreased sense of hearing or distorted hearing

耳聋 [ěr lóng]

deafness: lack or loss, complete or partial, of the sense of hearing

干聋 [gān lóng]

dry deafness: deafness due to impacted earwax

耵聍 [dīng níng]

cerumen: earwax

耵耳 [dīng ěr]

impacted cerumen: accumulated cerumen forming a solid mass that adheres to the wall of the external auditory meatus

耳眩晕 [ěr xuàn yūn]

aural vertigo: vertigo due to otopathy

脓耳眩晕 [nóng ěr xuàn yūn]

otopyorrheal vertigo: vertigo due to suppurative otitis media

耳瘘 [ěr lòu]

ear fistula: fistula in front of or behind the ear with exudation

耳菌 [ěr jūn]

ear polyp: polyp of the external auditory meatus, also called 耳蕈 [ěr xùn]

耳蕈 [ěr xùn]

mushroom-like vegetation of the ear: synonym for ear polyp (耳菌 [ěr jūn])

耳挺 [ěr tǐng]

protruding vegetation from the earhole: a long-stemmed papilloma of the external auditory meatus

耳痔 [ěr zhì]

nodular vegetation of the ear; ear pile: nodular papilloma of the external auditory meatus

耳疳 [ěr gān]

ulcered ear: chronic suppurative otitis media

聤耳 [tíng ěr]

ear with purulent discharge: suppurative otitis media

耳后发 [ěr hòu fā]

postauricular phlegmon: acute suppurative or gangrenous mastoiditis

耳聋口哑 [ěr lóng kǒu yǎ]

deaf-mutism: absence both of the sense of hearing and the ability to speak

鼻科 [bí kē]

rhinology: a branch of medicine that deals with the nose and its diseases

明堂 [míng táng]

(1) prominent part for inspection: an ancient term for the nose, especially the apex of the nose; **(2) point marks:** marks for acupuncture points on a model

畜门 [xù mén]

nostril: an ancient term for nostril

鼻尖 [bí jiān]

nose tip: tip of the nose

鼻准 [bí zhǔn]

apex of the nose; apex nasi: tip of the nose, the most distal portion of the nose

山根 [shān gēn]

root of the nose; radix nasi: upper portion of the nose, which is attached to the frontal bone

頞 [è]

(1) radix nasi: root of the nose; **(2) nose stem**: dorsal middle part of the nose as a whole

鼻柱 [bí zhù]

nose stem: dorsal middle part of the nose, also called 鼻梁 [bí liáng]

鼻梁 [bí liáng]

nose bridge: a popular name for the nose stem (鼻柱 [bī zhù])

鼻翼 [bí yì]

ala nasi: wing of the nose

鼻前孔 [bí qián kǒng]

anterior naris; nostril: either of the two openings in the nose

鼻前庭 [bí qián tíng]

nasal vestibule: cavity of the nose

鼻病 [bí bìng]

nasal disease: disease of the nose

鼻塞 [bí sè]

nasal congestion; nasal obstruction: inability to breathe through the nose

鼻窍不利 [bí qiào bù lì]

same as 鼻塞 [bí sè]

鼻燥 [bí zào]

(1) dryness of the nasal cavity; (2) rhinitis sicca: atrophic rhinitis without secretions

鼻涕 [bí tì]

nasal discharge

不辨香臭 [bù biàn xiāng chòu]

anosmia: loss or impairment of the sense of smell

鼻疔 [bí dīng]

nasal boil: boil occurring at the nasal vestibule, or at the tip or wing of the nose

鼻疮 [bí chuāng]

nasal sore: a disease marked by recurrent inflammation of the nasal vestibule with ulceration, crusting, itching and pain, also called 鼻疳 [bī gān]

鼻疳 [bī gān]

nasal vestibulitis, same as nasal sore 鼻疮 [bī chuāng]

伤风鼻塞 [shāng fēng bí sè]

wind-affected nasal obstruction; acute rhinitis: a disease marked by acute nasal congestion due to wind affliction

鼻窒 [bí zhì]

chronic rhinitis: a chronic nasal disease marked by recurrent nasal obstruction, sometimes accompanied by impairment of the sense of smell

鼻槁 [bí gǎo]

atrophic rhinitis: a disease of the nose characterized by dry mucous membrane with atrophy, enlarged nasal passages and foul smell, progressing to ozena

鼻藁 [bí gǎo]

same as 鼻槁 [bí gǎo]

鼻臭证 [bí chòu zhèng]

ozena: atrophic rhinitis with fetid smell

鼻鼽 [bí qiú]

sniveling nose, allergic rhinits: a disease characterized by sudden and recurrent attacks of nasal itching, sneezing, thin discharge and stuffed nose, also known as 鼽嚏 [qiú tì]

鼽嚏 [qiú tì]

sniveling nose with sneezing, same as 鼻鼽 [bí qiú]

鼻渊 [bí yuān]

rhinorrhea with turbid discharge; sinusitis: a nasal disease characterized by persistent excessive flow of turbid nasal discharge, often seen in inflammation of a paranasal sinus, also called 脑漏 [nǎo lòu], 脑渗 [nǎo shèn] and 控脑砂 [kòng nǎo shā]

脑漏 [nǎo lòu]

another name for sinusitis (鼻渊 [bí yuān])

脑渗 [nǎo shèn]

another name for sinusitis (鼻渊 [bí yuān])

控脑砂 [kòng nǎo shā]

another name for sinusitis (鼻渊 [bí yuān])

鼻息肉 [bí xī ròu]

nasal polyp: protruding growth from the nasal mucous membrane, also called 鼻痔 [bí zhì] or 鼻菌 [bí jūn]

鼻痔 [bí zhì]

another name for nasal polyp (鼻息肉 [bí xī ròu])

鼻菌 [bí jūn]

another name for nasal polyp (鼻息肉 [bí xī ròu])

鼻赘 [bí zhuì]

(1) nasal polyp: same as 鼻息肉 [bí xī ròu]; **(2) rhinophyma:** rosacea at the hypertrophic stage involving the lower half of the nose

鼻息肉病 [bí xī ròu bìng]

nasal polyposis: the development of multiple polyps on the nasal mucosa

鼻衄 [bí nǜ]

nosebleed; epistaxis: attack of bleeding from the nose

鼻洪 [bí hóng]

profuse nasal bleeding

脑衄 [nǎo nǜ]

severe epistaxis: severe attack of bleeding from the nose

鼻梁骨折 [bí liáng gǔ zhé]

fracture of the nose bridge

咽喉科 [yān hóu kē]

laryngology: a branch of medicine that deals with the throat, pharynx, larynx, nasopharynx and their diseases

喉核 [hóu hé]

tonsils: either of a pair of prominent masses that lie one on each side of the throat between the anterior and posterior pillars of the fauces

喉关 [hóu guān]

isthmus of the fauces: the passage between the cavity of the mouth and the pharynx

喉嗌 [hóu yì]

pharynx: the passage between the mouth and the posterior nares and the esophagus

颃颡 [háng sǎng]

nasopharynx: the part of the pharynx above the soft palate

喉底 [hóu dǐ]

retropharynx: the posterior part of the pharynx

蒂丁 [dì dīng]

uvula: pendulum of the palate

乳蛾 [rǔ é]

tonsillitis: redness and swelling of the painful tonsils, resembling a moth, sometimes covered with a yellowish white secretion like milk, hence the Chinese name which literally means "milky moth", also known as "throat moth" (喉蛾 [hóu é])

喉蛾 [hóu é]

"throat moth": another name for tonsillitis (乳蛾 [rǔ é])

单蛾 [dān é]

unilateral tonsillitis: inflammation of the tonsil of only one side

双蛾 [shuāng é]

bilateral tonsillitis: inflammation of the tonsils of both sides

风热乳蛾 [fēng rè rǔ é]

wind-heat tonsillitis: acute tonsillitis caused by attack of wind-heat

虚火乳蛾 [xū huǒ rǔ é]

deficiency-fire tonsillitis: chronic tonsillitis caused by fire of deficiency type

石蛾 [shí é]

"stony moth"; hypertrophy of the tonsil: hard hypertrophied tonsils in children with no inflammation

咽喉肿痛 [yān hóu zhǒng tòng]

sore throat: painful swelling of the throat

喉痹 [hóu bì]

inflammation of the throat: redness, swelling and pain of the throat, also called 咽痹 [yān bì]

咽痹 [yān bì]

inflammation of pharynx: same as inflammation of the throat (喉痹 [hóu bì])

风热喉痹 [fēng rè hóu bì]

wind-heat pharyngitis: acute pharyngitis caused by wind-heat

风寒喉痹 [fēng hán hóu bì]

wind-cold pharyngitis: acute pharyngitis caused by wind-cold, occasionally occurring in a debilitated person

虚火喉痹 [xū huǒ hóu bì]

deficiency-fire pharyngitis: chronic pharyngitis caused by fire of deficiency type

帘珠喉痹 [lián zhū hóu bì]

granular pharyngitis: chronic pharyngitis with granules on the posterior wall of the pharynx

喉痈 [hóu yōng]

throat abscess: abscess of the throat, including retropharyngeal abscess and peritonsillar abscess

猛疽 [měng jū]

ominous (throat) abscess: abscess of the laryngopharynx that causes obstruction of breathing and is often fatal if not properly treated in time

喉关痈 [hóu guān yōng]

(1) faucial abscess; (2) peritonsillar abscess

咽后痈 [yān hòu yōng]

retropharyngeal abscess: suppurative inflammation in the posterior wall of the pharynx, also called 里喉痈 [lǐ hóu yōng]

里喉痈 [lǐ hóu yōng]

retropharyngeal abscess, same as 咽后痈 [yān hòu yōng]

颌下痈 [hé xià yōng]

submaxillary abscess: suppurative inflammation beneath the maxilla

喉癣 [hóu xuǎn]

tinea-like erosion of throat: the ulceration of the laryngopharyngeal mucosa resembling tinea, often referring to laryngeal tuberculosis

喉喑[瘖] [hóu yīn]

aphonia: loss of voice

急喉喑[瘖] [jí hóu yīn]

acute aphonia: acute loss of voice

暴喑[瘖] [bào yīn]

sudden aphonia: sudden loss of voice, also called 卒喑 [cù yīn]

卒喑[瘖] [cù yīn]

same as sudden aphonia (暴喑 [bào yīn])

慢喉喑[瘖] [màn hóu yīn]

chronic aphonia: chronic loss of voice

悬雍肿 [xuán yōng zhǒng]

swelling of the uvula: uvulitis

悬痈 [xuán yōng]

(1) uvular abscess: abscess of the uvula; **(2) pyogenic infection of**

perineum

悬旗小舌 [xuán qí xiǎo shé]

uvular hematoma: hematoma on the uvula, also called 悬旗风 [xuán qí fēng]

悬旗风 [xuán qí fēng]

uvular wind: another name for uvular hematoma (悬旗小舌 [xuán qí xiǎo shé])

喉风 [hóu fēng]

throat wind: a general term for serious conditions of swelling and pain in the throat with difficulty in breathing and swallowing

急喉风 [jí hóu fēng]

acute throat wind; acute throat infection: acute laryngitis with difficulty in breathing and speaking

紧喉风 [jǐn hóu fēng]

constrictive throat wind; constrictive throat infection: acute laryngitis mainly manifested as a sensation of suffocation, difficulty in breathing and swallowing

缠喉风 [chán hóu fēng]

entwining throat wind; entwining throat infection: a severe throat infection with redness entwining the fauces in the interior and swelling surrounding the neck at the exterior

锁喉风 [suǒ hóu fēng]

obstructive throat wind: acute throat infection with obstruction or closure of the larynx

喉痹 [hóu bì]

throat blockage; pharyngitis: inflammation of the pharynx with marked painful swelling that causes difficulty in breathing and swallowing

急喉痹 [jí hóu bì]

acute pharyngitis: acute inflammation of the pharynx, also called 卒喉痹 [cù hóu bì]

卒喉痹 [cù hóu bì]

sudden onset of pharyngitis: same as acute pharyngitis (急喉痹 [jí hóu bì])

喉疳 [hóu gān]

throat necrosis: ulcerative necrosis of the throat

梅核气 [méi hé qì]

plum-stone syndrome; globus hystericus: subjective sensation of choking with a lump in the throat

骨鲠 [gǔ gěng]

bone sticking: sticking of a fishbone or other type of bone in the throat or esophagus

喉瘤 [hóu liú]

tumor in the throat: new growth of the throat, unilateral or bilateral

喉岩 [hóu yán]

carcinoma of throat, also called 喉菌 [hóu jūn]

喉菌 [hóu jūn]

another name for carcinoma of the throat (喉岩 [hóu yán])

口齿科 Diseases of the Mouth and Teeth

口齿科 [kǒu chǐ kē]

dentistry: that branch of medicine that deals with the teeth, oral cavity, and associated structures, as well as their diseases

真牙 [zhēn yá]

wisdom tooth: third molar that is the last tooth to erupt

齿更 [chǐ gēng]

dental transition: eruption of permanent teeth to replace deciduous teeth

齿落 [chǐ luò]

dedentition: shedding or loss of teeth

齿齘 [chǐ xiè]

teeth grinding: grinding of teeth during sleep, also called 齘齿[xiè chǐ]

牙痛 [yá tòng]

toothache: pain in a tooth or teeth

风热牙痛 [fēng rè yá tòng]

wind-heat toothache: paroxysmal attacks of toothache ameliorated by cold and aggravated by heat, accompanied by redness and swelling of the gums

风火牙痛 [fēng huǒ yá tòng]

wind fire toothache, same as wind-heat toothache (风热牙痛 [fēng rè yá tòng])

风寒牙痛 [fēng hán yá tòng]

wind-cold toothache: paroxysmal attacks of toothache aggravated by cold

胃火牙痛 [wèi huǒ yá tòng]

stomach-fire toothache: intense toothache with marked gingival redness, swelling, and discharge of pus or oozing of blood

虚火牙痛 [xū huǒ yá tòng]

deficiency-fire toothache: slight, dull toothache with mild gingival redness and swelling or even atrophy

齿龋 [chǐ qǔ]

dental caries: localized destruction of the tooth leading to cavity formation

齿蠹 [chǐ dù]

dental decay, same as dental caries (齿龋 [chǐ qǔ])

龋齿 [qǔ chǐ]

carious tooth: tooth or teeth with caries

龋齿牙痛 [qǔ chǐ yá tòng]

carious toothache: toothache due to dental caries

龋脱 [qǔ tuō]

carious odonpotosis: loss of teeth due to caries

牙痈 [yá yōng]

gingival abscess: localized, painful, inflammatory lesion of the gums with pyorrhea

牙蛟痈 [yá yǎo yōng]

distal gingival abscess: gingival abscess occurring at the most distal end, accompanied by difficulty in opening the mouth

牙宣 [yá xuān]

gingival recession: exposure of the root surfaces of teeth due to the drawing back of gingivae from the necks of teeth, also known as 齿龈宣露 [chǐ yín xuān lù], 齿挺 [chǐ tǐng] or 食床 [shí chuáng]

齿龈宣露 [chǐ yín xuān lù]

another name for gingival recession (牙宣 [yá xuān])

齿挺 [chǐ tǐng]

another name for gingival recession (牙宣 [yá xuān])

食床 [shí chuáng]

an ancient name for gingival recession (牙宣 [yá xuān])

牙疳 [yá gān]

ulcerative gingivitis: a disease marked by painful inflammation of the gums with necrosis and fetid discharge

风热牙疳 [fēng rè yá gān]

wind-heat ulcerative gingivitis: acute ulcerative gingivitis

走马牙疳 [zǒu mǎ yá gān]

noma; cancrum oris: ulcerative gingivitis with development as rapid as a "horse running", spreading to large-area destruction of buccal mucosa and tissues of the face (hence the Chinese name with the literal meaning of "horse-running" ulcerative gingivitis), often abbreviated as 走马疳 [zǒu mǎ gān]

走马疳 [zǒu mǎ gān]

same as noma (走马牙疳 [zǒu mǎ yá gān])

飞扬喉 [fēi yáng hóu]

diffuse palatitis: wide-spreading inflammation of the palate

口疮 [kǒu chuāng]

aphtha: a superficial small ulcer on the buccal mucosa, also called 口疳 [kǒu gān]

口疳 [kǒu gān]

same as aphtha (口疮 [kǒu chuāng])

口糜 [kǒu mí]

oral erosion: a condition marked by multiple spots of erosion on the buccal mucosa

唇风 [chún fēng]

exfoliative cheilitis: persistent exfoliation of the lip caused by inflammation of the mucous membrane

骨槽风 [gǔ cáo fēng]

osteomyelitis of the jaw: an infectious inflammatory disease of the jaw bone with local death and separation of tissue

重舌 [chóng shé]

double tongue: hypertrophy of the bilateral sublingual glands, making a shape of doubled tongue

莲花舌 [lián huā shé]

lotus tongue: a form of hypertrophy of the sublingual glands, making a shape of a lotus flower

绊舌 [bàn shé]

ankyloglossia: restricted movement of the tongue, often resulting from short lingual frenum

舌痈 [shé yōng]

tongue abscess: suppurative inflammation of the tongue

舌疔 [shé dīng]

tongue boil: localized painful swelling and inflammation of the tongue, having a hard core, and forming pus

舌疮 [shé chuāng]

tongue sore: a sore occurring on the tongue with local cracking and swelling and discharge of blood, accompanied by foul breath and constipation

唇疮 [chún chuāng]

lip sore: sore occurring on the lip, itching or painful, sometimes with purulent discharge

唇疔 [chún dīng]

lip pustule: furuncle on the lip or at the corner of the mouth, small but deep-rooted, with pustule formation

唇疽 [chún jū]

lip abscess: an infectious inflammation of the lip leading to abscess formation

痰包 [tán bāo]

phlegm cyst: retention cyst of the floor of the mouth, also called 舌下痰包 [shé xià tán bāo]

舌下痰包 [shé xià tán bāo]

sublingual cyst, same as phlegm cyst (痰包 [tán bāo])

鹅口疮 [é kǒu chuāng]

thrush: disease usually in infants, marked by milky-white adhesion in the mouth and throat, with pus formation

齿龈肿痛 [chǐ yín zhǒng tòng]

painful swollen gum: inflammation of the gum

齿龈结瓣 [chǐ yín jié bàn]

petaloid gum: inflammation of the gum with the appearance of valves

雀舌 [què shé]

sparrow's tongue: a lingual vegetation that looks like a sparrow's tongue, with pain at the beginning and then erosion

唇菌 [chún jūn]

lip cancer

舌菌 [shé jūn]

carcinoma of the tongue

骨伤科 Orthopedics and Traumatology

骨折与脱位 Fractures and Dislocations

正骨（科） [zhèng gǔ (kē)]

orthopedics: a branch of medicine concerned with the preservation and restoration of the function of the skeletal system, its articulation and associated structures

伤科 [shāng kē]

traumatology: a branch of medicine that deals with wounds and disability from injuries

骨伤科 [gǔ shāng kē]

traumato-orthopedics: a branch of medicine that includes orthopedics and traumatology

疡医 [yáng yī]

traumato-orthopedist: an ancient name for a specialist in traumato-orthopedics

折疡 [zhé yáng]

trauma and fracture: an ancient name for various traumatic conditions

金创 [jīn chuāng]

incised wound: wound made by a metallic cutting instrument, also called 金疡 [jīn yáng]

金疡 [jīn yáng]

incised wound: same as 金创 [jīn chuāng]

踠跌 [wǎn diē]

fracture from a fall: fracture of a limb or limbs caused by a fall

折骨绝筋 [zhé gǔ jué jīn]

fracture with broken tendon; closed fracture: breaking of the bone that produces tendon rupture but no open wound on the skin

折骨列肤 [zhé gǔ liè fū]

fracture with split skin; open fracture: breaking of the bone producing an open wound on the skin

断端移位 [duàn duān yí wèi]

displacement of fractured ends: movement of fractured ends from the usual or correct place

骨折 [gǔ zhé]

fracture: the breaking of a bone. The terms for various types of fracture commonly used in contemporary Chinese traumatology are the same as those used in Western medicine, and are listed in the following table.

锁骨骨折	suǒ gǔ gǔ zhé	**clavicle fracture**
肩胛骨骨折	jiān jiá gǔ gǔ zhé	**scapula fracture**
肱骨外科颈骨折	gōng gǔ wài kē jǐng gǔ zhé	**humerus surgical neck fracture**
肱骨干骨折	gōng gǔ gàn gǔ zhé	**humerus shaft fracture**
肱骨髁上骨折	gōng gǔ kē shàng gǔ zhé	**humerus supracondylar fracture**
肱骨髁间骨折	gōng gǔ kē jiān gǔ zhé	**humerus intercondylar fracture**
肱骨外髁骨折	gōng gǔ wài kē gǔ zhé	**humerus external condyle fracture**
肱骨内上髁骨折	gōng gǔ nèi shàng kē gǔ zhé	**humerus internal epicondyle fracture**
尺骨鹰嘴骨折	chǐ gǔ yīng zuǐ gǔ zhé	**ulna coronoid process fracture**
桡骨头骨折	ráo gǔ tóu gǔ zhé	**radius head fracture**
尺骨干骨折	chǐ gǔ gàn gǔ zhé	**ulna shaft fracture**
尺骨上1/3骨折合并桡骨头脱位	chǐ gǔ shàng 1/3 gǔ zhé hé bìng ráo gǔ tóu tuō wèi	**ulna (upper third) fracture with radius proximal end dislocation**
桡骨下1/3骨折合并下桡尺骨关节脱位	ráo gǔ xià 1/3 gǔ zhé hé bìng xià ráo chǐ gǔ guān jié tuō wèi	**radius (lower third) fracture with distal radio-ulnar dislocation**
桡骨下端骨折	ráo gǔ xià duān gǔ zhé	**radius lower end fracture**
腕舟骨骨折	wàn zhōu gǔ gǔ zhé	**hand scaphoid fracture**
掌骨骨折	Zhǎng gǔ gǔ zhé	**metacarpal fracture**
指骨骨折	zhǐ gǔ gǔ zhé	**phalanx fracture**
股骨颈骨折	gǔ gǔ jǐng gǔ zhé	**femur neck fracture**
股骨粗隆间骨折	gǔ gǔ cū lóng jiān gǔ zhé	**femor intertrochanteric fracture**
股骨干骨折	gǔ gǔ gàn gǔ zhé	**femur shaft fracture**
股骨髁上骨折	gǔ gǔ kē shàng gǔ zhé	**femur epicondyles fracture**

股骨髁部骨折	gǔ gǔ kē bù gǔ zhé	**femur condyles fracture**
髌骨骨折	bìn gǔ gǔ zhé	**patella fracture**
胫骨髁骨折	jìng gǔ kē gǔ zhé	**tibia condyles fracture**
胫腓骨干双骨折	jìng féi gǔ gàn shuāng gǔ zhé	**tibia and fibula shaft fracture**
腓骨干骨折	féi gǔ gàn gǔ zhé	**tibia shaft fracture**
踝骨骨折	huái gǔ gǔ zhé	**ankle bone fracture**
距骨骨折	jù gǔ gǔ zhé	**astragalus fracture**
跟骨骨折	gēn gǔ gǔ zhé	**calcaneous fracture; heel bone fracture**
足舟骨骨折	zú zhōu gǔ gǔ zhé	**foot navicular fracture; foot scaphoid fracture**
跖骨骨折	zhí gǔ gǔ zhé	**metatarsal bone fracture**
趾骨骨折	zhǐ gǔ gǔ zhé	**toe fracture**
胫骨干折	jìng gǔ gàn zhé	**tibia shaft fracture**
脊柱骨折	jǐ zhù gǔ zhé	**vertebral column fracture**
寰、枢椎骨折	Huán、shū zhūi gǔ zhé	**atlas-axis vertebral fracture**
颈椎单纯骨折	jìng zhuī dān chún gǔ zhé	**cervical vertebral simple fracture**
胸腰椎骨折	Xiōng yāo zhuī gǔ zhé	**thoraco-lumbar vertebral fracture**
外伤性截瘫	wài shāng xìng jié tān	**traumatic paraplegia**
骨盆骨折	gǔ pén gǔ zhé	**pelvic fracture**
肋骨骨折	lèi gǔ gǔ zhé	**rib fracture**
裂缝骨折	liè fèng gǔ zhé	**fissured fracture**
青枝骨折	qīng zhī gǔ zhé	**greenstick fracture**
骨骺分离	gǔ hóu fēn lí	**epiphyseal dissociation; epiphyseal separation**

脱位 [tuō wèi]

dislocation; luxation: the displacement of a bone. The terms for various types of dislocation commonly used in contemporary Chinese traumatology are the same as those used in Western medicine and are listed in the following table.

脱臼 [tuō jiù]

another name for dislocation (脱位 [tuō wèi])

脱骱 [tuō jiè]

an ancient term for dislocation (脱位 [tuō wèi])

脱髎 [tuō liáo]

an ancient term for dislocation (脱位 [tuō wèi])

下颌关节脱位	xià hé guān jié tuō wèi	**mandible dislocation**
胸锁关节脱位	xiōng suǒ guān jié tuō wèi	**sternoclavicular dislocation**
肩关节脱位	jiān guān jié tuō wèi	**shoulder dislocation**
肩锁关节脱位	jiān suǒ guān jié tuō wèi	**acromioclavicular dislocation**
肘关节脱位	zhǒ guān jié tuō wèi	**elbow dislocation**
桡骨头半脱位	Ráo gǔ tóu bàn tuō wèi	**radius head subluxation**
月骨前脱位	yuè gǔ qián tuō wèi	**lunate anterior dislocation**
拇指腕掌关节脱位	mǔ zhǐ wàn zhǎng guān jié tuō wèi	**thumb carpometacarpal dislocation**
拇指掌指关节脱位	mǔ zhǐ zhǎng zhǐ guān jié tuō wèi	**thumb metacarpophalangeal dislocation**
掌指关节脱位	zhǎng zhǐ guān jié tuō wèi	**metacarpophalangeal dislocation**
指间关节脱位	Zhǐ jiān guān jié tuō wè i	**interphalangeal dislocation**
髋关节脱位	Kuān guān jié tuō wèi	**hip dislocation**
髌骨脱位	Bìn gǔ tuō wèi	**patella dislocation**
膝关节脱位	xī guān jié tuō wèi	**knee dislocation**
踝关节脱位	huái guān jié tuō wèi	**ankle dislocation**
距骨脱位	jù gǔ tuō wèi	**astragalus/talus dislocation**
跖跗关节脱位	Zhí fū guān jié tuō wèi	**tarsometatarsal dislocation**
跖趾关节脱位	Zhí zhǐ guān jié tuō wèi	**metatarsophalangeal dislocation**
足趾间关节脱位	zú zhǐ jiān guān jié tuō wèi	**foot interphalangeal dislocation**

正骨手法 [zhèng gǔ shǒu fǎ]

manipulation of bone setting: manual correction of a fracture or dislocation

正骨八法 [zhèng gǔ bā fǎ]

eight bone-setting manipulations: the commonly used manipulations in bone-setting, – palpating, rejoining, hold-carrying, lifting, pressing, circular rubbing, pushing, and grasping

断骨接整 [duàn gǔ jié zhěng]

reduction of fracture: reunion of a fracture in its normal position

平整复元 [píng zhěng fù yuán]

correction and reduction: restoration the original normal position of the fractured bone in bone-setting, often called reduction (整复 [zhěng fù]) for short

整复 [zhěng fù]

reduction: correction of a fracture, an abbreviation of correction and reduction (平整复元 [píng zhěng fù yuán])

手摸心会 [shǒu mō xīn huì]

understanding tacitly by touching: understanding the condition of a fracture such as the location of the fractured ends by careful palpation

拔伸牵引 [bá shēn qiān yǐn]

pulling and traction: the basic procedure for fracture reduction by pulling the limb along its long axis, and traction in the proper direction

旋转屈伸 [xuán zhuǎn qū shēn]

rotating, bending and stretching: the manipulative procedure for reduction of a fracture near a uniaxial joint with an angulation deformity, i.e., restoring the normal physiological axis first by rotating the distal part, and then correcting the dislocated bone by bending and stretching

提按端挤 [tí àn duān jǐ]

lifting, pressing, holding, and squeezing: the manipulative procedure for reduction of dislocation after the overlapping, rotation and angulation deformities have been corrected, lifting and pressing for reduction of upper-lower dislocation, and holding and squeezing for right-left dislocation

摇摆触碰 [yáo bǎi chù pèng]

rocking and tapping: the manipulative procedure for further reduction of a transverse, serrated fracture, rocking to make close contact of the broken ends, and tapping after splintage to make the proper embedment

夹挤分骨 [jiā jǐ fēn gǔ]

separating bones by squeezing: the manipulative procedure for reducing a fracture of two long bones in parallel, such as ulnar and radial dual fracture

端法 [duān fǎ]

hold-carrying: a manipulation used in massotherapy and bone setting performed by carrying the diseased extremity upward and downward with its distal end held in one or both hands of the operator

提法 [tí fǎ]

lifting: a manipulation of bone fracture reduction by lifting the broken bone upwards and outwards with the hand or a rope so as to obtain a complete reduction directly or indirectly

拉法 [lā fǎ]

traction: a basic reduction manipulation for overlapping and displacement of fractured bones, also called 牵拉法 [qiān lā fǎ]

牵拉法 [qiān lā fǎ]

traction, same as 拉法 [lā fǎ]

接法 [jiē fǎ]

rejoining: a method of rejoining the broken ends or fragments of a fractured bone

接骨续筋 [jiē gǔ xù jīn]

reunion of bone, muscle and ligament: rejoining of the fractured bone and restoration of the soft tissue

折顶 [zhé dǐng]

turning to the opposite: manipulative procedure for reducing a transverse or serrated fracture when traction force is inadequate to completely correct the overlapping displacement, i.e., increasing the angulation by pressing to make the broken ends touch each other, and then placing them in the correct position by turning the angulation in the opposite direction

回旋 [huí xuán]

reverse rotation: manipulative procedure for reducing oblique or spiral fracture with dorsal displacement by holding the proximal and distal parts and rotating them in the direction opposite to the displacement

足蹬 [zú dēng]

pressing down with the foot: a procedure for reducing forward dislocation of the shoulder, elbow and hip joint by pressing down with the foot while pulling with the hands

膝顶 [xī dǐng]

pushing with the knee: a procedure for reducing dislocation of the shoulder and elbow by pushing with a knee while pulling with the hands

杠杆支撑 [gàng gǎn zhī chēng]

propping with a lever: a procedure with the aid of a lever for a long-standing dislocation difficult to reduce by the hands alone

端提捺正 [duān tí nà zhèng]

holding, lifting, and restoring to the right location: comprehensive or individual application of holding, lifting, squeezing and pressing manipulations for reduction of dislocation

捺正 [nà zhèng]

manual correction: a therapeutic method of restoring the dislocated ends of a fracture or luxation with the hands

续筋接骨 [xù jīn jiē gǔ]

reunion of fractured bone and tendon: reuniting of fractured bone and restoring the normal function of injured muscles and tendons

拔伸复位 [bá shēn fù wèi]

pulling-extending reduction: reduction by exerting a pulling force along the long axis of a bone

拔伸牵引 [bá shēn qiān yǐn]

pulling-extension traction: traction along the long axis of a bone

拔伸捏正 [bá shēn niē zhèng]

reduction by pulling and kneading: a manipulation in traumatology by pulling the fractured bone and kneading the displaced ends simultaneously for restoration

挺腿拔伸 [tǐng tuǐ bá shēn]

straightening traction: a manipulation in bone-setting accomplished by first straightening the leg and then applying traction

顺骨捋筋 [shùn gǔ lǚ jīn]

tendon-stroking along the bone: a manipulation in bone-setting performed by stroking the tendons and muscles along the long axis of the bone

欲合先离 [yù hé xiān lí]

reunion preceded by separation: a manipulation of bone-setting, by which the overlapping fracture ends are separated and then restored along the axis

离而复合 [lí ér fù hé]

osteodiastasic reduction: a reduction manipulation by separating the fractured ends first and then restoring them to the normal position

纳入原位 [nà rù yuán wèi]

manual restoration: restoration of the dislocated bone to its normal position by the hands

外固定 [wài gù dìng]

external fixation: the immobilization of the parts of a fractured bone by the use of attachments from outside

夹板固定 [jiā bǎn gù dìng]

splintage: application of splints for fixation

夹板固定疗法 [jiā bǎn gù dìng liáo fǎ]

splintage therapy: fixation treatment by the use of splints and pads between the skin and the splint for the fixation of fracture, also called 固定垫 [gù dìng diàn]

托板 [tuō bǎn]

supporting board: a rectangular wooden board used to support the diseased part in bone-setting

后侧夹板 [hòu cè jiā bǎn]

posterior splint: a splint fixed at the posterior aspect of an extremity

鼎式夹板固定 [dǐng shì jiā bǎn gù dìng]

tripod-shaped splint fixation: fixation beyond the joint with a tripod-shaped splint

棉枕固定 [mián zhěn gù dìng]

cotton-pad fixation: stabilization of a fractured bone by means of cotton pads

固定垫 [gù dìng diàn]

fixation pad: a pad made of paper or cotton to be placed between the skin and the splint for fixing the fractured ends after reduction, also called 压垫 [yā diàn]

压垫 [yā diàn]; **压力垫** [yā lì diàn]

pressure pad: a synonym for fixation pad (固定垫 [gù dìng diàn])

平垫 [píng diàn]

flat pad: a square or rectangular pad, 4 – 8 cm long and 1.5 – 4 cm thick, suitable for the flat part of a limb and often used for fixation of a shaft fracture

高低垫 [gāo dī diàn]

high-low pad: a pad thick on one side and thin on the other side, used for fixation of clavicle fractures

葫芦垫 [hú lú diàn]

calabash pad: a pad with two bigger ends and a narrow middle part of the same thickness, in the shape of a calabash or a dumbbell, useful for a radius head fracture or dislocation

横垫 [héng diàn]

transverse pad: a strip of pad about 6-7cm long and 1.5 – 2cm wide and about 0.3cm thick, useful for the lower end fracture of the radius

抱骨垫 [bào gǔ diàn]

peri-bony pad: a semilunar-shaped pad useful for fixation of fractured bone such as ulna coronoid process fracture and patella fracture

分骨垫 [fēn gǔ diàn]

bone-separating pad: a pressing pad used to separate the double fracture of two parallel bones

合骨垫 [hé gǔ diàn]

bone-combining pad: a pad with thicker sides and a thinner middle part, suitable for the fixation of lower ulna-radial joint separation

大头垫 [dà tóu diàn]

megacaput pad: a kind of fixation pad with cotton wrapped on one end of the splint, forming a mushroom-shaped pad, used for the fixation of the fractured surgical neck of the humerus

一垫固定法 [yī diàn gù dìng fǎ]

fixation with one pad: a fixation method by using a single pad at the site of a fracture

二垫固定法 [èr diàn gù dìng fǎ]

fixation with two pads: a fixation method for fracture with lateral displacement by using two pads each on the displacement side of the two broken ends in order to prevent recurrence

三垫固定法 [sān diàn gù dìng fǎ]

fixation with three pads: a fixation method for fracture with angulation deformity by placing one pad at the prominence of the angle and the other two on the counter side close to the two broken ends

抱膝器 [bào xī qì]

peripatellapexor: an appliance for patellapexy

扎带 [zhā dài]

bandage: a strip of cloth for binding the splint

内固定 [nèi gù dìng]

internal fixation: the immobilization of the parts of a fractured bone by the use of attachments from inside

复位 [fù wèi]

reduction: correction of a fracture or dislocation

坐式复位 [zuò shì fù wèi]

sitting reduction: reduction of a dislocated shoulder joint by traction in the sitting position

慢性复位 [màn xìng fù wèi]

gradual reduction: a manipulation of gradual restoration of a fractured bone by traction or raising the pillow-pad

入臼 [rù jiù]

joint reduction: the restoration of a joint to its normal position by manipulation

熨药 [yùn yào]

hot-compressing drug: drug used for hot compress

手法牵引 [shǒu fǎ qiān yǐn]

manual traction: pulling with the hands

牵推法 [qiān tuī fǎ]

pull-push technique: a manual reduction of the temporomandibular joint

攀索叠砖 [pān suǒ dié zhuān]

holding a rope and standing on a pile of bricks: an ancient method of traction for lumbar or thoracic injury (fracture or dislocation) wherein the patient is asked to stand on a pile of bricks (usually three under each foot), holding a rope hanging above, while the practitioner takes away the bricks one by one for gradual traction

牵引疗法 [qiān yǐn liáo fǎ]

traction therapy: treatment of bone disorders by applying a pulling force. In contemporary Chinese medicine most of the terms for various traction therapies are the same as those in Western medicine, and the rest are self-explanatory from the Western medical point of view. The commonly used ones are listed in the following table.

皮肤牵引	Pí fū qiān yǐn	**skin traction**
骨牵引	Gǔ qiān yǐn	**bone traction**

颅骨牵引	Lú gǔ qiān yǐn	**skull traction**
尺骨鹰嘴牵引	chǐ gǔ yīng zuǐ qiān yǐn	**traction through ulnar olecranon**
股骨下端牵引	Gǔ gǔ xià duān qiān yǐn	**traction through femoral distal end**
胫骨结节牵引	jìng gǔ jié jié qiān yǐn	**traction through tibial tubercle**
跟骨牵引	gēn gǔ qiān yǐn	**transcalcaneal traction**
肋骨牵引	Lèi gǔ qiān yǐn	**rib traction**
布托牵引	Bù tuō qiān yǐn	**cloth-wrapping traction**
颌枕带牵引	Hé zhěn dài qiān yǐn	**madibulo-occipital bandage traction**
骨盆悬吊牵引	gǔ pén xuán diào qiān yǐn	**pelvic sling traction**
骨盆牵引带牵引	gǔ pén qiān yǐn dài qiān yǐn	**pelvic bandage traction**

筋伤 Soft Tissue Injuries

筋断 [jīn duàn]

musculotendinous rupture: complete or partial disruption of muscle and tendon

筋缩 [jīn suō]

(1) muscle contracture: permanent shortening of muscle with deformity and dysfunction; **(2)** ***jinsuo*** **(GV 8)**

筋痿 [jīn wěi]

(1) muscle flaccidity: weakness and softness of muscle; **(2) impotence**

筋粗 [jīn cū]

musculotendinous thickening: thickening of tendon and muscle after injury, due to blood stasis, or due to regeneration, degeneration or spasm of the tissue

筋结 [jīn jié]

musculotendinous nodulation: occurrence of a cystic mass on the muscle or tendon due to stagnation of *qi* and blood after soft tissue injury

筋柔 [jīn róu]

musculotendinous softening: relaxation and weakness of the joint after soft tissue injury

筋伤 [jīn shāng]

soft tissue injury: injury of soft tissue, including muscle, muscle tendon, tendon sheath, ligament, joint capsule, synovial bursa, intervertebral disc, peripheral nerve, and blood vessel. The terms for various soft tissue injuries used in contemporary Chinese traumatology are basically the same as those used in Western medicine and are listed in the following table.

Soft tissue injuries of the shoulder		
肩部扭挫伤	jiān bù niǔ cuò shāng	**shoulder sprain and contusion**
肩凝症	jiān níng zhèng	**frozen shoulder**
肩袖损伤	Jiān xiù sǔn shāng	**rotator cuff injury**
肱二头肌长头肌腱炎	gōng èr tóu jī cháng tóu jī jiàn yán	**brachial biceps long head tendonitis**
肱二头肌短头肌腱捩伤	gōng èr tóu jī duǎn tóu jī jiàn liè shāng	**brachial biceps short head tendon sprain**
肱二头肌腱断裂	gōng èr tóu jī jiàn duàn liè	**rupture of brachial biceps tendon**
肩关节周围炎	jiān guān jié zhōu wéi yán	**periarthritis of shoulder**
肩峰下滑液囊炎	jiān fēng xià huá yè náng yán	**subacromial bursitis**
Soft tissue injuries of the elbow		
肘关节扭挫伤	zhǒu guān jié niǔ cuò shāng	**elbow sprain and contusion**
肱骨外上髁炎	gōng gǔ wài shàng kē yán	**external humeral epicondylitis**
肱骨内上髁炎	gōng gǔ nèi shàng kē yán	**internal humeral epicondylitis**
旋前圆肌综合征	xuán qián yuán jī zōng hé zhēng	**round pronator syndrome**
旋后肌综合征	xuán hòu jī zōng hé zhēng	**supinator syndrome**
肘关节骨化性肌炎	zhǒu guān jié gǔ huá xìng jī yán	**ossifying myositis of elbow**
尺骨鹰嘴滑膜囊炎	chǐ gǔ yīng zuǐ huá mó náng yán	**bursitis of olecranon**
Soft tissue injuries of the wrist and hand		
腕关节扭伤	wàn guān jié niǔ shāng	**wrist sprain**

桡侧伸腕肌腱周围炎	ráo cè shēn wàn jī jiàn zhōu wéi yán	**radial extensor perimyotenositis of wrist**
腕管综合征	wàn guǎn zōng hé zhēng	**carpal tunnel syndrome**
指伸、指屈肌腱断裂	zhǐ shēn、zhǐ qū jī jiàn duàn liè	**tendinous rupture of digital flexor or extensor muscle**
腱鞘囊肿	jiàn qiào náng zhǒng	**ganglion cyst**
桡骨茎突狭窄性腱鞘炎	ráo gǔ jìng tū xiá zhǎi xìng jiàn qiào yán	**tenosynovitis stenosans [of processus styloideus radii]**
指屈肌腱鞘炎	zhǐ qū jī jiàn qiào yán	**tenosynovititis of digital flexor muscle**
Soft tissue injuries of the hip and thigh		
股四头肌损伤	gǔ sì tóu jī sǔn shāng	**injury of quadriceps femoris**
股内收肌群损伤	gǔ nèi shōu jī qún sǔn shāng	**injury of femoral adductors**
髋关节一过性滑膜炎	kuān guān jié yī guò xìng huá mó yán	**transient bursitis of hip joint**
弹响髋	tán xiǎng kuān	**snapping hip**
股骨大转子滑膜囊炎	gǔ gǔ dà zhuàn zǐ huá mó náng yán	**trochanteric bursitis of femur**
Soft tissue injuries of the knee and shin		
膝关节内、外侧副韧带损伤	xī guān jié、wài cè fù rèn dài sǔn shāng	**injury of medial/lateral collateral ligament of knee joint**
膝交叉韧带损伤	xī jiāo chā rèn dài sǔn shāng	**cruciate ligament injury of knee**
半月板损伤	bàn yuè bǎn sǔn shāng	**meniscus injury**
膝关节创伤性滑膜炎	xī guān jié chuāng shāng xìng huá mó yán	**traumatic synovitis of knee**
髌腱断裂	bìn jiàn duàn liè	**rupture of patellar tendon**
髌前、髌下滑膜囊炎	bìn qián、bìn xià huá mó náng yán	**prepatellar or infrapatellar bursitis**
髌骨软化症	bìn gǔ ruǎn huà zhèng	**chondromalacia patellae**
髌下脂肪垫肥厚	bìn xià zhī fáng diàn féi hòu	**hypertrophy of subpatellar fat pad**
腘窝囊肿	guó wō náng zhǒng	**popliteal cyst**
腓肠肌损伤	Féi cháng jī sǔn shāng	**injury of gastrocnemius muscle**

Soft tissue injuries of the ankle and foot		
距小腿关节内、外侧韧带损伤	jù xiǎo tǔi guān jié nèi、wài cè rèn dài sǔn shāng	**injury of medial or lateral ligament of talocrural joint**
跗跖关节扭伤	fū zhí guān jié niǔ shāng	**tarsometatarsal sprain**
跟腱断裂	gēn jiàn duàn liè	**rupture of Achilles tendon**
跟腱滑膜囊炎	gēn jiàn huá mó náng yán	**Achilles bursitis**
跟腱炎	gēn jiàn yán	**Achilles tendinitis**
踝管综合征	huái guǎn zōng hé zhēng	**tarsal tunnel syndrome**
腓骨长、短肌腱滑脱	féi gǔ cháng、duǎn jī jiàn huá tuō	**olisthy of long or short peroneal tendon**
跟痛症	gēn tòng zhèng	**heel pain**
跖痛症	zhí tòng zhèng	**metatarsal pain**
蹞跖滑膜囊炎	mǔ zhí huá mó náng yán	**hallucal bursitis**
Soft tissue injuries of the chin and neck		
颞颌关节紊乱症	niè hé guān jié wěn luàn zhèng	**disorder of temporomandibular joint**
颈部急性扭挫伤	jǐng bù jí xìng niǔ cuò shāng	**acute sprain and contusion of neck**
落枕	lào zhěn	**stiff neck**
颈椎病	jǐng zhuī bìng	**cervical spondylosis**
肌性斜颈	Jī xìng xié jìng	**myogenic torticollis**
颈椎关节突关节错缝	jǐng zhuī guān jié tū guān jié cuò fèng	**fissured fracture of cervical vertebral process**
Soft tissue injuries of the chest and back		
胸部扭挫伤	xiōng bù niǔ cuò shāng	**thoracic sprain and contusion**
项背急性扭挫伤	xiàng bèi jí xìng niǔ cuò shāng	**acute nuchal sprain and contusion**
胸廓出口综合征	xiōng kuò chū kǒu zōng hé zhēng	**thoracic outlet syndrome**
胸椎小关节错缝	xiōng zhuī xiǎo guān jié cuò fèng	**minor joint dislocation of thoracic vertebrae**

Soft tissue injuries of the lumbosaccral region		
急性腰扭伤	Jí xìng yāo niǔ shāng	**acute lumbar sprain**
慢性腰肌劳损	màn xìng yāo jī láo sǔn	**chronic lumbar muscle strain**
第三腰椎横突综合征	dì sān yāo zhuī héng tū zōng hé zhēng	**transverse process syndrome of third lumbar vertebra**
腰椎间盘突出症	yāo zhuī jiān pán tū chū zhèng	**protrusion of lumbar intervertebral disc**
腰椎椎管狭窄症	yāo zhuī zhuī guǎn xiá zhǎi zhèng	**lumbar spinal canal stenosis**
骶髂关节损伤	dǐ qià guān jié sǔn shāng	**sacro-iliac injury**
腰椎退行性滑脱	yāo zhuī tuì xíng xìng huá tuō	**lumbar retrograde spondylolisthesis**
腰臀部筋膜炎	yāo tún bù jīn mó yán	**lumbogluteal fasciitis**
臀肌挛缩症	tún jī luán suō zhèng	**contraction of gluteal muscles**
梨状肌综合征	lí zhuàng jī zōng hé zhēng	**periform muscle syndrome**
坐骨结节滑膜囊炎	zuò gǔ jié jié huá mó náng yán	**bursitis of ischial tuberosity**
尾骶部挫伤	wěi dǐ bù cuò shāng	**sacrococcygeal contusion**
Peripheral nerve injuries		
正中神经损伤	zhèng zhōng shén jīng sǔn shāng	**median nerve injury**
尺神经损伤	chǐ shén jīng sǔn shāng	**ulnar nerve injury**
桡神经损伤	ráo shén jīng sǔn shāng	**radial nerve injury**
臂丛神经损伤	bì cóng shén jīng sǔn shāng	**brachial plexus nerve injury**
坐骨神经损伤	zuò gǔ shén jīng sǔn shāng	**sciatic nerve injury**
腓神经损伤	Féi shén jīng sǔn shāng	**peroneal nerve injury**
腓总神经损伤	Féi zǒng shén jīng sǔn shāng	**common peroneal nerve injury**
胫神经损伤	jìng shén jīng sǔn shāng	**tibial nerve injury**

撕裂伤 [sī liè shāng]

laceration; lacerated wound: a torn and ragged wound

断裂伤 [duàn liè shāng]

rupture; ruptured wound: a wound with disruption of tissue

骨错缝 [gǔ cuò fèng]

fissured fracture: a crack extending from the surface into, but not through a long bone

扭伤 [niǔ shāng]

sprain: a sudden or violent twist or wrench of a joint causing stretching or tearing of ligaments

挫伤 [cuò shāng]

contusion: an injury of the subcutaneous or deeper tissues without a break in the skin

碾挫伤 [niǎn cuò shāng]

crushing-contusion: a crushed and contused wound

牵拉肩 [qiān lā jiān]

dragged shoulder: sprain of the short head tendon of the brachial biceps

弹响指 [tán xiǎng shāng]

snapping finger: another name for tenovaginitis of the flexor digitorum. It is so called because the finger is liable to have a momentary spasmodic arrest of flexion of extension followed by a snapping into place.

理筋手法 [lǐ jīn shǒu fǎ]

soft-tissue injury manipulation: a collective term for various manipulations for restoring and treating injured soft tissues, including pressing, rubbing, kneading, pinching, pushing, grasping, lifting, plucking and shaking

理筋 [lǐ jīn]

tendon-regulation: a manipulation in traumatology performed by pressing and pushing the injured tendon along its course with the fingers slowly and repeatedly to regulate and soothe the tendon and promote the flow of *qi* and blood

分筋 [fēn jīn]

tendon-separation: a manipulation in traumatology performed by pressing deeply with the tip of the thumb close to the nodulation or tender point of the tendon, and slowly kneading and plucking for separating adhesion or relieving spasm

筋正 [jīn zhèng]

tendon restoration: restoration of the tendon or soft tissue to its normal position

筋合 [jīn hé]

tendon reunion: reuniting of the tendon and muscle after injury

搓法 [cuō fǎ]

twisting (manipulation): a manipulation of giving an injured limb twists with two palms in the direction opposite each other

揉法 [róu fǎ]

kneading (manipulation): a manipulation involving pressing and moving to and fro or circularly on an affected area with the flat of the thumb, the tips of the index, middle and ring finger, the thenar or the root of the palm

指揉法 [zhǐ róu fǎ]

finger kneading (manipulation): a manipulation involving kneading with the index and middle fingers or with the index, middle and ring fingers

掌揉法 [zhǎng róu fǎ]

palm kneading (manipulation): a manipulation involving kneading with palm in a circular motion

拳揉法 [quán róu fǎ]

fist kneading (manipulation): a manipulation involving kneading with the ulnar aspect of the fist in a circular motion

肘揉法 [zhǒu róu fǎ]

elbow kneading (manipulation): a manipulation involving kneading the deep muscle with the olecranon of the elbow on the body surface of an affected area

抱踝手法 [bào huái shǒu fǎ]

peri-ankle manipulation: a manipulation involving kneading the ankle

撙令平正 [zǔn nà píng zhèng]

kneading restoration: a manipulation for the restoration of a local injury to its normal condition by kneading

撙捺皮相 [zǔn nà pí xiàng]

observation after kneading-pressing: observing a fractured bone after kneading and pressing the fractured ends

撙捺相近 [zǔn nà xiāng jìn]

kneading-pressing close: a manipulation in bone-setting performed by kneading and pressing the fractured ends close to each other

推法 [tuī fǎ]

pushing (manipulation): pushing and squeezing the muscles with the fingers, palms, or elbow forward, apart or spirally, with force

一指禅推法 [yī zhǐ chán tuī fǎ]

single-finger meditation pushing: a manipulation involving pushing the tissue with the tip, the flat or the outer side of the thumb, on which the operator's *qi* is concentrated by meditation, also called single-finger meditation pushing therapy (一指禅推拿疗法 [yī zhǐ chán tuī ná liáo fǎ])

一指禅推拿疗法 [yī zhǐ chán tuī ná liáo fǎ]

single-finger meditation pushing therapy: same as single-finger meditation pushing (一指禅推法 [yī zhǐ chán tuī fǎ])

指推法 [zhǐ tuī fǎ]

finger pushing (manipulation): a manipulation of pushing with the ventral side of the thumb while the other fingers are slightly bent, usually along the course of a meridian or the muscle fibers

掌推法 [zhǎng tuī fǎ]

palm pushing (manipulation): a manipulation of pushing with the root of a palm or with the root of a palm which is overlapped by the other palm

肘推法 [zhǒu tuī fǎ]

elbow pushing (manipulation): a manipulation of pushing forcefully with the olecranon of the elbow

滚法 [gǔn fǎ]

rolling (manipulation): moving by turning a hollow fist with the thumb bent over the fingers over the skin back and forth continuously with moderate force and small amplitude

拍击法 [pāi jī fǎ]

patting-striking (manipulation): combination of patting manipulation and striking manipulation

击法 [jī fǎ]

striking: a manipulation performed by striking the affected limb with the palm, fist, or a specially made rod

拳击法 [quán jī fǎ]

fist striking (manipulation): a manipulation involving striking the body surface with the ulnar side of a fist or fists

掌击法 [zhǎng jī fǎ]

palm striking (manipulation): a manipulation involving striking the body surface with the root of a palm

指节拍法 [zhǐ jié pān fǎ]

knuckle patting (manipulation): a manipulation involving patting a certain part of the body with the dorsal side of the finger joints when the fingers are slightly bent

劈法 [pī fǎ]

vertical palm striking (manipulation): a manipulation involving striking a certain area of the body surface by using the ulnar side of the palms with the fingers extended, as if splitting the treated area

啄法 [zhuó fǎ]

pecking (manipulation): a manipulation involving tapping an area of the body surface with the finger tips when the fingers are slightly bent, resembling pecking by a bird

棒击法 [bàng jī fǎ]

rod striking (manipulation): a manipulation involving striking the body surface with a mulberry branch

摩法 [mā fǎ]

circular rubbing (manipulation): rubbing the affected part with the ventral aspect of the finger tips or the palm in a circular motion with moderate force and frequency

掌摩法 [zhǎng mā fǎ]

palmar circular rubbing (manipulation): circular rubbing performed on the body surface of the affected area by using the palm

指摩法 [zhǐ mā fǎ]

digital circular rubbing (manipulation): rotary rubbing performed on the body surface of the affected area by using the ventral aspect of the thumb, index finger and middle finger in combination

擦法 [cā fǎ]

rubbing (manipulation): a manipulation performed by rubbing with the flat of the finger, the thenar, or the palm to and fro over the skin continuously with a high frequency

掌擦法 [zhǎng cā fǎ]

palm rubbing (manipulation): rubbing the treated area of the body surface with the whole palm

鱼际擦法 [yú jì cā fǎ]

eminence rubbing (manipulation): rubbing the treated area of the body surface with the thenar eminence

侧擦法 [cè cā fǎ]

side rubbing (manipulation): rubbing the treated area of the body surface with the ulnar side of the palm

抖法 [dǒu fǎ]

shaking (manipulation): a manipulation by which the distal end of the affected extremity is held and pulled outwards by the operator and shaken up and down within the limit of movement

弹法 [tán fǎ]

flicking (manipulation): a manipulation performed by hitting the affected area with the back of the index fingertip or middle fingertip by flicking it against the thumb

弹筋法 [tán jīn fǎ]

tendon-plucking (manipulation): a manipulation performed by repeatedly pulling up the tendon or muscle and immediately releasing it

按法 [àn fǎ]

pressing (manipulation): a manipulation involving pushing steadily in a direction vertical to the body surface

指按法 [zhǐ àn fǎ]

finger pressing (manipulation): a manipulation involving pressing with the ventral part of the thumb or with the ventral part of the index, middle and ring fingers in combination

掌按法 [zhǎng àn fǎ]

palm pressing (manipulation): a manipulation involving pressing the treated area with the radial eminence, ventral surface or root part of the palm. An overlapping hand may be added if forceful pressing is necessary.

肘按法 [zhǒu àn fǎ]

elbow pressing (manipulation): a manipulation involving pressing with the olecranon of the elbow

拿法 [ná fǎ]

grasping (manipulation): a manual treatment for soft-tissue injury by lifting and squeezing or lifting and rapidly releasing the affected muscles with the thumb and the index and middle fingers or with the thumb and the other four fingers of one or both of the operator's hands

捏法 [niē fǎ]

pinching (manipulation): a manipulation performed by holding and lifting the superficial tissues by using the thumb with the index and middle fingers or the thumb with the other four fingers, and squeezing and pushing forward

合指捏法 [hé zhǐ niē fǎ]

finger-combining pinching (manipulation): pinching with three fingers (the thumb with the index and middle fingers) or with five fingers (the thumb with the other four fingers)

双手捏法 [shuāng shǒu niē fǎ]

bimanual pinching (manipulation): pinching with the fingers of both hands or the roots of both palms

屈指捏法 [qū zhǐ niē fǎ]

finger-bending pinching (manipulation): pinching the muscle firmly with the thumb and index finger bent like a pair of pliers and kneading

踩跷法 [cǎi qiào fǎ]

treading (manipulation): a manipulation rarely used at present, performed by treading on the affected area for reduction, e.g., treading on the back for the reduction of a protruded intervertebral disc

摇法 [yáo fǎ]

rotating (manipulation): a manipulation performed by turning the patient's head and neck, or shoulder, wrist, hip joint, knee joint, and ankle to and fro to relieve rigidity

扳法 [bān fǎ]

counterpulling (manipulation): a manipulation of extending, bending or rotating the spine or a limb by pulling with two hands in an opposite direction beyond a limited range instantaneously

扳颈椎法 [bān jǐng zhuī fǎ]

cervical counterpulling (manipulation): a manipulation involving reducing a dislocated cervical vertebra by counterpulling

颈椎单人旋转复位法 [jǐng zhuī dān rén xuán zhuǎn fù wèi fǎ]

single-handed rotating reduction of cervical vertebra: a reduction manipulation often used for treating dislocation of an upper cervical vertebra

颈椎角度复位法 [jǐng zhuī jiǎo dù fù wèi fǎ]

angular reduction of cervical vertebra: a reduction manipulation often used for treating dislocation of a middle cervical vertebra

颈椎侧旋复位法 [jǐng zhuī cè xuán fù wèi fǎ]

laterally-rotating reduction of cervical vertebra: a reduction manipulation often used for treating dislocation of a lower cervical vertebra

扳胸椎法 [bān xiōng zhuī fǎ]

thorcic counterpulling (manipulation): a manipulation involving reducing a dislocated thoracic vertebra by counterpulling

掌推扳胸椎法 [zhǎng tuī bān xiōng zhuī fǎ]

thoracic counterpulling with palm pushing (manipulation): a manipulation of reducing a displaced thoracic vertebra by placing the palm root of one hand on the spinous process of affected vertebra while the patient is lying prone, pushing forward and upward with the aid of the other hand at the end of the patient's deep exhalation with a nimble action which causes a click

膝顶扳胸椎法 [xī dǐng bān xiōng zhuī fǎ]

thoracic counterpulling with knee pushing (manupilation): a method of reducing a displaced thoracic vertebra by pushing upward and forward with the operator's right knee and pressing simultaneously the upper chest backward and downward with the operator's hands at the end of the patient's inspiration with a nimble action which causes a click

扳腰椎法 [bān yāo zhuī fǎ]

lumbar counterpulling (manipulation): a manipulation to reduce a dislocated lumbar vertebra by counterpulling

斜扳腰椎法 [xié bān yāo zhuī fǎ]

oblique lumbar counterpulling (manipulation): a manipulation to reduce a dislocated lumbar vertebra by placing one hand on the anterior aspect of the patient's shoulder and the other hand on the patient's buttock, and pulling in opposite directions with a nimble forceful action which causes a click

腰椎旋转复位法 [yāo zhuī xuán zhuǎn fù wèi fǎ]

lumbar rotating reduction (manipulation): a manipulation to reduce a dislocated lumbar vertebra by rotating the lumbar spine

后伸扳腰法 [hòu shēn bān yāo fǎ]

extending lumbar counterpulling (manipulation): a manipulation to reduce a dislocated lumbar vertebra by pressing the patient's waist with one hand and lifting the patient's legs with the other hand to cause a lumbar extension

拔伸法 [bá shēn fǎ]

pulling and stretching (manipulation): a manipulation involving pulling and stretching in combination

屈伸法 [qū shēn fǎ]

flexing and stretching (manipulation): a manipulation consisting of alternate flexing and stretching

背法 [bēi fǎ]

back-carrying (manipulation): a manipulation to reduce a protruded lumbar intervertebral disc by carrying the patient on the operator's back while the two are standing back to back

肩臂功 [jiān bì gōng]

acromiobrachial functional training: functional training of the shoulder and forearm

腿功 [tuǐ gōng]

leg training: a method of training the lower limb in convalescence after bone-setting

双手攀足式 [shuāng shǒu pān zú shì]

grasping the foot with the hands: a posture for lumbar training by grasping one's foot with both hands

双手托天式 [shuāng shǒu tuō tiān shì]

pushing upwards with both hands: a posture for training the functional activity of the upper limbs by pushing the hands upward as if lifting a weight

拧拳反掌式 [nǐng quán fǎn zhǎng shì]

clenching the fist, turning over and opening the hand: an exercise for training the carpal joint

振挺 [zhèn tǐng]

small wooden stick: a stick, 2-3 cm in diameter, used as a patting device for dispersing swelling and dissipating ecchymosis in traumatology

通利关节 [tōng lì guān jié]

easing the joint: making the joint movement easy

骨病 Osteopathy

骨病 [gǔ bìng]
osteopathy: disease of a bone

Suppurative inflammation of bone		
急性化脓性骨髓炎	jí xìng huà nóng xìng gǔ suí yán	**acute suppurative osteomyelitis**
慢性化脓性骨髓炎	màn xìng huà nóng xìng gǔ suí yán	**chronic suppurative osteomyelitis**
化脓性关节炎	huà nóng xìng guān jié yán	**suppurative arthritis**
硬化性骨髓炎	yìng huà xìng gǔ suí yán	**sclerosing osteomyelitis**
Bone tuberculosis		
脊柱结核	jǐ zhù jié hé	**tuberculosis of spine**
髋关节结核	kuān guān jié jié hé	**tuberculosis of hip joint**
膝关节结核	xī guān jié jié hé	**tuberculosis of knee joint**
骶髂关节结核	dǐ qià guān jié jié hé	**tuberculosis of sacro-iliac joint**
骨干结核	gǔ gàn jié hé	**diaphysial tuberculosis**
Osteoarthiritis		
类风湿性关节炎	lèi fēng shī xìng guān jié yán	**rheumatoid arthritis**
强直性脊柱炎	jiāng zhí xìng jǐ zhù yán	**ankylosing spondylitis**
髋关节骨性关节炎	kuān guān jié gǔ xìng guān jié yán	**osteoarthritis of hip**
膝关节骨性关节炎	xī guān jié gǔ xìng guān jié yán	**osteoarthritis of knee**
牛皮癣性关节炎	niú pí xuǎn xìng guān jié yán	**psoriatic arthritis**
痛风性关节炎	tòng fēng xìng guān jié yán	**gouty arthritis**
神经性关节炎	shén jīng xìng guān jié yán	**neuropathic arthritis**

Atrophy-flaccidity of bone		
骨质疏松症	gǔ zhì shū sōng zhèng	**osteoporosis**
佝偻病	Gōu lóu bìng	**rickets**
骨软化症	gǔ ruǎn huà zhèng	**osteomalacia**
Sequelae of poliomyelitis		
臀肌瘫痪	Tún jī tān huàn	**paralysis of gluteal muscles**
股四头肌瘫痪	gǔ sì tóu jī tān huàn	**paralysis of quadriceps femoris**
小腿肌瘫痪	xiǎo tuǐ jī tān huàn	**paralysis of crural muscles**
Osteonecrosis		
股骨头缺血性坏死	gǔ gǔ tóu quē xuè xìng huài sǐ	**ischemic necrosis of caput femoris**
胫骨结节骨骺炎	jìng gǔ jié jié gǔ hóu yán	**epiphysitis of tibial tuberosity**
脊椎骨骺骨软骨炎	jǐ zhuī gǔ hóu gǔ ruǎn gǔ yán	**osteochondritis of epiphysis of spine**
距骨缺血性坏死	jù gǔ quē xuè xìng huài sǐ	**ischemic necrosis of talus**
Congenital osteoarticular deformities		
先天性斜颈	xiān tiān xìng xié jǐng	**congenital torticollis**
颈肋	Jǐng lèi	**cervicle rib**
脊柱侧凸症	jǐ zhù cè tū zhèng	**scoliosis**
脊柱裂	jǐ zhù liè	**rachischisis; spina bifida**
先天性高肩胛症	xiān tiān xìng gāo jiān jiǎ zhèng	**congenital elevation of scapula**
先天性桡骨缺如	xiān tiān xìng ráo gǔ quē rú	**congenital absence of radius**
先天性髋关节脱位	xiān tiān xìng kuān guān jié tuō wèi	**congenital hip luxation**
膝内翻	xī nèi fān	**genu varum**
膝外翻	xī wài fān	**genu valgum**
先天性胫骨假关节	xiān tiān xìng jìng gǔ jiǎ guān jié	**congenital tibia pseudoarthrosis**
先天性马蹄内翻足	xiān tiān xìng mǎ tí nèi fān zú	**congenital equinovarus**
Developmental disturbances of bone		

成骨不全	chéng gǔ bù quán	**osteogenesis imperfecta**
软骨发育不全	ruǎn gǔ fā yù bù quán	**achondroplasia**
石骨症	shí gǔ zhèng	**marble bone; osteopetrosis**
Bone tumors		
骨瘤	gǔ liú	**osteoma**
软骨瘤	ruǎn gǔ liú	**chondroma**
骨软骨瘤	gǔ ruǎn gǔ liú	**osteochondroma**
骨样骨瘤	gǔ yàng gǔ liú	**osteoid osteoma**
骨巨细胞瘤	gǔ jù xì bāo liú	**bone giant cell tumor**
骨血管瘤	gǔ xuè guǎn liú	**hemangioma of bone**
骨肉瘤	gǔ ròu liú	**osteosarcoma**
软骨肉瘤	ruǎn gǔ ròu liú	**chondrosarcoma**
纤维肉瘤	xiān wéi ròu liú	**fibrosarcoma**
骨髓瘤	gǔ suí liú	**myeloma**
骨转移瘤	gǔ zhuǎn yí liú	**metastic tumor of bone**
Endemic and professional osteo-articular diseases		
大骨节病	dà gǔ jié bìng	**Kaschin-Beck disease**
氟骨病	fú gǔ bìng	**skeletal fluorosis**
振动病	zhèn dòng bìng	**vibration disease**
Syphilis of bone and joint		
骨梅毒	gǔ méi dú	**syphilis of bone**
关节梅毒	guān jié méi dú	**syphilis of joint**

内翻 [nèi fān]

inversion: the condition of being turned inward (as of the foot)

外翻 [wài fān]

eversion: the condition of being turned outward (as of the foot)

附骨疽 [fū gǔ jū]

"bone-attaching abscess": suppurative osteomyelitis including osteomyelitits and tuberculosis of bone

骨痨 [gǔ láo]

bone phthisis: osteoarticular tuberculosis

医学史 MEDICAL HISTORY

名医 Distinguished Physicians

岐伯 [qí bó]

Qi Bo: famous physician in the reign of Huangdi (2698-2589 B.C.). He was asked by the emperor to taste various kinds of herbs and to study medicine and pharmacy. The first and greatest medical work produced in China — the *Huangdi Nei Jing* (黄帝内经), or *Huangdi's Internal Classic*, or *Canon of Medicine* — mainly consists of questions and answers between Huangdi and Qi Bo on medical issues.

雷公 [léi gōng]

Lei Gong: (1) a famous physician in the reign of Huangdi. Discussions between Huangdi and Lei Gong on medicine and pharmacy, acupuncture and moxibustion are recorded in the *Canon of Medicine*; (2) the style name of 雷敩 [léi xiào], a pharmacist in the period of the Northern and Southern Dynasties who wrote the *Lei Gong Pao Zhi Lun* (雷公炮炙论), or *Lei's Method of Preparing Drugs* (c5th century)

医和 [yī hé]

Yi He: famous physician in the Spring and Autumn Period (c600 B.C.), who put forward the theory that abnormality in the six climatic conditions, namely, cloudy, sunny, windy, rainy, gloomy, and bright, would lead to various illnesses

扁鹊 [biǎn què]

Bian Que: another name of Qin Yueren (秦越人) (c500B.C.), the earliest Chinese physician versed in diagnosis and treatment, especially in pulse taking and acupuncture. To him was ascribed the authorship of such medical works as *Bian Que Nei Jing* (扁鹊内经), or *The Internal Classic of Bian Que,* and *Bian Que Wai Jing* (扁鹊外经), or *The External Classic of Bian Que*, both of which have been lost.

秦越人 [qín yuè rén]

Qin Yueren: the original name of Bian Que (扁鹊 [biǎn què])

淳于意 [chún yú yì]

Chunyu Yi: famous physician (c205-? B.C.) styled Cang Gong (仓公),

the Reverend Master of Granary, for having been put in charge of the public granary of the State of Qi (齐国). He was said to have attached great importance to pulse taking and keeping complete clinical records.

仓公 [cāng gōng]

Cang Gong: style of Chunyu Yi (淳于意)

张机 [zhāng jī]

Zhang Ji: one of the most influential physicians in the history of Chinese medicine (150?-219?), also called Zhang Zhongjing (张仲景). He was the first to advocate the differentiation of syndromes (identification of patterns) in accordance with the six meridians and the eight principal syndromes and the principle of treating diseases according to syndrome differentiation (pattern identification). To him is ascribed the authorship of several medical books on various topics, the most important of which now extant are the *Shang Han Za Bing Lun* (伤寒杂病论), or *Treatise on Cold-induced and Miscellaneous Diseases,* and the *Jin Kui Yao Lue Fang Lun* (金匮要略方论), or *Synopsis of Prescriptions of the Golden Chamber.*

张仲景 [zhāng zhòng jǐng]

Zhang Zhongjing: another name of Zhang Ji (张机)

华佗 [huà tuó]

Hua Tuo: famous surgeon and at the same time master of all branches of medicine, also known as Hua Fu (华旉 or Hua Yuan-hua (华元化) (?-203). He was said to have performed many major operations including abdominal section with herbal anesthesia and to be the first to recommend therapeutic gymnastics called *Wu Qin Xi* (五禽戏), or *the Frolics of Five Animals*. The book *Zhong Zang Jing* (中藏经), or *Treasured Classic* was once ascribed to him but it was in fact compiled by an unknown author during the Six Dynasties.

华旉 [huà fū]

Hua Fu: another name of Huo Tuo (华佗)

王熙 [wáng xī]

Wang Xi: commissioner of the Imperial Academy of Medicine, also called Wang Shuhe (王叔和) (c210-285). He was well versed in pulse-taking, and was the author of the *Mai Jing* (脉经), or *The Pulse Classic*, the easrliest comprehensive book on sphygmology now extant in China. He perfected and systemized the art of pulse-taking, yet emphasized the use of all the other methods of diagnosis as well. He rearranged Zhang Zhongjing's *Treatise on Cold-induced and Miscellaneous Diseases,* and thus contributed much to preserving that important classic of medicine.

王叔和 [wáng shū hé]

Wang Shuhe: another name of Wang Xi (王熙)

皇甫谧 [huáng fǔ mì]

Huangfu Mi: also called Huangfu Shi-an (皇甫士安) (215-282), who suffering from rheumatism, studied medicine and became a famous acupuncturist and compiled the book *Zhen Jiu Jia Yi Jing* (针灸甲乙经), or *The ABC Classic of Acupuncture and Moxibustion*, the first monograph exclusively on the subject, in which the art of acupuncture is explained minutely

皇甫士安 [huáng fǔ shì ān]

Huangfu Shian: another name of Huangfu Mi (皇甫谧)

葛洪 [gě hóng]

Ge Hong: famous physician and world-renowned alchemist (283-343), popularly known as Ge Zhichuan (葛稚川) or Bao Pu Zi (抱朴子), author of the *Bao Pu Zi* (抱朴子), a treatise on alchemy, dietetics and magical practices, and the *Zhou Hou Bei Ji Fang* (肘后备急方), or *A Handbook of Prescriptions for Emergencies*, which includes many valuable descriptions and records of diseases

葛稚川 [gě zhì chuān]

Ge Zhichuan: another name of Ge Hong (葛洪)

抱朴子 [bào pǔ zǐ]

Bao Pu Zi: alias of Ge Hong (葛洪)

龚庆宣 [gōng qìng xuān]

Gong Qingxuan: expert in the Northern and Southern Dynasties (in the late 5th century) who compiled the *Liu Juanzi Gui Yi Fang* (刘涓子鬼遗方), or *Liu Juanzi's Ghost-Bequeathed Prescriptions*, the earliest extant book on external medicine

陶弘景 [táo hóng jǐng]

Tao Hongjing: Taoist who specialized in the study of herbs, also called Tao Tongming (陶通明) (456-536), who compiled the *Ben Cao Jing Ji Zhu* (本草经集注), or *Commentary on Sheng Nong's Herbal*, one of the most valuable books on materia medica in China, describing 730 varieties of medical substances, including vegetable, animal and mineral drugs. Tao was also the author of the *Yang Xing Yan Ming Lu* (养性延命录) *Recordings of the Art of Health and Life Preservation*.

陶通明 [táo tōng míng]

Tao Tongming: another name of Tao Hongjing (陶弘景)

徐之才 [xǘ zhī cái]

Xu Zhicai: a well known physician, also called Xu Shimao (徐士茂) (505-572). He was especially proficient in the preparation of drugs, and wrote the *Yao Dui* (药对), or *Pharmacy and Compatibility* on the basis of (雷公药对) *Lei's Pharmacy and Compatibility*.

徐士茂 [xǘ shì mào]

Xu Shimao: another name of Xu Zhicai (徐之才)

雷敩 [léi xiào]

Lei Xiao: great pharmacist and author of the *Lei Gong Pao Zhi Lun* (雷公炮炙论), or *Lei's Treatise on the Preparation of Drugs* (c500), a standard work dealing with the processing of drugs

甄权 [zhēn quán]

Zhen Quan (c540-643): physician in the Tang Dynasty, who was a leading expert at acupuncture and the author of the *Zhen Fang* (针方) *Needling Prescriptions,* and the *Ming Tang Ren Xing Tu* (明堂人形图), or *Figures of the Human Body*

巢元方 [cháo yuán fāng]

Chao Yuanfang (550-630): imperial physician of Emperor Yangdi (炀帝) of the Sui Dynasty, who took charge of the compilation of the *Zhu Bing Yuan Hou Zong Lun* (诸病源候总论), or *Treatise on Causes and Symptoms of Diseases*, the first Chinese work in this category and still a valuable reference book

杨上善 [yáng shàng shàn]

Yang Shang-shan (585-670): physician at the turn of the Sui and Tang dynasties, imperial physician from 605-616 and one of the earliest physicians who made notes and commentaries on the *Internal Classic* or *Canon of Medicine* and was the author of *Huangdi Nei Jing Tai Su* (黄帝内经太素), or *Fundamentals of Huangdi's Internal Classic*, an important reference book for studying the *Internal Classic*

孙思邈 [sūn sī miǎo]

Sun Simiao (581-682): prominent physician of the Tang Dynasty and the author of the *Qian Jin Yao Fang* (千金要方), or *Invaluable Prescriptions* (652), and the *Qian Jin Yi Fang* (千金翼方), or *Supplement to the Invaluable Prescriptions* (682), which have been considered compilations of the medical achievements before the 7th century

苏敬 [sū jìng]

Su Jing (599-674): court official of the Tang Dynasty, also known as Su Gong (苏恭). He was ordered by the emperor to review traditional herbals with a staff of 22 scholars and physicians. As a result of their work, in 659, the *Xin Xiu Ben Cao* (新修本草), or *Newly Compiled Materia Medica (of Tang)* or *Tang Ben Cao* (唐本草), or *The Tang Materia Medica* was published as the first official pharmacopoeia in China.

苏恭 [sū gōng]

Su Gong: another name of Su Jing (苏敬)

孟诜 [mèng shēn]

Meng Shen (621-713): herbalist of the Tang Dynasty, author of the *Shi Liao Ben Cao* (食疗本草), or *A Dietetic Materia Medica.* The original has been lost, but the text can be found in the *Lei Zheng Ben Cao* (类证本草), or *Classified Materia Medica.*

鉴真 [jiàn zhēn]

Jian Zhen (688-763): outstanding Buddhist monk as well as a physician. He introduced Chinese medicine to Japan.

王焘 [wáng tāo]

Wang Tao (c670-755): distinguished physician of the Tang Dynasty. Trying to cure his sick mother, he made up his mind to go in for medicine. Having worked in the imperial library for twenty years and read a lot of medical books, he compiled a book of his own, titled *Wai Tai Mi Yao* (外台秘要), or *Medical Secrets of an Official* (752), an exhaustive study of every branch of medicine, up to that time.

陈藏器 [chén cáng qì]

Chen Zangqi: famous herbalist of the 8th century, who compiled the *Ben Cao Shi Yi* (本草拾遗), or *A Supplement to the Herbal*

王冰 [wáng bīng]

Wang Bing (c710-805): physician specializing in the art of healing and health preservation, who spent twelve years rearranging and revising the *Su Wen* (素问), or *Plain Questions*, one of the two component parts of

Huangdi's Internal Classic, into 24 volumes, with notes, commentaries and supplements.

昝殷 [zǎn yīn]

Zan Yin (c797-860)**:** specialist in women's diseases and the author of the *Jing Xiao Chan Bao* (经效产宝), or *Tested Treasures of Obstetrics*, written 852-856, and one of the earliest extant books on obstetrics

王维一 [wáng wéi yī]

Wang Weiyi (c987-1067)**:** distinguished acupuncturist of the Northern Song Dynasty who sponsored the casting of two life-sized, hollow bronze figures, on the surface of which were marked the courses of the meridians and the exact location of the acupuncture points. He also took charge of the compilation of a very important book entitled *Tong Ren Shu Xue Zhen Jiu Tu Jing* (铜人俞穴针灸图经), or *Illustrated Manual of Acupoints on Bronze Figures* (published in 1027), which facilitated the locating of acupuncture points and the teaching of acupuncture.

王惟德 [wáng wéi dé]

Wang Weide: another name of Wang Wei-yi (王维一)

苏颂 [sū sòng]

Su Song (1020-1101)**:** official who compiled the *Tu Jing Ben Cao* (图经本草), or *Illustrated Herbal* (1062) in 21 volumes, with the appended pictures collected from different provinces by the order of the emperor. This was the first complete herbal with detailed pictorial illustrations of each medicament.

沈括 [shěn kuò]

Shen Kuo (1030-1095)**:** also called Shen Cunzhong (沈存中). Though more famous as a scientist, Shen was renowned in medical circles for a treatise on therapeutics and medicine titled *Su Shen Liang Fang* (苏沈良方), or *Best Formulas Collected by Su Shi and Shen Kuo*.

沈存中 [shěn cún zhōng]

Shen Cunzhong; another name for Shen Kuo (沈括)

苏轼 [sū shì]

Su Shi: a scholar and physcian, one of the two authors of the *Su Shen Liang Fang* (苏沈良方), or *Best Formulas Collected by Su Shi and Shen Kuo*

钱乙 [qián yǐ]

Qian Yi (c1032-1113)**,** also called Qian Zhongyang (钱仲阳), appointed court physician in 1090, whose experience as a pediatrician for more than 40 years was summed up by his student Yan Xiaozhong (阎孝忠) in the book *Xiao Er Yao Zheng Zhi Jue* (小儿药证直诀), or *Key to Therapeutics of Children's Diseases* (1119) in 3 volumes. One of the earliest pediatric books in ancient China, it had a profound influence upon the development of this subject. Qian was the first to give valuable definitions of measles, scarlatina, fever, chickenpox and smallpox, and point out the peculiar features of pediatrics. He also forward new methods of diagnosis and treatment.

钱仲阳 [qián zhòng yáng]

Qian Zhongyang: another name of Qian Yi (钱乙)

庞安时 [páng ān shí]

Pang Anshi (c1043-1100)**:** physician noted for several medical works, among which the most widely read was a detailed and comprehensive treatise on various kinds of fever under the title of *Shang Han Zong Bing Lun* (伤寒总病论), or *General Discourse on Cold-induced Diseases* (1100)

寇宗奭 [kòu zōng shì]

Kou Zongshi: an expert on materia medica in the Song Dynasty, author of the Ben Cao Yan Yi (本草衍义), or *Amplified Materia Medica* (1116), which lists 460 commonly used medicines with valuable records of identification, pharmacology, and process of preparation

刘昉 [liú fǎng]

Liu Fang (c1080-1150)**:** official of the Southern Song Dynasty, interested in the art of healing, especially pediatrics, and researcher into old prescriptions and remedies. Together with Wang Li (王历), compiled the You You Xin Shu (幼幼新书), or *A New Book of Pediatrics* (1132), one of the earliest monographs of its kind, with substantial content.

唐慎微 [táng shèn wēi]

Tang Shenwei, also called Tang Shenyuan (唐审元), a physician especially proficient in therapeutics, who declined the offer of an official post to devote his life to medical practice and collecting folk recipes. He wrote the *Jing Shi Zheng Lei Bei Ji Ben Cao* (经史证类备急本草), or *Classic Classified Materia Medica for Emergencies* (1108), a work in 31 volumes, and submitted it to the emperor who changed the title to *Da Guan Ben Cao* (大观本草), or *Daguan Herbal*.

唐审元 [tάng shěn yuάn]

Tang Shenyuan: another name of Tang Shen-wei (唐慎微)

成无己 [chéng wú jǐ]

Cheng Wuji (1066-1155?)**:** leading physician of the Jin Dynasty, known for his assiduous study of and commentary on Zhang Zhongjing's classical work *Treatise on Cold-induced and Miscellaneous Diseases.* His *Zhu Jie Shang Han Lun* (注解伤寒论), *Commentary on the Treatise on Cold-induced Diseases* (1142), is considered the earliest of its kind in Chinese medical literature.

许叔微 [xǔ shū wēi]

Xu Shu-wei (1079-1154?)**:** leading physician of the Song Dynasty and a disciple of Zhang Zhongjing. He prepared graphic illustrations of 36 varieties of the pulse based on Zhang Zhongjing's work, and propounded the theory of using drugs in relation to the intensity of the disease. Xu was the author of several medical works, among which the *Lei Zheng Pu Ji Ben Shi Fang* (类证普济本事方), or *Classified Effective Prescriptions for Universal Relief* (1132?) in 10 volumes has been one of his most widely read.

陈言 [chén yάn]

Chen Yan: leading physician of the Song Dynasty, also called Chen Wuze (陈无择), author of the *San Yin Ji Yi Bing Zheng Fang Lun* (三因极一病证方论), or *Treatise on the Three Categories of Pathogenic Factors and Prescriptions*, a work in 18 volumes published in 1174, in which causes of diseases are grouped under three headings in accordance with Zhang Zhongjing's theory

陈无择 [chén wú zé]

Chen Wuze: another name of Chen Yan (陈言)

王执中 [wάng zhí zhōng]

Wang Zhizhong: physician of the Song Dynasty skilled in acupuncture and moxibustion, author of the *Zhen Jiu Zhi Sheng Jiug* (针灸资生经), or *Classic of Nourishing Life with Acupuncture and Moxibustion* (1220)

齐仲甫 [qí zhòng fǔ]

Qi Zhongfu: physician of the Song Dynasty with rich experience in treating women's diseases, author of the very popular medical work *Nü Ke Bai Wen* (女科百问), or *Hundred Questions on Women's Diseases* (1220 A.D.)

张元素 [zhāng yuán sù]

Zhang Yuansu: physician of the 12th century, also called Zhang Jiegu (张洁古). He made the bold announcement that in view of the different conditions between ancient and modern times it was impossible to treat new diseases with old methods, discarded obsolete traditional formulas and devised a system of his own. Most of the doctors of the Jin-Yuan period (1115-1368) were influenced by his teachings. He was the author of the *Zhen Zhu Nang* (珍珠囊), or *The Pearl Bag* and other medical works. Among his disciples were such eminent doctors as Li Gao (李杲) and Wang Hao-gu (王好古).

张洁古 [zhāng jié gǔ]

Zhang Jiegu: another name of Zhang Yuansu (张元素)

刘完素 [liú wán sù]

Liu Wansu: also called Liu Shouzhen (刘守真) (c1120-1200). He propounded the theory that diseases were caused by excessive heat in the body, and advocated the use of medicines of cold nature, thus starting the Cold School of Medicine. He was the author of the *Su Wen Xuan Ji Yuan Bing* (素问玄机原病), or *Etiology Based on Plain Questions* and other medical works, and had much influence on the School of Epidemic Febrile Diseases in the Ming and Qing Dynasties.

刘守真 [liú shǒu zhēn]

Liu Shouzhen: another name of Liu Wansu (刘完素)

张从正 [zhāng cóng zhèng]

Zhang Congzheng: also called Zhang Zihe (张子和) (c1156-1228). Once a court physician, with rich experience in various branches of medicine, he compared a disease to a foreign substance in the organism which should be attacked and driven out by drastic drugs, such as diaphoretics, emetics and purgatives and thus started the Attack or Purgation School. He was the author of the *Ru Men Shi Qin* (儒门事亲), or *The Scholars' Care of Their Parents*, which was completed by his disciple Ma Zhiji (麻知己).

张子和 [zhāng zǐ hé]

Zhang Zihe: another name of Zhang Congzheng (张从正)

李杲 [lǐ gǎo]

Li Gao: also called Li Mingzhi (李明之) or Li Dongyuan (李东垣) (1180-1251), a disciple of Zhang Yuansu, who held that diseases, apart from external changes, were mainly caused by internal injury to the spleen and stomach (i.e., by intemperance in drinking and eating or overwork) and advocated cure by regulating the spleen and the stomach and nourishing the original *qi*. He was considered to be the founder of the School for Strengthening the Spleen and Stomach. His masterpiece was the *Pi Wei Lun* (脾胃论), or *Treatise on the Spleen and Stomach.*

李东垣 [lǐ dōng yuán]

Li Dongyuan: another name of Li Gao (李杲)

李明之 [lǐ míng zhī]

Li Mingzhi: another name of Li Gao (李杲)

宋慈 [sòng cí]

Song Ci: also called Song Huifu (宋惠父) (1186-1249 A.D.), author of the *Xi Yuan Ji Lu* (洗冤集录), or *Instructions to Coroners*, a treatise on forensic medicine written on the basis of his personal experience as a judge and his profound knowledge of previous works on the subject, which exerted a great influence on Chinese jurisprudence.

宋惠父 [sòng huì fù]

Son Huifu: another name of Song Ci (宋慈)

陈自明 [chén zì míng]

Chen Ziming: also called Chen Liangfu (陈良甫) (c1190-1270), a distinguished gynecologist from a family of medical practitioners for many generations and the author of two important books – *Fu Ren Da Quan Liang Fang* (妇人大全良方), or *The Complete Book of Effective Prescriptions for Women* and *Wai Ke Jing Yao* (外科精要), or *Essence of External Medicine*

陈良甫 [chén liáng fǔ]

Chen Liangfu: another name of Chen Ziming (陈自明)

陈文中 [chén wén zhōng]

Chen Wenzhong, noted pediatrist in the 13th century, and author of the *Chen Shi Xiao Er Dou Zhen Fang* (陈氏小儿痘疹方), or *Chen's Prescriptions for Smallpox and Measles in Children* (1241), and *Xiao Er Bing Yuan Fang Lun* (小儿病源方论), or *Treatise on Etiology of Children's Diseases* (1253)

严用和 [yán yòng hé]

Yan Yonghe: physician (c1206-1268), author of the *Yan's Ji Sheng Fang* (严氏济生方), or *Yan's Prescriptions for Succouring the Sick* or *Ji Sheng*

Fang (济生方) *Prescriptions for Succouring the Sick* for short.

危亦林 [wēi yì lín]

Wei Yilin: also called Wei Dazhai (危达斋) (1277-1347), famous for bone-setting. Based on the his own experience and the findings of his ancestors, he compiled a large number of prescriptions in the book titled *Shi Yi De Xiao Fang* (世医得效方), or *Effective Formulas Tested by Physicians for Generations*.

危达斋 [wēi dá zhāi]

Wei Dazhai: another name of Wei Yilin (危亦林)

齐德之 [qí dé zhī]

Qi Dezhi: court academician and surgeon of the Imperial Academy in the Yuan Dynasty, who emphasized taking the organism as a whole while treating carbuncles and sores and was the author of *Wai Ke Jing Yi* (外科精义), or *Essentials of External Medicine*

罗天益 [luó tiān yì]

Luo Tianyi: also called Luo Qianfu (罗谦甫), a physician in the Yuan Dynasty (1279-1368 A.D.) who studied medicine under Li Gao (李杲) for more than ten years and was once an imperial doctor. On the basis of Li Gao's theories, as well as those of other schools and his own experience, he wrote the *Wei Sheng Bao Jian* (卫生宝鉴), or *Precious Mirror of Hygiene*.

罗谦甫 [luó qiān fǔ]

Luo Qianfu: another name of Luo Tianyi (罗天益)

王好古 [wáng hào gǔ]

Wang Haogu: distinguished physician in the 13th century, also called Wan Jinzhi (王进之), or Wang Hai-zang (王海藏), whose chief contribution was the explanation of yin syndromes and the use of warming tonics in the later stage of cold-induced diseases. Five of his publications are exstant, including the *Tang Ye Ben Cao* (汤液本草), or *Materia Medica of Decoction* (1289).

王进之 [wáng jìn zhī]

Wang Jinzhi: another name of Wang Haogu (王好古)

王海藏 [wáng hǎi zàng]

Wang Haizang: another name of Wang Haogu (王好古)

曾世荣 [zēng shì róng]

Zeng Shirong: specialist in children's diseases with over fifty years of experience, author of the *Huo You Kou Yi* (活幼口议), or *Discussions on Saving the Lives of Infants and Children* (1283) and the *Huo You Xin Shu* (活幼新书), or *A New Book for Saving the Life of Infants and Children* (1294). His special contribution to pediatrics lay in his skill in grouping the different natures and forms of what was in fact a single disease, thus aiding diagnosis.

朱震亨 [zhū zhèn hēng]

Zhu Zhenheng: also called Zhu Danxi (1282-1358), he took indulgence as the root of all troubles and stressed the value of tonics for the purpose of making up the deficit yin. He advocated the theory that yang was always in excess while yin was often deficient, and thus belonged to the Yin-Nourishing School. He was the author of the *Ge Zhi Yu Lun* (格致余论), or *Supplementary Treatise on Knowledge from Practice*, and the *Ju Fang Fa Hui* (局方发挥), or *Expounding on the Formularies of the Bureau of Pharmacy*.

朱丹溪 [zhū dān xī]

Zhu Danxi: another name of Zhu Zhenheng (朱震亨)

忽思慧 [hū sī huì]

Hu Si-hui: a great dietitian of Mongolian nationality in the 14th century. He was the imperial chef of the Yuan Dynasty for more than ten years before he compiled the *Yin Shan Zheng Yao* (饮膳正要), or *Principles of Correct Diet*.

滑寿 [huá shòu]

Hua Shou: also called Hua Boren (滑伯仁) (1304-1386), author of a very useful treatise on acupuncture, the *Shi Si Jing Fa Hui* (十四经发挥), or *Elaboration of the Fourteen Meridians*. Hua was good at differential diagnosis and particularly skilful in acupuncture. His study of the meridians and points contributed much to the development of this branch of medicine.

滑伯仁 [huá bó rén]

Hua Boren: another name of Hua Shou (滑寿)

葛乾孙 [gě qián sūn]

Ge Qiansun: also called Ge Ke-jiu (葛可久) (1305-1353), a noted physician who treated diseases effectively with herbal medicines, needling and massage. He was the author of the *Shi Yao Shen Shu* (十药神书), or *Miraculous Book of Ten Recipes*, a record of diagnosis and treatment of pulmonary tuberculosis.

葛可久 [gě kě jiǔ]

Ge Kejiu: another name of Ge Qiansun (葛乾孙)

倪维德 [ní wéi dé]

Ni Weide: also called Ni Zhongxian (倪仲贤) (1307-1377), an eye specialist and author of a valuable book on the causes and mechanism of eye diseases, called the *Yuan Ji Qi Wei* (元机启微), or *Revealing the Mystery of the Origin*

倪仲贤 [ní zhòng xián]

Ni Zhongxian: another name of Ni Weide (倪维德)

楼英 [lóu yīng]

Lou Ying: also called Lou Gongshuang (楼公爽) or Lou Quan-shan (楼全善) (1332-1402), author of the *Yi Xue Gang Mu* (医学纲目), or *Compendium of Medicine*, in which diseases were classified into various types and categories according to yin-yang and viscera. This system of classification was very helpful in diagnosis and treatment.

楼公爽 [lóu gōng shuǎng]

Lou Gongshuang: another name of Lou Ying (楼英)

戴思恭 [dài sī gōng]

Dai Sigong: also called Dai Yuanli (1324-1405), a court physician of the Ming Dynasty and president of the Imperial College of Physicians, author of the *Zheng Zhi Yao Jue* (证治要诀), or *Principles of Diagnosis and Treatment*, and *Zheng Zhi Yao Jue Lei Fang* (证治要诀类方), or *Classified Prescriptions According to the Principles of Diagnosis and Treatment*. He well expounded his master Zhu Zhenheng's theory of nourishing yin.

戴原礼 [dài yuán lǐ]

Dai Yuanli: another name of Dai Sigong (戴思恭)

熊宗立 [xióng zōng lì]

Xiong Zongli: physician of the Ming Dynasty, author of the *Ming Fang Lei Zheng Yi Shu Da Quan* (名方类证医书大全), or *Complete Medical Work of Proved Recipes*, also called *Yi Shu Da Quan* (医书大全), or *Complete Work of Medical Books* (1446)

寇平 [kòu píng]

Kou Ping: an outstanding pediatrician of the 15th century, the author of the *Quan You Xin Jian* (全幼心鉴), or *Directions in Pediatrics* (1451), in which indigestion or unsuitable food is held to be mainly responsible for children's illnesses

虞抟 [yú tuán]

Yu Tuan: also called Yu Tianmin (虞天民) (1438-1517), adapted over thirty precious medical works and edited his own *Yi Xue Zheng Zhuan* (医学正传), or *Orthodox Medical Record*

虞天民 [yú tiān mín]

Yu Tianmin: another name of Yu Tuan (虞抟)

韩懋 [hán mào]

Han Mao: physician of the Ming Dynasty, author of the *Han Shi Yi Tong* (韩氏医通), or *Han's Book of Medicine* (1522), in which the importance of diagnosis in the treatment of disease is stressed and improvements in case recording with more comprehensive regulations are shown

薛铠 [xuē kǎi]

Xue Kai: also called Xue Liangwu (薛良武), a distinguished imperial physician, especially well known in pediatrics, author of the *Bao Ying Cuo Yao* (保婴撮要), or *Essentials for the Care of Infants* (1556), in which he stresses the importance of giving the right dosage of drugs according to age and recommends the severing of the umbilical cord by cautery

薛良武 [xuē liáng wǔ]

Xue Liangwu: another name of Xue Kai (薛铠)

王纶 [wáng lún]

Wang Lun: physician who wrote the *Ming Yi Za Zhu* (明医杂著) *Collection of Physicians' Experiences in the Ming Dynasty* (1549)

汪机 [wāng jī]

Wang Ji: also called Wang Xingzhi (汪省之) (1463-1539), author of several medical books, such as the *Zhen Jiu Wen Da* (针灸问答), or *Catechism on Acupuncture and Moxibustion*, which is clear, simple and keeps to essentials, and is very useful for beginners, the *Wai Ke Li Li* (外科理例), or *External Medicine with Illustrations*, and *Yi Xue Yuan Li* (医学原理), or *Principles of Medicine* etc.

汪省之 [wāng xǐng zhī]

Wang Xingzhi: another name of Wang Ji (汪机)

薛己 [xuē jǐ]

Xue Ji: also called Xue Xinfu (薛新甫) (c1487-1559), son of Xue Kai

(薛铠). As a famous physician versed in various aspects of medicine, he compiled many medical works, such as *Nü Ke Cuo Yao* (女科撮要), or *Essentials of Obstetrics and Gynecology* and *Wai Ke Shu Yao* (外科枢要), or *Essentials of External Medicine*. His and his father's works were edited by Wu Guan (吴琯) and titled *Xue Shi Yi An* (薛氏医案), or the *Xues' Medical Records.*

薛新甫 [xuē xīn fǔ]

Xue Xinfu: another name of Xue Ji (薛己)

卢和 [lú hé]

Lu He: distinguished herbalist of the 16th century, author of the *Shi Wu Ben Cao* (食物本草), or *Dietary Materia Medica*, in which he gives explanations on the laxative value of vegetables and their good effect on health. He advocates a vegetable diet, advising that meat should be eaten sparingly.

沈之问 [shěn zhī wèn]

Shen Zhiwen: expert in the diagnosis and treatment of leprosy in the 16th century, compiler of the *Jie Wei Yuan Sou* (解围元薮), or *Source of Relief* (1550), a monograph on leprosy.

孙一奎 [sūn yī kuí]

Sun Yikui: also called Sun Wenyuan (孙文垣) or Sun Dong-su (孙东宿) (1520-1600), author of the Chi Shui Xuan Zhu (赤水玄珠), or *Black Pearl of the Red River*, *Yi Zhi Xu Yu* (医旨绪余), or *Supplement to the Principles of Medicine* and *Yi An* (医案), *Medical Records*, collected by his sons, in which he advocates the combination of various schools and maintains that a doctor should be conversant with all the theories in order to master the whole art of healing

孙文垣 [sūn wén yuán]

Sun Wenyuan: another name of Sun Yikui (孙一奎)

孙东宿 [sūn dōng sù]

Sun Dongsu: another name of Sun Yikui (孙一奎)

徐春甫 [xú chūn fǔ]

Xu Chunfu: also called Xu Ru-yuan (徐汝元), the author of the *Gu Jin Yi Tong Da Quan* (古今医统大全), or *A Complete Work of Ancient and Modern Medicine* (1556), in which rich and valuable materials in various fields of medicine are accumulated. Xu warns that healthy people should avoid patients with consumptive diseases, particularly pulmonary tuberculosis.

徐汝元 [xú rǔ yuán]

Xu Ruyuan: another name of Xu Chunfu (徐春甫)

李梴 [lǐ yán]

Li Yan: also called Li Jianzhai (李健斋), a physician of the 16th century who summarized the prescriptions used at that period and divided them into 18 different kinds. Li was the author of the *Yi Xue Ru Men* (医学入门), or *Introduction to Medicine* and the *Xi Yi Gui Ge* (习医规格), or *Rules for Medical Study.*

李濂 [lǐ lián]

Li Lian: literary man of the Ming Dynasty, who had been an official in Shanxi Province and was famous for his command of ancient Chinese language and literature. He wrote the *Yi Shi* (医史), or *History of Medicine* (1513), which records the lives of distinguished physicians. Li was the earliest biographer of ancient medical professionals.

万全 [wàn quán]

Wan Quan: also called Wan Mi-zhai (万密斋) (c1495-1585), a distinguished pediatrist from a family of physicians for three generations, who inherited their rich clinical experience, especially in pediatrics. He advocates that a child should be frequently exposed to sunlight and fresh air, trained to resist cold and protected from being frightened, and should not be overfed or given too much drug treatment. He was the author of the *Dou Zhen Shi Yi Xin Fa* (痘疹世医新法), or *Experience in the Treatment of Smallpox and Rashes Handed Down through Generations*, the *You Ke Fa Hui* (幼科发挥), or *Expounding on Pediatrics* and the *Yu Ying Jia Mi* (育婴家秘), or *Family Secrets in Child Care*.

万密斋 [wàn mì zhāi]

Wan Mizhai: another name of Wan Quan (万全)

李时珍 [lǐ shí zhēn]

Li Shizhen: also called Li Dongbi (李东壁) or Li Bin-hu (李濒湖) (1518-1593), a great physician and naturalist. His father Li Yan-wen (李言闻) was an accomplished medical practitioner. Carrying on his father's profession, Li concentrated on medical studies, and his medical skill gained wide recognition among his contemporaries. He wrote a dozen medical works, among which the *Ben Cao Gang Mu* (本草纲目), or *Compendium of Materia Medica* is the greatest. His other works include the *Bin Hu Mai Xue* (濒湖脉学), or *Binhu's Sphygmology* and *Qi Jing Ba Mai Kao* (奇经八脉考), or *A Study of the Eight Extra Meridians*.

李濒湖 [lǐ bīn hú]

Li Binhu: another name of Li Shizhen (李时珍)

李东壁 [lǐ dōng bì]

Li Dongbi: another name of Li Shi-zhen (李时珍)

马莳 [mǎ shì]

Ma Shi: physician of the Ming Dynasty, author of the *Huangdi Nei Jing Su Wen Zhu Zheng Fa Wei* (黄帝内经素问注证发微), or *An Elaboration on the Spiritual Pivot of Huangdi's Internal Classic* and the *Huangdi Nei Jing Ling Shu Zhu Zheng Fa Wei* (黄帝内经灵枢注证发微), or *An Elaboration on Spiritual Pivot of Huangdi's Internal Classic* (1589)

张三锡 [zhāng sān xī]

Zhang Sanxi, physician of the Ming Dynasty, who emphasized the six aspects of medical work, i.e. meridians, diagnostic methods, pathogenesis, principles and methods of treatment, materia medica, and *qi* circulation. He wrote the *Yi Xue Liu Yao* (医学六要), or *Six Essentials of Medicine* (1609), which exerted a great influence on medical professionals of later generations.

杨继洲 [yáng jì zhōu]

Yang Jizhou: also called Yang Jishi（杨济时）(1522-1620). His grandfather had been an imperial physician. He succeeded his grandfather as a physician, being paticularly skilful in acupuncture. He compiled a very comprehensive and practical book, called the *Zhen Jiu Da Cheng* (针灸大成), or *Great Compendium of Acupuncture and Moxibustion* (1601), a work serving as a link between the past and the future.

杨济时 [yáng jì shí]

Yang Jishi: another name of Yang Jizhou (杨继洲)

王肯堂 [wáng kěn táng]

Wang Kentang: also called Wang Yutai (王宇泰) or Wang Sun-an (王损庵) (1549-1639). Having served as a court official for some years, Wang returned to his native place and devoted most of his time to studying medicine until he became a famous physician. He was the author of the *Liu Ke Zheng Zhi Zhun Sheng*（六科证治准绳）, or *Standards of Diagnosis and Treatment in Six Branches of Medicine*, which had the largest circulation of all medical books in the 17th century in China.

王宇泰 [wáng yǔ tài]

Wang Yutai: another name of Wang Kentang (王肯堂)

王损庵 [wáng sǔn ān]

Wang Sun'an: another name of Wang Kentang (王肯堂)

李中立 [lǐ zhōng lì]

Li Zhongli: also called Li Zhengyu (李正宇), author of the *Ben Cao Yuan Shi* (本草原始), or *Origin of Materia Medica* (1612), a practical book for pharmacists. Li did the illustrations of the medical substances himself, with their properties and methods of preparation described in detail. His book may be considered as one of the earliest works in the field of pharmacognosy.

李正宇 [lǐ zhèng yǔ]

Li Zhengyu: another name of Li Zhongli (李中立)

高武 [gāo wǔ]

Gao Wu: also called Gao Mei-gu (高梅孤), a famous acupuncturist of the Ming Dynasty who compiled the *Zhen Jiu Jie Yao* (针灸节要), or *Extracts of the Principles of Acupuncture and Moxibustion*, and the *Zhen Jiu Ju Ying* (针灸聚英), or *A Collection of Gems of Acupuncture and Moxibustion*. To help locate the acupoints, he made three bronze figures as models – a man, a woman and a child.

高梅孤 [gāo méi gū]

Gao Meigu: another name of Gao Wu (高武)

赵献可 [zhào xiàn kě]

Zhao Xianke: also called Zhao Yangkui (赵养葵), a physician of the Ming Dynasty and the author of the *Yi Guan* (医贯), or *Key Link of Medicine.* He developed the "life gate" theory, attaching special importance to the function of this organ, and stressed the significance of reinforcing the fire of the "life gate".

赵养葵 [zhào yǎng kúi]

Zhao Yangkui: another name of Zhao Xianke (赵献可)

陈实功 [chén shí gōng]

Chen Shigong: also called Chen Yuren (陈毓仁) (1555-1636), a distinguished doctor of internal medicine, with 40 years practical experience summarized in his book *Wai Ke Zheng Zong* (外科正宗), or *Orthodox Manual of External Medicine*

陈毓仁 [chén yù rén]

Chen Yuren: another name of Chen Shigong (陈实功)

缪希雍 [miào xī yōng]

Miao Xiyong: also called Miao Zhongchun (缪仲淳) (1556-1627?), a physician of the Ming Dynasty, who often treated the poor free of charge. As an expert on materia medica, Miao was the author of the *Sheng Nong Ben Cao Jing Shu* (神农本草经疏), or *Annotation on Sheng Nong's Herba* and the *Xian Xing Zhai Yi Xue Guang Bi Ji* (先醒斋医学广笔记), or *Miao's Extensive Notes on Medicine*, which impresses the readers with his rich knowledge and clinical experience in internal medicine, external medicine, gynecology and pediatrics.

缪仲淳 [miào zhòng chún]

Miao Zhongchun: another name of Miao Xiyong (缪希雍)

龚廷贤 [gōng tíng xián]

Gong Tingxian: also called Gong Yunlin (龚云林 [gōng yún lín]) a physician of the Ming Dynasty in the 16th century, author of *Wan Bing Hui Chun* (万病回春), or *Restoration from All Illnesses,* and *Shou Shi Bao Yuan* (寿世保元), or *Longevity and Life Preservation*. Gong was also a famous massotherapist and the author of the *Xiao Er Tui Na Mi Zhi* (小儿推拿秘旨), or *Secret Principles of Massotherapy for Children*.

龚云林 [gōng yún lín]

Gong Yunlin: another name of Gong Tingxian (龚廷贤)

张介宾 [zhāng jiè bīn]

Zhang Jiebin: also called Zhang Jingyue (张景岳) (c1563-1640), author of several books on subjects such as sphygmology, gynecology, pediatrics and external medicine. Being especially versed in the *Internal Classic*, Zhang was the author of the Lei Jing (类经), or *Systematic Compilation of the Internal Classic*. His complete works, known as the *Jing Yue Quan Shu* (景岳全书), or *Jing Yue's Complete Works,* appeared in 1624.

张景岳 [zhāng jǐng yuè]

Zhang Jingyue: another name of Zhang Jiebin (张介宾)

吴有性 [wú yǒu xìng]

Wu Youxing: also called Wu Youke (吴又可) (1582-1652), a pioneer epidemiologist, author of the *Wen Yi Lun* (温疫论), or *Treatise on Pestilence* (1642), a book devoted to the special study of several kinds of epidemic diseases then prevalent in many parts of China. Wu put forward the theory of pestilential factors, and made a great contribution to the development of knowledge about epidemic infectious diseases.

吴又可 [wú yòu kě]

Wu Youke: another name of Wu Youxing (吴有性)

喻昌 [yù chāng]

Yu Chang: also called Yu Jiayan (喻嘉言) (c1585-1664), a well-known skilful medical practitioner and the author of the *Shang Lun Zhang Zhong Jing Shang Han Lun* (尚论张仲景伤寒论), *A Critical study of Zhang Zhongjing's Treatise on Cold-induced Diseases* (simply *Shang Lun Pian* (尚论篇), or *Critical Study*) and the *Yi Men Fa Lü* (医门法律), or *Principles and Prohibitions of Medical Profession*, in which Yu made a new categorization of cold-induced diseases and expounded his original ideas on some subjects, such as autumn dryness

喻嘉言 [yù jiā yán]

Yu Jia-yan: another name of Yu Chang (喻昌)

武之望 [wǔ zhī wàng]

Wu Zhiwang: also called Wu Shuqing (武叔卿) (?-1629 A.D.), a physician who compiled the *Ji Yin Gang Mu* (济阴纲目), or *Compendium of Therapies for Women's Diseases* (1620), which was circulated far and wide. He also wrote the *Ji Yang Gang Mu* (济阳纲目), or *Compendium of Therapies for Men's Diseases.*

武叔卿 [wǔ shū qīng]

Wu Shuqing: another name of Wu Zhiwang (武之望)

陈司成 [chén sī chéng]

Chen Sicheng: also called Chen Jiushao (陈九韶), a physician of the Ming Dynasty, specialized in treating syphilis, who wrote the Mei Chuang Mi Lu (霉疮秘录), or *Secret Records of Syphilis* (1632), which not only summed up the experiences of his physician ancestors but also provided new records of diagnosis and treatment of the disease as the first monograph on syphilology in China.

陈九韶 [chén jiǔ sháo]

Chen Jiushao: another name of Chen Sicheng (陈司成)

李中梓 [lǐ zhōng zǐ]

Li Zhongzi: also called Li Shicai (李士材) (1588-1655), a physician who wrote and compiled many books, such as the *Nei Jing Zhi Yao* (内经知要), or *Essentials of Internal Classic*, the *Yi Zong Bi Du* (医宗必读), or *Essential Readings in Medicine* on the basis of *Internal Classic* and the

Treatise on Cold-induced Diseases, with reference to works written by other distinguished physicians and without neglecting his own experience in clinical practice

李士材 [lǐ shì cái]

Li Shicai: another name of Li Zhongzi (李中梓)

傅仁宇 [fù rén yǔ]

Fu Renyu, also called Fu Yunke (傅允科), a famous oculist in the Ming Dynasty and author of the *Shen Shi Yao Han* (审视瑶函), or *A Precious Work of Ophthamology*, also known as the *Yan Ke Da Quan* (眼科大全), or *A Complete Book of Ophthalmology* (1644), which contains detailed descriptions of the symptoms, diagnosis and treatment of eye diseases.

傅允科 [fù yǔn kē]

Fu Yunke: another name of Fu Renyu (傅仁宇)

傅山 [fù shān]

Fu Shan: also called Fu Qingzhu (傅青主) (1607-1684), was a well-known poet, painter, calligrapher and distinguished physician. After the fall of the Ming Dynasty, he resigned his post to fight against the new Qing regime. In the field of medicine, he left such books as the *Bian Zheng Lu* (辨证录), *Notes on Diagnosis*, the *Shi Shi Mi Lu* (石室秘录), or *Secret Records in Stone House*, the *Dong Tian Ao Zhi* (洞天奥旨), or *Mysterious Teachings in Cave*. Since the author was persecuted by the government, his real name was not made known. The above-mentioned books were rearranged and republished by Chen Shiduo (陈士铎) under the name of Xian Shou (仙授), or God's Teaching. Certain parts of the book were extracted and published again in the middle of the 19th century, titled *Fu Qing Zhu Nü Ke* (傅青主女科), *Fu Qingzhu's Works on Women's Diseases* or *Fu Qing-zhu's Obstetrics and Gynecology* and *Fu Qing Zhu Nan Ke* (傅青主男科), *Fu Qing-zhu's Works on Men's Diseases*.

傅青主 [fù qīng zhǔ]

Fu Qingzhu: another name of Fu Shan (傅山)

汪昂 [wāng ɑ́ng]

Wang Ang: also called Wang Renan (汪讱安) (1615-?), a physician of the Qing Dynasty who wrote a number of medical books such as the *Yi Fang Ji Jie* (医方集解), or *Collection of Prescriptions with Exposition*, *Tang Tou Ge Jue* (汤头歌诀), or *Prescriptions in Rhymes*. Wang held a correct and broad-minded attitude toward the introduction of Western medicine to China at the end of Ming Dynasty, and wrote that it was the brain, not the heart that was the seat of mental activities.

汪讱安 [wāng rèn ān]

Wang Renan: another name of Wang Ang (汪昂)

张璐 [zhāng lù]

Zhang Lu: also called Zhang Luyu (张路玉) or Zhang Shiwan (张石顽) (1617-1699), author of many medical works. His most famous work, the *Yi Tong* (医通), or *Treatise on General Medicine* (1695), in 16 volumes, took him fifty years to complete. In it, various methods of vaccination or variolation and the spread of this practice in China at that time were given in detail. Zhang emphasized the good points of the Warm Tonic School and was one of its chief protagonists.

张路玉 [zhāng yù lù]

Zhang Luyu: another name of Zhang Lu (张璐)

张石顽 [zhāng shí yán]

Zhang Shiwan: another name of Zhang Lu (张璐)

张志聪 [zhāng zhì cōng]

Zhang Zhicong: physician of the Qing Dynasty, author of the *Huang Di Nei Jing Su Wen Ji Zhu* (黄帝内经素问集注), or *Variorum of the Plain Questions of the Internal Classic* (1670)

李惺庵 [lǐ xīng ān]

Li Xing'an, also called Li Yongcui (李用粹) or Li Xiuzhi (李修之), a physician of the Qing Dynasty, who compiled the *Zheng Zhi Hui Bu* (证治汇补), or *Supplement to Diagnosis and Treatment*, a book of limpid style and practical value

李用粹 [lǐ yòng cuì]

Li Yongcui: another name of Li Xing'an (李惺庵)

李修之 [lǐ xiū zhī]

Li Xiuzhi: another name of Li Xing'an (李惺庵)

萧赓六 [xiāo gēng liù]

Xiao Gengliu: physician of the Qing Dynasty, author of the *Nü Ke Jing Lun* (女科经纶), or *Principles of Gynecology and Obstetrics* (1684)

柯琴 [kē qín]

Ke Qin: also called Ke Yunbo (柯韵伯) (1662-1735), a physician at the beginning of the Qing Dynasty, who wrote the Shang Han Lun Zhu (伤寒

论注), or *Annotations of the Treatise on Cold-induced Diseases*, the *Shang Han Lun Yi* (伤寒论翼), or *Supplementary Treatise on Cold-induced Diseases*, and the *Shang Han Fu Yi* (伤寒附翼), or *Additions to the Treatise on Cold-induced Diseases*. The three books combined were called *Shang Han Lai Su Ji* (伤寒来苏集), or *Renewal of the Treatise on Cold-induced Diseases*.

柯韵伯 [kē yùn bó]

Ke Yunbo: another name of Ke Qin (柯琴)

魏之琇 [wèi zhī xiù]

Wei Zhixiu: also called Wei Liuzhou (魏柳洲) (1722-1772), a physician of the Qing Dynasty, compiler of the *Xu Ming Yi Lei An* (续名医类案), or *Supplement to the Classified Medical Records of Distinguished Physicians,* with medical records of many distinguished physicians of the early Qing Dynasty. He was also the author of the *Liu Zhou Yi Hua* (柳州医话), *Liu-zhou's Medical Essays*, published in the middle of the 19th century.

魏柳洲 [wèi liù zhōu]

Wei Liuzhou: alias of Wei Zhixiu (魏之琇)

叶桂 [yè guì]

Ye Gui: also called Ye Tianshi (叶天士) or Ye Xiang-yan (叶香岩) (1667-1746), a physician renowned for his remarkable methods of diagnosis and treatment, and a recognized leader of the School of Epidemic Febrile Diseases, advocating the scheme of four-level syndrome or pattern (defense, *qi*, nutrient, and blood) differentiation. Ye also introduced the use of aromatic stimulants in the treatment of epidemic fevers, with great success. His lectures and teachings were edited by his disciples in a book titled *Wen Re Lun* (温热论), or *On Epidemic Febrile Diseases* (1746).

叶天士 [yè tiān shì]

Ye Tianshi: another name of Ye Gui (叶桂)

叶香岩 [yè xiāng yán]

Ye Xiangyan: alias of Ye Gui (叶桂)

尤怡 [yóu yí]

You Yi: also called You Zaijing (尤在泾) (?-1749 A.D.), a physician of the Qing Dynasty, who made detailed studies of the *Treatise on Cold-induced Diseases* and *Synopsis of Prescriptions of the Golden*

Chamber, and wrote the *Shang Han Guan Zhu Ji* (伤寒贯珠集), or *A String of Beads from the Treatise on Cold-induced Diseases*, the *Jin Kui Yi* (金匮翼), or *Supplements to the Commentaries on the Synopsis of the Golden Chamber*, etc. The medical records of his patients were arranged in order by his descendants in book form, titled *Jing Xiang Lou Yi An* (静香楼医案), or *Medical Case Records by the Master of the Quiet Fragrant Chamber*.

尤在泾 [yóu zài jīng]

You Zaijing: another name of You Yi (尤怡)

陈复正 [chén fù zhèng]

Chen Fuzheng: also called Chen Feixia (陈飞霞) (c1736-1795), a physician of the Qing Dynasty, who studied Taoism and the art of medicine, and excelled as a pediatrist, being particularly good at treating contagious eruptive fevers and infantile convulsions. He was the author of the *You You Ji Cheng* (幼幼集成), or *Collection of Works on Pediatrics*, with a comprehensive description of children's diseases and a collection of simple and useful prescriptions.

陈飞霞 [chén fēi xiá]

Chen Feixia: another name of Chen Fuzheng (陈复正)

薛雪 [xuē xuě]

Xue Xue: also called Xue Shengbai (薛生白) (1681-1770), who was as famous a physician as his contemporary Ye Tianshi (叶天士) and specially skilful in treating epidemic febrile diseases. He was the author of the *Shi Re Tiao Bian* (湿热条辨), or *Detailed Analysis of Damp-Heat*, which made contributions to the study of epidemic febrile diseases.

薛生白 [xuē shēng bái]

Xue Shengbai: another name of Xue Xue (薛雪)

徐大椿 [xú dà chūn]

Xu Dachun: also called Xu Lingtai (徐灵胎) or Xu Da-ye (徐大业) (1693-1771), the author of numerous books, such as the Nan Jing Jing Shi (难经经释), or *Explanation of Difficult Classics*, the *Yi Guan Bian* (医贯砭), or *A Critique on Key Link of Medicine* and *Yi Xue Yuan Liu Lun* (医学源流论), or *On the Origin and Source of Medicine*. He did not cling to conventional methods, and opposed the abuse of drastic drugs hot in nature and pungent in flavour as tonics.

徐灵胎 [xú líng tāi]

Xu Lingtai: another name of Xu Dachun (徐大椿)

徐大业 [xú dà yè]

Xu Daye: another name of Xu Dachun (徐大椿)

何梦瑶 [hé mèng yáo]

He Mengyao: also called He Xichi (何西池) (1693-1763), an official as well as a literary man and physician, author of a number of books, inclding the *Yi Bian* (医碥), or *Fundamentals of Medicine*, the *Ben Cao Yun Yu* (本草韵语), or *Herbal in Rhymes*, the *Shen Xiao Jiao Qi Mi Fang* (神效脚气秘方), or *Wonderful Recipes for Beriberi*, *Fu Ke Liang Fang* (妇科良方), or *Prescriptions for Gynecology*, *You Ke Liang Fang* (幼科良方), or *Prescriptions for Pediatrics*, and *Dou Zhen Liang Fang* (痘疹良方), or *Prescriptions for Poxes and Measles*

何西池 [hé xī chí]

He Xichi: alias of He Mengyao (何梦瑶)

程国彭 [chéng guó péng]

Cheng Guopeng: also called Cheng Zhongling (程钟龄) (1679-?), a celebrated physician and the author of the *Yi Xue Xin Wu* (医学心悟), or *Medicine Comprehended*, which is both concise and practical, and consequently is often referred to by medical practitioners. Cheng was also the author of the *Wai Ke Shi Fa* (外科十法), or *Ten Methods of External Medicine*.

程钟龄 [chéng zhōng líng]

Cheng Zhongling: another name of Cheng Guopeng (程国彭)

沈金鳌 [shěn jīn áo]

Shen Jin'ao: also called Shen Qianlü (沈芊绿) (1717-1776), the author of the *Shen Shi Zun Sheng Shu* (沈氏尊生书), or *On the Importance of Life Preservation* which deals with various branches of medicine as well as *qigong* therapy. The book is rich in content and has long been very popular.

沈芊绿 [shěn qiān lǜ]

Shen Qianlü: another name of Shen Jinao (沈金鳌)

赵学敏 [zhào xué mǐn]

Zhao Xuemin: (1719-1805), also called Zhao Shuxuan (赵恕轩) (1719-1805), a physician and famous pharmacist, author of the *Ben Cao Gang Mu Shi Yi* (本草纲木拾遗), or *Supplement to the Compendium of Materia Medica* (1765), in which all the new drugs that had come into use since the Ming Dynasty are listed. He also collected and systemized the folk healer Zhao Baiyun's (赵伯云) experiences in two books titled *Chuan Ya Nei Bian* (串雅内编), or *Treatise on Folk Medicine* and *Chuan Ya Wai Bain* (串雅外编), or *Extra Treatise on Folk Medicine*.

赵恕轩 [zhào shù xuān]

Zhao Shuxuan: another name of Zhao Xuemin (赵学敏)

郑宏纲 [zhèng hóng gāng]

Zheng Honggang: also called Zheng Meijian (郑梅涧) (c1727-1787), a laryngologist. His widely read book *Chong Lou Yu Yao* (重楼玉钥), or *Jade Key to the Secluded Chamber* deals exclusively with laryngology. It involves the physiology and pathology of the larynx and pharynx, as well as the diagnosis, treatment and prognosis of related diseases. The treatment includes needling, manipulation, gargling, topical insufflation, and external application.

郑梅涧 [zhèng méi jiàn]

Zheng Meijian: another name of Zheng Honggang (郑宏纲)

郑瀚 [zhèng hàn]

Zheng Han: also called Zheng Ruoxi (郑若溪) (c1746-1813), son of Zheng Honggang (郑宏纲), also an expert in laryngology, who compiled the *Chong Lou Yu Yao Xu Bian* (重楼玉钥续编), or *Sequel to the 'Jade Key to the Secluded Chamber'*

郑若溪 [zhèng ruò xī]

Zheng Ruoxi: another name of Zheng Han (郑瀚)

余霖 [yú lín]

Yu Lin, physician of the Qing Dynasty with rich experience in the treatment of epidemic febrile diseases. He compiled the *Zhen Yi Yi De* (疹疫一得), or *A View of Epidemic Febrile Diseases with Rashes* (1785). He initiated the use of large doses of gypsum with success.

陈念祖 [chén niàn zǔ]

Chen Nianzu: also called Chen Xiuyuan (陈修圆) or Chen Shenxiu (陈慎修) (c1753-1823). He compiled many popular works which have been widely read both by professionals and laymen, such as the *Shang Han Lun Qian Zhu* (伤寒论浅注), or *Simplified Commentary on the Treatise on Cold-induced Diseases*, *Yi Xue San Zi Jing* (医学三字经), or *The A.B.C. of Medicine*, *Jin Kui Yao Lue Qian Zhu* (金匮要略浅注), or *Simplified Commentary on the Synopsis of the Golden Chamber*,

Changsha Fang Ge Kuo (长沙方歌括), or *Formulas by Zhang Zhong-jing in Verse*, and the *Shi Fang Ge Kuo* (时方歌括), or *Popular Recipes in Verse.*

陈修圆 [chén xiū yuán]

Chen Xiuyuan: another name of Chen Nianzu (陈念祖)

陈慎修 [chén shèn xiū]

Chen Shenxiu: another name of Chen Nianzu (陈念祖)

吴瑭 [wú táng]

Wu Tang: also called Wu Jutong (吴鞠通) (1758-1836), an authority on acute epidemic febrile diseases, author of the *Wen Bing Tiao Bian* (温病条辨), or *Analysis of Warm Diseases* (1798), in which he summarizes his own experience in the treatment of epidemic febrile diseases, makes distinctions between different fevers and devises new methods of treatment

吴鞠通 [wú jū tōng]

Wu Jutong: another name of Wu Tang (吴瑭)

王清任 [wáng qīng rèn]

Wang Qingren: also called Wang Xunchen (王勋臣) (1768-1831). He stressed the importance of studying the internal organs, and was famous for being the author of the Yi Lin Gai Cuo (医林改错), or *Correction of the Errors of Medical Works,* in which he drew sketches of the internal organs and corrected a number of mistakes in the previous conceptions on the basis of personal observation of exposed bodies in public cemeteries. There are also quite a few new conceptions and some effective formulas for moving *qi*, activating blood and removing stasis in this book.

王勋臣 [wáng xūn chén]

Wang Xunchen: another name of Wang Qingren (王清任)

章楠 [zhāng nán]

Zhang Nan, a physician of the Qing Dynasty, author of the *Yi Men Bang He* (医门棒喝), or *Medical Alarms* (1825), which made contributions to the theory and treatment of epidemic febrile diseases

林佩琴 [lín pèi qín]

Lin Peiqin: also called Lin Yunhe (林云和) or Lin Xitong (林羲桐) (1772-1839). Integrating the strong points of various medical schools with his own clinical experience, he compiled the *Lei Zheng Zhi Cai* (类证治裁), or *Classified Treatment*, in which he emphasizes the importance of syndrome (pattern) differentiation for treatment. The theories of different medical schools he quotes are well selected and are of practical value.

林云和 [lín yún hé]

Lin Yunhe: another name of Lin Peiqin (林佩琴)

林羲桐 [lín xī tóng]

Lin Xitong: another name of Lin Peiqin (林佩琴)

吴其浚 [wú qí jùn]

Wu Qijun: also called Wu Yuezhai (吴瀹斋) (1789-1847), an official as well as a botanist. Having devoted his whole life to the study of plants, he compiled the *Zhi Wu Ming Shi Tu Kao* (植物名实图考), or *An Illustrated Book on Plants*. It served as a supplement to Li Shi-zhen's *Compendium of Materia Medica* and made significant contributions to the study of medicinal plants and general botany, in both China and abroad.

吴瀹斋 [wú yuè zhāi]

Wu Yuezhai: another name of Wu Qijun (吴其浚)

王泰林 [wáng tài lín]

Wang Tailin: also called Wang Xugao (王旭高) (1798-1862), at first good at treating wounds, later specialized in internal medicine and made a detailed study of liver troubles. Wang was the author of the *Yi Fang Zheng Zhi Hui Bian* (医方证治汇编), or *A Collection of Classified Prescriptions with Diagnosis and Treatment,* and *Yi Xue Chu Yan* (医学刍言), or *Preliminary Remarks on Medicine*. His case records were collected by his disciple in book form, titled *Wang Xugao Yi An* (王旭高医案), or *Medical Case Records by Wang Xugao*.

王旭高 [wáng xù gāo]

Wang Xugao: another name of Wang Tailin (王泰林)

朱沛文 [zhū pèi wén]

Zhu Peiwen: physician of the 19th century, who advocated that traditional Chinese and Western medicine should complement each other. He compiled the *Hua Yang Zang Fu Tu Xiang Yue Zuan* (华洋脏腑图象约纂), or *A Brief Account of the Chinese and Western Anatomy* (1892), in which knowledge of Western anatomy and physiology was introduced and used as a commentary on the *Canon of Medicine*.

吴尚先 [wú shàng xiān]

Wu Shangxian: also called Wu Shiji (吴师机) or Wu Anye (吴安业)

(c1806-1886), who advocated external therapies, such as ointment and plaster application, hydrotherapy and kerotherapy for those who could not afford high charges for oral medication and also for those who did not wish to drink decoctions. He was the author of the *Li Yue Pian Wen* (理瀹骈文), or *A Rhymed Discourse on New Therapeutics* (1870).

吴师机 [wú shī jī]

Wu Shiji: another name of Wu Shangxian (吴尚先)

吴安业 [wú ān yè]

Wu Anye: another name of Wu Shangxian (吴尚先)

王士雄 [wáng shì xióng]

Wang Shixiong: also called Wang Mengying (王孟英) (1808-1866), a well-known specialist in epidemic febrile diseases. He compiled the *Wen Re Jing Wei* (温热经纬), or *An Outline of Epidemic Febrile Diseases*, and the *Huo Luan Lun* (霍乱论), or *On Diseases with Sudden Vomiting and Diarrhea*, and put all the case records of his patients in the book *Wang Shi Yi An* (王氏医案), or *Wang's Medical Case Records*.

王孟英 [wáng mèng yīng]

Wang Mengying: another name of Wang Shixiong (王士雄)

张筱衫 [zhāng xiǎo shān]

Zhang Xiaoshan: also called Zhang Zhengjun(张振鋆), a physician and well-known massotherapist of the Qing Dynasty, author of the *Li Zheng An Mo Yao Shu* (厘正按摩要术), or *Revised Techniques of Massage* (1898)

张振鋆 [zhāng zhèn jūn]

Zhang Zhenjun: another name of Zhang Xiaoshan (张筱衫)

陆懋修 [lù mào xiū]

Lu Maoxiu: also called Lu Jiu-zhi (陆九芝) (1818-1886), a physician who wrote the *Shi Bu Zhai Yi Shu* (世补斋医书), or *A Book of Medicine*, clung closely to the old tradition, particularly to the doctrine of Zhang Zhongjing

陆九芝 [lù jiǔ zhī]

Lu Jiuzhi: another name of Lu Maoxiu (陆懋修)

唐宗海 [táng zōng hǎi]

Tang Zonghai: also called Tang Rongchuan (唐容川) (1847-1897), a physician at the end of the Qing Dynasty, who was one of the first to try to unite traditional Chinese medicine and Western medicine, and the author of the *Zhong Xi Hui Tong Yi Jing Jing Yi* (中西汇通医经精义), or *Essentials of Confluent Traditional Chinese and Western Medicine.* He tried to prove that traditional Chinese medicine was not unscientific, and pointed out that both the Chinese and Western systems of medicine were worthy of note. He was also the author of the *Xue Zheng Lun* (血证论), or *Treatise on Blood Syndromes,* in which some special methods of treating hemorrhagic diseases are recommended.

唐容川 [táng róng chuān]

Tang Rongchuan: another name of Tang Zonghai (唐宗海)

何炳元 [hé bǐng yuán]

He Bingyuan: also called He Lianchen (何廉臣) (1861-1929). He studied both traditional Chinese and Western medicine. Comparing the two, he came to the conclusion that Western medicine was not perfect, and that traditional Chinese medicine should not be neglected. He was the author of a number of books, such as the *Zhong Feng Xin Quan* (中风新诠), or *A New Exposition of Apoplexy*, the *Xin Yi Zong Bi Du* (新医宗必读), or *A New Selection of Required Readings for Medical Professional*, the *Nei Ke Zheng Zhi Quan Shu* (内科证治全书), or *A Complete Book of Diagnosis and Treatment of Internal Medicine*, the *Quan Guo Ming Yi Yan An Lei Bian* (全国名医验案类编), or *A Classified Collection of Successful Medical Case Records of Noted Chinese Physicians*.

何廉臣 [hé lián chén]

He Lianchen: another name of He Bingyuan (何炳元)

陆以湉 [lù yǐ tián]

Lu Yitian, physician of the late Qing Dynasty, author of the *Leng Lu Yi Hua* (冷庐医话), or *Deserted House Medical Talks* (1897)

雷丰 [léi fēng]

Lei Feng: also called Lei Shaoyi (雷少逸), a physician at the end of the Qing Dynasty, specialized in treating epidemic febrile diseases. He wrote the Shi Bing Lun (时病论), or *Treatise on Seasonal Diseases*, which was widely read because the methods of treatment and prescriptions recommended proved highly effective.

雷少逸 [léi shào yì]

Lei Shaoyi: another name of Lei Feng (雷丰)

丁甘仁 [dīng gān rén]

Ding Ganren: also called Ding Zezhou (丁泽周) (1865-1926). He set up the Shanghai Institute of Traditional Chinese Medicine in 1916, the Women's Institute of Traditional Chinese Medicine, and the Guangyi Hospital of Traditional Chinese Medicine, and made great contributions to the training of physicians of the traditional school. He was the author of the *Hou Sha Zheng Zhi Gai Yao* (喉痧证治概要), or *An Outline of Diagnosis and Treatment of Scarlet Fever.* The book *Ding Gan Ren Yi An* (丁甘仁医案), or *Ding Gan-ren's Medical Case Records* was compiled by his students.

丁泽周 [dīng zé zhōu]

Ding Zezhou: another name of Ding Ganren (丁甘仁)

张锡纯 [zhāng xī chún]

Zhang Xichun: also called Zhang Shoufu (张寿甫) (1860-1933). He researched ancient medical books and advocated the combination of traditional Chinese and Western medicine, and was the author of the *Yi Xue Zhong Zhong Can Xi Lu* (医学衷中参西录), or *Records of Traditional Chinese and Western Medicine in Combination*, which is widely read.

张寿甫 [zhāng shòu fǔ]

Zhang Shoufu: another name of Zhang Xichun (张锡纯)

张寿颐 [zhāng shòu yí]

Zhang Shouyi: also called Zhang Shanlei (张山雷) (1872-1934), a physician of the modern age versed in treating internal and external diseases, author of a series of medical books on various subjects, such as *Zhong Feng Jiao Quan* (中风斠诠), or *Treatise on Stroke*, and the *Yang Ke Gang Yao* (疡科纲要), or *An Outline of Traumatolocy* and an educationist of traditional Chinese medicine

张山雷 [zhāng shān léi]

Zhang Shanlei: another name of Zhang Shouyi (张寿颐)

恽铁樵 [yùn tiě qiáo]

Yun Tieqiao, also called Yun Shujue (恽树珏) (1878-1935), a student of literature at first, who later, because of his poor health and the death of his children, went in for Chinese and Western medicine. Yun ran medical schools and took part in the campaign to oppose the defamation and extermination of tradtional Chinese medicine. He advocated supplementing Chinese medicine with Western medical theories. He wrote more than 20 books, such as *Qun Jing Jian Zhi Lu* (群经见智录),

or *Wisdom Exposed in the Medical Classics*, *Shang Han Lun Yan Jiu* (伤寒论研究), or *Research into Treatises on Cold-induced Diseases*, and *Mai Xue Fa Wei* (脉学发微), or *Detailed Study of Pulse Lore*.

恽树珏 [yùn shù jué]

Yun Shujue: another name of Yun Tieqiao (恽铁樵)

谢观 [xiè guān]

Xie Guan: modern physician (1878-1950) who compiled the *Zhong Guo Yi Xue Da Ci Dian* (中国医学大词典), or *A Dictionary of Traditional Chinese Medicine* (1921), which includes more than 70,000 entries, and *Zhong Yi Yi Xue Yuan Liu Lun* (中医医学源流论), or *Origin and Development of Traditional Chinese Medicine*

陆渊雷 [lù yuān léi]

Lu Yuanlei: modern physician (1894-1955) and educationalist of traditional Chinese medicine, who, being influenced by the school of confluent traditional Chinese and Western medicine, tried to quote Western medicine to prove ancient Chinese medical theories

承澹盦 [chéng dàn ān]

Cheng Dan'an: a famous acupuncturist (1899-1957), who set up a society of acupuncture research and then a special school for training acupuncturists. His chief writings include the *Zhong Guo Zhen Jiu Zhi Liao Xue* (中国针灸治疗学), or *Chinese Acupuncture-Moxibustion Therapy*, the *Zhen Jiu Jing Hua* (针灸精华), or *Quintessence of Acupuncture and Moxibustion*, and the *Zhong Guo Zhen Jiu Xue* (中国针灸学), or *Chinese Acupuncture and Moxibustion*.

名著 Well-known Medical Works

黄帝内经 [huáng dì nèi jīng]

***Huang Di Nei Jing*, or *Huangdi's Internal Classic*, or *Huangdi's Canon of Medicine*:** the oldest and greatest medical classic extant in China, with its authorship ascribed to the ancient Emperor Huangdi (2698-2589 B.C.). Actually the work was a product of various unknown authors in the Warring States Period (475-221 B.C.). The book consists of two parts: *Su Wen* (素问), or *Plain Questions*, and *Ling Shu* (灵枢), or *Spiritual Pivot* or *Divine Axis*, the latter also known as the *Canon of Acupuncture*.

内经 [nèi jīng]

Nei Jing, or ***Internal Classic*** or ***Canon of Medicine*****:** an abbreviation for *Huangdi's Canon of Medicine*

黄帝内经素问 [huáng dì nèi jīng sù wèn]

Huang Di Nei Jing Su Wen, or ***Plain Questions of Huangdi's Canon of Medicine*****,** also called *Su Wen*, or *Plain Questions* for short, one of the two parts of the *Canon of Medicine*, originally consisting of 9 volumes, with 81 articles. After the Wei and Jin Dynasties only 8 volumes were left. In the Tang Dynasty while making notes and commentaries on the book, Wang Bing (王冰) divided it into 24 volumes and made up for some of the lost articles. In the Northern Song Dynasty Lin Yi (林亿) et al, read proofs and made notes on it again, and all later extant editions were based on this one. The book deals with a variety of subjects, such as human anatomy and physiology, causes of diseases, pathology, diagnosis, syndrome differentiation, treatment, disease prevention, health preservation, man and nature, the application of the theories of yin and yang, the five elements and the circulation of *qi*, etc. The book has been prized by physicians of all generations.

素问 [sù wèn]

Su Wen, or ***Plain Questions*****:** abbreviation for *Huang Di Nei Jing Su Wen* (黄帝内经素问), or *Plain Questions of Huangdi's Canon of Medicine*

黄帝内经灵枢经 [huáng dì nèi jīng líng shū jīng]

Huang Di Nei Jing Ling Shu Jing, or ***Spiritual Pivot of Huangdi's Canon of Medicine*****,** also called *Ling Shu* (灵枢), or *Spiritual Pivot* or *Divine Axis* for short, one of the two parts of the *Canon of Medicine*. The subjects of *Spiritual Pivot* are similar to those of *Plain Qestions*, but the former has a more detailed description of meridians and needling and is less detailed in theories concerning the circular movement of the five elements. In introducing basic theories and clinical practice, the two books supplement each other. This book is also titled *Zhen Jing* (针经), or *Canon of Acupuncture*.

灵枢 [líng shū]

Ling Shu, or ***Spiritual Pivot*** or ***Divine Axis*****:** abbreviation for *Huang Di Nei Jing Ling Shu Jing*, or *Spiritual Pivot of Huangdi's Canon of Medicine*

黄帝内经素问注证发微 [huáng dì nèi jīng sù wèn zhù zhèng fā wēi]

***Huang Di Nei Jing Su Wen Zhu Zheng Fa Wei*, or *An Elaboration on Plain Questions of Huangdi's Internal Classic*,** also called *An Elaboration on Plain Questions* for short, written by Ma Shi (马莳) of the Ming Dynasty (1586)

黄帝内经灵枢注证发微 [huáng dì nèi jīng líng shū zhù zhèng fā wēi]

***Huang Di Nei Jing Ling Shu Zhu Zheng Fa Wei*, or *An Elaboration on Spiritual Pivot of Huangdi's Internal Classic*,** also called *An Elaboration on Divine Axis* for short, written by Ma Shi (马莳) of the Ming Dynasty (1586)

类经 [lèi jīng]

***Lei Jing*, or *Classified Canon* or *Systematic Compilation of the Internal Classic*,** compiled by Zhang Jiebin (张介宾) and published in 1624. It is a rearrangement of the *Nei Jing* or *Canon of Medicine*. The book consists of 12 categories, including hygiene, yin-yang, organ pictures, pulse, meridians, sapours, theories of treatment, acupuncture, etc. It has been considered by students of the *Nei Jing*, or *Canon of Medicine*, as one of the most important reference books for the study of this classic.

类经图翼 [lèi jīng tú yì]

Lei Jing Tu Yi*, or *Illustrated Supplementary to the Classified Canon (1624), a supplementary to the *Classified Canon* with illustrations, compiled by Zhang Jiebin (张介宾)

内经知要 [nèi jīng zhī yào]

Nei Jing Zhi Yao*, or *Essentials of the Internal Classic* or *Essentials of the Canon of Medicine (1642), compiled by Li Nian'e (李念莪). The book is divided into 8 parts, including yin-yang, pulse, meridians, principles of treatment, etc. Combining basic with clinical theories, the author takes extracts from and makes expositions of the *Internal Classic*. The book is clearly written and well organized.

难经 [nán jīng]

Nan Jing*, or *Difficult Classic* or *Classic of Medical Problems, a book which appeared in the 1st or 2nd century B.C., authorship unknown, though it is often ascribed to Qin Yueren (秦越人). It deals with fundamental medical theories and expounds the main points of the *Nei Jing* or *Internal Classic* in the form of questions and answers. The points for acupuncture and moxibustion, the method of needling, the physiological and pathological conditions related to the meridians and collaterals, and the method of pulse-taking are all discussed.

难经本义 [nán jīng běn yì]

Nan Jing Ben Yi, or ***The Genuine Meaning of the Difficult Classic,*** compiled by Hua Shou (滑寿) and published in 1366, a most influential book among commentatorial works on the *Nan Jing*, or *Difficult Classic*

伤寒杂病论 [shāng hán zá bìng lùn]

Shang Han Za Bing Lun, or ***Treatise on Cold-induced and Miscellaneous Diseases***, written by Zhang Zhongjing (张仲景) at the beginning of the 3rd century, in which diagnosis and treatment of fevers and other miscellaneous diseases are dealt with. The book was rearranged by Wang Shuhe (王叔和) in the Jin Dynasty, and later in the Song Dynasty it was divided by Jiao Zheng Yi Shu Ju (校正医书局), or Bureau for Rectifying and Publishing Medical Books into two parts: *Shang Han Lun* (伤寒论), or *Treatise on Cold-induced Diseases* and *Jin Kui Yao Lue Fang Lun* (金匮要略方论), or *Synopsis of Prescriptions of the Golden Chamber.*

伤寒论 [shāng hán lùn]

Shang Han Lun, or ***Treatise on Cold-induced Diseases***, a new edition of Zhang Zhongjing's (张仲景) *Treatise on Cold-induced and Miscellaneous Diseases,* rearranged by Wang Shuhe (王叔和) in 10 volumes, in which acute febrile diseases induced by cold are analysed and differentiated in accordance with the theory of the six meridians. This book has been one of the most influential works in the history of Chinese medicine.

伤寒明理论 [shāng hán míng lǐ lùn]

Shang Han Ming Li Lun, or ***Concise Exposition of Cold-induced Diseases*** (1156), written by Cheng Wuji (成无已) of the Jin Dynasty, a concise reference book for beginners to study the *Treatise on Cold-induced Diseases* in which compatibility of ingredients is stressed

伤寒来苏集 [shāng hán lái sū jí]

Shang Han Lai Su Ji, or ***Renewal of the Treatise on Cold-induced Diseases***, in 8 volumes, compiled by Ke Qin (柯琴) of the Qing Dynasty, a good commentary on the *Treatise on Cold-induced Diseases*

伤寒类方 [shāng hán lèi fāng]

Shang Han Lei Fang, or ***Classified Prescriptions from the Treatise on***

Cold-induced Diseases (1759), written by Xu Dachun (徐大椿) of the Qing Dynasty, in which the 113 prescriptions recommended in the *Treatise on Cold-induced Diseases* are classified into 12 categories with discussions of their indications

伤寒贯珠集 [shāng hán guàn zhū jí]

Shang Han Guan Zhu Ji, or ***A String of Beads from the Treatise on Cold-induced Diseases*** (1810), compiled by You Yi (尤怡) of the Qing Dynasty, a rearrangement of the *Treatise on Cold-induced Diseases* in the order of the six pairs of meridians, with various methods of treatment

金匮要略方论 [jīn kuì yào lüè fāng lùn]

Jin Kui Yao Lue Fang Lun, or ***Synopsis of Prescriptions of the Golden Chamber***, or simply *Jin Kui Yao Lue*, or *Synopsis of the Golden Chamber*, by Zhang Zhongjing (张仲景) at the beginning of the 3rd century. It was rearranged by Wang Shuhe (王叔和) in three volumes, dealing mainly with miscellaneous diseases of internal medicine, and some surgical and women's diseases in 25 chapters, including 262 prescriptions.

金匮要略 [jīn kuì yào lüè]

Jin Kui Yao Lue, or ***Synopsis of the Golden Chamber***, same as *Jin Kui Yao Lue Fang Lun*, or *Synopsis of Prescriptions of the Golden Chamber*

金匮要略心典 [jīn kuì yào lüè xīn diǎn]

Jin Kui Yao Lue Xin Dian, or ***Commentaries on the Synposis of the Golden Chamber*** written by You Yi (尤怡) of the Qing Dynasty and published in 1729. It comments on *Synopsis of the Golden Chamber* briefly and to the point, with all the theories and major problems clearly explained and some mistakes corrected. The unintelligible places in the original book are left untouched rather than wrongly interpreted.

金匮翼 [jīn kùi yì]

Jin Kui Yi, or ***Supplements to Commentaries on the Synopsis of the Golden Chamber***, written by You Yi (尤怡) and published in 1768 to supplement the *Jin Kui Yao Lue Xin Dian*, or *Commentaries on Synopsis of the Golden Chamber*. It deals exclusively with miscellaneous diseases of internal medicine, which are divided into 48 groups. It is succinct in wording, and the prescriptions chosen are of practical value.

脉经 [mài jīng]

Mai Jing, or ***The Pulse Classic***, written by Wang Shuhe (王叔和) in the 3rd century, generally acknowledged as the standard work on the subject and the earliest comprehensive work dealing with sphygmology extant

诊家枢要 [zhěn jiā shū yǎo]

Zhen Jia Shu Yao*,** or ***Essentials for Diagnosticians (1359), a monograph on the pulse written by Hua Shou (滑寿), in which 30 kinds of pulse conditions with their corresponding diseases are described

濒湖脉学 [bīn hú mài xué]

***Bin Hu Mai Xue*,** or ***Binhu's Sphygmology*,** written by Li Shizhen (李时珍) in 1564, in which 27 kinds of pulses and their diagnostic value are given in detail in lucid verses. This book has been very popular for centuries.

四诊抉微 [sì zhěn jué wēi]

Si Zhen Jue Wei*,** or ***The Essentials of Four Diagnostic Examinations （1723）, written by Lin Zhihan (林之翰), an influential monograph on diagnostics

诸病源侯总论 [zhū bìng yuán hóu zǒng lùn]

Zhu Bing Yuan Hou Zong Lun*,** or ***Treatise on Causes and Symptoms of Diseases (610), compiled by Chao Yuanfang (巢元方) et al. in 50 volumes with detailed discussions on the etiology and symptomology of various diseases. It consists of 67 categories with 1, 720 entries and many brilliant expositions frequently cited by authors of later generations.

三因极一病证方论 [sān yīn jí yī bìng zhèng fāng lùn]

San Yin Ji Yi Bing Zheng Fang Lun*,** or ***Treatise on the Three Categories of Pathogenic Factors and Prescriptions, written by Chen Yan (陈言) in 1174. It classifies the causes of diseases into external, internal and miscellaneous ones which are regarded as neither external nor internal.

神农本草经 [shén nóng běn cǎo jīng]

Shen Nong Ben Cao Jing*,** or ***Shen Nong's Herbal or ***The Herbal*,** China's earliest materia medica, believed to be a product of the 1st century B.C. with its authorship attributed to the ancient emperor "the Divine Peasant" Shen Nong, in which 365 kinds of drugs are listed and divided into three classes: superior, common and inferior

名医别录 [míng yī bié lù]

Ming Yi Bie Lu*,** or ***Miscellaneous Records of Famous Physicians, a book on pharmacology compiled on the basis of *Shen Nong's Herbal* by Tao Hongjing (陶弘景), who expounded *Shen Nong's Herbal*, and supplemented it with 365 kinds of medicinal substances

食疗本草 [shí liáo běn cǎo]

Shi Liao Ben Cao, or ***Materia Medica of Diet Therapy***, a monogrph recording herbs which can be used as both food and drugs by Meng Shen (孟诜) of the Tang Dynasty. The original has been lost, but its text can be found in *Lei Zheng Ben Cao* (类证本草) or *Classified Materia Medica* and *Ishinpo* (医心方) by Yasuriri Tanba (丹波康赖 912-995), a noted Japanese physician.

唐本草 [táng běn cǎo]

Tang Ben Cao, or ***The Tang Materia Medica*** (659), also called *Xin Xiu Ben Cao* (新修本草), or *Newly Compiled Materia Medica (of Tang)*, compiled by Su Jing (苏敬) and 22 other scholars. It lists 844 medical substances. Since it was sponsored by the Tang court, it is considered to be the earliest pharmacopoeia published officially in the world.

新修本草 [xīn xīu běn cǎo]

Xin Xiu Ben Cao, or ***Newly Compiled Materia Medica of Tang***: another name of Tang Ben Cao, or *The Tang Materia Medica*

本草拾遗 [běn cǎo shí yí]

Ben Cao Shi Yi, or ***A Supplement to the Herbal***, in 10 volumes by Chen Cangqi (陈藏器) of the Tang Dynasty (8th century). It mainly adds medicinal substances not included in *Xin Xiu Ben Cao*, or *Newly Compiled Materia Medica of Tang*.

经史证类备急本草 [jīng shǐ zhèng liè bèi jí běn cǎo]

Jing Shi Zheng Lei Bei Ji Ben Cao, or ***Classic Classified Materia Medica for Emergencies***, or *Zheng Lei Ben Cao* (证类本草), or *Classified Materia Medica* for short, compiled by Tang Shen-wei (唐慎微) at the end of the 11th century. It lists 1, 746 kinds of medicine with directions for use and preparation, and many new prescriptions. The book laid a solid foundation for the development of Chinese materia medica.

证类本草 [zhèng lèi běn cǎo]

Zheng Lei Ben Cao, or ***Classified Materia Medica***: abbreviation for *Jing Shi Zheng Lei Bei Ji Ben Cao*, or *Classic Classified Materia Medica for Emergencies*

汤液本草 [tāng yè běn cǎo]

Tang Ye Ben Cao, or ***Materia Medica of Decoction***, written by Wang Haogu (王好古) and published in 1289, with a list of 238 kinds of drugs, in which the flavor, taste and therapeutic properties as well as the mutual influences of medicines when used in combination are given in detail

救荒本草 [jiù huāng běn cǎo]

Jiu Huang Ben Cao*, or *Herbal for the Relief of Famines, compiled by Zhu Su (朱橚) in 1406, listing 414 plants which might be used for food in times of famine

本草纲目 [běn cǎo gāng mù]

Ben Cao Gang Mu*, or *Compendium of Materia Medica, compiled by Li Shizhen (李时珍), a gigantic and most comprehensive work published in 1596, in 52 volumes which took the author 30 years to complete. It lists 1,892 medical substances, more than 1,000 illustrations and over 10,000 prescriptions with detailed descriptions of the appearance, properties, methods of collection and preparation and use of each substance. This book is far more than a pharmaceutical compendium, it is also a comprehensive work on various branches of natural science, including botany, zoology, mineralogy and metallurgy.

本草备要 [běn cǎo bèi yào]

Ben Cao Bei Yao*, or *Essentials of Materia Medica, written by Wang Ang (王昂) and published in 1694, a simple but important book on materia medica, dealing first with the nature of drugs and then describing the properties and tastes, uses and indications of 470 kinds of commonly used drugs, with over 400 illustrations

本草纲目拾遗 [běn cǎo gāng mù shí yí]

Ben Cao Gang Mu Shi Yi*, or *A Supplement to the Compendium of Materia Medica, written by Zhao Xuemin (赵学敏) in 1765, and listing 716 medical substances not included in Li Shi-zhen's *Compendium of Materia Medica*, with some imported from abroad.

珍珠囊药性赋 [zhēn zhū náng yào xìng fù]

Zhen Zhu Nang Yao Xing Fu*, or *Nature of the Drugs of the Pearl Bag in Songs, also known as *Lei Gong Yao Xing Fu* or *Lei's Nature of Drugs in Songs*, written by Yuan Shan Dao Ren (元山道人) at the beginning of the Ming Dynasty, which describes in detail the indications and cautions for the use of 90 kinds of common drugs, and introduces 1,406 medical substances in the form of songs and notes

雷公药性赋 [léi gōng yào xìng fù]

Lei Gong Yao Xing Fu*, or *Lei's Nature of Drugs in Songs: another name of *Zhen Zhu Nang Yao Xing Fu*, or *Nature of the Drugs of the Pearl Bag in Songs*

用药法象 [yòng yào fǎ xiàng]

Yong Yao Fa Xiang, or ***Rules for the Use of Drugs***, written by Li Gao (李杲), in which drugs are classified according to their therapeutic properties into 4 kinds: ascending, descending, floating and sinking

雷公炮炙论 [léi gōng páo zhì lùn]

Lei Gong Pao Zhi Lun, or ***Lei's Treatise on the Preparation of Drugs***, written by Lei Xiao (雷斅) in the 5th century, in which the fundamental processes of preparing drugs are dealt with. It is one of the earliest books extant on this subject.

炮炙大全 [páo zhì dà quán]

Pao Zhi Da Quan, or ***A Complete Handbook on the Preparation of Drugs*** (1622), compiled by Miao Xiyong (缪希雍) and Zhuang Ji-guang (庄继光) on the basis of Lei's work on the subject, with some additions made of the new methods then popular among the people

饮膳正要 [yǐn shàn zhèng yào]

Yin Shan Zheng Yao, or ***Principles of Correct Diet*** (1330) written by Hu Sihui (忽思慧). It lists the food and drink of the royal family and the nobility, and describes with illustrations, the nature, taste and indications of about 200 different kinds of medicinal herbs which can be used as food.

植物名实图考 [zhí wù míng shí tú kǎo]

Zhi Wu Ming Shi Tu Kao, or ***An illustrated Book of Plants***, written by Wu Qijun (吴其濬) in 38 volumes and published in 1848, a book on botany which includes no less than 1,714 plant species. The author gives a comparatively detailed description of the shape, color, nature, taste, uses and habitat of each plant, with vivid and true-to-life drawings of them.

植物名实图考长编 [zhí wù míng shí tú kǎo cháng biān]

Zhi Wu Ming Shi Tu Kao Chang Bian, or ***A Lengthy Compilation of Plants with Illustrations***, written by Wu Qijun (吴其濬) in 22 volumes and published in 1848 on the basis of data from ancient literature, to form a pair with the *Zhi Wu Ming Shi Tu Kao*, or *An Illustrated Book of Plants*, with 788 plant substances listed

全国中草药汇编 [quān guó zhōng cǎo yào huì biān]

Quan Guo Zhong Cao Yao Hui Bian, or ***A Compilation of Chinese Medicinal Herbs***, in two volumes with a list of about 2,200 herbal medicines. The names, sources, morphology, environment, cultivation, collection and preparation, chemistry, pharmacology, nature, taste, uses, indications and administration of each medicine are given in detail, with pictures of the living plants, published in 1975 by the People's Health Publishing House.

肘后备急方 [zhǒu hòu bèi jí fāng]

Zhou Hou Bei Ji Fang, or ***A Handbook of Prescriptions for Emergencies***, written by Ge Hong (葛洪 283-343), in which the prescriptions recorded are simple and the drugs used are common and effective and many valuable descriptions of diseases and treatments are recorded

备急千金要方 [bèi jí qiān jīn yào fāng]

Bei Ji Qian Jin Yao Fang, or ***Invaluable Prescriptions for Emergencies*** or Qian Jin Yao Fang (千金要方), or *Invaluable Prescriptions* for short, compiled by Sun Simiao (孙思邈) at the end of the 7th century in 30 volumes, with a general introduction, prescriptions of various clinical branches, diet, pulse-taking, acupuncture, etc.

千金要方 [qiān jīn yào fāng]

Qian Jin Yao Fang, or ***Invaluable Prescriptions***: abbreviation for *Bei Ji Qian Jin Yao Fang*, or *Invaluable Prescriptions for Emergencies*

千金翼方 [qiān jīn yì fāng]

Qian Jin Yi Fang, or ***Supplement to the Invaluable Prescriptions***, compiled by Sun Simiao (孙思邈) at the end of the 7th century in 30 volumes, including various medical branches such as herbal lore, febrile diseases, obstetrics and gynecology, pediatrics, miscellaneous diseases of internal medicine, pulse-taking, acupuncture and diet, which, together with *Qian Jin Yao Fang*, or *Invaluable Prescriptions*, is considered a compendium of the medical achievements made before the Tang Dynasty

外台秘要 [wài tái mì yào]

Wai Tai Mi Yao, or ***Medical Secrets of an Official*** (752), compiled by Wang Tao (王焘) in 40 volumes in which a comprehensive and exhaustive study of medicine is made, with 1,104 issues of medical problems discussed and over 6,000 prescriptions recorded

太平圣惠方 [tài píng shèng huì fāng]

Tai Ping Sheng Hui Fang, or *Taiping Sacred Remedies* (992) or simply *Sheng Hui Fang*, or *Sacred Remedies*, compiled by Wang Huaiyin (王怀隐) in ten volumes, recording 16,834 prescriptions of various medical branches with discussions of the diagnosis and pathology of various diseases

圣惠方 [shèng huì fāng]

Sheng Hui Fang, or ***Sacred Remedies*****:** abbreviation for *Tai Ping Sheng Hui Fang,* or *Taiping Sacred Remedies*

太平惠民和剂局方 [tài píng huì mín hé jì jú fāng]

Tai Ping Hui Min He Ji Ju Fang, Formularies of the Bureau of People's Welfare Pharmacy or simply *He Ji Ju Fang*, or *Formularies of the Bureau of Pharmacy*, compiled by Chen Shiwen (陈师文) et al., in 1151, in 10 volumes, consisting of 788 prescriptions in 14 categories which were popular and effective. Most of the medicines are in pill or powder form, ready for use and storage

和剂局方 [hé jì jú fāng]

He Ji Ju Fang, or ***Formularies of the Bureau of Pharmacy*****:** abbreviation for Tai Ping Hui Min He Ji Ju Fang, *Formularies of the Bureau of People's Welfare Pharmacy*

普济本事方 [pǔ jì běn shì fāng]

Pu Ji Ben Shi Fang, or ***Effective Prescriptions for Universal Relief***, also called *Ben Shi Fang*, or *Effective Prescriptions* for short, a book in 10 volumes, written by Xu Shuwei (许叔微) of the Southern Song Dynasty and published in the middle of the 12th century. It mainly deals with common diseases related to internal medicine, listing 23 kinds of treatment with more than 300 prescriptions. At the end of each prescription are attached the author's proved case records.

本事方 [běn shì fāng]

Ben Shi Fang, or ***Effective Prescriptions*****:** abbreviation for *Pu Ji Ben Shi Fang*, or *Effective Prescriptions for Universal Relief*

济生方 [jì shēng fāng]

Ji Sheng Fang, or ***Prescriptions for Succouring the Sick***, also called *Yan Shi Ji Sheng Fang* or *Yan's Prescriptions for Succouring the Sick*, a book in 10 volumes, written by Yan Yonghe (严用和) in 1253, which consists of 79 articles dealing with diseases of internal medicine, surgery and gynecology and includes over 450 prescriptions, all proved effective by the author

严氏济生方 [yán shì jì shēng fāng]

***Yan Shi Ji Sheng Fang*, or *Yan's Prescriptions for Succouring the Sick*:** the full name of *Ji Sheng Fang*, or *Prescriptions for Succouring the Sick*

世医得效方 [shì yī dé xiào fāng]

Shi Yi De Xiao Fang*, or *Effective Formulas Tested by Physicians for Generations (1345), compiled by Wei Yilin (危亦林) on the basis of the author's family experiences as physicians for five successive generations, in which are listed prescriptions for children's diseases, internal medicine, ophthalmology, oral diseases, dentistry, bone-setting, war wounds, ulcers and carbuncles

局方发挥 [jú fāng fā huī]

Ju Fang Fa Hui*, or *An Expounding of the Formularies of the Bureau of Pharmacy, written by Zhu Zhenheng (朱震亨) in the 14th century. Zhu pointed out and criticized the mechanical and indiscriminate use of the formularies of the Bureau of the People's Welfare Pharmacy which were popular at that time.

普济方 [pǔ jì fāng]

Pu Ji Fang*, or *Prescriptions for Universal Relief, a most complete collection of prescriptions (61,739 prescriptions and 239 illustrations) in 168 volumes, written by Teng Hong (滕弘) et al. under the patronage of Zhu Su (朱橚), and issued in 1406

奇效良方 [qí xiào liáng fāng]

Qi Xiao Liang Fang*, or *Wonderful Well-tried Prescriptions （1470）, a book in 69 volumes with authorship ascribed to Dong Su (董宿) and Fang Xian (方贤). According to the principles of treatment, it divides recipes into 64 families, such as wind, cold, heat, etc., which are subdivided into still smaller groups with a list of more than 7,000 prescriptions, chiefly passed down from the Song and Ming Dynasties, and including methods of needling and bone-setting.

医方集解 [yī fāng jí jiě]

Yi Fang Ji Jie*, or *Collection of Prescriptions with Expositions, written by Wang Ang (汪昂) in the Qing Dynasty and published in 1682. It lists about 700 prescriptions, divided into 21 classes, such as tonifying, exterior-releasing, vomiting-inducing, harmonizing, *qi*-regulating, blood-regulating, etc., and describes in detail the combination of ingredients, properties, and indications of each recipe with reference to the theories of various schools.

汤头歌诀 [tāng tóu gē jué]

Tang Tou Ge Jue*, or *Prescriptions in Rhymes written by Wang Ang (汪昂) of the Qing Dynasty and published in 1694. Over 300 prescriptions are selected and written in the form of more than 200 songs. To each song are appended simple notes to make it easier for the beginners to learn them by heart. This book was very popular.

串雅内、外编 [chuàn yǎ nèi、wài biān]

Chuan Ya Nei Wai Bian*, or *Bound Volume of Treatises on Folk Medicine, a joint edition of the two books *Treatise on Folk Medicine* and *Extra Treatise on Folk Medicine* written by Zhao Xuemin (赵学敏) in 1759 on the basis of employed by folk healers and reference materials in medical works concerned. Each consists of 4 volumes including simple, handy, cheap yet effective prescriptions, as well as methods of making drugs and of treating diseaeses of animals and plants.

时方歌括 [shí fāng gē kuò]

Shi Fang Ge Kuo*, or *Popular Prescriptions in Verse (1801), written by Chen Nianzu (陈念祖) of the Qing Dynasty with 108 popular and practical prescriptions recommended in verse

理瀹骈文 [lǐ yuè pián wén]

Li Yue Pian Wen*, or *A Rhymed Discourse on New Therapeutics, written by Wu Shangxian (吴尚先), who was famous for practising folk medicine and advocating external therapies such as ointment and plasters, hydrotherapy, breathing therapy, cautery and moxibustion

温疫论 [wēn yì lùn]

Wen Yi Lun*, or *Treatise on Pestilence (1642), written by Wu Youke (吴又可), a study of etiology and pathology of epidemic febrile diseases. The author points out it is pestilential factors that get into the human body through the mouth and nose and cause epidemic febrile diseases.

温热论 [wēn rè lùn]

Wen Re Lun*, or *Treatise on Epidemic Febrile Diseases, comprising lectures by Ye Tianshi (叶天士) and edited by his disciple Gu Jingwen (顾景文) in 1746, a book on the diagnosis and treatment of epidemic febrile diseases in which the theory of development or transmission of disease among the four systems (superficial defense, *qi*, nutrient and blood) of the body is introduced

温病条辨 [wēn bìng tiáo biàn]

Wen Bing Tiao Bian, or ***Analysis of Warm Diseases***, written by Wu Tang (吴瑭) in 1798, a development of Ye Tian-shi's *Treatise on Epidemic Febrile Diseases*, in which differential diagnosis of diseases according to pathological changes of the triple energizer is given in detail

温热经纬 [wēn rè jīng wěi]

Wen Re Jing Wei, or ***An Outline of Epidemic Febrile Diseases***, written by Wang Mengying (王孟英) in 1852 in 5 volumes, which throw light on the cause of epidemic febrile diseases, their signs and symptoms, and methods of treatment on the basis of the theories set out in the *Internal Classic* and *Treatise on Cold-induced and Miscellaneous Diseases,* and with reference to the viewpoints of distinguished physicians of the Qing Dynasty such as Ye Gui (叶桂), Xue Xue (薛雪), Chen Pingbo (陈平伯) and Yu Shiyu (余师愚).

时病论 [shí bìng lùn]

Shi Bing Lun, or ***Treatise on Seasonal Diseases***, written by Lei Feng (雷丰) in 1882, a book of practical value, mainly dealing with febrile diseases of the four seasons, stating the causes, symptoms and treatment of the diseases and introducing the author's own prescriptions

脾胃论 [pí wèi lùn]

Pi Wei Lun, or ***Treatise on the Spleen and Stomach***, written by Li Gao (李杲) and published in 1249. Based on the nutritional viewpoint expressed in the *Internal Classic*, the author emphasizes and explaines the importance of nourishing the spleen and the stomach. For curing spleen and stomach troubles caused by improper diet or fatigue, he recommendes *Bu Zhong Yi Qi Tang*, or Decoction for Reinforcing the Middle and Replenishing Qi and *Sheng Yang Yi Wei Tang*, or Decoction for Activating Yang and Replenishing the Stomach.

十药神书 [shí yào shén shū]

Shi Yao Shen Shu, or ***A Miraculous Book on Ten Recipes***, written by Ge Qiansun (葛乾孙) in 1348, containing 10 recipes, namely, three remedies for hemoptysis, three for cough, one hypnotic and three nutrients, all of which are said to be sound remedies for treating consumption, especially pulmonary tuberculosis

证治汇补 [zhèng zhì huì bǔ]

Zheng Zhi Hui Bu**,** or ***Supplement to Diagnosis and Treatment***, in 8 volumes, written by Li Yongcui (李用粹) and published in 1687, which mainly deals with miscellaneous diseases of internal medicine, recording more than 80 kinds of diseases with their diagnoses, methods of treatment and prescriptions

类证治裁 [lèi zhèng zhì cái]

Lei Zheng Zhi Cai**,** or ***Classified Treatment***, written by Lin Peiqin (林佩琴) in 1839. The author differentiates and analyzes various diseases of internal medicine, gynecology and surgery according to their causes and clinical manifestations, and introduces concrete therapy and prescriptions. To many diseases are appended case records for reference. This book integrates the good points of various schools, and has been quite influential in medical circles.

血证论 [xuè zhèng lùn]

Xue Zheng Lun**,** or ***Treatise on Blood Syndromes*** (1884), written by Tang Rongchuan (唐容川). This book deals with the diagnosis and treatment of various blood troubles, including a general introduction and descriptions over 170 diseases. The author breaks fresh ground in this field.

经效产宝 [jīng xiào chǎn bǎo]

Jing Xiao Chan Bao**,** or ***Tested Treasures of Obstetrics***, or simply *Chan Bao*, or *Treasures of Obstetrics* written by Zan Yin (昝殷) in 852-856. It is the earliest book exclusively on obstetrics in which diseases during pregnancy, at the time of parturition and after delivery are diagnosed and treated.

产宝 [chǎn bǎo]

Chan Bao**,** or ***Treasure of Obstetrics*****:** abbreviation of *Jing Xiao Chan Bao*, or *Tested Treasures of Obstetrics*

卫生家宝产科备要 [wèi shēng jiā bǎo chǎn kē bèi yào]

Wei Sheng Jia Bao Chan Ke Bei Yao**,** or ***A Precious Manual of Obstetrics for Home Use*** (1184), a valuable book on obstetrics compiled by Zhu Duanzhang (朱端章). The author pools knowledge of obstetrics and of nursing infants from all previous medical works.

女科百问 [nǚ kē bǎi wèn]

Nü Ke Bai Wen**,** or ***One Hundred Questions on Women's Diseases*** (1220), written by Qi Zhongfu (齐仲甫) of the Song Dynasty, in which the main problems of gynecology and obstetrics are dealt with in the form of questions and answers

妇人大全良方 [fù rén dà quán liáng fāng]

Fu Ren Da Quan Liang Fang or ***Fu Ren Liang Fang Da Quan*****, or** ***The Complete Book of Effective Prescriptions for Women*** or simply *Fu Ren Liang Fang*, or *Effective Prescriptions for Women* (1237), written by Chen Ziming (陈自明). This is the first and most important book on gynecology and obstetrics

妇人良方 [fù rén liáng fāng]

Fu Ren Liang Fang**, or** ***Effective Prescriptions for Women*****:** abbreviation for *Fu Ren Da Quan Liang Fang* or *Fu Ren Liang Fang Da Quan*, or *The Complete Book of Effective Prescriptions for Women*

万氏女科 [wàn shì nǚ kē]

Wan Shi Nü Ke**, or** ***Wan's Gynecology and Obstetrics*** (1549), written by Wan Quan (万全) of the Ming Dynasty, with discussions on problems of various kinds of gynecological and obstetric diseases

济阴纲目 [jì yīn gāng mù]

Ji Yin Gang Mu**, or** ***Compendium of Therapies for Women's Diseases***, a book on obstetrics and gynecology in 5 volumes, written by Wu Zhiwang (武之望) and published in 1620. In 1665, Wang Qi (汪琪) made commentaries on the book and re-edited it into 14 volumes. Troubles with menstruation, leukorrhea, pregnancy and parturition are discussed with prescriptions of practical value.

女科经纶 [nǚ kē jīng lún]

Nü Ke Jing Lun**, or** ***Principles of Gynecology and Obstetrics*** (1684), compiled by Xiao Gengliu (萧庚六) of the Qing Dynasty, substantial in content, with notes and annotations attached

傅青主女科 [fù qīng zhǔ nǚ kē]

Fu Qing Zhu Nü Ke**, or** ***Fu Qing-zhu's Obstetrics and Gynecology***, also known as *Nü Ke* (女科) or *Obstetrics and Gynecology*, a book in 2 volumes written by Fu Shan (傅山), in the 17th century and first published in 1827. The book consists of 77 articles dealing with the diagnosis and treatment of diseases of obstetrics and gynecology, with simple language and practical prescriptions. The author also wrote the *Chan Hou Bian* (产后编), or *Postpartum Care*, dealing with the diagnosis and treatment of 43 kinds of diseases within the scope of obstetrics. The combined edition of the two books is called *Fu Shi Nü Ke Da Quan* (傅氏女科大全) or *Fu's Complete Works of Obstetrics and Gynecology.*

小儿药证直诀 [xiǎo ér yào zhèng zhí jué]

Xiao Er Yao Zheng Zhi Jue, or ***Key to the Therapeutics of Children's Diseases***, written by Qian Yi (钱乙), generally acknowledged as the greatest pediatrist in Chinese medicine. It was edited and published by his pupil Yan Jizhong (阎季忠) in 1119 in three volumes – one on diagnosis, one on case recording and one on prescriptions. The author emphasizes the peculiarities of pediatrics and the characteristics of children's physiology and pathology.

幼幼新书 [yòu yòu xīn shū]

You You Xin Shu, or ***A New Book of Pediatrics*** (1132), a comprehensive treatise on children's diseases in 40 volumes compiled by Liu Fang (刘昉), Wang Li (王历) and Wang Shi (王湜), dealing with the etiology, diagnosis and therapies of various kinds of children's diseases, child care, etc.

小儿痘疹方论 [xiǎo ér dòu zhěn fāng lùn]

Xiao Er Dou Zhen Fang Lun, or ***Treatise on Smallpox and Measles in Children*** (1241), written by Chen Wenzhong (陈文中), a noted pediatrist of the 13th century

幼科铁镜 [yòu kē tiě jìng]

You Ke Tie Jing, *Iron Mirror of Pediatrics* (1695), a medical book on Pediatrics written by Xia Ding (夏鼎) in the Qing Dynasty, in which the diagnosis and treatment of common diseases of children were discussed and massotherapy recommended

幼幼集成 [yòu yòu jí chéng]

You You Ji Cheng, or ***Collection of Works on Pediatrics*** (1750), written by Chen Fuzheng (陈复正), who collected and reorganized the main contents of ancient books on pediatrics, adding his own views on some theoretical problems concerning therapy for certain diseases, e.g. infantile convulsions

小儿推拿秘旨 [xiǎo ér tuī ná mì zhǐ]

Xiao Er Tui Na Mi Zhi, or ***Secret Principles of Massotherapy for Children***, written by Gong Yunlin (龚云林) of the Ming Dynasty and edited with a supplement and published by Yao Guozhen (姚国桢) in 1604. It is one of the earliest works on this subject.

小儿推拿广意 [xiǎo ér tuī ná guǎng yì]

Xiao Er Tui Na Guang Yi, or ***Elucidation of Massotherapy for Children***, also called *Tui Na Guang Yi*, or *Elucidation of Massotherapy* for short, written by Xiong Yingxiong (熊应雄) about 1676 in the Qing Dynasty

推拿广意 [tuī ná guǎng yì]

Tui Na Guang Yi, or ***Elucidation of Massotherapy***: abbreviation of *Xiao Er Tui Na Guang Yi*, or *Elucidation of Massotherapy for Children*

刘涓子鬼遗方 [liú juān zǐ guǐ yí fāng]

Liu Juan-zi Gui Yi Fang, or ***Liu Juan-zi's Ghost-Bequeathed Prescriptions***, the earliest medical work on surgery, written by Gong Qingxuan (龚庆宣) in 496-499, dealing mainly with the treatment of traumatic wounds, carbuncles, mastitis, burns, eczema and scabies, with excellent remarks on surgical nursing, drainage and sterilization. The book is titled "ghost-bequeathed" in order to emphasize the marvelous effect of the prescriptions.

理伤续断秘方 [lǐ shāng xù duàn mì fāng]

Li Shang Xu Duan Mi Fang, or ***Secrets of Treating Wounds and Rejoining Fractures***, also called *Xian Shou Li Shang Xu Duan Mi Fang*, or *Secrets of Treating Wounds and Rejoining Fractures Handed Down by the Fairy*, the earliest book on bone-setting, written by Taoist Priest Lin (蔺道人) in about 846 A.D., with remarks on traction, reunion and fixation of fractured and dislocated bones

仙授理伤续断秘方 [xiān shòu lǐ shāng xù duàn mì fāng]

Xian Shou Li Shang Xu Duan Mi Fang, or ***Secrets of Treating Wounds and Rejoining Fractures Handed Down by a Fairy***: the full name of the *Li Shang Xu Duan Mi Fang*, or *Secrets of Treating Wounds and Rejoining Fractures*

外科精要 [wài kē jīng yào]

Wai Ke Jing Yao, or ***Essence of External Medicine*** (1263), written by Chen Ziming (陈自明), one of the earliest books on external medicine with differential diagnosis and treatment of furuncles, carbuncles, gangrene, ulcers and wounds

外科精义 [wài kē jīng yì]

Wai Ke Jing Yi, or **Essentials of External Medicine** (1335), written by Qi Dezhi (齐德之) of the Yuan Dynasty, consisting of 35 articles on external medicine, 145 prescriptions for making decoctions, boluses, plaster and pills, the process of preparing drugs, and the main indications of single-item prescriptions

秘传外科方 [mì chuán wài kē fāng]

Mi Chuan Wai Ke Fang, or ***Secret Methods of External Medicine*** by Zhao Yizhen (赵宜真), which appeared in 1395, with 24 surgical illustrations

解围元薮 [jiě wéi yuáng sǒu]

Jie Wei Yuan Sou, or ***Source of Relief***, a book specially devoted to leprosy, written by Shen Zhiwen (沈之问) in 1550, which deals with the cause of leprosy, its various manifestations, and relations to meridians, and lists 249 prescriptions

疮疡经验全书 [chuāng yáng jīng yàn quán shū]

Chuang Yang Jing Yan Quan Shu, or ***A Complete Manual of Experiences in the Treatment of Sores***, usually attributed to Dou Hanqing (窦汉卿) but was actually written by Dou's grandson. The book appeared in 1569, and deals with all diseases requiring surgical treatment, classified according to the various parts of the body.

外科启玄 [wài kē qǐ xuán]

Wai Ke Qi Xuan, or ***Revealing the Mysteries of External Medicine***, written by Shen Gongchen (申拱宸) and published in 1604. It begins with a general exposition of the various forms of therapy and then deals with different types of cases requiring surgical treatment, with illustrations

外科正宗 [wài kē zhèng zōng]

Wai Ke Zheng Zong, or ***Orthodox Manual of External Medicine***, written by Chen Shigong (陈实功) on the basis of forty years of personal experience, in which each disease is dealt with separately, with diagnosis, therapeutic methods and operations, as well as case records and prescriptions. It was published in 1617 and has ever since been one of the most influential books on external medicine.

外科大成 [wài kē dà chéng]

Wai Ke Da Cheng, or ***A Complete Book of External Medicine***, written by Qi Kun (祁坤) in 1665. It gives an exhaustive description of diagnosis and treatment of surgical diseases and is the book upon which *Yi Zong Jin Jian Wai Ke Xin Fa Yao Jue* (医宗金鉴外科心法要诀) or *Golden Mirror of Medicine: Essentials of External Diseases* is based.

外科证治全生集 [wài kē zhèng zhì quán shēng jí]

Wai Ke Zheng Zhi Quan Sheng Ji**,** or ***Life-saving Manual of Diagnosis and Treatment of External Diseases*** (1740), written by Wang Weide (王惟德) of the Qing Dynasty, emphasizing the use of the elimination method in treating ulcers and carbuncles

伤科补要 [wài kē bǔ yào]

Shang Ke Bu Yao**,** or ***Supplement to Traumatology*** (1803), written by Qian Xiuchang (钱秀昌) of the Qing Dynasty dealing with treatment of trauma and bone-setting as well as tested prescriptions used in this field, in rhymes

伤科汇纂 [shāng kē huì zuǎn]

Shang Ke Hui Zuan**,** or ***Compilation of Traumatology*** (1817), written by Hu Tingguang (胡廷光) of the Qing Dynasty, dealing with differential diagnosis and treatment of fractures and dislocation of bones

银海精微 [yín hǎi jīng wēi]

Yin Hai Jing Wei**,** or ***Essence of the Silvery Sea***, a book on ophthalmology in 2 volumes, which appeared in the 13th century, with its authorship attributed to Sun Simiao (孙思邈). "Silvery sea" is a metaphorical expression for the eyes.

秘传眼科龙木论 [mì chuán yǎn kē lóng mù lùn]

Mi Chuan Yan Ke Long Mu Lun**,** or ***Long Mu's Secret Treatise on Ophthalmology***, an anonymous book in ten volumes which appeared in the 13th century, including 72 kinds of eye diseases, with glaucoma and cataracts as the two chief ailments

原(元)机启微 [yuán jī qǐ wēi]

Yuan Ji Qi Wei**,** or ***Revealing the Mystery of the Origin (of Eye Diseases)*** (1370), written by Ni Weide (倪维德), which gives a systematic exposition of eye diseases not only as a local affliction but as part of defective functioning of the whole body, and often due to unhygienic conditions

审视瑶函 [shěn shì yáo hán]

Shen Shi Yao Han**,** or ***A Precious Work on Ophthalmology***, also titled *Yan Ke Da Quan*, or *A Complete Work on Ophthalmology*, a comprehensive and exhaustive treatise on eye diseases by Fu Yunke (傅允科), which appeared in 1644 in seven volumes, listing 108 kinds of eye troubles and their treatment

眼科大全 [yǎn kē dà quán]

***Yan Ke Da Quan*, or *A Complete Book of Ophthalmology*:** another name of *Shen Shi Yao Han*, or *A Precious Work on Ophthalmology*

针灸甲乙经 [zhēn jiǔ jiǎ yǐ jīng]

Zhen Jiu Jia Yi Jing*, or *The ABC Classic of Acupuncture and Moxibustion (c259), written by Huangfu Mi (皇甫谧), the earliest exclusive and systemized book on acupuncture and moxibution, in which the names and number of points of each meridian and their exact locations are defined. It also deals with the properties and indications of each point and the methods of needle manipulation.

铜人俞穴针灸图经 [tóng rén shù xué zhēn jiǔ tú jīng]

Tong Ren Shu Xue Zhen Jiu Tu Jing*, or *Illustrated Manual of Acupoints on the Bronze Figure, written by Wang Weiyi (王惟一), first published in 1027 in 3 volumes. The author made detailed studies of the acupuncture points and marked out a total of 657 points on the famous bronze figure.

针灸资生经 [zhēn jiǔ zī shēng jīng]

Zhen Jiu Zi Sheng Jing*, or *Classic of Nourishing life with Acupuncture and Moxibustion (1220), written by Wang Zhizhong (王执中), a systematic presentation of acupuncture and moxibustion including the location of meridians and points, and 46 illustrations, based on the author's clinical experience.

十四经发挥 [shí sì jīng fā huī]

Shi Si Jing Fa Hui*, or *Elaboration of the Fourteen Meridians (1341), written by Hua Shou (滑寿), a marked development in meridian theory

针灸聚英 [zhēn jiǔ jù yīng]

Zhen Jiu Ju Ying*, or *A Collection of Gems of Acupuncture and Moxibustion (1529), written by Gao Wu (高武), in which the author brings together the theories of various schools concerning acupuncture and moxibustion.

针灸问答；针灸问对 [zhēn jiǔ wèn dá; zhēn jiǔ wèn duì]

Zhen Jiu Wen Da [Dui]*, or *Catechism of Acupuncture and Moxibustion (1530), written by Wang Ji (汪机), in which the theories and principles of acupuncture and moxibustion are expounded

针灸大成 [zhēn jiǔ dà chéng]

Zhen Jiu Da Cheng*, or *Great Compendium of Acupuncture and

Moxibustion (1601), written by Yang Jizhou (杨继洲), who clarifies confusion over points and meridians and unifies the divergent views concerning them

针刺麻醉 [zhēn cì má zuì]

Zhen Ci Ma Zui*,** or ***Acupuncture Anesthesia, published in 1972, in which the history, characteristics, theories and methods of acupuncture and anesthesia, and the points most commonly used for this purpose, as well as the application of this art in various operations and the electro-acupuncture anaesthesia devices in common use are given in detail. It is a preliminary summing-up of the results of scientific reserch in this field.

洗冤集录 [xǐ yuān jí lù]

Xi Yuan Ji Lu*,** or ***Instructions to Coroners (1247), a book on forensic medicine written by Song Ci (宋慈). The original book had 10 volumes, but after the Ming Dynasty, only four remained. It systematically sums up the achievements made before the Song Dynasty in this field, and introduces tests for and identifications of toxicity, and measures for emergency treatment. It also deals with anatomy, pathology, bone-setting, surgical operations, etc. This book is of great value, and has been translated into many languages.

周易参同契 [zhōu yì cān tóng qì]

Zhou Yi Can Tong Qi*,** or ***Analogism of Principles of Changes Formulated in the Zhou Dynasty, written by Wei Boyang (魏伯阳) of the Han Dynasty, in which along with teachings about making elixers (pills) of immortality externally through alchemy, the art of internal exercise for immortality is dealt with, and the part of the human body where *qi* was believed to be stored was thus called *dantian* (elixir field), analogous to the furnace in alchemy

养性延命录 [yǎng xìng yán mìng lù]

Yang Xing Yan Ming Lu*,** or ***Recordings of the Art of Health and Life Preservation, written by Tao Hongjing (陶弘景) of the Jin Dynasty, in which many forms of *qigong* exercise are recorded

黄庭经 [huáng tíng jīng]

Huang Ting Jing*,** or ***Classic of the Yellow Yard, a book on *qigong* exercise written by Wei Huacun (魏华存) of the Jin Dynasty, in which concentration on the 'yellow yard', breathing and swallowing of saliva are stressed in *qigong* exercise. The "yellow yard" is equivalent to *dantian*

(elixir field), part of the human body on which the mind should be concentrated during *qigong* exercise.

修习止观坐禅法要 [xiū xí zhǐ guān zuò chán fǎ yào]

Xiu Xi Zhi Guan Zuo Chan Fa Yao, or ***Principles of Buddhist Cultivation***, written by Zhi Kai (智𫖮), a famous Buddhist monk of the Sui Dynasty, in which methods of adjustment of posture, breathing and mentality are dealt with

内功图说 [nèi gōng tú shuō]

Nei Gong Tu Shuo, or ***Illustrated Internal Qigong Exercise***, compiled by Wang Zuyuan (王祖源) of the Qing Dynasty, in which several forms of *qigong* exercise are described, with illustrations

中藏经 [zhōng zàng jīng]

Zhong Zang Jing, or ***Treasured Classic***, a comprehensive book on medicine, ascribed to Hua Tuo (华佗) but most probably written by an unknown author during the Six Dynasties. The book includes 49 articles on diagnosis and treatment, pulse, internal organs, deficiency and excess syndromes, cold and heat syndromes, etc, as well as a list of prescriptions.

儒门事亲 [rú mén shì qīn]

Ru Men Shi Qin, or ***The Scholars' Care of Their Parents***, Zhang Zihe (张子和), whose classification of diseases is based on Liu Wan-su's (刘完素) theory of six exogenous pathogenic factors and whose three methods of treatment are diaphoresis, emesis and purgation

兰室秘藏 [lán shì mì cáng]

Lan Shi Mi Cang, or ***A Secret Book Kept in the Chamber*** (1276), a comprehensive book on medicine written by Li Gao (李杲), which deals with various kinds of diseases classed into 21 groups. In the book the author's *Treatise on Diseases of the Spleen and Stomach* was especially prized by physicians of later generations; the prescriptions listed were mostly created by the author himself.

丹溪心法 [dān xī xīn fǎ]

Dan Xi Xin Fa, or ***Danxi's Experiental Therapy***, written by Zhu Zhenheng (朱震亨) of the Yuan Dynasty, but rearranged and edited by his disciples. In 1481, the book was re-edited, with supplements and corrections by Cheng Chong (程充), with 6 treatises on medical theories at the beginning and then 100 articles dealing with various diseases, most of which are concerned with internal medicine. The author's theory that "yang was ever excessive and yin ever deficient" is reflected in the whole book.

格致余论 [gé zhì yú lùn]

Ge Zhi Yu Lun*, or *Supplementary Treatise on Knowledge from Practice (1347), by Zhu Zhenheng (朱震亨). The author further expounds the theory of "ever excessive yang with deficient yin" in this book.

明医杂著 [míng yī zǎ zhù]

Ming Yi Za Zhu*, or *Collection of Physicians' Experiences in the Ming Dynasty (1549), written by Wang Lun (王纶) and annotated by Xue Ji (薛己) in the Ming Dynasty

医门法律 [yī mén fǎ lǜ]

Yi Men Fa Lü*, or *Principles and Prohibitions of the Medical Profession, (1658) by Yu Chang (喻昌). It explains the principles of diagnosis and treatment based on syndrome differentiation, points out the errors usually made, and suggests prohibitions in this respect, hence the title.

医林改错 [yī lín gǎi cuò]

Yi Lin Gai Cuo*, or *Corrections of the Errors in Medical Works (1830), by Wang Qingren (王清任), who insisted on making anatomical observations and had made studies for dozens of years on the internal organs of the human body. In this book the author corrected certain mistakes made by past generations concerning the internal organs, and suggested new methods of treating blood stasis and hemiplegia. His method of activating the blood and removing stasis is still of practical value.

冷庐医话 [lěng lú yī huà]

Leng Lu Yi Hua*, or *Deserted House Medical Talks (1897), by Lu Yitian (陆以湉), including informal essays, short sketches and notes dealing with medical problems

医学衷中参西录 [yī xué zhōng zhōng cān xī lù]

Yi Xue Zhong Zhong Can Xi Lu*, or *Records of Traditional Chinese and Western Medicine in Combination, by Zhang Xichun (张锡纯) and published from 1918 to 1934. There were altogether 30 volumes in seven issues. The revised edition consists of five parts, viz, prescriptions, medical substances, medical theories, notes and case records. The author attempted to integrate traditional Chinese medicine with Western medicine.

名医类案 [míng yī lèi àn]

Ming Yi Lei An, or ***Classified Medical Records of Distinguished Physicians,*** compiled by Jiang Guan (江瓘) and his son, and completed in 1552. Later Wei Zhixiu (魏之琇) revised the book. The book deals with acute and chronic infectious diseases, and miscellaneous diseases concerned with internal medicine, external medicine, gynecology, pediatrics, etc., with detailed medical case records and well chosen methods of treatment and prescriptions. Occasional notes and commentaries are made by the authors.

续名医类案 [xù míng yī lèi àn]

Xu Ming Yi Lei An, or ***Supplement to the Classified Medical Records of Distinguished Physicians*** (1770), compiled by Wei Zhixiu (魏之琇), a sequel to the *Ming Yi Lei An*, or *Classified Medical Records of Distinguished Physicians* by Jiang Guan (江瓘) of the Ming Dynasty, with a supplement of medical records of distinguished physicians of the early Qing Dynasty, most of which deal with acute infectious diseases

古今医案按 [gǔ jīn yī àn àn]

Gu Jin Yi An An, or ***Comments on Medical Records: Ancient and Modern***, a collection of medical records of various authors compiled by Yu Zhen (俞震) in 1776, with comments and elucidations attached

医贯 [yī guàn]

Yi Guan, or ***Key Link of Medicine***, a book of medical theories, written in 1687 by Zhao Xianke (赵献可), who supported Xue Ji's (薛己) views, advocating that the "life gate fire" was in charge of the whole body, and emphasizing the importance of "genuine fire" and "genuine water". It is an important reference book for studying the "life gate".

临证指南医案 [lín zhèng zhǐ nán yī àn]

Lin Zheng Zhi Nan Yi An, or ***Medical Records as a Guide to Practice*** (1766), by Ye Gui (叶桂), in 10 volumes, rearranged by Hua Xiuyun (华岫云) et al. Of the 10 volumes, eight are devoted to miscellaneous diseases of internal medicine, one to gynecology and one to pediatrics.

圣济总录 [shèng jì zǒng lù]

Sheng Ji Zong Lu, or ***Complete Record of Holy Benevolence***, a monumental work consisting of 200 volumes (only 26 volumes are extant) compiled by a staff of physicians under imperial orders and completed around 1111-1117. It covers every branch of the healing arts, with about 20,000 prescriptions recorded.

医学正傳 [yī xué zhèng fù]

Yi Xue Zheng Zhuan*, or *Orthodox Medical Record (1515), a comprehensivc medical book compiled by Yu Tuan (虞抟). At the beginning of the book are listed 51 issues that were not fully elucidated by the author's predecessors. The text was written in the light of various medical works of the past generations as well as the author's own experience .

古今医统 [gǔ jīn yī tǒng]

Gu Jin Yi Tong*, or *Ancient And Modern Medicine, compiled by Xu Chunfu (徐春甫) and completed in 1556. It sums up and classifies the contents of more than 100 medical and related works of the previous generations

古今医统大全 [gǔ jīn yī tǒng dà quán]

Gu Jin Yi Tong Da Quan*, or *A Complete Work of Ancient and Modern Medicine: the full name of the *Gu Jin Yi Tong*, or *Ancient And Modern Medicine*

医学入门 [yī xué rù mén]

Yi Xue Ru Men*, or *Introduction to Medicine (1575), compiled by Li Yan (李梴), a comprehensive medical book dealing with various branches of medicine. It not only presents the views of various schools, but also expounds the author's own ideas.

证治准绳 [zhèng zhì zhǔn shéng]

Zheng Zhi Zhun Sheng*, or *Standards for Diagnosis and Treatment (1602), written by Wang Kentang (王肯堂). It gives a detailed and exhaustive description of symptoms and treatment methods. The whole series consists of six branches, namely miscellaneous diseases of internal medicine, cold-induced diseases, ulcers and boils, pediatrics, gynecology, and classified prescriptions. The work sums up the rich experiences of the doctors of previous generations and had its widest circulation in the 17th century.

六科证治准绳 [liù kē zhèng zhì zhǔn shéng]

Liu Ke Zheng Zhi Zhun Sheng*, or *Standerds of Diagnosis and Treatment in the Six Branches of Medicine: the full name of the *Zheng Zhi Zhun Sheng*, or *Standards for Diagnosis and Treatment*

景岳全书 [jǐng yuè quán shū]

Jing Yue Quan Shu*, or *Jingyue's Complete Works (1624), in 64 volumes, written by Zhang Jiebin (张介宾), styled Jingyue (景岳). The book includes studies of theories, pulse, cold-induced diseases, internal medicine, gynecology, pediatrics, external medicine, materia medica, modern prescriptions, ancient prescriptions, etc. The author extracted the essence of various schools and made a systematic analysis of the diagnosis and treatment of diseases based on syndrome differentiation. Advocating the theory "yang is ever in excess and yin never sufficient", he recommends using warm tonifying drugs, and wrote two whole volumes of new prescriptions.

医宗必读 [yī zōng bì dú]

Yi Zong Bi Du*, or *Essential Readings in Medicine (1637), compiled by Li Zhongzi (李中梓) in 10 volumes, and one of the most influential introductory books of medicine, including medical history, physiology, *zang-fu* organs, diagnostic methods, materia medica, syndrome differentiation and treatment of various internal diseases

张氏医通 [zhāng shì yī tōng]

Zhang Shi Yi Tong*, or *Zhang's Treatise on General Medicine (1695), a comprehensive medical work by Zhang Lu (张璐), dealing with diagnosis and treatment of diseases of various branches of medicine, with case records and prescriptions attached

古今图书集成医部全录 [gǔ jīn tú shū jí chéng yī bù quán lù]

Gu Jin Tu Shu Ji Cheng Yi Bu Quan Lu*, or *Collection of Ancient and Modern Books, Section on Medicine (1726), in 520 volumes, compiled by Jiang Tingxi (蒋廷锡) et al. It includes the *Internal Classic* and over 100 other medical works written up to the beginning of the Qing Dynasty, with commentaries on ancient medical works, diagnosis and treatment of various diseases, biographies of physicians, etc.

医学心悟 [yī xué xīn wù]

Yi Xue Xin Wu*, or *Medicine Comprehended (1732), one of the most influential books of clinical medicine, compiled by Cheng Guopeng (程国彭) in 5 volumes, dealing with the diagnostic methods, eight principles of syndrome differentiation, eight therapeutic methods, syndrome differentiation and treatment of internal diseases, external diseases, women's diseases, diseases of the sense organs, etc.

医宗金鉴 [yī zōng jīn jiàn]

Yi Zong Jin Jian*, or *Golden Mirror of Medicine (1742), in 90 volumes, one of the best treatises on general medicine, written by a staff of 80 persons headed by Wu Qian (吴谦) in compliance of an imperial order. A considerable part of the book is made up of extracts, revisions and corrections of previous works.

陈修圆医书十六种 [chén xiū yuán yī shū shí liù zhǒng]

Chen Xiu Yuan Yi Shu Shi Liu Zhong*, or *Sixteen Medical Works of Chen Xiuyuan (1865), a series of practical medical works compiled by Chen Nianzu (陈念祖) styled Xiuyuan (修圆), also known as *Nan Ya Tang Yi Shu Quan Ji*, or *Complete Medical Works of Nan Yan Tang*

南雅堂医书全集 [nán yǎ táng yī shū quán jí]

***Nan Yan Tang Yi Shu Quan Ji*, or *Complete Medical Books of Nan Yan Tang*:** another title of the *Chen Xiu Yuan Yi Shu Shi Liu Zhong*, or *Sixteen Medical Works of Chen Xiuyuan*

中国医学大辞典 [zhōng guó yī xué dà cí diǎn]

Zhong Guo Yi Xue Da Ci Dian*, or *A Dictionary of Chinese Medicine (1921), compiled by Xie Guan (谢观) et al. and published in 1921. It has more than 37,000 entries.

中国药学大辞典 [zhōng guó yào xué dà cí diǎn]

Zhong Guo Yao Xue Da Ci Dian*, or *A Dictionary of Chinese Pharmaceuticals Published in 1935, and including all kinds of medicinal substances recorded in the medical literature of previous generations

珍本医书集成 [zhēn běn yī shū jí chéng]

***Zhen Ben Yi Shu Ji Cheng*, or *Collection of Precious Medical Works*,** a collection of medical works compiled by Qiu Qingyuan (裘庆元), and published in 1936. Of more than 3,000 books on medicine, the author chose 90, which were classified into 12 subjects, viz, medical classics, herbals, pulses, cold-induced diseases, internal medicine, external medicine, gynecology, pediatrics, general treatment, prescriptions, medical case records and miscellaneous.

中国医学大成 [zhōng guó yī xué dà chéng]

Zhong Guo Yi Xue Da Cheng*, or *A Great Collection of Chinese Medical Works (1936), compiled by Cao Bingzhang (曹炳章) on the basis of 128 important medical works. The collection covers 13 subjects, including medical classics, medical substances, diagnoses, prescriptions, general treatment, various clinical subjects, medical case records and miscellaneous topics, with abstracts and notes attached to each book

附录一 中文笔划索引

Appendix I Chinese Character Stroke Index

四画

[一]

[丶]

五画

[一]

六画

[一]

[|]

[ㄱ]

八画

[一]

九画

[一]

[丿]

十画

[ㄱ]

十一画

[一]

[ㄱ]

十二画

[一]

[丶]

[ㄱ]

十三画

[一]

[丨]

[┐]

十四画

[一]

[丨]

[丿]

附录二 中文拼音索引
Appendix II Chinese Character Phonetic Index

附录三 引文索引（按中文笔划顺序排列）
Appendix III Index of Citations

附录四 英文索引

Appendix IV Index of Terms in English

(including Latin and Romanized Chinese)

766
acupuncture 针法, 424
acupuncture-moxibustion 针灸, 424
acupuncturist 针灸医生, 424
acute aphonia 急喉喑[瘖], 682
acute appendicitis 肠痈, 588
acute conjunctivitis 风火眼, 667
acute dacryocystitis 漏睛疮, 667
acute infantile convulsion 急惊风, 620
acute keratoconjunctivitis 暴赤生翳, 668
acute lymphangitis 红丝疔, 642
acute mastitis 乳痈, 646
acute pharyngitis 急喉痹, 683
acute rhinitis 伤风鼻塞, 679
acute throat infection 急喉风, 683
acute throat wind 急喉风, 683
acute thyroiditis 瘿痈, 648
adaptation to seasonal changes 顺应四时, 13, 546
addiction 癖嗜, 70
adhesive plaster 膏药, 280
adhesive-plaster dermatitis 膏药风, 655
adjusting *qi* 调气, 250
adjuvant [assistant] ingredient 佐药, 376
advanced periods 月经提前, 135
adverse ascent of *qi* 上气, 565
adverse transmission to the pericardium 逆传心包, 76
aerial infection 天受, 551
afterbirth 胞衣, 胎衣, 598
afternoon (tidal) fever 午后潮热, 121
agalactia 乳汁不行, 乳汁不通, 619
Agastache 藿香, 325
aggregation syndrome 积证, 589
aggregation-accumulation masses 癥瘕积聚, 积聚 589
agitated pulse 脉躁, 143
Agkistrodon 蕲蛇, 321
agonizing arthralgia 痛痹, 582
Agrimonia Bud 鹤草芽, 371
Aifu Nuangong Pills 艾附暖宫丸, 420
air 大气, 50
air-borne 天受, 551
Airpotato Yam 黄药子, 302
ala nasi 鼻翼, 32, 678
alarm point 募穴, 486
Albizia Flower 合欢花, 347
alchemy 炼丹, 535
alcohol addiction 酒癖, 70
alcohol fire cupping 滴酒法, 500
all joints 百节, 49
allergic rhinits 鼻鼽, 679
alleviating pain 止痛, 265
All-inclusive Grand Tonic Decoction 十全大补汤, 394
All-inclusive Grand Tonic Pills 十全大补丸, 414
Aloe 芦荟, 369
Aloes 芦荟, 369
alopecia areata 斑秃, 654
alopecia seborrheica 发蛀脱发, 654
alopecia 发落, 油风, 654
Alpinia-Cyperus Pill 良附丸, 398
alternating fever and chills 寒热往来, 121
alternative preponderance of yin and yang 阴阳胜复, 5
Alum 白矾, 明矾, 372

白丑, 332
Black Catechu 儿茶, 373
black coating 黑苔, 110
black discoloration 黑色, 100
Black Nightshade Herb 龙葵, 317
black of the eye 黑睛, 661
Black Pharbitis Seed 黑丑, 331
Blackberrylily Rhizome 射干, 318
Blackened Swallowwort Root 白薇, 310
blackening the hair and beard 乌须发, 269
Black-tailed Snake 乌梢蛇, 321
bladder 膀胱, 19; 胞, 597
bladder damp-heat syndrome 膀胱湿热证, 205
bladder deficiency-cold syndrome 膀胱虚寒证, 205
bladder heat retention syndrome 热结膀胱证, 205
bladder meridian (BL) (足太阳)膀胱经, 440
bladder meridian of foot *taiyang* 足太阳膀胱经, 440
blanch 渾, 277
blazing of both *qi* and blood 气血两燔, 77
blazing of both *qi* and nutrient 气营两燔, 77
"bleating convulsion" 羊痫风, 575
bleeding following sinking of *qi* 血随气陷, 90
bleeding from the gums 齿衄, 113
blepharitis angularis 眦帷赤烂, 665
blepharoptosis 胞睑下垂, 废睑, 103; 上胞下垂, 睑皮垂缓, 666
blindness in ophathalmosteresis 瞽症, 674
blindness 目盲, 663
Blister Beetle 斑蝥, 373
block pattern of wind-stroke 中风闭证, 576
blockage disease 痹(病), 581
blockage of bladder *qi* 膀胱气闭, 89
block-rejection 关格, 585
blood 血, 54
blood accumulation 蓄血, 592
blood chamber 血室, 21, 598
blood deficiency 血虚, 168
blood deficiency producing wind 血虚生风, 79
blood deficiency syndrome 血虚证, 168
blood failing to circulate in vessels 血不循经, 90
blood fever 血热, 630
blood flooding 血崩, 604
blood heat transforming into dryness 血热化燥, 165
blood heat with raging wind 血热风盛, 165
"blood orbiculus" 血轮, 39, 659
blood prostration 血脱, 593
blood *qi* 血气, 54
blood stasis due to *qi* deficiency 气虚血瘀, 90
blood stasis due to *qi* stagnation 气滞血瘀, 90
blood stasis infertility 血瘀不孕, 610
blood stranguria 血淋, 594
blood syncope 血厥, 579
blood system 血分, 53
blood system syndrome 血分证, 165

edema syndrome 水气证, 172
edema under the eyes 目下肿, 102
edema-alleviating diuretic (drug [medicinal]) 利水消肿药, 288
edematous disease 水肿病, 590
edge of the tongue 舌边, 33
Effective Formulas Tested by Physicians for Generations 世医得效方, 756
Effective Prescriptions for Universal Relief 普济本事方, 755
Effective Prescriptions for Women 妇人良方, 760
Effective Prescriptions 本事方, 755
Egg Capsule of Mantid 桑螵蛸, 366
"egret's cough" 鹭鸶咳, 634
eight bone-setting manipulations 正骨八法, 692
eight confluence points 八脉交会穴, 486
eight extra meridians 奇经八脉, 443
eight influential points 八会穴, 486
eight joints 八溪, 49
eight principal therapeutic methods 八法, 215
eight principles 八纲, 147
eight regions of the eye 八廓, 39, 659
eight signs of infantile convulsion 惊风八候, 620
eight-diagram walking 八卦步, 532
eighteen antagonisms 十八反, 378
Eight-ingredient Rectification Powder 八正散, 405
Eight-Precious Motherwort Pills 八珍益母丸, 420
eight-principle pattern identification 八纲辨证, 147
eight-principle syndrome differenttiation 八纲辨证, 147
eight-section brocade 八段锦, 540
Eight-Treasure Decoction 八珍汤, 394
Eight-Treasure Pills 八珍丸, 413
Elaboration of the Fourteen Meridians 十四经发挥, 765
elbow kneading (manipulation) 肘揉法, 704
elbow pressing (manipulation) 肘按法, 707
elbow pushing (manipulation) 肘推法, 705
electric ophthalmia 电光伤目, 672
electric stimulator 电针仪, 501
electro-acupuncture anesthesia 电针麻醉, 501
electro-acupuncture, galvano-acupuncture 电针, 501
electro-exploratory method 电测法, 501
elevating formula 升剂, 379
elevating the middle *qi* 升提中气, 240
elevating yang to cure drooping 升阳举陷, 240
elevating yang 升阳, 241
eliminating stagnant blood by catharsis 攻下逐瘀, 230
eliminating summer-heat and resolving dampness 祛暑化湿, 清暑化湿, 224
eliminating the stale and the stagnant 去菀陈莝, 230
elimination and tonification in

exterior-excess and interior-deficiency syndrome 表实里虚证, 152
exterior-heat and interior-cold syndrome 表热里寒证, 151
exterior-interior releasing formula 表里双解剂, 387
exterior-interior transmission 表里传, 163
exterior-releasing drug [medicinal] 解表药, 285
exterior-releasing formula 解表剂, 380
exterior-releasing therapy 解表法, 215
external acoustic meatus 耳道, 41
external affection 外感, 60, 557
external application 外敷, 敷, 270, 271
external auditory meatus 耳窍, 41
external cold 外寒, 62
external contraction 外感, 60
external damp(ness) 外湿, 63
external disease 外证, 640
external dryness 外燥, 64
external dryness syndrome 外燥证, 178
external exercise 外功, 526
external fixation 外固定, 695
external genitals 阴器, 45
external hemorrhoid 外痔, 649
external malleolus 外踝, 核骨, 47
external opening of the ear 外耳门, 505
external ophthalmopathy 外障, 663
external therapy 外治法, 270
external treatment 外治, 270
external urethral orifice (of the female) 廷孔, 45
external wind 外风, 62
external wind syndrome 外风证, 173
externally contracted cough 外感咳嗽, 564
externally contracted headache 外感头痛, 573
externally contracted lumbago 外感腰痛, 596
extinguishing wind and arresting epilepsy 熄风定痫, 264
extinguishing wind and arresting spasm 息风定痉, 263
extinguishing wind and relieving spasm 熄风解痉, 263
extinguishing wind and resolving phlegm 息风化痰, 255
extinguishing wind 息[熄]风, 263
extra conductant ingredient 药引子, 377
extra points 经外穴, 487
extracorporeal cosmic cycle 离体周天, 537
extracorporeal heavenly circuit 离体周天, 537
Extractum Malti 饴糖, 355
extraordinary organs 奇恒之腑, 19
extreme heat producing wind syndrome 热极生风证, 186
extreme heat producing wind 热极生风, 186
extreme heat producing wind 热极生风, 79
extremely abnormal pulse 脉悬绝, 144
extremely poisonous, moderately

Heche Dazao Pills 河车大造丸, 414
heding (EX-LE2) 鹤顶, 493
heel 踵, 47
hegu (LI4) 合谷, 448
heliao (LI19) 禾髎, 449
heliao (TE22) 和髎, 473
helix 耳轮, 41, 503
helix cauda 耳轮尾, 504
helix crus 耳轮脚, 503
helix notch 轮屏切迹, 505
helix tubercle 耳轮结节, 503
helminthic amenorrhea 虫积经闭, 602
hemangioma 血瘤, 648
hematemesis 呕血, 吐血, 130, 592
hematemesis and epistaxis during menstruation 经行吐衄, 606
hematemesis during menstruatio 经行吐血, 606
Hematite 赭石, 代赭石, 351
hematochezia 便血, 592
hematuria 尿血, 溲血, 128, 592
hemihidrosis 半身汗多, 123
hemilateral headache 偏头痛, 123
hemiplegia 半身不遂, 偏枯, 578
hemiplegia with wry mouth 喎僻不遂, 578
hemoptysis 咯血, 113
hemoptysis with coughing 咳血, 592
hemoptysis without coughing 咯血, 592
hemorrhagic syndrome 血证, 591
hemorrhoid 痔, 649
hemospermia 血精, 595
hemostatic (drug [medicinal]) 止血药, 290
Hemp Seed 火麻仁, 369
Hemp-seed Pill 麻子仁丸, 385
Henbane Seed 天仙子, 莨菪子, 306
henggu (KI11) 横骨, 44, 468
Herba Abri 鸡骨草, 312
Herba Agastachis 藿香, 325
Herba Agrimoniae 仙鹤草, 337
Herba Andrographitis 穿心莲, 317
Herba Artemisiae Annuae 青蒿, 310
Herba Artemisiae Scopariae 茵陈, 茵陈蒿, 313
Herba Asari 细辛, 296
Herba Capsellae 荠菜, 339
Herba Centipedae 鹅不食草, 297
Herba Cirsii 小蓟, 337
Herba Cistanchis 肉苁蓉: 大芸, 360
Herba Commelinae 鸭跖草, 317
Herba Cymbopogonis 芸香草, 307
Herba Cynomorii 锁阳, 361
Herba Dendrobii 石斛, 356
Herba Dianthi 瞿麦, 329
Herba Ecliptae 墨旱莲, 339
Herba Elshotziae 香薷, 296
Herba Ephedrae 麻黄, 295
Herba Epimedii 淫羊藿, 仙灵脾, 361
Herba Equiseti Hiemalis 木贼, 308
Herba Erodii seu Geranii 老鹳草, 322
Herba Eupatorii 佩兰, 325
Herba Houttuyniae 鱼腥草, 316
Herba Humuli Scandentis 葎草, 319
Herba Leonuri 益母草, 坤草, 344
Herba Lobeliae Chinensis 半边莲, 318
Herba Lophatheri 淡竹叶, 竹叶,

interior heat syndrome 里热证, 150
interior heat 里热, 150
interior retention of water-fluid syndrome 水饮内停证, 171
interior syndrome 里证, 148
interior-exterior interspace 膜[募]原, 36
interior-warming drug [medicinal] 温里药, 289
interior-warming formula 温里剂, 391
interlocking of cold and heat 寒热错杂, 81
intermenstrual bleeding 经间期出血, 603
intermittent dysentery 休息痢, 561
intermittent pulse 代脉, 141
internal abscess 内痈, 642
Internal Classic 内经, 746
internal cold 内寒, 62
internal damage headache 内伤头痛, 573
internal damp(ness) 内湿, 64
internal deflagration of heart fire 心火内焚, 181
internal deflagration of heart fire 心火内焚, 86
internal dryness 内燥, 64
internal exercise *tuina* [massage] 内功推拿, 524
internal exercise 内功, 526
internal fixation 内固定, 697
internal flaming of heart fire 心火内炽, 86, 181
internal hemorrhoid 内痔, 649
internal injury 内伤, 68
internal malleolus 内踝, 合骨, 47
internal ophthalmopathy 内障, 663
internal stirring of liver wind 肝风内动, 185
internal wind 内风, 62
internally damaged cough 内伤咳嗽, 564
internally damaged feve 内伤发热, 569
internally injured lumbago 内伤腰痛, 596
interposed moxibustion 间隔灸, 497
interrogation 问诊, 120
interstitial keratitis 混睛障, 670
intertragic notch 屏间切迹, 505
intestinal parasitosis 虫积, 629
intestinal *qi* colic 盘肠气痛, 637
intestine-astringing antidiarrheal formula 涩肠固脱剂, 397
intolerance of cold 畏寒, 120
intolerance of the five *zang* organs 五脏所恶, 21
intradermal needle 皮内针, 428
intradermal needling 皮内针法, 428
intramammary abscess 乳疽, 647
Introduction to Medicine 医学入门, 770
intruding pathogen 客邪, 59
Inula Flower 旋覆花, 300
Inula-Haematite Decoction 旋复代赭汤, 399
"invalid eyelid" 睑废, 666
Invaluable Prescriptions for Emergencies 备急千金要方, 754
Invaluable Prescriptions 千金要方, 754
invasion of white membrane into the cornea 白膜侵睛, 669

producing fluid with sweet-cold 甘寒生津, 261
profuse clear urine 尿清长, 128
profuse nasal bleeding 鼻洪, 680
profuse sputum 痰多, 113
profuse sweating 大汗, 122
prolapse of the rectum 脱肛, 650
prolapse of uterus 阴挺, 609
prominent muscle 肿, 42
prominent part for inspection 明堂, 677
promoting blood circulation 通利血脉, 266
promoting digestion and relieving distension 消食下气, 247
promoting digestion and removing (food) stagnancy 消食导滞, 消导, 247
promoting digestion and resolving (food) stagnation 消食化滞, 246
promoting digestion to harmonize the stomach 消食和胃, 247
promoting eruption 透疹, 219
promoting granulation 生肌, 268
promoting lactation 下乳, 266, 266
promoting pus discharge 托疮, 267
promoting suppuration 攻溃, 268
promoting tissue regeneration and wound healing 生肌敛疮, 268
promoting tissue regeneration 生肌, 268
property and flavor 气味, 性味, 278
proportional body *cun* 同身寸, 424
propping with a lever 杠杆支撑, 694
prostatic hypertrophy 精癃, 651
prostatitis 精浊, 650
prostration of blood with (*qi*) collapse 血脱气脱, 90
prostration pattern of stroke 中风脱证, 577
protective *qi* 卫气, 51
protracted dysentery 迁延痢, 561
protruding and moving tongue 吐弄舌, 109
protruding tongue 吐舌, 109
protruding vegetation from the earhole 耳挺, 677
protrusion of the eyeballs 眼球突出, 103
protrusion of the navel 脐突, 625
proved formula 验方, 374
pruritus cutis 风瘙痒, 655
Pseudobulbus Cremastrae seu Pleiones 山慈菇, 302
pseudo-cold 假寒, 158
pseudo-heat 假热, 158
pseudopterygium 流金凌木, 667
psoriasis 白疕, 654
pterygium 胬肉攀睛, 667
Pu Ji Ben Shi Fang 普济本事方, 755
Pu Ji Fang 普济方, 756
pubes margin 毛际, 44
Pubescent Angelica and Loranthus Decoction 独活寄生汤, 401
Pubescent Holly Root 毛冬青, 345
pubic bone 横骨, 44
pubic symphysis 曲骨, 44
pucan (BL61) 仆参, 466
Pueraria-Scutellaria-Coptis Decoction 葛根黄芩黄连汤, 387
puerperal epidemic febrile disease 产后病温, 617

stir-bake with adjuvant 加辅料炒, 276
stir-bake with fluid adjuvant 炙, 276
stirring the tongue 搅舌, 522
stomach 胃, 18
stomach cavity 胃脘, 18
stomach crisis due to putrid blood 败血冲胃, 616
stomach deficiency-cold syndrome 胃虚寒证, 195
stomach diabetes 胃消, 593
stomach disharmony 胃不和, 87
stomach excess-cold syndrome 胃实寒证, 195
stomach failing to send downward harmoniously 胃失和降, 87
stomach fire 胃火, 196
stomach fluid consumption 胃津亏损, 170
stomach fluid insufficiency syndrome 胃燥津亏证, 170
stomach fluid 胃津, 19
stomach heat 胃热, 195
stomach insufficiency 胃虚, 194
stomach meridian (ST) (足阳明)胃经, 437
stomach meridian of foot *yangming* 足阳明胃经, 437
stomach *qi* 胃气, 18, 52
stomach *qi* deficiency 胃气虚, 194
stomach *qi* deficiency syndrome 胃气虚证, 194
stomach *qi* disharmony 胃气不和, 86
stomach *qi* failing to descend 胃气不降, 87
stomach *qi*, vitality, and root 胃、神、根, 143
stomach stuffiness 胃痞, 583
stomach yang 胃阳, 18
stomach yang deficiency syndrome 胃阳虚证, 195
stomach yang deficiency 胃阳虚, 194
stomach yin 胃阴, 19
stomach yin deficiency syndrome 胃阴虚证, 194
stomach yin deficiency 胃阴虚, 194
stomach yin insufficiency 胃阴不足, 194
stomachache 胃痛, 129
Stomach-clearing Powder 清胃散, 389
stomach-fire syndrome 胃火证, 196
stomach-fire toothache 胃火牙痛, 685
stomach-heat vomiting 胃热呕吐, 635
stomach-insufficiency sweating 胃虚汗, 634
Stomach-pacifying Powder 平胃散, 403
stone needle 砭石, 428
stony goiter 石瘿, 648
"stony moth" 石蛾, 681
stool sometimes loose and sometimes hard 溏结不调, 127
stopping bleeding, hemostasis 止血, 254
stopping hiccups 止呃, 265
storage of five *zang* organs 五脏所藏, 21
Storax Pills 苏合香丸, 418
Storax 苏合香, 346

subcutaneous fluid retention 溢饮, 566
subcutaneous node 结核, 641
subduing yang and extinguishing wind 潜阳熄风, 262
subduing yang 潜阳, 262
Suberect Spatholobus Stem 鸡血藤, 342
subjugation in five elements 五行相乘, 9
sublingual cyst 舌下痰包, 687
sublingual vein 舌下脉络, 106
submaxillary abscess 颌下痈, 682
subperiosteal abscess of the mastoid 耳后附骨痈, 675
subsidiary bone 辅骨, 47
Succinum 琥珀, 347
suction cup 抽气罐, 499
suction cupping 抽气罐法, 500
sudamina crystalline 晶痦, 116
sudden aphonia 暴喑[瘖], 卒喑[瘖], 682
sudden asthmatic attack 马脾风, 634
sudden attack of wind-heat on the eye 暴风客热, 668
sudden blindness 暴盲, 672
sudden diarrhea (disease) 暴泻(病), 586
sudden epilepsy 暴痫, 638
sudden illness 暴病, 552
sudden infantile diarrhea 小儿卒利, 小儿暴泻, 635
sudden onset of pharyngitis 卒喉痹, 683
sudden peeling of coating 光剥舌, 111
sudden protrusion of the eyeball 突起睛高, 睛高突起, 674
sudden redness of the bulbar conjunctiva 白睛暴赤, 663
Suhexiang Pills 苏合香丸, 418
suited to person 因人制宜, 208
suited to time, place and person 因时、因地、因人制宜, 208
Sulfur, Sulfur 硫黄, 371
suliao (GV25) 素髎, 481
summer affliction 苦夏, 629
summer boil 暑疖, 641
summer consumption 疰夏, 629
summer consumptive disease 疰夏病, 630
summer convulsion 暑痉, 555
summer convulsive seizur 暑痫, 555
summer fever disease 夏季热病, 630
summer fever 夏季热, 630
summer filth disease 暑秽病, 554
summer filth 暑秽, 554
summer phthisis 暑瘵, 555
summer *qi* 暑气, 63
summer warm disease 暑温病, 555
summer warm 暑温, 555
summer-damp 暑湿, 63
summer-heat 暑, 暑热, 63
summer-heat affection 感暑, 554
summer-heat affliction 伤暑, 冒暑, 554
summer-heat disease 暑病, 554
summer-heat dizziness [vertigo] 感暑眩晕, 572
summer-heat into *yangming* 暑入阳明, 555
summer-heat malaria 暑疟, 559

Treasure of Obstetrics 产宝, 759
Treasured Classic 中藏经, 767
treating diarrhea with diuretics 利小便, 实大便, 258
treating disease from the root 治病求本, 209
treating disease of the left with points on the right, and vice versa 左病右取, 右病左取, 212
treating the fundamental 治本, 209
treating the incidental 治标, 209
treating the incidental and fundamental simultaneously 标本兼[同]治, 209
treating the lower for the upper, and treating the upper for the lower 上病下取, 下病上取, 211
treating yang for yin diseases 阴病治阳, 211
treating yin for yang diseases 阳病治阴, 211
Treatise on Blood Syndromes 血证论, 759
Treatise on Causes and Symptoms of Diseases 病源侯总论, 750
Treatise on Cold-induced and Miscellaneous Diseases 伤寒杂病论, 748
Treatise on Cold-induced Diseases 伤寒论, 748
Treatise on Epidemic Febrile Diseases 温热论, 757
Treatise on Pestilence 温疫论, 757
Treatise on Seasonal Diseases 时病论, 758
Treatise on Smallpox and Measles in Children 小儿痘疹方论, 761
Treatise on the Spleen and Stomach 脾胃论, 758
Treatise on the Three Categories of Pathogenic Factors and Prescriptions 三因极一病证方论, 750
Tui Na Guang Yi 推拿广意, 762
treatment in the opposite direction 从治, 211
treatment in the same direction 逆治, 211
Tree Peony Bark 牡丹皮, 309
Tree-of-heaven Bark 椿皮, 椿根白皮, 313
trembling of the extremities 手足颤动, 101
trembling of the lips 口振, 112
trembling tongue 颤动舌, 108
tremor 颤震[振], 振掉, 581
tremor of the tongue 舌战, 108
triangular fossa 三角窝, 504
trichiasis 倒睫, 睫毛倒入, 664
trichiasis and entropion 倒睫拳毛, 664
Trichosanthes-Allium-Pinellia Decoction 瓜蒌薤白半夏汤, 398
tri-monthly menstruation 居经, 599
triple energizer 三焦, 19
triple energizer meridian (TE) (手少阳)三焦经, 441
triple energizer meridian of hand *shaoyang* 手少阳三焦经, 441
triple-energizer pattern identification 三焦辨证, 166
triple-energizer syndrome differ entiation 三焦辨证, 166
tripod-shaped splint fixation 鼎式夹

nal] 祛风湿药, 287
wind-dryness 风燥, 67
wind-dryness cough 风燥咳嗽, 564
wind-extinguishing and spasm-controlling drug [medicinal] 息风止痉药, 293
wind-extinguishing formula 熄风剂, 401
wind-fire 风火, 66
wind-fire attack on the eye 风火眼, 667
wind-fire painful eye 风火眼痛, 668
wind-fire toothache 风火牙痛, 684
wind-heat 风热, 66
wind-heat affliction 风热感冒, 553
wind-heat attack on the eye 风热眼, 668
wind-heat attacking the lung syndrome 风热犯肺证, 197
wind-heat cough 风热咳嗽, 564
wind-heat dispersing drug [medicinal] 发散风热药, 285
wind-heat dizziness [vertigo] 风热眩晕, 572
wind-heat exterior syndrome 风热表证, 175
wind-heat headache 风热头痛, 573
wind-heat lumbago 风热腰痛, 596
wind-heat pathogen 风热邪气, 66
wind-heat pharyngitis 风热喉痹, 681
wind-heat syndrome 风热证, 175
wind-heat tinnitus 风热耳鸣, 676
wind-heat tonsillitis 风热乳蛾, 681
wind-heat toothache 风热牙痛, 684
wind-heat ulcerative gingivitis 风热牙疳, 686
wind-phlegm 风痰, 61
wind-phlegm dizziness [vertigo] 风痰眩晕, 572
wind-phlegm headache 风痰头痛, 574
wind-phlegm syndrome 风痰证, 172
wind *qi* 风气, 61
wind-stroke, apoplexy 中风, 576
wind-treating formula 治风剂, 401
wind-warm 风温, 65
wind-warm (disease) 风温, 553
wind-warm (syndrome) 风温, 553
wind-warm disease 风温病, 553
wind-warm pathogen 风温邪气, 65
winter warm 冬温, 557
wiping the forehead 抹前额, 520
wiping 抹法, 515
wiry pulse 弦脉, 141
wisdom tooth 真牙, 33, 684
withdrawal of needle 引针, 431
withering of the helix 耳轮干枯, 104
withering of the teeth 齿槁, 113
Wolfberry-Chrysanthemum Rehmannia Pills 杞菊地黄丸, 415
womb 女子胞, 20
Wonderful Well-tried Prescriptions 奇效良方, 756
wood fire torturing metal 木火刑金, 10
wood restricting earth 木克土, 9
wood subjugating asthenic earth 土虚木乘, 10
wood subjugating earth 木乘土, 9
wooden tongue 木舌, 109, 626
word-articulating breathing 吐字呼吸, 534

yin edema 阴水, 591
yin epilepsy 阴痫, 575, 638
yin exhaustion 亡阴, 157
yin fluids 阴液, 56
Yin Hai Jing Wei 银海精微, 764
yin heel vessel (YinHV) 阴跷脉, 444
yin impairment involving yang 阴损及阳, 5
yin jaundice 阴黄, 562
yin link vessel (YinLV) 阴维脉, 444
yin macula 阴斑, 115
yin malaria 牝疟, 560
yin meridians 阴经, 436
yin pathogens 阴邪, 61
yin preponderance with yang insufficiency 阴盛阳衰, 74
yin preponderance 阴盛, 74
yin prostration 脱阴, 75
yin *qi* 阴气, 52
Yin Qiao Powder 银翘散, 381
Yin Shan Zheng Yao 饮膳正要, 753
yin summer affliction 阴暑, 554
yin sweating 阴汗, 123
yin syndrome 阴证, 147
yin syndrome resembling yang 阴证似阳, 158
yin tonic 补阴药, 294
yin zang-organs 阴脏, 15
yinbai (SP1) 隐白, 456
yinbao (LR9) 阴包, 478
Yinchenhao Decoction 茵陈蒿汤, 404
yin-collapse syndrome 阴脱证, 157
yin-deficiency colds 阴虚感冒, 553
yin-deficiency fever 阴虚发热, 569
yindu (KI19) 阴都, 468
yin-exhaustion syndrome 亡阴证, 157
yin-fluid insufficiency syndrome 阴液亏虚证, 156
yingchuang (ST16) 膺窗, 452
yingu (KI10) 阴谷, 468
yingxiang (LI20) 迎香, 449
yin-heel vessel syndrome 阴跷脉病证, 207
yinjiao (CV7) 阴交, 482
yinjiao (GV28) 龈交, 481
yinlian (LR11) 阴廉, 478
yinlingquan (SP9) 阴陵泉, 456
yin-link vessel syndrome 阴维脉病证, 207
yinmen (BL37) 殷门, 464
Yin-nourishing and Lung-clearing Decoction 养阴清肺汤, 403
yin-nourishing drug [medicinal] 养阴药, 294
Yin-nourishing Lung-clearing Extract 养阴清肺膏, 409
yin-nourishing moistening formula 滋阴润燥剂, 402
Yinqiao Jiedu Pills [Tablets] 银翘解毒丸[片], 407
yin-replenishing drug [medicinal] 滋阴药, 294
yin-replenishing formula 补阴剂, 395
Yin-restoring Pill 左归丸, 395
yinshi (ST33) 阴市, 454
yintang (EX-HN3) 印堂, 37, 487
yin-tonifying drug [medicinal] 补阴药, 294
yinxi (HT6) 阴郄, 458
yin-yang balance 阴阳平衡, 4

Acknowledgement

I am indebted to Ms. Li Ning (李宁) for her devoted and untiring help in preparing the typescript and marking the phonetic symbols, Ms. Liu Rongzhen (刘荣珍) for drawing the illustrations, and Mr. Xie Ping (谢平) for careful proof-reading of the manuscript.

图书在版编目（CIP）数据

新编汉英中医药分类词典 / 谢竹藩 编著.
—北京：外文出版社，2002.9
ISBN 7-119-03126-0
I. 新… II. 谢… III. 中国医药学—词典—汉、英 IV. R2—61
中国版本图书馆 CIP 数据核字（2002）第 056577 号

责任编辑 胡开敏
装帧设计 蔡 荣
印刷监制 张国祥

新编汉英中医药分类词典

谢竹藩 编著

*

外文出版社出版
(中国北京百万庄大街 24 号)
邮政编码 100037
外文出版社网址 http://www.flp.com.cn
外文出版社电子信箱: info@flp.com.cn
sales@flp.com.cn

三河市汇鑫印务有限公司印刷
中国国际图书贸易总公司发行
(中国北京车公庄西路 35 号)
北京邮政信箱第 399 号 邮政编码 100044
2002 年(大 32 开)第 1 版
2002 年 9 月第 1 版第 1 次印刷
(英)
ISBN 7-119-03126-0/R·186(外)
09800
14-E-3509 S